[redacted]

Chemical And Biological Aspects Of Drug Dependence

Editors:

S. J. Mulé, Ph.D., Chief
New York State
Narcotic Addiction Control Commission
Testing and Research Laboratory
Brooklyn, New York

Henry Brill, M.D., Director
Pilgrim State Hospital
West Brentwood, New York

published by:

CRC PRESS

THE CHEMICAL RUBBER CO.
18901 CRANWOOD PARKWAY
CLEVELAND, OHIO 44128

CRC UNISCIENCE SERIES

Another information program recently initiated by CRC is the "Uniscience" Series. The function of "Uniscience" has been defined as the publication of highly authoritative scientific reference works dealing with those subjects for which there exists an urgent necessity for published information due to significant new developments.

To achieve this function, the "Uniscience" program utilizes the conventional reference book format, but with one, all-important difference: it has radically reduced the traditional lag between completion of the manuscript and publication of the printed book. Utilizing newly developed editorial procedures together with newly perfected computerized type-setting equipment, the time-span normally required from manuscript to printed book has been dramatically shortened to a matter of only a few months.

This very real "break-through" in production time makes it possible for the Uniscience Series to provide a new dimension in the distribution of scientific information.

B. J. Starkoff, President
THE CHEMICAL RUBBER CO.

CONTRIBUTORS

Dr. M. M. Baden
New York University
School of Medicine
New York, New York 10016

Dr. Henry Brill
Pilgrim State Hospital
P. O. Box 22
West Brentwood, New York 11717

Dr. S. T. Christian
NIMH Addiction Research Center
P. O. Box 2000
Lexington, Kentucky 40507

Dr. Doris H. Clouet
New York State
NACC Testing & Research Laboratory
80 Hanson Place
Brooklyn, New York 11217

Dr. B. M. Cox
Department of Pharmacology
Chelsea College of Science & Technology
Manresa Road
London, S. W. 3, England

Dr. W. L. Dewey
Department of Pharmacology
University of North Carolina
School of Medicine
Chapel Hill, North Carolina 27514

Dr. Seymour Ehrenpreis
New York State Research Institute
for Neurochemistry & Drug Addiction
Ward's Island, New York 10035

Mr. B. Eisenberg
Department of Neuropathology
N.Y.S. Psychiatric Institute
722 West 168th Street
New York, New York 10032

Dr. Max Fink
New York Medical College
5 East 102nd Street
New York, New York 10029

Dr. H. F. Fraser
1131 Merrick Drive
Merrick Place
Lexington, Kentucky 40502

Dr. Robert George
Department of Pharmacology
University of California
Los Angeles, California 90024

Dr. M. Ginsburg
Department of Pharmacology
Chelsea College of Science & Technology
Manresa Road
London, S. W. 3, England

Dr. S. Hashimoto
N. Y. State Psychiatric Institute
722 West 168th Street
New York, New York 10032

Dr. M. Helpern
New York University
School of Medicine
New York, New York 10016

Dr. Carl C. Hug, Jr.
Dept. of Anesthesiology & Pharmacology
Emory University, School of Medicine
69 Butler Street, S. E.
Atlanta, Georgia 30303

Dr. Arthur Jacobson
Section on Medicinal Chemistry
National Institutes of Health
Bldg. 4, Room 136
Bethesda, Maryland 22014

Dr. Reese T. Jones
The Langley Porter Neuropsychiatric Institute
401 Parnassus Avenue
San Francisco, California 94122

Dr. H. Kalter
Department of Pediatrics
Childrens Hospital Research Foundation
Elland Avenue & Bethesda
Cincinnati, Ohio 45229

Dr. M. Kaufman
N.Y.S. Psychiatric Institute
722 West 168th Street
New York, New York 10032

Dr. Charles S. Lieber
Mt. Sinai School of Medicine (CUNY)
Section of Liver Disease & Nutrition
Veterans Administration Hospital
130 West Kingsbridge Road
Bronx, New York 10468

Mr. J. C. Liu
Department of Neuropathology
N.Y. State Psychiatric Institute
722 West 168th Street
New York, New York 10032

Dr. Peter Lomax
Department of Pharmacology
University of California
Los Angeles, California, 90024

Dr. Anand L. Misra
New York State NACC
Testing & Research Laboratory
80 Hanson Place
Brooklyn, New York 11217

Dr. S. J. Mulé, Chief
New York State NACC
Testing & Research Laboratory
80 Hanson Place
Brooklyn, New York 11217

Dr. Leon Roizin
Psychiatric Research
N.Y. State Psychiatric Institute
722 West 168th Street
New York, New York 10032

Dr. Maurice H. Seevers
Department of Pharmacology
University of Michigan
School of Medicine
Ann Arbor, Michigan 48104

Dr. Alexander T. Shulgin
1483 Shulgin Road
Lafayette, California 94549

Dr. Eric J. Simon
New York University School of Medicine
New York, New York 10016

Dr. Charles B. Smith
Department of Pharmacology
University of Michigan
School of Medicine
Ann Arbor, Michigan 48104

Dr. Solomon H. Snyder
Department of Pharmacology
Johns Hopkins School of Medicine
725 North Wolfe Street
Baltimore, Maryland 21205

Dr. D. N. Teller
New York State Research Institute
for Neurochemistry & Drug Addiction
Ward's Island, New York 10035

Dr. E. O'F. Walsh
Department of Biochemistry
University of Hong Kong
Hong Kong

Dr. Abraham Wikler
Center for Advanced Study
in the Behavioral Sciences
202 Junipero Serra Blvd.
Stanford, California 94305

PREFACE

Drug dependence has reached epidemic proportions affecting all strata of our society. Since the etiology of drug dependence is complex and largely unknown, its treatment and prevention have proceeded on a "trial and error" basis with mainly disappointing results. A major alternative would be a task force attack at the cellular level to uncover the molecular basis for the development of drug dependence. Such knowledge would lead to rational, effective, and successful programs, to cure and/or prevent drug dependence.

It is the purpose, indeed the objective, of this monograph to provide the scientist with a reference text that provides the basic knowledge and background information that currently defines the chemical and biological basis of drug dependence. The approach being a logical extension of the purpose, the nature of drug dependence and drug abuse must first be clearly defined and characterized. Since many drugs of various chemical formulations induce physical and/or psychic dependence, the characteristics of drug dependence of each pharmacological class of drugs must be described. The importance of quantitative screening tests and procedures for determining drug dependence in man and in animals and the abuse potential of the drug must be understood. Certainly a drug may be defined by its chemical structure as well as by the altered function that follows an interaction with the endogenous receptor. Therefore, the chemical characteristics of such a seemingly disparate group of compounds must be defined and, where possible, correlated with their capacity to induce drug dependence. This relationship may further be viewed through similarities in receptor activity, disposition, and biotransformation as well as detection and identification of these drugs in the biological medium. The foregoing knowledge now allows the presentation of the touchstone of the text, i.e., the theories related to tolerance development and physical dependence. Since these drugs act primarily within the central nervous system, it seemed most logical to include in this section the electrophysiology, neuropathology, teratology, embryolethality, and mutagenicity of these compounds. Finally, full attention to biochemical mechanisms associated with such biological strata as enzymes, proteins, nucleic acids, carbohydrates, neurohumors, lipids, and hormones was explained in relationship to drug dependence. The monograph appropriately ends with a bonus providing insight into theoretical biochemical mechanisms related to physical and/or psychic dependence.

The unusually broad nature of the subject matter demanded the expertise that could only be provided through multiple authorship. The group of "super" contributors brought such outstanding backgrounds, knowledge, and experience to bear on their specific chapters that the editorial task was practically reduced to mere proofreading. Of course, regardless of the effort, it is impossible in a multiauthored text to be fully aware of omitted data or to eliminate all duplication of information.

Special acknowledgment is made to Ms. Mary Gatsoulis and Earleen Ryan for cheerfully and effectively attending to the mundane tasks of record keeping, letter and manuscript typing, filing, and copying. The absence of such effective assistance certainly would have prevented the final publication of this book.

S. J. Mulé
H. Brill
New York, N. Y.

THE EDITORS

S. J. Mulé, Ph.D., is Chief of the New York State Narcotic Addiction Control Commission Testing and Research Laboratory, New York.

Dr. Mulé received his B.A. degree in Chemistry in 1954 from College of Wooster, Wooster, Ohio; the M.S. degree in Biochemistry and Physiology in 1955 from Rutgers University, New Brunswick, New Jersey; and the Ph.D. degree in Pharmacology in 1961 from the University of Michigan, Ann Arbor, Michigan. Dr. Mulé subsequently received postdoctoral training in the Departments of Physiological Chemistry and Pharmacology at the University of Wisconsin. He continued his research at the Addiction Research Center of the National Institute of Mental Health, Lexington, Kentucky. His present research concerns the disposition and biotransformation of narcotic analgesics, the detection and identification of drugs subject to abuse, and the biochemical mechanisms of drug dependence.

Dr. Mulé has published extensively in the scientific literature and is a member of pharmacological, chemical, and forensic societies.

Henry Brill, M.D., is Director, Pilgrim State Hospital, West Brentwood, Long Island, New York.

Dr. Brill is a graduate of Yale College and Yale School of Medicine. He is a member of Phi Beta Kappa and Sigma Xi.

As First Deputy Commissioner of the New York State Department of Mental Hygiene, Dr. Brill was instrumental in developing the state's narcotic addiction program and the alcoholic program from 1954 to 1964. He was formerly Vice Chairman of the New York State Narcotic Addiction Control Commission. Since 1971 Dr. Brill has been a member of the National Commission on Marihuana and Drug Abuse.

Dr. Brill is a diplomate or member of numerous professional societies, among which is the Expert Panel of Drug Dependence of the WHO. He has authored some 50 papers on drug dependence.

TABLE OF CONTENTS

INTRODUCTION

INTRODUCTION

H. Brill

It is perhaps appropriate to devote the introduction to a volume on the chemical and biological aspects of drug dependence to a discussion of some of the background of this group of problems. In this process we shall see how the history of chemistry and of technology has been entangled with the development of drug dependence and shall review some of its psychosocial, legal, and human aspects. Finally, we shall examine some of the reasons why we may hope that further work in the laboratory sciences may at long last contribute to a breakthrough to effective treatment and prevention. It seems that nothing which relates to the problem of drug dependence is simple, probably because we do not really understand it. As a result, this background discussion will be complex; it may even seem contradictory in some respects, but this will not be a contrived complexity. It is inherent in the nature of the topic.

This will not be a review of technical history, sociology, or psychosocial and social issues, but rather a general discussion of relevant material drawn from these and other fields with a view to providing something of a backdrop or perspective for the specific and technical material which follows. In addition, it may serve as an indication that the broader, human issues involved in drug dependence are considered important in relation to the scientific work in this field. From considerable personal contact with those doing such work I know this to be true.

In the course of the discussion we shall see that in the past, chemistry and pharmacology have actually provided the drugs which created the major part of modern drug dependence. In this sense, dependence is an unexpected and unwanted by-product of a series of chemical advances which began at the close of the 18th century. We shall also note that the tide has turned, and recent chemical advances are now contributing to the treatment of opiate addiction, giving promise of much more to come. This direction of affairs amounts to a chemical solution for a problem which was created by chemistry. At first glance, it seems somewhat illogical, but it has good precedent and is really very logical, even if some wag has insisted on quoting the following jingle in this context.

There was a man in our town
and he was wondrous wise;
He jumped into a bramble bush
and scratched out both his eyes
And when he saw his eyes were out
with all his might and main
He jumped into another bush
and scratched them in again. (Anon.)

THE DERIVATION OF THE TERM DRUG DEPENDENCE

Let us begin with a note about a basic science contribution which is not often recognized as such; that is, the creation of a name for the condition under discussion. This story will provide a minor but illuminating example of the effectiveness of the basic science approach as compared with other, more direct methods. A bitter and fruitless debate had gone on for many years about the proper use of such terms as addiction, habituation, abuse, and misuse. However, no consensus was ever reached about the exact meaning or specific application of these terms, all of which were based on a mixture of value judgments, simple logic, and direct clinical observation. None of them had a clear well-defined, objective meaning. This situation was finally corrected not by the exercise of a more acute logic but by the introduction of the new laboratory-based term "drug dependence" which refers to an objective pattern of drug-seeking behavior that can be experimentally demonstrated in animals as well as man and is thus of general applicability. Two further advantages are that it is not unencumbered by the stigma of previous associations and is flexible in form since it permits the addition of modifying phrases to specify subtypes such as the morphine type, the cocaine type, etc. To balance this, is the disadvantage that it can be misinterpreted and misused by debaters who insist that it is descriptive of that aspect of the condition that is harmful or objectionable which opens the door to rhetoric about all the harmless or necessary forms of human dependence. Nevertheless, the term is operationally defined, and it has proved to be a significant contribution to a clearer understanding of this subject.

HISTORICAL NOTE

As previously mentioned, the history of modern drug dependence can be seen as beginning with the chemical advances of the late 18th century and continuing with the introduction of a series of new substances, each of which gave rise to a social problem. The chemical isolation of the alkaloid morphine at the beginning of the 19th century eventually changed the Western world's minor opium eating problem into the major one of morphinism and the invention of the syringe opened the way, first for hypodermic addiction and later for the intravenous form, each more serious than its predecessor. Further chemical advance at the end of the 19th century led to the acetylation of morphine to make heroin, which has taken such a toll in death, disability, and crime. During the 19th century period of scientific advance, cocaine was extracted from the coca leaf and as a result a rural problem of the Andes Mountain Indians became a world-wide issue. Advances in chemistry led also to the production of a series of fully synthetic dependence-producing substances, including the barbiturates, the non-barbiturate sedatives, the stimulants, and most recently, the hallucinogens. A more complete list of syntheic drugs that produce dependence would have to include such older drugs as paraldehyde and chloralhydrate, as well as the anesthetics, ether and nitrous oxide, and an interminable array of industrial chemicals.

While such advances in chemistry and pharmacology had much to do with the development of the current drug-dependence problem, they were by no means the only technical and scientific factors. Much was also contributed by advances in science and technology in general and the operation of the latter factors can be discerned throughout the course of recorded history chiefly because they created the means for diffusion of the drugs. Thus, we can attribute a large share of the responsibility for the current situation to advances in communication and transportation which have carried these drugs and information about them around the world with an efficiency that made possible such mass phenomena as the recent explosive increase in the use of cannabis, a drug which in less than a decade has touched an estimated 24 million in the U.S. alone, has swept over Europe, and is even now in process of erupting on the Japanese drug scene for the first time in the history of that country. The early part of this story, however, unfolds with extreme slowness over many centuries.

DRUG DEPENDENCE–A RELATIVELY NEW PROBLEM

It is an interesting and unexplained historical fact that drug dependence (aside from alcoholism) was not described in any records before the Middle Ages. Cannabis and opium were known to certain ancient peoples, and had extensive medical use, but were scarcely mentioned in euphoriants. Their earliest spread was for medical purposes and, in the case of cannabis, for fiber. This spread can be traced to advances in technology which opened ancient trade routes that stretched across Southern Asia from China to Europe; it was along these routes that traders carried opium and cannabis. By the Middle Ages, opium had found its way into China, Southern Asia, North Africa, and Europe; it came to America also as a medicine in colonial times. By the early Middle Ages cannabis and opium had finally begun to emerge as social problems in parts of Asia and in the Muslim World, but Europe still remained curiously immune to all drugs except alcohol until the 19th century even though opium continued to have wide medical application and cannabis was a prominent fiber plant with some medical use.

Advances in science and technology also helped

to usher in the Age of Exploration which led to the discovery of America and the opening up of vast areas in Asia, Africa, and the islands of the South Pacific. European explorers reported finding a long series of locally-used social and recreational drugs which were in this way added to what might be called the world-wide pharmacopoeia of pleasure. Notable among these additions was tobacco and with it came the technique of smoking, a method hitherto unknown in Europe and Asia. Tobacco smoking was introduced by European traders into China in the 16th century and within a relatively short time, smoking was adapted to opium and replaced opium eating. This laid the foundation of a problem which was not brought under control until our own time, although reports from Communist China now indicate that it has been virtually eradicated. Most of the new drugs found during this period of exploration have remained in local use only and are inactive entries in world pharmacology. These include a number of crude natural products such as khat, kava, and betel. Others, however, subsequently emerged on the international drug scene and here we would list cocaine and a number of hallucinogens.

While opium for social use was an important article of commerce by the 18th century and was the cause of two military interventions by Britain in China in the middle of the 19th century, cannabis as a social drug had a more insidious history. Such use spread gradually from East Central Asia, where it seems to have originated, and by the 10th century had reached all of Southeast Asia, the Middle East, and North Africa; it was finally brought to Central and South America during the colonial period. The spread from Spanish America into the U.S. began very gradually in the 1920's and was marked by a brief spell of great activity in the 1930's followed by over two decades of relative quiescence which ended in the 1960's with the current wave which has carried it to Europe, Japan, and Australia. It is significant that the essence of the spread has been the propagation of an idea because the plant itself had long been present in virtually all countries including China, where it is still not used as a social drug. Incidentally, one may note that the indigenous sources of new psychoactive drugs may not be completely exhausted as shown by Wasson's discoveries of new hallucinogenic mushrooms in Mexico as late as the 1950's.

LAG TIME IN IDENTIFYING DEPENDENCE POTENTIAL

As we review this history, it is important to remember that the dependence-producing effects of all of these drugs were an unexpected by-product and for the most part were not recognized until the drugs had been in use for long periods of time. Moreover, virtually all of these substances were introduced or synthesized for valid medical purposes. The older drugs were essential parts of the pharmacopoeia, and the modern ones were a small fraction of a new system of treatment that has, within the space of our own lifetime, revolutionized the practice of medicine, extended the useful lives of millions, and saved untold millions more.

Yet, when we examine the facts we must concede that so far the spectacular advances have dealt only with the somatic aspects of human existence. Progress has been less than spectacular in the case of the psychoactive agents, those drugs which deal with the most personal and intimate aspects of life, where man deals not with external factors, but with his own psyche and its disorders. Much has, of course, been accomplished even here. For example, the functional psychoses can now be alleviated or altogether suppressed, and this is no small matter when we remember that it was this therapy which initiated a trend toward the emptying of the great mental hospitals. In addition, the newer drugs offer some help for those psychic disorders which are misnamed "minor" and here we would include the neurotic anxieties and such symptoms as insomnia which, like the toothache, are a source of comedy only for those who have not suffered from them. Even so, the psychotropic drugs have long been viewed with considerable suspicion by the public, and as we have seen, recent history provides considerable justification for such suspicion. We can see how deep-seated is this attitude about the psychotropic drugs from the wave of concern which was touched off about phenothiazines and rauwolfia products when they were introduced in the 1950's for the treatment of major mental disorder. There was fear that these were "happy pills" which might subvert those who took such medication, and make addicts out of them. As it turned out, these particular suspicions were unjustified, but one must admit that these drugs were an exception in the history of psychoactive substances which have so often been found finally to have the quality of reinforcement, which can produce dependence. It is, incidentally, not reassuring to note that each major type of dependence has been discovered first in the street, and this discovery was only later confirmed medically, sometimes only after a long period of controversy and doubt, as in the case of the barbiturates and the amphetamines. The determination may not be an easy one outside of the laboratory and even the great Freud was misled into using cocaine as a treatment for morphine addiction. The lag between medical introduction and identification of dependence potential is consistent for almost all of the drugs of dependence, although by a curious coincidence, two of the inhalants, ether and nitrous oxide, were used for social purposes before they were used for anesthesia.

THE HUMAN FACTOR

Even though the creation of new powerful agents and their diffusion throughout the world have intensified the problem of dependence, the human factor has played a fundamental role since the propensity to find and use such substances appears to be universal if one includes such minor items as tea, coffee, tobacco, kava, khat, and betel. Such universality indicates some deep human need, which may be partly biological since it is satisfied by a biological agent which must initiate its action at the somatic level. If it is biological, research has as yet given us not the slightest inkling as to the mechanism. We know only that virtually wherever humans have been found or adequate records of their past uncovered there is evidence of the use of such substances. The underlying drive appears to be the pleasure-pain principle which is the mainspring of all motivation, and governs the behavior of living things generally. This principle guides them away from harm and draws them toward biologically-favorable situations. It has an obvious survival value since it produces necessary adjustments to the environment which in turn give pleasure or reduce pain. Human beings have long known that they can, in a sense, outwit this principle and produce the same or similar subjective effects with drugs. In the course of history man has found a profusion of substances which enable him to short-circuit the environmental adjustment since they act directly on the pleasure-pain system, even converting social anxiety into social enjoyment, a quality that has always been a major drug-taking motive as might be expected in a social animal. Man shares with lower forms the ability to react with pleasure to such drugs, but only man has had the ingenuity to identify these pleasure-producing substances by his own initiative, and what is more important, to pass on this information as a part of his cultural heritage. This story may be seen as nothing more than a manifestation of an evil or weak part of human nature that makes harmful things out of good ones. On the other hand, it may also be seen as evidence of an overwhelming need. Man must somehow meet the drive for social contentment and must control his reactions to problems which grow out of social pressures and the demands of an increasingly complex world; these reactions can be self-defeating. Evaluation of the motivational side of drug dependence is further complicated by the fact that such motivational aspects are not homogeneous. Indeed an important typology of drug dependence is based essentially on differences in the motivations of the users. The type that has always roused social concern is using psychoactive drugs for social and recreational purposes, while taking the same drugs even in the same amounts for medical purposes is seen very differently. Both types may involve drug dependence, but the medical type lacks the contagious quality of social drug use, and there are other behavioral differences which account for differences in social attitudes about them. A third category that may also be identified on the basis of motivation is the religious type; this too is generally regarded with little social concern probably because it tends to be more rigorously controlled, although some explain the negative attitudes about social drug-taking in terms of anhedonic elements in society.

CONTROL BY LAW AND BY EDUCATION AND THE NEED FOR RESEARCH

The first reaction to the appearance of social use of new drugs or substances has traditionally been one of profound suspicion. This will eventually lead to attempts to try to check it by law and/or by educational efforts. Such efforts have been directed against tobacco and coffee, as well as opium, morphine, and cocaine. With some notable exceptions, these efforts have proven to be of limited value and have failed to reach their goal. For this reason, attention is now shifting to a third alternative which is a technical solution based on better understanding of the phenomenon itself. This approach has been reinforced by the fact that efforts at legal control have recently been colliding for the first time with strong trends toward an increasing sensitivity concerning the rights of the individual with respect to his private behavior. This has produced an unprecedented resistance to many forms of legal drug control measures; even where there is no outright resistance, there is now increasing criticism of types of controls that were not previously questioned. It is unfortunate that in the heat of this debate many liberals have left the impression that they see such drug taking as a positive good, whereas this is in fact the view of only a minority; the others attack the laws as bad but still do not recommend drug taking.

There is little debate about the educational approach which may be seen as the second of three major approaches. Historically speaking, antidrug education has often proven effective in maintaining the status quo with respect to substances which have not yet come into general vogue or which are generally condemned even when the educational methods are unsophisticated and take the form of reinforcing unsubstantiated folklore. This was the case with antidrug education in the U.S. a few decades ago. It has, however, been far less effective with respect to control of drugs which have already come into wide social use. This is exemplified in the current anti-tobacco campaign which has had only a small impact even though it is well organized, well substantiated in content, sophisticated in presentation, and well organized in operation. The plain fact is that educational drug campaigns in our society have been of limited power except to reinforce existing tendencies. We still know too little about the dynamics of these types of large group behavior to pretend to influence them in any specific way. We can only aim to contain as far as possible those that are considered unfavorable and hope that they will prove to be passing fads. At this time, we must acknowledge that the drugs are a part of modern life, and even the idea of formally adding to the current limited list of approved social and recreational drugs has influenced people throughout the world. It may or may not be a passing fad, and at this time no one can state with assurance what will be the price of such an extension. Some hold that all fears are unfounded, while others see evil omens in the experience of countries where drugs have been uncontrolled as in the case of China with opium. Similarly, there is much concern about the reports of current experience of mass use of "white drugs" and "soft drugs" in various parts of Asia, the Middle East, and Africa.

LIMITS OF DEBATE AND DIALECTIC

Emotions originally generated about laws and law enforcement now run high with respect to many other aspects of drug taking. Rivers of ink have been spilled in debate on this subject, and the ingenuity of armies of debaters has exhausted the resources of dialectic and rhetoric, but to no avail since the dialectic has proven only that contradictory gambits of logic may be constructed out of the same bits of fact. The rhetoric has only deepened the feelings of the debaters. If one can judge by the reactions of recent audiences, there is reason to believe that the general public has, for the moment at least, reached a sort of satiety on the subject. Yet, whether the public is aroused or apathetic and regardless of the debate, the real problems and questions remain unanswered. These are questions rooted in biological fact and because of their very nature, one would expect to find answers in scientific demonstration rather than logic or debate; experience is that debate has not provided answers. Unlike most questions about the psyche and social problems, this one has a large visible biological element, one that is subject to the experimental method. There are indications that this state of affairs has been generally recognized. Both sides in the drug controversy, those who seek to prohibit and those who are opposed to prohibitions, agree on one point, namely that we need a better understanding of drug dependence itself and all of the associated phenomena. In other words, they may disagree on the law and education, but they agree on a third approach, research. This has created a strong pressure for drug-dependence research, and more importantly, has insured sources of funds for such work. This has had the effect of diverting research effort away from other areas and into drug studies because it has come at a time when other types of research have been experiencing reduced fiscal and public support.

SOME THOUGHTS RELATED TO RESEARCH

In approaching drug dependence from a technical and research point of view, a useful model to consider describes the condition due to the interaction of three sets of factors: those which have to do with the individual, those which have to do with the drug, and those of the environment. This model is, of course, a modification of the public health model for contagious disease, where the elements are the host, agent, and environment. The relative influence of each in the totality which we call drug dependence is likely to be variable for different drugs, individuals, and environments. In the past, much effort has been expended trying to settle this issue by logic built upon clinical observation and statistical retrospective studies. Because the presenting syndrome is one of mass human behavior, the emphasis has been largely on the social, psychiatric, and psychological aspects, while the biological aspects have been overshadowed. We have even heard comments to the effect that the problem is a people problem and not a drug problem. This last formulation may have value in clinical treatment and in educational programs, but it appears inadequate for research since it ignores the interactional aspects. A full discussion of this issue alone would involve a highly complex and theoretical consideration of the relative place of biological and psychosocial factors in drug dependence. In turn, this is a special instance of the general question of body-mind relationships, all of which is well beyond the scope of this introduction. For our purposes it would seem adequate to confine our discussion to the practical side of studying a condition which involves the interaction of psyche, soma, drug, and environment. We can, of course, only assume that there exists a somatic correlate for each psychic and behavioral aspect of drug dependence, which includes all reactions of social significance. Furthermore, it still remains to be shown how much of what we call physical dependence is physical in the usual sense and how much is due to nonspecific conditioning or social conditioning. Even more important, one cannot be sure to what extent solutions of drug dependence problems will be somatic and biological and to what extent they must be social and/or psychic. There are those who assert that drug dependence problems are not due to drugs at all, but due to such environmental factors as antidrug laws and social rejection, while others assert that the problem is not specific but lies in the underlying propensities of the person which would inevitably lead him to other and even worse alternatives if there were no drugs. A more practical and tangible question to be settled is to what extent the complications of the drug life are intrinsic and direct drug effects and to what extent they are secondary to exposure, poverty, malnutrition, infection, and other stresses. Finally, it remains to be proven in a rigorous fashion that the benefits of taking drugs do not outweigh the harm – at least for some drug takers and for some drugs. This question is particularly active with respect to cannabis and even some of the other hallucinogens.

Years of world-wide discussion and debate on these issues have failed to resolve them, and it is generally conceded that the stalemate of discussion must be broken by specific new information. It seems unlikely that purely epidemiological data will accomplish this because it is generally acknowledged that retrospective statistical studies cannot provide proof of a causal relationship in an association. An important alternative lies in direct laboratory and basic science studies even though drug dependence expresses itself as a form of human behavior which is willed and purposeful, and is a group activity which spreads by social contact. Until the last few years this type of research has been sparse indeed and has had little attention with a few notable exceptions such as at Lexington and Ann Arbor where an amazing amount of work has been done by a handful of investigators.

Now the time has come for an expansion of such basic studies. This is under way on an unprecedented scale, with a new understanding of the biological aspects of drug dependence emerging. The results of such work are likely to be comparatively slow and as a rule not spectacular, but the laboratory approach has demonstrated the power of seemingly small discoveries to change the larger social picture and to have a massive impact on larger events. This has been demonstrated in the related field of therapeutic psychopharmacology where the phenothiazines have revolutionized psychiatric practice within less than two decades. In drug dependence, the introduction of the antagonists as therapy has been an important step in principle; although limited in scope it points to an important potential for the future. Methadone maintenance has had a significant practical impact. It is also promising in principle because it has shown that the morphine-type of physical dependence by itself may not be as damaging as was once thought, providing that the reinforcement of the drug experience is somehow withheld or blocked. This phenomenon is a fertile source of study.

Until now, advances have been on a relatively superficial level. Studies of the more fundamental biological events in drug dependence have barely begun, but it would seem that no other approach has the potential to provide essential components for the necessary solutions. Such potential is to be found in a study of the pharmacodynamics of these drugs and of the biological elements in the causal nexus as well as the pathology associated with drug dependence. This is true even though the basic scientific approach may seem circuitous and indirect as compared to the direct attack by logic and by social approaches, which seek to attack the problem as it is seen in the field.

Finally, we can expect that basic studies will illuminate more than drug dependence because this is a fundamental attack on a problem of body-mind interaction. It is the only example of such interaction in which the agent is objective, quantifiable, and subject to chemical manipulation, and an important part of the reaction is capable of demonstration in the animal model.

In closing this discussion it might be well to take cognizance of the recent reemergence of a deep-seated ambivalence toward research, a feeling that has long been in abeyance but still is embedded in our culture and expresses a fear of the unforeseen consequences of newly found information. On a practical level this concern has a basis in reality since increased scientific knowledge does confer increased power both for evil as well as for good. The cultural expression of this feeling contains a large component that is less intellectualized and involves a strong element of guilt. This is seen in the Biblical story about Adam's expulsion from the Garden for eating the forbidden fruit from the tree of knowledge and in the story of Prometheus who suffered eternal punishment for having brought mankind the forbidden knowledge of fire. Icarus, too, is a mythological symbol who was destroyed for literally flying too high in his inventive drives. A variation on this theme is found in the medieval legends about Dr. Faustus who bartered his soul to the devil in exchange for forbidden knowledge and the power which it conferred. This exemplified the deep fear of a superstitious age about the forces which such knowledge might bring down upon the populace.

These stories have often been regarded as cultural remnants of a bygone era. This era seemed particularly distant during the enthusiasm for research that marked the early days of atomic energy, Sputnik, space exploration, the wonder drugs, and computer technology. Today, things look somewhat different and there is again some suspicion about the value of man's efforts in exploring and conquering the unknown. Much attention is being paid to books like Rachel Carson's *Silent Spring* and *The Mirage of Health* by Rene Dubos. Concern about the environment includes the thought that not all new discoveries may be good; enthusiasm for research has diminished, and some are even calling for a moratorium on all research, although basic research seems to be the main target. This attitude seems, however, to be more an emotional position than a real policy. When faced with intractable problems, society still turns to research for an answer and demands more information with which to proceed. This has been the case with respect to drug dependence and demands for such research are stronger today than ever before. What is more important, the support is financial as well as moral.

The urgent needs of society represent an opportunity for the kind of scientific contribution which is called "relevant." I know of no public health problem in the psychosocial area which is so amenable to laboratory techniques and so promising with respect to its immediate goals and to broader problems of mental health and illness. The technical papers which make up this volume strongly indicate that the challenge of this opportunity is now being met.

SIGNIFICANCE AND CHARACTERISTICS OF DRUG DEPENDENCE

CHARACTERISTICS OF DEPENDENCE ON AND ABUSE OF PSYCHOACTIVE DRUGS

M. H. Seevers

TABLE OF CONTENTS

DEFINITION OF DRUG AS APPLIED TO DEPENDENCE AND ABUSE OF PSYCHOACTIVE SUBSTANCES

If a drug is defined as any substance used in the prevention, cure, or mitigation of disease, many of the commonly used psychoactive substances, LSD, other hallucinogens, volatile solvents and others, do not comply with this definition. Some semanticists, therefore, object to designating them as drugs. The term chemical is not generally applicable. It does not apply to marijuana, opium, peyote, or any other plant materials or their extractives. Lacking a more apt term, *drug* will be used here arbitrarily to apply to all psychoactive substances. It is a common and usual designation which is generally understood by most classes of society.

Non-medical use of drugs[1] has been avoided here purposely since it conveys the tacit implication that medical usage is free from dependence and abuse. It identifies drug abuse specifically with self-administration. Who is to determine whether an individual self-administers psychoactive substances excessively for nonmedical or for medical purposes? Furthermore, if applied literally, it would characterize only a fraction of the drugs of use and abuse, and exclude those which have no established medical use, cannabis, hallucinogens, volatile solvents, and so forth.

DRUG DEPENDENCE

General Considerations as a Scientific Phenomenon

Many terms have been utilized to characterize what is currently termed drug dependence by an increasing majority of the scientific and legal communities. The German sücht, Möller's[2] euphomania, and Lindesmith's[3] craving, are inadequate to encompass the total picture since they ignore the importance of physical dependence as a secondary reinforcer. Bejerot[4] has recently revived the discarded French "toxicomania." Psychoactive drugs he calls "toxicotics" and presents an elaborate and confusing classification involving pharmacology, law, medical diagnosis, sociology, etc. His subdivision of toxicomanias into benign and banal is difficult to harmonize with the generally accepted meaning of the term mania.

The most commonly used terms prior to 1965 were habituation and addiction. Habituation usually characterized drug use without serious harmful effects to the individual and especially to society. Addiction, by contrast, implies compulsive abuse associated with physical dependence. It is often used as a synonym for this phenomenon. It usually implies dire effects on the individual and on society. In common parlance the term addiction also carries moral implications, without regard to the relative capacity of the drug to induce dependence, or to its relative effects on the individual and society. For example, some crusaders against tobacco apply the term addiction with equal force and stigma to cigarette smokers as to heroin-dependent persons. It is a common lay term and it has by no means disappeared from use even by scientists. It is a common designation by those in the communications media and public forum who wish to stir the emotions or exploit the spectacular by painting a grim picture of all drug use.

The writer[5] was in part responsible for identifying physical dependence with the term addiction. It became apparent 30 years later that the genesis of drug-seeking behavior involved psychological reinforcement as the primary stimulus to compulsive drug use. Physical dependence, if it exists, may serve as a secondary strengthening factor. In 1962, I suggested[6] that habituation and addiction should be abandoned as scientific terms in view of the multiplicity and nonspecificity of meanings in scientific, as well as in lay use. In 1965, this suggestion was implemented by the World Health Organization[7] which proposed the term dependence to characterize both the psychological and physical aspects of individual-psychoactive drug interactions.

Major criticism of the term dependence has taken two courses; first, that it lacks specificity since it is no different from innumerable habits which regulate life, second, that vitamin deficient, diabetic, and cardiac insufficient patients are "dependent" on drugs. Both of these arguments are scientifically fatuous because they ignore the fact that the term is limited here to drugs that are psychoactive. Furthermore, psychoactive drugs are reinforcing by a direct effect on the nervous system. They do not correct a deficiency or imbalance, or any existing pathologic state. Moreover, they modify the capacity of the nervous system to react to and to interpret the nature of the reward.

Neither does the fact that the term dependence has been used with considerable latitude in other scientific terminology detract from its use in relationship to psychoactive drugs. Microbiologists have used it to denote adaptation of bacteria to chemical inhibitors of growth. This type of adaptation can be easily differentiated from drug dependence since it has been shown to be largely genetic, rather than phenotypic, adaptation. Dependence has also been used to describe the increased demand of an organism for one of the normal metabolites such as pyridoxine. Neither of these scientific uses of the term conflicts with drug dependence as it applies to psychoactive drugs since they clearly involve different mechanisms of action.

Definition of Dependence

Drug dependence may be defined in scientific terminology as follows: *Repeated use of psychoactive drugs leading to a conditioned pattern of drug-seeking behavior. A characteristic, predictable and reproducible syndrome is associated with each drug (or drug type). It may be modified or reinforced by drug-induced physical and/or pathological components. The intensity of response varies with the nature and amount of the drug and the method, frequency, and duration of administration.*

Psychological Dependence

Definition

Several adjectives, psychic, psychogenic, in addition to psychological have been used to characterize this type of dependence. Psychologists use the term positive reinforcement. Positive reinforcement involves the behavioral responses to many types of reward, food, drink, sex, and the like. In this instance, the specific reinforcer is a drug whose effects are sufficiently attractive and psychologically rewarding at the first trial to initiate the desire and motivate the user to repeat the experience. One reinforcement is obviously inadequate to constitute psychological dependence. As the term is applied to drugs, neither is it necessary to satisfy the strict requirements commonly used to define habit, repetition of acts with sufficient frequency or duration to become involuntary.

Determination of the existence of psychological dependence on drugs therefore requires an arbitrary decision relating to the frequency and duration of reinforcements. This is difficult to accomplish since the strength of the reinforcement is critical, a factor that varies not only with the chemical, physical, and pharmacological characteristics of the drug, but also with the dose, method, frequency, and duration of administration.[8]

Types and Patterns of Use

If "psychological dependence" is acceptable as a useful biological term, it seems pertinent to describe a few general types as a basis for assessing their significance as it relates to the individual and to society. This cataloguing is descriptive and arbitrary. Innumerable patterns exist even with a single drug. When multiple drug use is involved, exceedingly complex situations may emerge which defy simple characterization. Some are unwilling to accept the more benign and intermittent patterns of use as evidence of psychological dependence.

Occasional use – There may be long periods between use. Such use may be light or heavy and commonly involves a social setting with hedonistic features. It may be either of minor or major significance, depending on the drug, the dosage, and the previous condition of the individual. Examples are LSD and other hallucinogens, marijuana, glue sniffing, "joy-popping" with heroin, and so forth.

Continued frequent use at irregular intervals – Short term, for instance, several days of spree use (to the point of severe intoxication). Examples include alcohol, amphetamines, hashish, and cocaine.

Regular long term use to the point of continuous intoxication with periodic free intervals of several days' duration – Examples are amphetamines, cocaine, sometimes alcohol, and barbiturates.

Regular daily use with long free intervals – For example, alcohol (heavy social drinker), barbiturates, oral amphetamines, and tranquilizers.

Compulsive continuous chronic use, with few, if any, free intervals – Examples are alcohol, barbiturates, heroin (and other narcotics), tranquilizers, oral amphetamines and other stimulants, and hashish. Even tobacco, coffee, and aspirin may be included in this category.

In my opinion, two types of psychological dependence which should be excluded in considering psychoactive drug dependence as it relates to drug abuse are: a) the placebo effect which may be a psychological component of any drug use and b) drugs which are psychologically rewarding because they increase or decrease sensory input by peripheral action. Some examples are aspirin, other antipyretic analgesics, antacids, and others.

Even though heavy chronic use may induce toxic and pathologic effects in the individual, for example, renal pathology with phenacetin, such drugs do not constitute a significant social hazard and should be categorized in terms of chronic toxicity rather than as drug abuse.

Physical Dependence

Definition

Physical dependence may be defined as follows: *The state of latent hyperexcitability which develops in the central nervous system of higher mammals following frequent and prolonged administration of the morphine-like analgesics, alcohol, barbiturates, and other depressants. It is not manifest subjectively or objectively during drug administration. Specific symptoms and signs, the abstinence syndrome, occur upon abrupt termination of drug administration; or with the morphine-like agonists by administering the specific antagonists.*

Types of Physical Dependence

Morphine agonist type – Whereas morphine is the classical prototype of this type of physical dependence, it occurs with all of the morphine-like agonists. This currently includes several thousand individual compounds of ten or more different molecular configurations.

Physical dependence to morphine-like narcotic analgesics is highly specific and characterizes a unique biologic phenomenon. It is readily reproducible in primates and higher mammalian forms, less so in lower mammals, and not at all in the lowest animal species. It has specific and clearly defined parameters, being characterized by high grade drug specificity as well as cell specificity, since it apparently may be induced in only one type of cell, the neuron. Mutual cross tolerance and dependence exist between all morphine-like agonists. This is specific and does not occur with other depressant drugs.

Morphine-antagonist type – Most known antagonists are not pure pharmacological entities. They contain both antagonist and agonist components; the ratio between the two varying with the substance under consideration. This type of physical dependence represents the reaction to the agonist component of the mixed agonist-antagonists such as nalorphine, cyclazocine, pentazocine, and others. The abstinence syndrome bears certain similarities to the classic morphine agonist syndrome, but is much less intense. It would appear to represent the cellular response of only a fraction of the neuronal centers involved in the total mosaic which comprises the morphine agonist syndrome. Pure antagonists like naloxone which lacks the agonist component produce no detectable evidence of physical dependence.

Alcohol-barbiturate type – This type of physical dependence is clearly distinguishable from the morphine-type. It is characterized by an all-or-none dose response relationship, as well as a specific time-response effect. Its induction requires large doses of alcohol or barbiturates, administered with such frequency that the brain is never completely drug free. The major signs of alcohol abstinence resemble the effects produced by convulsive drugs; severe motor hyperreflexia, generalized tremors, and grand mal convulsions. These are associated with a psychosis-like state with disorders of cognition and hallucinations. It is produced not only by ethanol, but also higher alcohols, organic solvents, and other depressant substances with similar pharmacological properties. It is produced by all known barbiturates. Furthermore, cross tolerance and cross dependence exist in all of the classes of substances mentioned above, but not to morphine or morphine-like substances.

Psychoactive Substances Which Do Not Create Physical Dependence

Depressants – Physical dependence does not occur following chronic administration of the following depressants; phenothiazines, inorganic bromides, and bromide contain organic sedatives or antihistamines. Psychological dependence is also weak or nonexistent. Consequently, the dependence potential of these substances is low and abuse is uncommon.

Stimulants – Chronic administration of maximum tolerated quantities of the powerful stimulants, cocaine, all the psychomotor stimulants, amphetamines, methylphenidate, phenmetrazine, spa, and many others fail to create physical dependence in man and animals. In spite of this, they represent, as a class, the most psychologically reinforcing drugs and have the greatest abuse potential of all the psychoactive substances. Weak stimulants such as caffeine, nicotine, and betel also lack this capacity.

Hallucinogens – No psychotomimetic drug is known to produce physical dependence, including LSD, mescaline, and many others.

Although a mild withdrawal syndrome occurs in chronic hashish users, it has always been considered to be of psychological rather than physical origin. Recently Deneau and Kaymakcalan[9] have described a characteristic abstinence syndrome in rhesus monkeys who received .4

mg/kg delta-9 THC every 6 hours for a month. Further study of this phenomenon is essential before reaching conclusions concerning its significance in man.

Characteristics of Withdrawal of Drugs Which Do Not Create Physical Dependence

Following subacute or chronic administration of very large quantities of some of the drugs listed above, withdrawal may elicit severe symptoms and signs. This is especially the case with the stimulants. It is important to distinguish the nonspecific symptoms and signs of these classes of drugs from those of the specific abstinence syndrome of drugs which do induce physical dependence.

Clearly these symptoms and signs are in part psychogenic. They occur as an overlay to intensify the specific signs of physical origin in morphine and alcohol-barbiturate types of physical dependence. With the stimulants they derive largely from somatic changes relating to the intensity of the intoxication and the inability or the lack of desire of the user to follow the ordinary life routine required for maintenance of homeostasis, and even survival. For example, the "speed freak" who is under constant and unremitting stimulation for days, consumes little food and has absolute insomnia. The intense fatigue and weakness associated with withdrawal can be accounted for by the severe and rapid weight loss, acidosis, and disturbances in salt and water balance. The psychotic manifestations can be explained by the insomnia alone, since it is known to occur regularly with severe sleep deprivation.

It may appear to be only of academic interest to distinguish the origin of withdrawal symptoms and signs. But it must be borne in mind that the adverse effects of withdrawal from some drugs which fail to induce physical dependence, although severe, often do not have the same strength as secondary reinforcers leading to readministration of the drug. During withdrawal, the "speed freak" is so physically and emotionally debilitated that further drug administration is no longer rewarding. Further drug administration during withdrawal is incapable of reversing the situation, as would be the case with drugs which induce physical dependence. With tobacco the emotional reaction to breaking off of a long-established and continued habit pattern is adequate to explain the phenomenon.

DRUG ABUSE

Drug Abuse Defined as Societal Value Judgments

In contrast to drug dependence, the term drug abuse has no uniform connotation and cannot be characterized in simple or precise terms. The disapproval of innumerable "societies" relating to certain patterns of drug use by their members, is expressed as countless value judgments designated by the general term drug abuse.

Since these judgments are designed to distinguish acceptable from unacceptable use of a wide variety of drugs in any given "society," they may be expressed either in terms of societal concern for the welfare of the individual due to toxicity or pathology, or in terms of the hazards to society from the disordered behavior of the drugged individual. In many instances they are lumped together with no distinction between these two different facets of the problem. Efforts to find uniformity or consistency in these judgments with respect to logic, the mental or physical health of the individual, the present or future welfare of society, or general applicability to control of the problem as a basis for an acceptable definition of drug abuse are hopeless tasks.

The use and/or abuse of drugs is nearly universal. The complexities of individual-drug interactions touch every fabric of society. No member can escape its influences. Drug effects may be beneficial or harmful; use commonly implying benefits and abuse symbolizing harm. But no sharp line distinguishes use from abuse. Both are subject to innumerable interpretations and misinterpretations. More often than not, the sum total of drug effects on any individual is a mixture of benefits and harm; endless shades of gray, rarely black and white. Since individuals vary widely in their psychological and physical responses to a given drug, one man's use may be another's abuse - to paraphrase the old cliché.

Characterization of the term drug abuse has many variants; medical, legal, social, religious, moral, ethnic, political, and others, each representing a different point of view. However, most disregard the scientific facts concerning drug dependence, and almost invariably, without any discernible logic. The term drug abuse is often used as a synonym for drug dependence. Drug abuse is used to distinguish: *illegal* from legal use; *nonmedical* from medical use of any drug; *use of over-the-counter drugs* from prescription by physician; even *immorality* from morality. In addition, use in one ethnic subculture, religious group, nation, or political subdivisions, may be abuse in another.

Since this endless variety of meanings are almost invariably interpreted and applied as legal sanctions, the latter, like the term drug abuse, have no consistency whatsoever. Nor is there any established individual or social norm upon which to base a consistent public policy which would minimize the individual and social hazards of drug use. The term minimize is used here with purpose, since all knowledge, current and historical, establishes the fact that the only public policy which has any hope of success involves containment of the problem rather than the abolition of drug dependence and drug abuse. Drug abuse will be defined below in both scientific and medical terms.

Relation of Drug Abuse to Drug Dependence

Drug dependence does not lead invariably to drug abuse – Strong dependence may develop to many substances whose psychoactive properties are so minimal that they cannot be detected by objective methods. These include tobacco, coffee, betel, aspirin, and others. Some of these substances have potential for harm to the individual but have no potential for harm to society. Individual injury relates to chronic toxicity and can be distinguished clearly from abuse of psychoactive substances.

Drug abuse exists without any relation to drug dependence – The first trial of alcohol may result in a car crash involving several fatalities; the first involvement of the novice with cocaine or amphetamines may result in a psychosis-induced murder. This is certainly drug abuse, by any definition.

"Drug Culture" as a Cause of Drug Abuse

A very common misinterpretation of drug abuse is that it is an invariable sequel to drug dependence. Since nearly every individual is dependent upon some nonfood substance or drug, dependence is equated in societal terms as "drug culture." Such commonality of meaning lends admirably to the sequence: drug dependence (meaning self-administration of any drug) → "drug culture" (everyone dependent on something) → drug abuse (individual and social harm). With this illogic, "drug culture" becomes a wastebasket of banalities which is a convenient accounting device for explaining all of the ills which plague society.

So, the answer to drug abuse is simple. Eliminate drug dependence, "drug culture" will evaporate, and *presto chango* drug abuse with its attendant social evils, poverty, crime, and family disruption, will suddenly disappear. But how can drug dependence be eliminated? No problem at all. Abolish all advertising, drug cabinets will become bare, and the public will quit self-medication.

Such a simplistic interpretation of the place of drugs in the modern world is useful to those groups who would reorganize society to their own liking, especially those new groups which have taken upon themselves a responsibility of protecting the individual from industrial predators. It is also being used by individuals who would play on the emotions of the uninformed population for personal gain. *It is completely out of perspective with the scientific and medical facts concerning drug dependence, society's need for the indispensible place of self-medication in the scheme of health care, and the historical relationship of man to the ingestion of nonfood substances.*

Possibly this nonsense represents a reaction to the polar position of those who desire to "turn on" with drugs and develop the "drug culture" into a religion. In my opinion, it does not have such pure motives. In any case, the term "drug culture" as applied to either extreme position is unadulterated demogoguery. Furthermore, the tacit and naive assumption of those who favor this approach to the problem of drug abuse is that the public will no longer have any minor ills and complaints and will no longer need or seek medication unless it is prescribed by a physician.

Is Dependence on Psychoactive Drugs Incompatible with Mental Health?

Even when the term drug abuse is restricted, to psychoactive drugs, one only need raise the question, "Is the use of all psychoactive substances by self-medication inevitably incompatible with mental and/or physical health?" Expressed in more practical terms, "Does alcohol yield mental benefits to the ninety million drinkers who refrain from its abuse?" or "Do mental benefits occur to the great segment of the world population who regularly use tobacco, coffee, betel, minor analgesics, mild sedatives, and the like?"

If widespread dependence on these substances

is a measure of psychological reward which facilitates the ability to cope satisfactorily, a vast majority of the world population has answered this question in the affirmative. *Logic demands that mental health benefits of psychoactive substances, when used properly, be recognized as a scientifically established fact.*

What I am trying to say is that it is equally illogical, equally unsound scientifically and medically, and equally impractical to deny that the proper use of drugs may confer mental and physical benefits as a basis for damning the so-called "drug culture" as it is to propose that society shall abandon all constraints, "abuse" mind-altering drugs to its hearts content without regard to the consequences and establish a "psychedelic drug culture" as a basis for common understanding and international accord.

Unscientific Nature of "Soft" Drug – "Hard" Drug Concept

One other concept, equally absurd scientifically, categorizes psychoactive substances as "hard" or "soft." This malignant concept not only violates every pharmacological precept, but has contributed greatly to the unbelievable confusion among the public at large, among public officials, and even among scientists and physicians, who, if they took the trouble to become informed, should know better.

The plain, unvarnished and unemotional facts are that there are no hard or soft drugs in terms of their potential capacity for individual or social harm. *There is only hard and soft use.* Thus, any psychoactive drug may be administered without any harm whatsoever if the dose is small enough and the interval between doses permits detoxification of the previous dose.

One current classical example is "soft" marijuana and "hard" heroin. Marijuana is classified as soft because it is used occasionally, not regularly, and the yield of the active principle delta-9 THC from a "joint" is very small, often almost negligible. In consequence, not much happens. But delta-9 THC is of the same order of potency as most narcotics. And hashish can be as hard as any. Furthermore, heroin, or any narcotic, if used in small doses (for example, a therapeutic dose of 10 mg) once a day is also "soft" without the capacity to establish physical dependence or even significant psychological dependence. It is a fact of every day life in the therapeutic use of narcotics for the relief of pain.

One of the most striking examples is "hard" and "soft" alcohol. The alcoholic consumes large quantities of alcohol, dosing himself frequently, according to his subjective needs during the 24-hour diurnal-nocturnal cycle. At no time is his brain free of alcohol. Long continued use induces changes in the nervous system which elicit the specific behavioral characteristics of the alcoholic in abstinence, convulsive seizures, tremor, and delirium with hallucinations. These may be associated with clearly defined brain pathology. This hard pattern of use leads to behavioral disorders which are of great concern to society, representing one of our major medical problems.

By contrast, the heavy social drinker may consume half as much alcohol in a 24-hour period. But he limits consumption of alcohol to a single period of several hours, leaving an 18 to 20-hour interval between ingestion. This permits the brain to be alcohol-free and facilitates complete recovery. If the heavy social drinker adheres strictly to this drinking pattern, he will never reach the alcoholic state described above. Experimentally, these two human drinking models may be reproduced without fail in the rhesus monkey with identical results. In fact, by frequent intravenous administration of alcohol without interruption, behavioral changes of the "hard" alcoholic model may be produced in a matter of weeks.

Drug Abuse Potential Defined in Terms of Psychoactive Drug Induced Disorders of Behavior

The author believes,[10] as will be elaborated below, if the use of the term drug abuse is identified primarily with the disordered behavior induced by psychoactive drugs, a basis may be established for a more logical application of a social science which would deal specifically with the societal responses to such behavior.

Certain types of drug-induced behavior are more often than not, unacceptable to society. They may be separated into three broad categories: a) aggression or violence, b) loss of psychomotor control, and c) mental and emotional marasmus or shrivel.

Aggression or Violence

This may be of two general types: 1) release from normal inhibitions by depressants, alcohol, barbiturates, volatile solvents, and so forth, and 2) perceptual distortions leading to psychotic behavior patterns, LSD and other hallucinogens, amphetamines, and other stimulants.

Loss of Psychomotor Control

This involves mental and/or physical inability to perform perceptual motor tasks such as ambulation, driving motor vehicles, and handling machinery. It is one of the oldest social problems and it involves alcohol, barbiturates, and many kinds of sedatives.

Mental or Physical Marasmus or Shrivel

This involves syndromes which lead to inability or refusal to assume individual and/or social responsibility. It may occur with any class of drugs. Its outstanding characteristic is that the principal effort and time of the user is devoted to drug-seeking behavior and its consequences. It is most common with alcohol, hashish, narcotics, barbiturates and other sedatives, or in any situation where multiple drug use occurs.

Whereas these three categories are described separately, many psychoactive drugs are potentially capable of initiating behavior of all three types.

Drug Abuse Potential Not Correlated with Somatic Toxicity or Pathology

Placing the primary emphasis for assessing drug abuse potential on behavioral disorders to the exclusion of the acute and chronic effects of psychoactive drugs on the individual is purposeful for the following reasons:

a. The term drug abuse is misused widely and indiscriminately to describe any type of somatic toxicity or pathology from any drug without regard to the nature of its pharmacological action. Whereas society is obviously concerned with the toxicity of nonpsychoactive drugs, they do not induce any type of behavior which would constitute a threat to society since the brain is not involved. For example, the term drug abuse is applied to the long term excessive use of many OTC drugs, analgesic antipyretics (aspirin and phenacetin), cathartics, as well as tobacco, coffee and the like; substances which lack the capability of initiating disorders of behavior. Furthermore, although many efforts have been made to establish sanctions against the use of such substances in order to protect the individual, such a policy has had little public acceptance.

b. There is no correlation whatsoever between the capacity of a psychoactive drug to induce behavioral disorders and the capacity of these drugs to induce either brain or other somatic toxicity or pathology. *Of the six classes of substances with greatest abuse potential, only alcohol and barbiturates produce clearly established and reproducible brain pathology.* Cocaine, amphetamines, other stimulants, heroin, all morphine-like drugs, and cannabis, do not produce brain pathology. On the other hand, very heavy use of aspirin, which has no social abuse potential whatsoever, may produce renal damage.

Injury to the Individual Considered as a Separate but Related Problem

The principal, if not the sole purpose in any consideration of drug abuse, is to establish a basis for rational control of the problem which will protect both the individual and society. In the interests of clarity, and for the reasons mentioned above, individual-drug interactions which affect only the individual, should be considered separately from those which adversely affect society. Most societies fail to distinguish these two facets of the problem when dealing with methods of drug abuse control.

Adverse effects on the individual from psychoactive drugs may be separated into the following three categories:

1. *Specific drug-induced acute or chronic toxicity or pathology.* Among others, these may include acute lethal overdose, chronic liver, kidney, bone marrow injury, chromosome damage, and teratological effects. These injuries may be caused either by the drug of abuse or its adulterants. These effects are nonspecific for psychoactive drugs but occur with many drugs and chemicals.

Some psychoactive drugs, alcohol and barbiturates, may produce chronic brain pathology. Others, principally the hallucinogens and stimulants, may precipitate temporary or semipermanent psychotic episodes, or enhance preexisting emotional disorders.

2. *Related to drug administration.* Vascular thrombosis, blood borne infections such as malaria, hepatitis, or endocarditis and others.

3. *Related to the life style and unfavorable environment of the drug user.* Malnutrition, lowered resistance to bacterial and viral infections,

chronic diseases, tuberculosis, and the like. Many of these adverse effects are related to the economics of drug abuse. Many could be avoided if pure drugs are used, sanitation is observed, and proper nourishment is assured.

Clearly these adverse effects should be of concern to society. But it is much more difficult to mount the same degree of social pressure or to establish acceptable sanctions against influences which affect the individual than those which also affect others. This is well demonstrated in the existing situation with tobacco.

Can logic ever play a significant role in the decision making of society concerning problems like the self-administration of psychoactive substances where the principal element of concern involves the hedonistic desires and practices of its individuals? Even if this philosophical question is answered in the negative, the important facets of the problem as it affects both the individual and society should be kept in perspective if social justice shall prevail. This will never be possible unless the primary foundation for evaluating drug abuse potential is the pharmacological principles which dictate the psychological and behavioral responses to psychoactive drugs.

REFERENCES

1. Interim report of the Commission of Inquiry into the Non-Medical use of Drugs. Information Canada, Ottawa, 1970.

2. Möller, K. O., cited in Concepts, definitions, terminology, in *Addiction and Society,* Bejerot, N., Charles C Thomas, Springfield, Ill., 1970, 12.

3. Lindesmith, A. R., cited in Concepts, definitions, terminology, in *Addiction and Society,* Bejerot, N., Charles C Thomas, Springfield, Ill., 1970, 13.

4. Bejerot, N., *Addiction and Society,* Charles C Thomas, Springfield, Ill., 1970.

5. Tatum, A. L. and Seevers, M. H., Theories of drug addiction, *Physiol. Rev.*, 11, 107, 1931.

6. Seevers, M. H., Medical perspectives on habituation and addiction, *J.A.M.A.,* 181, 92, 1962.

7. Eddy, N. B., Halbach, H., Isbell, H., and Seevers, M. H., Drug dependence – its significance and characteristics, *Bull. WHO,* 32, 721, 1965.

8. Seevers, M. H., Psychopharmacological elements of drug dependence, *J.A.M.A.,* 206, 1263, 1968.

9. Deneau, G. A. and Kaymakcalan, S., Physiological and psychological dependence to synthetic delta-9 tetrahydrocannabinol (THC) in rhesus monkeys, *Pharmacologist,* 13, 246, 1971.

10. Seevers, M. H., Drug dependence vis-a-vis drug abuse, International Symposium on Drug Abuse, Ann Arbor, Michigan, November 9-13, 1970, Lea and Febiger, Inc., in press.

SIGNIFICANCE AND CHARACTERISTICS OF DRUG DEPENDENCE

Characteristics of Drug Dependence to:

NARCOTIC ANALGESICS AND ANTAGONIST

W. L. Dewey

TABLE OF CONTENTS

INTRODUCTION

The often overlapping, inaccurate, or at least confusing way in which such terms as dependence, addiction, habituation, and others were being used and interchanged, as well as the increasing number of drugs which were being abused prompted the World Health Organization to redefine a number of terms associated with drug abuse.[1] In essence, they suggested that one speak in more specific terms. The phrase "drug dependence of the morphine type" was suggested rather than "narcotic addiction" when referring to the syndrome observed due to repeated abuse of these agents. The repeated use of a number of drugs such as alcohol, barbiturates, minor tranquilizers, and others also produce a syndrome which is characterized by withdrawal. However, the withdrawal syndrome observed after the abrupt cessation of one drug type differs from that observed upon the abrupt cessation of repeated use of a drug of another class. By and large, it is the withdrawal syndrome that differentiates the physical dependence which develops from the repeated use of one type of drug from that of another. In addition, people become dependent on a number of drugs which do not produce a withdrawal syndrome when use is suddenly ceased. Nicotine, caffeine, amphetamines, and apparently marihuana are in this group. The dependence produced by these drugs is of a psychological nature. That is, the person thinks that he needs to continue taking the drug to carry out a normal or "withdrawal free" existence. A number of behavioral symptoms may occur, but these symptoms are controllable by the individual; whereas the physical withdrawal syndrome observed is uncontrollable. The presence or absence of withdrawal symptoms appears to be the principle difference between physical and psychological dependence.

Another characteristic of drug abuse that varies in intensity from one class of drugs to another is the craving that exists for repeated use of the drug. This craving may be due to a desire to experience the euphorogenic effect of the drug or to avoid the onset of the unpleasant withdrawal syndrome. Many suggest that this craving may be either all or a portion of the psychological dependence discussed above; however, if this craving is in fact due to a desire to avoid withdrawal, it could hardly be the major component of psychological dependence where one does not see a withdrawal syndrome. Upon repeated use of some drugs, an increase in the amount of drug is needed to produce an effect equivalent to that observed with the initial dose. This phenomenon is referred to as tolerance and is another component of drug abuse. The onset and magnitude of drug tolerance varies to some extent among drugs of the same class and to a greater degree among drugs of different classes. Each of the four characteristics discussed above, psychological dependence, craving, tolerance, and the withdrawal syndrome vary at least quantitatively, from one group of drugs that are abused to another. In fact, at least a temporal distinction in their appearance exists among different drugs of the same class, such as the difference in the severity and the onset of withdrawal after chronic methadone as opposed to that seen after chronic morphine.

Numerous reviews have appeared which describe a number of facets of the research involved in physical dependence to narcotic analgesics.[2-4] Most recently, the biochemical mechanisms involved in physical dependence on narcotic analgesics was reviewed by Schuster.[5] Rather than recapitulate that which has been reviewed, an attempt will be made to describe recent observations on the characteristics of the physical dependence syndrome observed in man and laboratory animals upon withdrawal of chronic treatment with narcotic analgesics. The phrase "physical dependence to opiates" will be used when discussing in general the overall syndrome observed with repeated use of morphine or one of its congeners, including diacetylmorphine (heroin), as well as such synthetic analgesics as meperidine, methadone, and others. When the characteristics of the syndrome of a specific drug are being considered, "physical dependence of that particular drug" will be used.

The compounds which are grouped in the broad classes of narcotic analgesics or antagonists constitute a spectrum of pharmacological activities. At one end of the spectrum are the compounds mentioned above, morphine, etc., which are pure analgesics, and at the other end is naloxone, which has relatively pure analgesic antagonistic activity. Between these extremes there are a number of agents which produce analgesia in man, yet also can inhibit or reverse the effects of one of the pure analgesics. Nalorphine, levallorphan, pentazocine, and cyclazocine are examples of drugs in this category which are referred to as narcotic-antagonist analgesics. In other words, these compounds have either agonistic or antagonistic activity depending on dose and presence or absence of other analgesics in the organism. It is the agonistic activity of these agents which must be considered in their dependence producing properties. The clinical use of the narcotic antagonists as analgesics was minimal in 1964 and the WHO committee did not direct themselves to the question of physical dependence to the narcotic antagonists. Extensive clinical trials and the ensuing marketing of pentazocine, the use of cyclazocine and naloxone in an attempt to treat persons dependent on narcotics, and clinical trials of other antagonists have all contributed to an increased knowledge of the effects of these drugs in man. In this chapter an effort will be made to describe that characteristics that have been observed in laboratory animals, as well as in persons who have received long-term administration of high doses of these drugs. Characteristics of the behavioral syndromes which were interpreted as a withdrawal syndrome when medication was abruptly discontinued will also be described.

PHYSICAL DEPENDENCE OF THE OPIATE TYPE IN MAN

Considerable information has been reported[6] concerning the characteristics of dependence to the narcotic analgesics. Drug dependence of the opiate type is characterized by a pronounced craving or psychological dependence and a marked tolerance to many of the effects of the opiates. The person does not become tolerant to the miosis produced by opiates and the "pin point" pupil differentiates the opiate-dependent individual from those who chronically abuse other drugs. The person dependent on these drugs seeks them for their euphorogenic effects, as well as to ward off the unpleasant withdrawal syndrome which occurs approximately 24 hours after the last dose. Initially, the seeking of the euphorogenic effects predominates the repeated use of the drug. However, only one of 88 female heroin addicts studied by d'Orban[7] was not a multiple drug user. This might suggest that the euphoric effects of heroin are not enough to satisfy all addicts and they misuse other drugs to obtain a high, which is reported to be different from that obtained from heroin. It has been reported[8] that some heroin addicts abuse barbiturates to potentiate the effects of poor heroin, while Hamburger[9] reported that seeking euphoria was not the motivation for barbiturate use by heroin addicts. The warding off of withdrawal as a possible reason for repeated use of the drug does not come into play until the person has taken a number of doses of the narcotic. Once the dependence is established, the fear of unpleasant withdrawal has more influence on the continued use. Often the opiate-dependent individual expends all of his energy to maintain his dependence and avoid withdrawal.

Interviews were conducted with 40 short-term heroin users in an attempt to determine what factors affected their cessation of drug usage.[10] Twenty-two of these cessations of heroin use were due to the physical separation of the user from his supply of drug (one or the other moved, etc.). The most significant finding of this research is that 9 of the 40 stopped using heroin because they knew they were physically dependent on the drug. This finding appears to be somewhat in contradiction with the idea that once a person becomes physically dependent on heroin he will find a way to continue its use to avoid the unpleasant withdrawal syndrome.

Often one thinks of the person dependent on opiates for a prolonged period of time as undernourished and generally in poor health. Such may be the case when the patient is dependent on heroin or another opiate which is obtained from illicit sources and quite possibly could be contaminated. This raises the question as to the source of the causative agent of the illness. Is it the primary effect of the opiate itself or is it the result of a contaminant in the drug or from the nonsterile needle used to inject the drug? Ball and Urbaitis[11] have recently reported that among 22 addicts who have been dependent on morphine (a drug which can be obtained in a sterile form) for some 35 years, 19 were in either fair or good health when examined on admission to the addiction research center in Lexington. The diseases of the three patients that were ill could not be attributed to the chronic use of morphine. These investigators concluded that these results suggested that opiates are not the primary cause of the illness. It is possible that the size of the sample is too small for such a conclusion. Moreover, one must question how these addicts obtained their drug in a pure and sterile form for such a long time. However, in checking the admission records at the hospital, they did find that the physical and mental conditions of these patients were not different from those of other patients.

The withdrawal syndrome can be precipitated by the injection of a narcotic antagonist, such as nalorphine, as well as abrupt cessation of the opiate. The withdrawal syndrome occurs almost immediately following the antagonist or begins about 24 hours after the last dose of an opiate.

The opiate withdrawal is characterized by abdominal pain, irritability, cold sweats, goose flesh, diarrhea, nausea, and vomiting. The severity of these symptoms has been described as being uncomfortable and comparable to a severe case of the flu; these effects are not usually life endangering in the otherwise healthy individual. The severity of the withdrawal syndrome is directly related to the quantity of drug consumed. The more drug to which the person is dependent, the more severe the withdrawal. In addition, a number of medical disorders can complicate matters and increase the severity or harmfulness of the withdrawal. These disorders include arthritis, cirrhosis of the liver, peptic ulcer, ulcerative colotis, hepatitis, epilepsy, and diabetes. A number of cardiovascular diseases, such as congestive heart failure, severe hypertension, and anginal syndrome, as well as the respiratory disease of asthma and pneumonia also can potentiate the severity of withdrawal.[12]

The onset of dependence is a function of the frequency and the magnitude of the dosage consumed. Opiates, such as morphine, can be used at therapeutic doses for many days without pronounced signs of withdrawal occurring on cessation of treatment. On the other hand, a number of injections during a short period of time may quickly render the patient dependent on the narcotic. The qualitative characteristics of dependence that occur with other opiates and with a number of synthetic agents such as meperidine and methadone are similar to those described above for morphine. As previously mentioned, temporal and quantitative differences exist among the drugs of this class.

Some reports concerning the dependence-producing propensity of analgesics which are not considered to be narcotics have appeared.[13] For example, the dependence producing property of *d*-propoxyphene is not well established; however, it partially suppressed the morphine abstinence syndrome in man,[14] and dependence on *d*-propoxyphene has been reported for at least one person.[15] This dependence was characterized by an extreme craving for the drug, as well as a pronounced tolerance and a withdrawal syndrome which appeared 1 to 2 days after the last dose. The withdrawal syndrome resembled that described above for morphine. On the other hand, dependence does not appear to occur to methotrimiprazine.[16]

TREATMENT OF OPIATE DEPENDENCE IN MAN

In 1965, Dole and Nyswander[17] reported that heroin addicts could be treated and rehabilitated on a high dosage regime of methadone. They suggested that although this treatment was based on the repeated use of a synthetic agent to which addiction would develop, certain benefits existed. These included the development of cross tolerance to other opiates, such as heroin, and the fact that methadone can be taken orally instead of intravenously; therefore removing the use of the needle which appears to be a psychological reinforcer in some addicts. These patients can work or attend school while being treated on the methadone maintenance program. This method of treatment is being used in many parts of the country. Although not a panacea, it is considered by some to be the best treatment available at the present time and should be made available to all addicts who wish to take part.[18]

Another approach which has been tried in the treatment of narcotic addiction is the administration of the narcotic antagonist, cyclazocine,[19-21] or more recently, naloxone. Both are active when given orally and will pharmacologically antagonize the effects of a dose of morphine or heroin for a period up to 24 hours. The duration of action of cyclazocine is longer than that of naloxone. Cyclazocine produces a number of pharmacological effects including dysphoria and sedation. The patient becomes tolerant to these effects of cyclazocine, but not to its antagonistic effects. Patients taking cyclazocine or naloxone, as opposed to those taking methadone, are not physically dependent on an opiate. One important difference in the method of treatment with cyclazocine or naloxone, as opposed to the treatment of addicts with methadone, is that the addict has to be completely withdrawn from the narcotic prior to the administration of the antagonist, or it will initiate abrupt withdrawal. Complete withdrawal from the narcotic is not necessary prior to the administration of methadone. The pharmacological basis for treatment of opiate dependence with cyclazocine or naloxone resides in their antagonistic activity; cross tolerance between methadone and other narcotics is the basis of its usefulness. A number of reviews[22-24] discuss the abuse potential of the narcotic-antagonist analgesics.

However, the considerable current interest in these compounds warrants further elaboration on their dependence-producing properties.

CHARACTERISTICS OF DEPENDENCE ON NALORPHINE IN MAN

In 1956, Isbell[25] reported that the abrupt withdrawal of nalorphine did not produce a morphine-like abstinence syndrome. The daily treatment of 150 mg/kg nalorphine produced a mild opiate withdrawal syndrome in one of two patients studied. This withdrawal syndrome was characterized by alternate feelings of hot and cold, a loss of body weight, restlessness, and poor sleep.[26] More recently, Martin and Gorodetzky[27] observed an abstinence syndrome after chronic nalorphine treatment which was characterized by diarrhea, rhinorrea, yawning, and scratching, as well as a number of possible sympathomimetic-type responses, such as loss of appetite, tachycardia, and increase in body temperature. These investigators concluded that the abstinence syndrome differed after the abrupt withdrawal of nalorphine from that observed with morphine. A significant difference between the characteristic of nalorphine dependence and morphine dependence is that during these chronic studies the patients did not "like" the nalorphine effects. It appears that tolerance and physical dependence exist to nalorphine, but due to the unpleasantness of many of its effects, it is not desired as are the opiates.

CHARACTERISTICS OF DEPENDENCE ON CYCLAZOCINE IN MAN

Cyclazocine often produced dysphoria and sedation in post addicts who frequently identified it as a barbiturate or an amphetamine, rather than an opiate.[28] Chronic treatment of 13.2 mg/70 kg/day cyclazocine produced tolerance to these effects and cross tolerance to nalorphine. Abrupt cessation of these injections produced an abstinence syndrome characterized by a loss of appetite and a decrease in body weight, as well as tachycardia, mydriasis, and an increase in body temperature. These withdrawal signs from cyclazocine appear to be sympathomimetic in origin, whereas the withdrawal signs from morphine are often interpreted as possibly the result of a cholinergic discharge. However, a decrease in caloric intake and a loss of body weight are also seen during withdrawal from opiates.

In 1966, Fraser and Rosenberg[29] reported that tolerance developed to the effects of cyclazocine to the extent that daily dosage could be increased from 2 doses of 0.4 mg on day one to a total daily dose of 9.2 mg on day 55. The patient was constipated throughout the study and reported that although he did not like the effects of cyclazocine, its effects did not disturb him. Medication was not continued after the 55th day, but the patient was observed for a possible withdrawal syndrome. The syndrome observed was characterized by an increase in body temperature, and an increase in blood pressure, but differed from withdrawal of opiates in that general body aches, restlessness, and insomnia were absent. As a matter of fact, sleep was increased. Also, nalorphine did not precipitate abstinence following chronic cyclazocine treatment.

CHARACTERISTICS OF DEPENDENCE ON PENTAZOCINE IN MAN

The initial study of the possible physical dependence properties of pentazocine in man was carried out by Fraser and Rosenberg[30] at the Addiction Research Center in Lexington, Kentucky. These investigators reported that pentazocine did not substitute for morphine in patients physically dependent on morphine and that chronic administration of pentazocine did not induce a morphine-like withdrawal syndrome after the injection of nalorphine. The other seven patients who had gone through morphine withdrawal some time earlier, asked to be taken off a chronic pentazocine injection schedule because they did not "like" the drug. A mild morphine-like abstinence withdrawal syndrome was observed in these patients when the drug was discontinued. The nonreliability of nalorphine to test for physical dependence to pentazocine has subsequently been questioned.[31] In later years, it was found that naloxone, not nalorphine or levallorphan, could antagonize the respiratory depression produced by pentazocine.[31-33] Had naloxone been available during the initial studies of pentazocine dependence potential, it may have induced a withdrawal syndrome. However, naloxone does not produce a withdrawal syndrome in mice implanted with a pellet of pentazocine, as it does in mice implanted with morphine or other opiates.[34] The results of these and other studies which showed dissimilar dependence-producing properties of pentazocine from morphine were considered when the drug was marketed in 1967 without restrictions. As the use of pentazocine increased, numerous cases of dependence to this drug have been reported. In 1969 the AMA Council on Drugs studied the evidence on the dependence-producing properties of pentazocine and published[35] their conclusion that the evidence available was not sufficient to suggest additional controls on this drug. However, they cautioned that physicians should prescribe pentazocine cognizant that dependence has been reported in certain cases and that refills and supplies should be carefully monitored, especially for the dependent-prone individual. The increased use of this analgesic since that time has again been accompanied by an increase in the number of papers which have appeared suggesting dependence on pentazocine. Weber and Rome[36] presented two case studies in which a dependence on pentazocine was apparent. A desire for repeated injections of the drug and withdrawal signs of a mild nature, compared to that seen during narcotic withdrawal, were observed. A number of the signs suggested by Kolb and Himmelsbach[37] to quantitate or evaluate the withdrawal syndrome from narcotics were observed in these patients. This syndrome was mild and brief. Both persons had easy access to large quantities of pentazocine, one being a physician and the other a pharmacology graduate student. Four patients who used pentazocine chronically tried to stop, but could not due to the withdrawal symptoms that ensued. When hospitalized, the pentazocine withdrawal syndrome was counteracted by methadone. The pentazocine withdrawal syndrome was reported to consist of "sweating, tremor, severe chills, muscle cramps (mainly leg muscles), followed by abdominal cramps, nausea, vomiting, itching and rhinorrhea."[38] Sandoval and Wang[31] reported two cases of expected pentazocine dependence. These cases appear to be somewhat complicated because one was a former meperidine addict and the other required psychiatric treatment. Withdrawal symptoms were observed in both patients and they were relieved by the injection of morphine or oral codeine. Profound craving for pentazocine was reported for one patient. This profound craving, which was the predominant characteristic observed on the seventh day of withdrawal, was eliminated by methadone.

In 1970, Jasinski and co-workers[39] reported that although pentazocine did not suppress the abstinence syndrome in patients dependent on morphine, it did produce a withdrawal syndrome which in some ways resembled that of morphine and in other respects that of nalorphine. In the same year, the Medical Letter reviewed the evidence for the propensity of pentazocine to produce dependence. They, like the AMA Council on Drugs two years earlier, suggested that pentazocine not be put under stricter controls, but that physicians and other medical personnel should be aware of the possible misuse of this agent. Wendel has recently reported an extensive review of the history of pentazocine abuse and concluded that the dependence risk of this drug is low.[40] Again, the Bureau of Narcotics and Dangerous Drug Act enacted in May of 1971, did not see fit to place pentazocine under control.

SUMMARY OF THE CHARACTERISTICS OF DEPENDENCE ON NARCOTIC ANALGESICS AND ANTAGONISTS IN MAN

Opiates, such as morphine and their analogues, as well as the synthetics (meperidine, methadone, etc.), which possess the ability to relieve severe pain in man, also have a significant propensity to produce dependence in man. Although some temporal and other quantitative differences may occur between the drugs in this class, by and large, their characteristics of dependence and withdrawal are qualitatively similar. The propensity of the narcotic antagonist analgesics such as nalorphine, cyclazocine, pentazocine, and others to produce dependence in man is less clear. A withdrawal syndrome is observed following abrupt cessation of chronic treatment with one of these agents. However, the characteristics of the dependence and the withdrawal syndrome observed with the narcotic antagonists appear to be strikingly different from that seen during opiate dependence and withdrawal. It is evident that pentazocine has been misused, and this fact should be considered when physicians or pharmacists are aware of repeated refills of prescriptions for this drug.

CHARACTERISTICS OF DEPENDENCE OF THE MORPHINE TYPE IN MICE

The use of pellets of morphine to induce tolerance and dependence was first reported by Maggiolo and Huidobro in 1961.[41] The abstinence signs consisted of a period of hyperactivity with increased activity and jumping followed by a period of neurological phenomena of tremors and occasional convulsions. They further reported[42] that the abstinence syndrome could be precipitated only by the injection of nalorphine and not by the removal of the pellet of morphine from the subcutaneous tissues. They found that the degree of the syndrome was directly related to the quantity of morphine implanted and that the pellet was better than repeated injections of the drug in inducing physical dependence. However, Cheney and Goldstein[43] recently reported that a certain amount of physical dependence can be detected in mice following a single injection of the opiate, levorphanol. The abstinence syndrome of pellet implanted mice was intensified if reserpine were given at least three hours prior to the injection of nalorphine. Other central nervous system depressants such as phenobarbital, chlorpromazine, etc. did not significantly alter the withdrawal syndrome. These observations prompted these investigators to suggest that an inverse relationship may exist between the abstinence syndrome in mice and level of catecholamines and/or serotonin in the brain. Recent studies by Way et al.[44] and Smith et al.[45] have further implicated the role of serotonin and catecholamines in the production of tolerance and physical dependence to morphine. Recently, Way and his co-workers[46] used a pellet implantation technique to quantitate tolerance and physical dependence in mice. The predominant characteristic of the withdrawal syndrome observed either 4 to 10 hours after abrupt withdrawal of the pellet or 5 minutes after an injection of the antagonist, naloxone, was the jumping observed in these mice when placed on a platform. Drug-naive mice would not jump from this platform. This jumping could be blocked by an injection of morphine or another potent narcotic analgesic but not by such CNS depressants as chlorpromazine or pentobarbital. This propensity to jump, observed during opiate withdrawal in mice, appears to be specific for this species. The reproducibility, the rapid onset, and the ability to quantitate physical dependence by using the mouse jumping test are distinct advantages over other methods.

CHARACTERISTICS OF PHYSICAL DEPENDENCE OF THE MORPHINE TYPE IN RATS

The abstinence syndrome observed following abrupt withdrawal of morphine or after the injection of an antagonist in rats chronically treated with morphine, differs considerably from that observed in man, monkey, or dog.[3] The most striking difference is that many of the characteristics observed in the higher species are not seen during opiate withdrawal in rats. Stretching, squealing when touched, chattering teeth, diarrhea, and hypersensitivity to noise were the most frequent withdrawal signs observed in rats. In 1963, Martin et al.[47] observed that during opiate withdrawal, rats would often violently shake their entire bodies for a short period of time. They described this phenomenon as "wet dog" shakes, due to the similarity between this behavior and that observed when a dog shakes off excess water. This characteristic of the opiate withdrawal syndrome ("wet dog" shakes) in the rat appears to be specific for this species.

The opiate withdrawal syndrome in rats has been described by some as predominantly depressant in nature, while others feel that stimulation is seen.[48] Khazan et al.[49] found that a state of depression was observed in rats for the first few hours after the last morphine injection, and this was followed by a period of stimulation which peaked approximately seven hours after the last morphine injection. Others[47] have also reported observing a two phase syndrome during opiate withdrawal in rats. The initial phase, which lasted from 8 to 16 hours after the last dose of morphine, was characterized by a fall in body weight and body temperature and an increase in activity (stimulation?). The second phase was characterized by a rapid increase in body weight and an increase in body temperature. This latter phase may last up to 72 hours after the last injection of morphine. Still other investigators[50] have used a fall in body weight as the principal criterion in quantitating opiate withdrawal in rats.

One of the characteristics of morphine dependence in rats is that these animals will perform a task to obtain injections of morphine from a syringe through an indwelling cannula. The animals made dependent on repeated doses of morphine prior to placement in the apparatus would perform the task to maintain their dose of morphine. If saline were then placed in the syringe instead of morphine or if an injection of nalorphine was given, a rapid increase in bar pressing was observed which was interpreted as a component of a withdrawal syndrome.[51,52]

CHARACTERISTICS OF PHYSICAL DEPENDENCE OF THE MORPHINE TYPE IN DOGS

In 1948 Wikler and Frank[53] demonstrated that a withdrawal syndrome characterized by restlessness, yawning, lacrimation, rhinorrhea, fever, and tremors, as well as an increase in the spontaneous activity of the hind limbs existed in dogs after the cessation of either chronic (every six hours) morphine or methadone in spinal dogs. They concluded that the production of physical dependence in spinal dogs implicated the spinal cord as a portion of the central nervous system that was involved with this phenomenon and that it probably was also involved with the withdrawal syndrome. The withdrawal syndrome could also be precipitated by an injection of nalorphine in these dogs.[54] This withdrawal syndrome could be precipitated by nalorphine in spinal dogs prior to the development of tolerance to the effects of morphine on these reflexes. This observation suggests that at least in spinal dogs, physical dependence occurred prior to the development of tolerance. It has been mentioned earlier that by using the mouse jump test some physical dependence was observed after the first injection of morphine. Martin and Eades[55] produced physical dependence in dogs within an eight-hour period by a constant intravenous infusion of morphine. The characteristics of the withdrawal syndrome produced by nalorphine following morphine infusion resembled those described above. Two differences were noted; namely, nalorphine produced neither hyperthermia nor as much of a stimulation of respiration in the morphine infused dog as it did in the dogs given morphine injections four times a day. These differences in the abstinence syndrome in acute intact and spinal chronically physically dependent dogs were investigated by carrying out infusion experiments in chronic spinal dogs.[56] Acute physical dependence to morphine develops more rapidly in supraspinal structures than in the spinal cord; however, chronic physical dependence to morphine does develop in the spinal cord and appears to involve certain cholinergic but not adrenergic mechanisms.[57]

CHARACTERISTICS OF DEPENDENCE OF THE MORPHINE TYPE IN MONKEYS

The behavior of rhesus monkeys during addiction to and withdrawal from opiates have been described in considerable detail by Seevers.[58] The monkey seldom vomits and does not appear to have the recurrent constipation and diarrhea often seen in dogs and man during addiction to opiates. Otherwise, few differences were observed between the syndrome during addiction in monkeys from that seen in man. This observation led to the establishment of the monkey as the laboratory animal of choice in studies designed to predict the propensity of addiction for new analgesics. The development of the self-adminstration technique[59] in which each monkey can control his own dose of compound has also been instrumental in establishing the popularity of the monkey in addiction studies. With this technique one can study addiction, craving, phenomenon, and either abrupt or antagonist induce withdrawal in the same animal.

CHARACTERISTICS OF DEPENDENCE ON NARCOTIC ANTAGONISTS IN LABORATORY ANIMALS

Few reports have appeared concerning the propensity of the narcotic antagonists to produce physical dependence in laboratory animals. Recently, Nuite[60] has shown that mice implanted with pellets of nalorphine, naloxone, cyclazocine, or pentazocine and challenged with a dose of naloxone did not show the jumping syndrome produced by naloxone in morphine-implanted mice. However, when pentazocine was injected intraperitoneally at increasing amounts 7 times in 2 days or 15 times in 4 days and challenged with naloxone 2 hours after the last injection of pentazocine, jumping from the platform was observed.[61] An injection of nalorphine did not induce the jumping syndrome in mice chronically given pentazocine, nor did mice chronically injected for two days with nalorphine show this phenomenon when injected with naloxone. A few jumps were observed in mice chronically treated with nalorphine for four days and then challenged with naloxone. Nalorphine did precipitate jumping in almost every mouse chronically treated with morphine in either the two or four day tests. These data indicate that if dependence on narcotic antagonists does occur in mice, it differs from that induced by narcotics such as morphine. Little work has been reported concerning the dependence producing effects of the antagonists using other laboratory species.

SUMMARY OF THE CHARACTERISTICS OF DEPENDENCE ON NARCOTICS AND NARCOTIC ANTAGONIST ANALGESICS IN LABORATORY ANIMALS

It appears that opiates, all of which produce dependence in man, also produce dependence in each animal species studied. In animals even more than in man, the characteristics of this dependence are best seen during withdrawal. Many similarities exist among the withdrawal syndrome observed in man, monkey, and dog. The rat is unique in its withdrawal syndrome to opiates in that "wet dog" shakes are observed. Mice, on the other hand, have an uncontrollable urge to jump during opiate withdrawal induced by cessation of treatment with the opiate or induced by the injection of an opiod antagonist. This characteristic jumping during withdrawal appears specific for this species. The many advantages of using mice: their lower cost, the relatively short duration of time needed to perform the experiment, its reproducibility, and the ease with which one can quantitate the results, make this observation a very useful tool in assessing dependence producing properties of new drugs. Possibly the mouse test could be used as a screening test prior to testing in monkeys. The similarities between the characteristics of opiate dependence and withdrawal in monkey and man indicate that the monkey is still the animal of choice for such determinations. However, the monkey test has a tendency to predict a different addiction liability for certain drugs than is seen in man. For example, the monkey test predicted a lower addiction liability for the benzomorphans such as phenazocine, etc. and a higher addiction liability for the piperidine type analgesic such as meperidine.

Few experiments have been reported concerning the characteristics of dependence of the narcotic-antagonist analgesics in laboratory animals. Monkeys will perform a task to self-administer pentazocine, cyclazocine, and nalorphine. The jumping syndrome, characteristic of opiate dependence, was observed in mice following a challenge of naloxone after chronic injections of pentazocine, but not after an injection of naloxone when pentazocine had been administered chronically in a pellet.

A number of researchers have been looking at various neurochemical systems, such as the role of nucleic acid or protein synthesis and to a greater extent the serotonergic, adrenergic, or cholinergic systems in an attempt to increase our knowledge of the biochemical systems involved in dependence. Possibly the important factor here may not be the effect of chronic administration of a drug such as morphine on any of these neurochemical systems in themselves, but how they effect the balance of one system to another. We have previously suggested this possibility for the mechanism of the analgesic activity of many of these drugs.[62,63] The complex syndrome observed during dependence and withdrawal suggests that more than one neurochemical system may be involved. Presently available analytical techniques do not allow us to simultaneously measure the effects of a drug on all of these systems. As a matter of fact, the technique used to measure any one of these systems is hardly sensitive enough to measure changes in small portions of brain tissue. Improvements in analytical procedures of the neurochemistry of the central nervous system, which hopefully will be developed in the near future, will be useful in increasing our knowledge about the mechanisms involved in the production of physical dependence to narcotics and narcotic antagonists in laboratory animals. The data accumulated from these experiments might be useful in extrapolating the mechanisms involved in the production of physical dependence to these agents in man.

REFERENCES

1. W.H.O. Expert Committee on Addiction-producing drugs, *W.H.O. Techn. Rep. Ser.*, 273, 1, 1964.

2. Wikler, A., Sites and mechanisms of action of morphine and related drugs in the central nervous system, *Pharmacol. Rev.*, 2, 435, 1950.

3. Seevers, M. H. and Deneau, G. A., Physiological aspects of tolerance and physical dependence, in *Physiological Pharmacology*, Vol. 1, Root, W. S. and Hofmann, H. G., Eds., Academic Press, New York, 1963, 565.

4. Halbach, H. and Eddy, N. B., Tests for addiction (chronic intoxication) or morphine type, *Bull. W.H.O.*, 28, 139, 1963.

5. Schuster, L., Tolerance and physical dependence, in *Narcotic Drugs Biochemical Pharmacology*, Clouet, D. H., Ed., Plenum Press, New York, 1971, 408.

6. Jaffe, J. H., Drug addiction and drug abuse, in *The Pharmacological Basis of Therapeutics*, Fourth ed., Goodman, L. S. and Gilman, A., Eds., The MacMillan Company, New York, 1970, 276.

7. d'Orban, P. T., Heroin dependence and delinquency in women - a study of heroin addicts in Halloway Prison, *Brit. J. Addict.*, 65, 67, 1970.

8. Cumberlidge, M. C., The abuse of barbiturates by heroin addicts, *Canad. Med. Ass. J.*, 98, 1045, 1968.

9. Hamburger, E., Barbiturate use in narcotic addicts, *J.A.M.A.*, 189, 366, 1964.

10. Schasre, R., Cessation patterns among neophyte heroin users, *Int. J. Addict.*, 1, 23, 1966.

11. Ball, J. C. and Urbaitis, J. C., Absence of major medical complications among chronic opiate addicts, *Brit. J. Addict.*, 65, 109, 1970.

12. Nelson, A. S., Medical problems associated with addiction to opioid drugs, *Int. J. Addict.*, 1, 50, 1966.

13. Cass, L. J., Joing, J. T., and Frederik, W. S., Physical dependence potentiality of analgesics, *Curr. Ther. Res.*, 3, 289, 1961.

14. Fraser, H. F. and Isbell, H., Pharmacology and addiction liability of *dl*- and *d*-propoxyphene, *Bull. Nar.*, 12, 9, 1960.

15. Elson, A. and Domino, E. F., Dextro propoxyphene addiction. Observations of a case, *J.A.M.A.*, 183, 482, 1963.

16. Fraser, H. F. and Rosenberg, D. E., Observations of the human pharmacology and addictiveness of methotrimeprazine, *Clin. Pharmacol., Ther.*, 4, 596, 1963.

17. Dole, V. P. and Nysander, M. A., Medical treatment of diacetylmorphine (heroin) addiction: A clinical trial, *J.A.M.A.*, 193, 646, 1965.

18. Kramer, J. C., Methadone maintenance for opiate dependence, *Calif. Med.*, 113, 6, 1970.

19. Martin, W. R., Gorodetzky, C. W., and McClane, T. K., An experimental study in the treatment of narcotic addicts with cyclazocine, *Clin. Pharmacol. Ther.*, 7, 455, 1966.

20. Freedman, A. M., Fink, M., Sharoff, R., and Zaks, A., Cyclazocine and methadone in narcotic addiction, *J.A.M.A.*, 202, 191, 1967.

21. Jaffe, J. H., Cyclazocine in the treatment of narcotic addiction, *Curr. Psychiat. Ther.*, 7, 147, 1967.

22. Fraser, H. F. and Harris, L. S., Narcotic and narcotic antagonist analgesics, *Ann. Rev. Pharmacol.*, 7, 277, 1967.

23. Martin, W. R., Opioid antagonists, *Pharmacol. Rev.*, 19, 463, 1967.

24. Eddy, N. B. and Martin, W. R., Drug dependence of specific opiate antagonist type, *Pharmakopsychiatric Neuro-Psychopharmakologie*, 3, 73, 1970.

25. Isbell, H., Attempted addiction to nalorphine, *Fed. Proc.*, 15, 442, 1956.

26. Schrappe, O., "Physical dependence" nach chronischer Verabreichung von *N*-allylnormorphin, *Arzniemittel-forschuy,* 9. 130, 1959.

27. Martin, W. R. and Gorodetzky, C. W., Demonstration of tolerance to and physical dependence on *N*-allylno-morphine (nalorphine), *J. Pharmacol. Exp. Ther.*, 150, 437, 1965.

28. Martin, W. R., Fraser, H. F., Gorodetzky, C. W., and Rosenberg, D. E., Studies of the dependence producing potential of the narcotic antagonist 2-cyclopropylmethyl-2′-hydroxy-5,9-dimethyl-6,7-benzomorphan (cyclazocine, Win 20,740, ARC II-C-3), *J. Pharmacol. Exp. Ther.*, 150, 426, 1965.

29. Fraser, H. F. and Rosenberg, D. E., Comparative effects of (1) chronic administration of cyclazocine (ARC-II-C-3), (II) substitution of nalorphine for cyclazocine and (III) chronic administration of morphine. Pilot crossover study, *Int. J. Addict.*, 1, 50, 1966.

30. Fraser, H. F. and Rosenberg, D. E., Studies on the human addiction liability of 2′-hydroxy-5,9-dimethyl-2-(3,3-dimethylallyl)-6,7-benzomorphan, *J. Pharmacol. Exp. Ther.*, 143, 149, 1964.

31. Sandoval, R. G. and Wang, R. I., Tolerance and dependence on pentazocine, *New Eng. J. Med.*, 280, 1391, 1969.

32. Keats, A. S. and Telford, J., Narcotic antagonists as analgesics; clinical aspects, in *Advances in Chemistry Series,* No. 45, 170, 1964.

33. Harris, L. S., Dewey, W. L., Howes, J. F., Voyda, C., Kennedy, J. S., Nuite, J. A., Snyder, J. W., and Porter, J. F., Studies of narcotic antagonist analgesics, Reported to Committee on Problems of Drug Dependence, February 21, 1968.

34. Nuite, J. A., personal communication.

35. Anonymous, The misuse of pentazocine. Its dependence-producing potential, *J.A.M.A.*, 209, 1518, 1969.

36. Weber, W. F. and Rome, H. P., Addiction to pentazocine – report of two cases, *J.A.M.A.*, 212, 1708, 1970.

37. Kolb, L. and Himmelsbach, C. K., Clinical studies of drug addiction: Critical review of withdrawal treatements with method of evaluating abstinence syndromes, *Amer. J. Psychiat.*, 94, 759, 1938.

38. Schoolar, J. C., Idanpaan-Heikkila, P., and Keats, A. S., Pentazocine addiction, *Lancet,* 1, 1263, 1969.

39. Jasinski, D. R., Martin , W. R., and Koeldtke, R. D., Effects of short- and long-term administration of pentazocine in man, *Clin. Pharmacol. Ther.*, 11, 383, 1970.

40. Wendel, H. A., Pentazocine dependence in medical practice, Reported to the Committee on Problems of Drug Dependence, February 16, 1971.

41. Maggiolo, C. and Huidobro, F., Administration of pellets of morphine to mice: abstinence syndrome, *Acta Physiol. Lat. Amer.*, 11, 201, 1961.

42. Huidobro, F. and Maggiolo, C., Some features of the abstinence syndrome to morphine in mice, *Acta Physiol. Lat. Amer.*, 11, 201, 1961.

43. Cheney, D. L. and Goldstein, A., Tolerance to opioid narcotics: time course and reversibility of physical dependence in mice, *Nature,* 232, 477, 1971.

44. Way, E. L., Loh, H. H., and Shen, F. H., Morphine tolerance, physical dependence, and synthesis of brain 5-hydroxytryptamine, *Science,* 162, 1290, 1968.

45. Smith, C. B., Villarreal, J. E., Bednarczyk, J. H., and Sheldon, M. I., Tolerance to morphine-induced increases in ^{14}C catecholamine synthesis in mouse brain, *Science,* 170, 1106, 1970.

46. Way, E. L., Loh, H. H., and Shen, F. H., Simultaneous quantitative assessment of morphine tolerance and physical dependence, *J. Pharmacol. Exp. Ther.*, 167, 1, 1969.

47. Martin, W. R., Wikler, A., Eades, C. G., and Pescor, F. G., Tolerance to and physical dependence on morphine in rats, *Psychopharmacologia*, 4, 247, 1963.

48. Gunne, L. M., Catecholamines and 5-hydroxytryptamine in morphine tolerance and withdrawal, *Acta Physiol. Scand.*, 58, Supplement 204, 37, 1963.

49. Khazan, N., Weeks, J. F., and Schroeder, L. A., Electroencephelographic, electromyographic, and behavioral correlates during a cycle of self-maintained morphine addiction in the rat, *J. Pharmacol. Exp. Ther.*, 1-5, 521, 1967.

50. Akera, T. and Brody, T. M., The addiction cycle to narcotics in the rat and its relation to catecholamines., *Biochem. Pharmacol.*, 17, 675, 1968.

51. Weeks, J. R., Self-maintained morphine "addiction" – a method for chronic programmed intravenous injections in unrestrained rats, *Fed. Proc.*, 20, 397, 1961.

52. Weeks, J. R., Experimental morphine addiction: method for autonomic intravenous injections in unrestrained rats, *Science*, 138, 143, 1962.

53. Wikler, A. and Frank, K., Hindlimb reflexes of chronic spinal dogs during cycles of addiction to morphine and methadone, *J. Pharmacol. Exp. Ther.*, 94, 382, 1948.

54. Wikler, A. and Carter, R. L., Effects of single doses of *N*-allylnormorphine on hindlimb reflexes of chronic spinal dogs during cycles of morphine addiction, *J. Pharmacol. Exp. Ther.*, 109, 92, 1953.

55. Martin, W. R. and Eades, C. G., Demonstration of tolerance and physical dependence in the dog following a short term infusion of morphine, *J. Pharmacol. Exp. Ther.*, 133, 262, 1961.

56. Martin, W. R. and Eades, C. G., A comparison between acute and chronic physical dependence in the chronic spinal dog, *J. Pharmacol. Exp. Ther.*, 146, 385, 1964.

57. Martin, W. R. and Eades, C. G., Pharmacological studies of spinal cord adrenergic and cholinergic mechanisms and their relation to physical dependence on morphine, *Psychopharmacologia*, 11, 195, 1967.

58. Seevers, M. H., Opiate addiction in the monkey 1. Methods of study, *J. Pharmacol. Exp. Ther.*, 56, 147, 1936.

59. Yanagita, T., Deneau, G. A., and Seevers, M. H., Evaluation of pharmacologic agents in the monkey by long term intravenous self or programmed administration, *Excerpta. Med. Int. Congr. Ser.*, 87, 453, 1966.

60. Nuite, J. A., Chronic effects of narcotic antagonists, *Fed. Proc.*, 30, 277, 1971.

61. Saelens, J. K., Granat, F. R., and Sawyer, W. K., A simple method for estimating the physical dependence capacity of analgesics in mice, Reported to Committee on Problems of Drug Dependence, February 17, 1971, 1311.

62. Dewey, W. L., Harris, L. S., Howes, J. F., and Nuite, J. A., The effect of various neurohumoral modulators on the activity of morphine and the narcotic antagonists in the tail flick and phenylquinone tests, *J. Pharmacol. Exp. Ther.*, 175, 435, 1970.

63. Harris, L. S., Central neurohumoral systems involved with narcotic agonists and antagonists, *Fed. Proc.*, 29, 28, 1970.

BARBITURATES, ALCOHOL, AND TRANQUILIZERS

R. Aston

TABLE OF CONTENTS

INTRODUCTION

Alcohol, barbiturates, nonbarbiturate hypnosedatives, and minor tranquilizers may all be considered to comprise a single pharmacological category of nonselective central nervous system depressants. They are characterized by progressive anxiolytic, sedative, and soporific effects with increasing doses. The minor tranquilizers, such as the benzodiazepines, may be differentiated from the hypnosedatives inasmuch as they display a wider dosage differential between anti-anxiety and hypnosedative activity.[1] Dependence to alcohol, barbiturates, and minor tranquilizers might, therefore, be grouped as dependence of the alcohol-hypnosedative type. There is no convincing evidence that major tranquilizers, such as the phenothiazines, can produce a dependent state.[1]

Alcohol-hypnosedative drug dependence includes a consideration of a diverse group of agents including ethanol and barbiturates, as well as drugs such as chloral hydrate, meprobamate, glutethimide, and chlordiazepoxide. Such drugs may be classed together on the basis of several criteria:[2,3]

1. in increasing doses, each drug will produce signs of progressive central nervous system depression, e.g., sedation and hypnosis;
2. overdosage with all of these agents elicits similar toxic signs, e.g., clouding of mental processes, ataxia, and eventual medullary paralysis;
3. chronic use of large doses of these agents leads to the production of a low-grade tolerance, so that there is persistent evidence of intoxication at higher doses;
4. mutual, though incomplete cross-tolerance is seen among the various agents in this class;
5. psychic dependence of varying degrees occurs to these drugs, i.e., the generation of a strong desire to continue using the drug. This craving may be, at least partially, suppressed by abusing another agent in the same class;
6. chronic use of large doses (not therapeutic doses) induces physical dependence, in which state the individual requires the drug continuously to maintain relatively normal physiological function, and, in which, precipitous withdrawal results in an abstinence syndrome which is similar for all agents in this group; and
7. mutual cross-dependence is observed between members of this class, e.g. barbiturates will suppress the alcohol abstinence syndrome, while opiates fail to suppress symptoms resulting from the withdrawal of hypnosedatives.

A frequent result of alcoholism is the development of pathology in various tissues and organs of the body, while similar associated pathological consequences have not been observed with hypnosedatives. This is, in part, due to the fact that, among the drugs in this dependence class, only alcohol can serve as food. The alcoholic may ingest the major portion of his dietary caloric intake in the form of ethanol. The resulting malnutrition and vitamin deficiency that occur contribute in a primary or secondary fashion to many of the pathophysiological consequences of chronic alcohol intoxication.

During a period of chronic intoxication with this category of drugs, the individual seeks escape from the harshness of reality and from his own feelings of inadequacy and anxiety by remaining in a continual state of drug-induced sedation and stupor typified by drowsiness, incoordination, ataxia, self-assertion, and a degree of euphoria. As a dose of the drug wears off, there is a return to depression and anxiety which can be relieved only by more drug. With continued use of large doses of the agent, physical dependence occurs, a state in which central adaptability to the drug precludes normal neuronal activity in the drug's absence. Symptoms resulting from abrupt abstinence from these agents are of an opposite nature to those produced by the drugs themselves. Withdrawal is characterized by signs of central excitation such as apprehension, tremor, hallucinations, and convulsions. These agents appear to induce a state of latent hyperexcitability during chronic abuse which is prevented from manifesting itself as long as the drug is being taken.

In the present review, characteristics of clinical intoxication and withdrawal of the hypnosedative class will be considered. In addition, emphasis will be placed upon the pathological sequelae of chronic alcoholism.

BARBITURATE DEPENDENCE

Nearly half a century elapsed between the introduction of barbiturates into clinical medicine in 1903 and the first definitive report of dependence to these agents in man.[4] This is even more surprising in view of the fact that several earlier reports appeared in the German literature describing the similarity of symptoms following barbiturate withdrawal and those of alcoholic delerium tremens.

The classic descriptions of chronic barbiturate intoxication and withdrawal provided by Isbell, Fraser, and their co-workers at Lexington[4,5] two decades ago, still represent the literature's most illuminating source for details of the characteristics of barbiturate dependence. A concise review of barbiturate abuse in relation to alcoholism has recently appeared,[6] and both Essig[7] and Wikler[8] have contributed valuable surveys of barbiturate dependence within the framework of general hypnosedative abuse. The following description of barbiturate intoxication and dependence is drawn largely from these sources.

Primary barbiturate dependence occurs especially in patients for whom these drugs are prescribed for chronic sedation. Barbiturates are frequently found also as components of a "mixed" dependence. This is especially true of alcoholics, amongst whom 20 to 40% are reported to abuse other drugs along with alcohol. In 50 to 70% of these cases, barbiturates are found to be taken. The alcoholic, introduced to barbiturates, finds their effects to be similar to, and to enhance those, of alcohol. The alcoholic may turn completely to barbiturates, finding them easier to conceal, and less upsetting to his stomach.

Barbiturates are classified, according to their duration of action, as ultra-short, intermediate, or long-acting compounds. The ultra-short acting agents are used as intravenous anesthetics and constitute no abuse problem. The intermediate group, such as pentobarbital (Nembutal®), secobarbital (Seconal®), amobarbital (Amytal®), and butabarbital (Butisol®), are frequently abused. Mixtures of intermediate barbiturates, such as Tuinal® (secobarbital and amobarbital) are frequently abused. Long-acting barbiturates, such as phenobarbital, are largely employed as anticonvulsants and dependence to this type of barbiturate is only occasionally seen.

Physical dependence to barbiturates rarely develops if the dose is less than 500 mg per day, although upon abrupt withdrawal of the drug, minor symptoms such as anorexia, insomnia, tremor, and anxiety may occur in a small proportion of individuals. With doses of less than 500 mg per day, for a period of two months, complete tolerance to the effects of such dosage is likely to develop. At daily doses of 500 to 800 mg per day physical dependence may occur, and if a dose of more than 800 mg per day is taken for a period of 60 days, withdrawal of the drug usually results in severe symptoms of delirium and grand mal type convulsive seizures.[9] Death may occur in this situation, which makes barbiturate withdrawal more dangerous than withdrawal from opiates.

Tolerance to barbiturates, though more marked than that to alcohol, never reaches the proportions observed in opiate dependence. As noted above, maximal tolerance is sufficient to render doses of 500 mg per day nearly ineffective, but at doses of 800 mg per day even maximal tolerance induction is insufficient to prevent signs of intoxication. Tolerance does not develop to the lethal effects of these drugs. Tolerance is ascribed by many authors to induction of hepatic enzyme activity, and by others to central neuronal adaptation. It is unlikely that either mechanism alone is responsible for tolerance in chronic barbiturate dependence. Cross-tolerance to other hypnosedatives and to ethanol occurs. When alcohol causes severe liver damage, however, the effects of barbiturates may be markedly enhanced.

Barbiturate Intoxication

Single doses of 150 mg of secobarbital in a fasted individual initially produce feelings of disinhibition, gregariousness, and light-headedness together with silliness and ataxia. Simple and complex reaction times are prolonged, and intellectual processes are impaired. These symptoms last for about two hours. The same doses given after a normal meal produce very minor effects. These effects are not unlike those of alcohol.

Large single doses of barbiturates in the drug-free individual, in the range of 0.4 to 0.7 g of secobarbital or pentobarbital, cause severe intoxication, and may even produce light coma. Difficulty in thinking, nystagmus, incoordination, and coarse tremor are common. The onset of symptoms is 30 to 45 minutes. Symptoms begin to abate in about two hours and disappear in about four to five hours. Individuals taking doses of this magnitude suffer the next day from nervousness, tremor, anorexia, and headache. Such individuals compare these symptoms to those of a post-alcoholic "hang-over".

The picture of chronic barbiturate intoxication is similar to that of ethanol. Barbiturates can cause drowsiness, impaired judgment, lack of emotional control, slurred speech, motor incoordination, and ataxia. Irritability, aggressive behavior, and paranoid ideation are observed. The individual loses interest in his personal appearance and becomes unkempt and dirty. No changes are observed during this period in respiratory minute volume, body temperature, or blood pressure, though a slight rise in pulse rate is seen. During the first month of chronic intoxication, enhanced delta wave activity (one to six cycles per second) is observed in electroencephalographic tracings. After this time, delta activity diminishes or may disappear, while beta wave activity (15 to 30 cycles per second) is greatly increased. Neither convulsions nor delirium are observed during chronic barbiturism.

During the period of intoxication, the total sleep time is increased only by about two hours a day. However, even with single daily hypnotic doses of barbiturates, a more rapid onset of sleep, a delay in the appearance of REM sleep, and a 40% reduction in the proportion of REM sleep are observed. After about five nights of barbiturate intake, the proportion of REM sleep returns to normal levels, indicating tolerance for this effect.[10]

Barbiturate Withdrawal Syndrome

Abrupt discontinuance of barbiturates, following prolonged chronic abuse, precipitates an abstinence syndrome not unlike that seen in alcohol withdrawal. No withdrawal symptoms occur during the first eight to sixteen hours following the last dose of barbiturate. During this time, symptoms of intoxication subside and the patient may be mistakenly assumed to be improving. Following this relatively asymptomatic period, the patient complains of anxiety, weakness, insomnia, and anorexia. Coarse tremor develops in the face and hands. After 24 to 30 hours of abstinence these symptoms become severe. In addition, muscle fasciculations and heightened deep reflexes are seen. Nausea and vomiting, enhanced startle response, mydriasis, and orthostatic hypotension occur.

Convulsions may occur from the second to about the eighth day of withdrawal. Usually one to four seizures, lasting less than three minutes, develop. These are generalized, tonic-clonic seizures of the grand mal variety. The patient usually regains consciousness within five minutes of the onset of the convulsion, and the whole episode appears subjectively as a "black-out".

The second major symptom of withdrawal is delerium. The onset is gradual, but is evident within two to four days after the last dose of drug, and usually lasts three to ten days. The main features of this psychotic episode are vivid auditory and visual hallucinations, disorientation as to time and place, and paranoid delusions occasioning extreme fear and agitation. Such barbiturate withdrawal psychoses may be related to the rebound increase in the proportion of REM sleep observed during early abstinence. Following four weeks of nightly soporofic doses of barbiturate, individuals have been shown to display this effect together with an abnormally rapid onset of REM sleep, a reduction in total sleep time, and a prolongation of the time required to fall asleep. In such studies, sleep patterns gradually return to normal after a period of about two weeks.[10] There is suggestive clinical evidence that the night terrors and delirium of withdrawal may reflect an intrusion of REM (dreaming) sleep into wakefulness.[11] Oswald[12] has suggested that REM sleep rebound may be indicative of increased protein synthesis in the brain associated with repair of neuronal damage caused by drug abuse.

Coincident with the symptoms of delerium are hyperventilation and an increase in pulse rate, blood pressure, and blood glucose level. During the delirious phase, rectal temperature is elevated. Marked hyperthermia may be prodromal to a fatal outcome, and requires immediate and vigorous treatment.

Following the acute manifestations of withdrawal, improvement is gradual. Weakness which persists longer than any other symptom, disappears after six to twelve weeks.

ALCOHOL DEPENDENCE

Alcohol is, by far, the most common intoxicant employed in Western Civilization. In the U.S. alone, the annual production of ethanol reaches 700,000,000 gal. Enough of this is manufactured in a potable form to supply the reported 65% of the adult population who use alcoholic beverages. It is conservatively estimated that there are about 6,500,000 alcoholics in the U.S. Some 8% of these are of the "skid row" type. In terms of numbers involved, alcohol dependence is unquestionably the major drug abuse problem in Western Culture.

The effects of alcohol on driving ability and traffic safety have been extensively reviewed in a 1968 publication of the American Medical Association.[13]

Alcohol Intoxication

The acute effects of alcohol ingestion have been either observed or experienced by everyone, and require little elucidation. The late Sir John Gaddum, with characteristic acumen and wit, divided intoxication into four stages correlated with increasing alcohol blood level ranges (expressed in mg per 100 ml blood); delightfully dizzy, 50 to 100; drunk and disorderly, about 200; dead drunk, about 300; and death's door, about 400.[14]

At lower blood levels, alcohol depresses inhibitions and repressions in the inebriate. There is loss of judgment, attention, efficiency, and logical thought. The individual becomes less self-critical and tends to overestimate his own abilities and performance. A sense of euphoria develops, and behavior becomes spontaneous and child-like.

With blood alcohol levels of 100 to 200 mg per 100 ml, common signs of frank intoxication or drunkenness appear. Slurring of speech, prolonged reaction times, and staggering gait occur. The experienced inebriate moves and acts with exaggerated care, while the inexperienced drinker loses self-control. Ability to control mood is lost and the drinker may become antic and silly, or may become quarrelsome, belligerent, and vicious.

In the range of 300 mg per 100 ml blood ethanol, approaching anesthesia is evident. Consciousness may be lost. There is sweating, mydriasis, a sluggish light reflex, and hyperemic conjunctivae. Respiration becomes irregular and sonorous. Body temperature declines as does blood pressure. The individual may lapse into a coma which, if it persists for more than five to ten hours, may terminate fatally.

Medullary paralysis and death occur at an average ethanol blood level of 400 mg per 100 ml. The LD50 (dose lethal in 50% of population) of alcohol is estimated to be 5 g/kg. Average lethal doses of alcohol range from 250 to 500 g, which is the equivalent of 22 to 46 fluid oz of 100 proof whiskey.

The correlation between blood alcohol concentration and the incidence of gross intoxication is of interest. The results of seven such studies, involving 6594 subjects, have been summarized.[13] For seven ranges of blood alcohol (as mg per 100 ml blood), the average percentage of individuals judged to be drunk were: 0 to 50, 4%; 51 to 100, 32%; 101 to 150, 62%; 151 to 200, 89%; 201 to 250, 95%; 251 to 300, 98%; and 301 to 350, 99%.

Pathologic Sequelae of Alcoholism

The use of alcohol presents a spectrum that ranges from social drinking through problem drinking to alcohol dependence. Unfortunately, there are no clearly defined criteria which can be used to define the point at which alcohol use becomes alcohol abuse. As with barbiturates, however, psychological dependence, tolerance, and withdrawal symptoms characterize the full blown dependent state. In addition, however, the alcoholic displays a syndrome of pathologies that result either from the cumulative toxicity of his drug or from extended periods of malnutrition. The pathological consequences of chronic alcohol abuse may be broadly categorized into neurological, myopathic, hepatic, hematological, and glucemic complications.[15]

Neurological Changes

Korsakoff's syndrome is a complex of symptoms which occurs with a much higher incidence in alcoholics than in the general population.[16] The main clinical symptoms of this neuropathy consist of amnesia, confabulation, disorientation, and peripheral neuritis. The state appears to be due to chronic thiamine deficiency in the alcoholic, but is not readily amenable to dietary thiamine supplements. Amnesia is the most characteristic symptom in Korsakoff's syndrome, involving registration, retention, and recall. Amnesia may be slight or profound and is principally related to events occurring after the onset of the syndrome. Confabulation (the relation of imaginary experiences to fill in gaps in memory) is most prominent in the early stages of the illness. Disorientation is usually related to time, but may also involve place and person.

The central lesions in this syndrome occur in the mamillary bodies, the region around the third ventricle and the aqueduct in 95 to 100% of cases. In about one half of the cases the dorsomedial nucleus of the thalamus is involved. It would appear that the mamillary damage is critically related to the memory defects observed in these patients.

Korsakoff's syndrome may develop slowly or it may, or may not, follow delirium tremens or *Wernicke's encephalopathy.* The latter illness is an acute form of Korsakoff's syndrome characterized by diplopia, muscular incoordination, mental confusion, and peripheral neuritis. The sites of central lesions in Wernicke's syndrome are the same as in Korsakoff's. The former illness is, however, improved clinically by thiamine administration.

Abstinence from alcohol and the institution of a well-balanced diet will reverse the clinical picture of Korsakoff's syndrome over a period of several months, though return of memory may be incomplete. Thiamine supplements do not appear to hasten recovery. After recovery patients may reexhibit the symptom complex if they return to their former drinking and eating habits.

Many alcoholics undergoing treatment display a symptom complex which has been termed *alcoholic dementia.* The syndrome includes disturbances of judgment and critical faculties, reduced memory and thought content, confabulation, perseveration, and loss of decorum. During treatment these symptoms regress and may disappear completely. In one study of hospitalized alcoholics displaying symptoms of dementia, it was found that a three-month course of treatment produced significant improvement in adjustment and intellectual functioning; however, evidence of an organic cerebral disorder still remained.[17] The mental deterioration of alcoholic dementia is correlated with a loss of cerebral cortical cells from the frontal lobes.

Alcoholic peripheral neuropathy is a relatively common condition characterized by reduced or absent deep tendon reflexes, and distal sensory impairment which most often involves the lower extremities.[15,18] It varies in severity from patchy sensory loss in the feet to total sensory loss in the legs. Distal wasting of muscle may be seen. Nerve conduction studies indicate slowing of motor and sensory conduction velocity, prolongation of latency to peak potential, and reduction in the amplitude of the action potential, in both sensory and motor nerves. There is a significant reduction in the mean fiber density of motor nerves. The major pathological finding is axonal or Wallerian degeneration, though less commonly, nerve fibers may display segmented demyelination. In patients with a history of acute onset of peripheral neuropathy, active axonal degeneration is extensive, while, in patients with a chronic history of neuropathy, numerous fibers exhibit regeneration and active degeneration is rare.

Continual degeneration and regeneration of peripheral nerve fibers appears to occur in alcoholics who maintain a nutritious diet, but sudden bouts of excess drinking, and resultant nutritional deficiency, may precipitate acute neuropathy. Thiamine deficiency appears to be of major importance in the etiology of this syndrome, inasmuch as in experimental studies in animals, thiamine deficiency alone can produce peripheral axonal degeneration.

Myopathic Changes

Skeletal muscle damage directly caused by alcohol was not recognized until recently. Alcoholic myopathy may be of either an acute or chronic nature.[19-21]

Acute alcoholic myopathy is always associated with recent ingestion of ethanol and is characterized by painful muscle cramps associated with acute necrosis of striated muscle. Weakness and tenderness of muscle is seen, often together with muscle or subcutaneous edema. Elevations in serum glutamic oxaloacetic transaminase, serum glutamic pyruvic transaminase, lactic dehydrogenase, and creatine phosphokinase are seen and may result from muscle necrosis.

Myoglobinuria, resulting from muscle degeneration, and renal failure are reported in 75 and 50% of these cases, respectively. The overall mortality in acute myopathy is 22%, with one half of those patients developing nephrosis dying. The cause of death in these cases is unclear. However, renal failure and hyperkalemia commonly precede death. It has been postulated that fatality results from the release of large quantities of potassium from necrotized striated muscle which, in the presence of oliguria or anuria, leads to hyperkalemia, culminating in fatal cardiac arrhythmias. In cases in which alcohol is withdrawn, however, recovery is the rule.

A benign form of acute myopathy has been described in which the main symptoms are spontaneous muscle cramps seen most often during exercise, myasthenia, and muscle swelling. These symptoms disappear after a few weeks of alcohol abstinence.

Chronic alcoholic myopathy is manifested as a slowly developing weakness, tenderness and atrophy of proximal muscles, mainly of the pelvic girdle and thighs, and, to a lesser extent, of the shoulder girdle. It is often associated with neuropathology, hepatic cirrhosis, or alcoholic psychosis. Conduction velocity in motor nerves is normal and no evidence of lower neuron damage is found. Serum creatine phosphokinase levels may be elevated, and the blood lactic acid rise due to ischemic exercise is commonly reduced. In these cases, clinical recovery of muscle strength requires weeks or months, and is seen in about one half of patients who abstain from alcohol.

Primary chronic alcoholic cardiomyopathy as a form of cardiac failure has been clearly established as a clinical entity. It often occurs in well-nourished individuals and does not respond to thiamine. There is suggestive evidence that alcoholic heart disease may be due to decreased serum and muscle magnesium levels seen in chronic alcoholism.[22] Sanders[23] has recently published an extensive critical review of alcoholic heart damage.

Alcoholic cardiomyopathy occurs in patients with a long history of excessive alcohol ingestion. These individuals most commonly notice dyspnea upon exertion, palpitations, night cough, weakness, and edema. In the early stages tachycardia or atrial fibrillation is seen. In later stages cardiomegaly with frank signs of heart failure develop. Among the electrocardiographic changes considered by some authorities to be distinctive in this form of heart failure are an early "spinous" T wave (needle-like spike), and a T wave which has either a shallow notch or deeper cleft at its summit. These effects may be due to progressive myocardial fibrosis which may eventually lead to inversion of the T wave. Electrocardiographic evidence of atrioventricular block is also common.

Post-mortem light microscopy of the myocardium reveals patchy areas of fibrosis, loss of striations in muscle fibers and varying degrees of edema, hyalinization, hydropic vacuolization, and nuclear abnormalities. Electron microscopic studies reveal swelling of the mitochondria and sarcoplasmic reticulum and disruption of cristae and myofibrillar disruption. Histochemical examination of alcoholic hearts reveals neutral lipid accumulation in myofibrils, and a marked decrease in the content of enzymes such as succinic, lactic, isocitric and malic dehydrogenases, cytochrome oxidase, and NAD-diaphorase. Such changes are even seen in the absence of cardiomyopathy and may represent the initial stages of alcohol-induced mitochondrial damage prodromal to myofibrillar damage and fibrosis.

Recent studies provide evidence that progressive diffuse interstitial myocardial fibrosis may cause alcoholic cardiomyopathy by producing mechanical restriction and low cardiac output. As a result, ventricular dilatation, increased intracardiac pressures and enhanced left ventricular end diastolic volume develop.[24] The usual post-mortem findings are moderate left ventricular hypertrophy with dilatation of the right ventricle and both atria.

The prognosis is poor unless drinking is stopped in the early stages of myocardial fibrosis. Treatment is the same as for congestive heart failure, i.e., digitalis, diuretics, and supplemental potassium.

Hepatic Changes

The hepatopathologic consequences of prolonged alcohol ingestion are usually divided into three syndromes: fatty liver, alcoholic hepatitis,[25] and Laennec's cirrhosis.[26]

Fatty infiltration of the liver regularly occurs in man after ethanol ingestion and is reversible. It is not understood what factors influence the incidence and severity of this disorder in the alcoholic. However, some relationship may hold between fatty infiltration of the liver and the immediate hypertriglyceridemia and a lactescent serum which lasts for about 17 to 20 hours after the last drink.[27] During this time, postalimentary lipidemia is enhanced. As the elevated triglyceride levels in serum return to normal, total lipids remain high, largely due to increased serum phospholipids and cholesterol. The excess plasma lipid may arise either through peripheral lipolysis of adipose tissue or through enhanced hepatic lipogenesis.[28]

Alcohol is known to enhance sympathetic activity in the body. Chronic alcohol ingestion has been shown to cause an increase in urinary dopamine, epinephrine, metanephrine, norepinephrine, and normetanephrine, which is proportionate to blood alcohol level.[29] Since catecholamines are known to induce lipolysis in adipose tissue, it may be that alcohol-induced hyperlipidemia and fatty liver are due to adrenergic and adrenal medullary activiation by ethanol.

There is no clear evidence that fatty liver is a necessary precursor to the development of either alcoholic hepatitis or cirrhosis. In controlled studies in man, fatty liver, in the absence of hepatic necrosis, has not lead to the production of cirrhosis.

Alcoholic hepatitis (steatonecrosis) appears to be prodromal to cirrhosis, although with hospital treatment, it may, or may not, progress to the latter state. Alcoholic hepatitis is an acute hepatic insufficiency characterized most frequently by symptoms of loss of appetite, nausea, vomiting, weakness, and jaundice. Hepatomegaly, ascites, spider angiomas, and splenomegaly are common. The severity of the disease ranges widely, some patients being essentially asymptomatic, while others are comatose. Patients with alcoholic hepatitis display, upon liver microscopy, hyaline deposition in the cytoplasm of liver cells (Mallory bodies), hepatocellular necrosis, and infiltration of liver with polymorphonuclear leukocytes. There is often, but not invariably, associated fatty infiltration of hepatocytes, fibrosis, and cirrhotic changes.

Advanced alcoholic hepatitis may progress, after variable periods of time, to *Laennec's cirrhosis,* which afflicts about 10% of chronic alcoholics. Studies in two human volunteers, fed one pint of ethanol daily for three to four weeks, with or without a normal diet, indicate that the initial hepatic changes which occur consist of mitochondrial swelling, vesiculation of the endoplasmic reticulum, and accumulation of neutral fat, as revealed by electron microscopy.[30] If such alcohol intake is continued for a period of two to three months, together with a balanced, vitamin-enriched diet, liver morphology has been reported to return to normal. If the dose of ethanol is gradually increased during this time, and a protein-poor diet introduced, there appear hepatocytic necrosis, inflammation, mesenchymal cell proliferation, and fibrosis.[26]

Therefore, it appears that with adequate nutrition, normal regenerative processes may reverse alcohol-induced hepatic degeneration. In the presence of protein deficiency, however, hepatocytic destruction can become predominant. Regenerative processes also increase the minimal requirements for vitamins and minerals. Folic acid, the most often deficient vitamin in alcoholics, is necessary for adequate nucleic acid synthesis, and its lack may inhibit liver regeneration. Such uncompensated hepatic cell damage can decrease alcohol dehydrogenase activity, so that a reduced rate of ethanol metabolism occurs, which exposes the liver to even greater insult. It has been shown that a correlation exists between severity of liver damage and decreases in alcohol dehydrogenase activity.[26] The latter enzyme requires NAD as coenzyme. Prolonged alcohol ingestion leads to hepatic accumulation of NADH due to ethanol oxidation. Fatty infiltration of the liver and hepatocytic damage have been attributed to such excess hepatic NADH content.

Fibrosis and nodular regeneration of liver cells observed in cirrhosis lead to gross deformation and lobular deformation causing deformation of vascular, lymphatic, and biliary networks. These changes, together with liver cell dysfunction, lead directly or indirectly, to the symptoms of hepatic cirrhosis which include hyperbilirubinemia, portal hypertension, ascites, mental changes, and renal failure.

The prognosis in this illness is good if the patient stops drinking before liver failure supervenes. The most important features of a therapeutic regimen are continued abstinence from alcohol and the use of a nutritious high-protein supplemented diet.

Hematological Changes

Prolonged ingestion of alcohol is commonly associated with *megaloblastic anemia,* and morphological changes in bone marrow smears. Vacuolation of erythroblasts and myelocytes occurs in proportion to the amount of ethanol taken. Such bone marrow changes may be related to a recently reported transient hemolysis associated with stomatocytosis (red cells in which the central area of pallor is replaced by a mouth-like unstained area) in acute alcoholics.[31] When alcohol replaces a significant proportion of the diet and folate deficiency occurs, ring sideroblasts (indicative of abnormal iron incorporation into haem) appear in bone marrow. Normoblastic erythropoiesis is converted to megaloblastic in about ten days. Suppression of bone marrow hemopoiesis appears to be a direct toxic effect of ethanol since alcohol can suppress the normal erthropoietic response to minimum dietary doses of folic acid.[32] Pyridoxine (vitamin B_6) utilization also appears to be affected by alcohol, inasmuch as parenteral pyridoxal phosphate, but not pyridoxine, has caused the disappearance of ring sideroblasts from the marrow of alcoholics while alcohol was being continued. Megaloblasts, however, persisted in marrow smears.[33]

Fifteen ounces of alcohol daily for ten days has been shown to suppress not only red cell formation, but also to produce *thrombocytopenia* and *leukopenia.* Moderate to severe reductions in platelet count were observed in 36% of consecutive hospital admissions of alcoholics in one reported study. The reduced platelet count was unrelated to hematocrit, white cell count, serum folate level or liver function, and appeared to be the result of a direct toxic effect of alcohol.[34]

Another effect alcohol has on blood, unrelated to bone marrow effects, is an increase in both serum iron levels and in the degree of saturation of the iron-binding capacity of the serum. Suppression of erythropoiesis, of course, reduces the utilization of dietary iron and indirectly, contributes to a rise in serum iron.

These effects of alcohol on the blood are reversed during abstinence. Serum iron levels decline as do serum folate levels during the first 48 to 72 hours of withdrawal from ethanol, as the utilization of these substances increases, and then return toward normal as physiological equilibrium is reached.[35] This is accompanied by a reticulocytosis, followed by a rise in hemoglobin to normal levels. If the platelet and granulocyte count were low, they return to normal. Thrombocytopenia reverts to normal after 5 to 18 days of abstinence from alcohol.[34] Bone marrow abnormalities are also reversed, with a decline in the number of ring sideroblasts and of vacuolated marrow cells to normal in 5 to 13 days after dosing with ethanol is stopped.[32]

Blood Glucose Changes

A condition of hypoglycemic coma, which may be fatal, can occur six to thirty-six hours following an alcohol bout in chronic alcoholics.[15,36] Post-alcoholic hypoglycemia occurs only after a fast period of 48 to 72 hours, apparently at a time when hepatic glycogen stores are low. In the fasting state, alcohol inhibits both glycogenolysis and peripheral utilization of glucose. Hypoglycemia occurs if the inhibition of hepatic glucose release is greater than the reduction in peripheral glucose utilization. There is evidence that in cirrhosis, which is associated with a diabetic glucose pattern, the hypoglycemic response to ethanol is reduced.[36]

Malabsorption Syndrome

Although a direct toxic effect of ethanol has been suggested in the etiology of myopathic, hematological, and hepatic pathologies, the neurological syndromes attendant upon chronic alcoholism appear to be primarily the result of malnutrition. Poor diet and hypovitaminosis are implicated in the development of overt cirrhosis as well. Hypovitaminosis results, of course, from the fact that alcohol replaces a large proportion of the normal diet in alcoholism. One study of 3000 alcoholics admitted to a large urban hospital, revealed that continuous dietary deficiency occurred in 35% of these patients, and periodic dietary deficiencies in 40%.[37] However, alcohol ingestion not only reduces dietary intake, but also causes a direct inhibition of absorption of many dietary constituents.

Thiamine malabsorption in the alcoholic is well substantiated. Alcoholics, with fatty liver or cirrhosis display a reduction in the absorption of orally- administered thiamine to about 30% of normal. Thiamine absorption returns to normal after six to eight weeks of high protein, vitamin-supplemented diet. In alcoholics free of liver disease, oral or parenteral administration of 1.5 g/kg ethanol reduced thiamine absorption from the gastrointestinal tract by 50% in 4 of 12 reported cases.[38]

Alcoholics appear to have a serum cyanocobalamin (vitamin B_{12}) level which is higher than normal. This has been explained as due to either leakage of the vitamin from damaged liver cells, or to an increased serum binding of cyanocobalamin in liver disease.[39] During early abstinence in alcoholics with no severe liver impairment, an abnormally low enteral absorption of the vitamin has been observed.[40]

Serum folate levels in early alcoholism have been reported to be higher than normal, due, perhaps, to a reduced folate utilization in hematopoiesis with resultant accumulation of the vitamin in the circulation. On the other hand, in long-term alcoholism with associated malnutrition, serum folate levels are reported to be below normal limits.[39] Other authors have found plasma and erythrocytic folate levels to be in the normal range in alcoholics with abnormal liver function tests, but exhibiting no malnutrition.[41]

Alcohol-induced malabsorption phenomena may be related to two factors. First, alcohol has been shown to stimulate pancreatic secretion and, at the same time, to produce obstruction to pancreatic outflow. This may be responsible for the high incidence of both acute and chronic subclinical pancreatitis in alcholics. Pancreatitis itself, however, does not appear to cause malabsorption unless accompanied by malnutrition, specifically a protein-deficient diet. Indeed, protein deficiency seems a prerequisite to pancreatic dysfunction in man, and both pancreatitis and intestinal malabsorption are reversed by dietary protein repletion.[42]

Vitamin deficiency has recently been reported to be the likely cause of a high incidence of red-green or blue-yellow *color blindness* in chronic alcoholics.[43,44] This defective color vision is temporary and after alcohol abstinence and a vitamin-rich, well-balanced diet, the incidence of this vision defect declines to that of the general population. The condition displays no correlation with either the incidence or severity of liver disease in alcoholics.

Acute Alcoholic Withdrawal Syndrome

The severity of the withdrawal symptoms seen during acute alcohol abstinence varies considerably in relation to both the preabstinent intake level and the duration of chronic intoxication. The mildest form of withdrawal is seen during a period of chronic drinking after a brief period of abstinence, e.g. after a night's sleep, and consists of tremulousness, nausea, and vomiting. Such symptoms are immediately checked by the alcoholic by taking another drink. The most severe withdrawal syndrome, i.e., delirium tremens, is usually associated with two to four days' abstinence following long-term, high intake alcohol abuse. Delirium tremens is most often seen when the daily intake exceeds 300 g of ethanol, the equivalent of about 15 pt of beer or 1 1/2 bottles of spirits per day. At this rate of intake, alcoholic abstinence symptoms can be precipitated after seven to fourteen days of continuous spree drinking.[45]

Upon cessation of drinking, the alcoholics' symptoms of intoxication subside over a period of six to eight hours. This is followed by the onset of a characteristic abstinence syndrome. The severity of acute withdrawal symptoms may be categorized in the following manner:

i. *mild to moderate:* primarily neuromuscular and gastrointestinal symptoms. The patient displays anorexia, nausea, epigastric distress, tremulousness, sweating, apprehension, and insomnia;

ii. *severe or impending delirium tremens:* diarrhea, vomiting, nightmares, and agitation occur in addition to those symptoms listed above. Autonomic hyperactivity is observed, as well, manifested as tachycardia, hyperpnea, and fever;

iii. *delirium tremens:* in addition to all the above symptoms, psychotic manifestations are seen. Hallucinations (tactile, auditory or visual), delusions, muttering delirium, and paranoia occur.[46] The hallucinations are usually of a threatening nature. A patient who exhibits only delusions and hallucinations, usually auditory, without signs of agitation, disorientation or autonomic hyperactivity, is usually described as exhibiting "alcoholic hallucinosis".[47] The patient displays incoordination, panic, disorientation, confusion, and clouded senses. Finally, grand mal seizures supervene, though occasionally they may be of the petit mal type.

The full-blown picture of delirium tremens, if it occurs, has an onset of 48 to 96 hours after the last drink, and is characterized by confusion, disorientation, psychomotor agitation, hallucinations, and delusions. This picture, however, may not emerge for as long as eight days after the initiation of abstinence. The incidence of true delirium tremens in abstinence is usually reported to be in the range of 5%. In a survey of 8606 alcoholic admissions to a state hospital over a period of five years ending in 1968, 98% showed definite symptoms of withdrawal. Among these, 278, or 4.8%, displayed symptoms of delirium tremens.[46] In this report, five patients died of alcohol-related problems (three of acute liver disease and two of acute hemorrhagic pancreatitis). No deaths were reported as due to delirium tremens. Others have reported up to 15% mortality during alcohol withdrawal, though only 6% of these were due solely to delirium tremens without other complicating factors.

It has been suggested that hallucinosis or delirium in alcohol withdrawal, as in barbiturate withdrawal, may be related to suppression of REM sleep during the phase of intoxication. Alcohol ingestion and abstinence appear to have marked effects upon sleep pattern and quality. During periods of chronic inebriation the total hours of sleep per day is increased, though the quality of sleep deteriorates due to prolonged onset of sleep, frequent movements and brief awakenings.[48] The duration of single sleep episodes decreases from six to eight hours to three to four hours.[49] There appear frequent shifts from one sleep stage to another with a marked reduction in stage 3 and 4 sleep, and numerous shifts to stage 1 sleep. The total amount of REM sleep is reduced during uncontrolled drinking. A significant reduction in REM sleep has even been observed in healthy nonalcoholics taking alcohol before bedtime.[48]

During withdrawal from alcohol, insomnia is a commonly reported problem. Fragmentation of sleep patterns, observed during inebriation, continues to occur. However, a rebound increase in the amount of REM sleep above the normal range of 20 to 25% of total sleep time is seen.[48] As much as 100% of sleep may be in the REM stage just prior to the onset of delirium tremens.[50] It has been suggested that when total REM sleep exceeds 50% of sleep time, REM activity tends to spill over into the awake state resulting in hallucinations.

A prominent feature of delirium tremens is gross autonomic hyperactivity, e.g. tachycardia, hyperhidrosis, and fever.[51,52] The most dangerous aspects of acute alcoholic withdrawal are hyperthermia and peripheral circulatory collapse.[52] Ogata et al.[29] have shown that alcohol ingestion enhances sympathetic activity, as indicated by a rise in urinary catecholamines and their metabolites. The highest urinary levels of catecholamines are observed during withdrawal. Urinary epinephrine is much more elevated than urinary norepinephrine. Such effects may be causally related to the symptoms of autonomic hyperactivity observed in the withdrawing patient.

The development of coarse tremor and subsequent convulsive seizure activity during withdrawal may be due to alterations of tissue levels of magnesium during intoxication and abstinence. Chronic alcohol intoxication can lead to a reduction in total body magnesium which is, however, not necessarily reflected in a reduced serum magnesium level.[51] It has been observed that an increase in urinary magnesium excretion occurs when blood levels of alcohol are rising, while urinary magnesium excretion may be normal, and serum levels constant, when blood ethanol levels are high but unchanging, as during periods of protracted intoxication. A marked positive magnesium balance is often observed in withdrawal, suggesting that magnesium depletion has occurred prior to abstinence.

Serum magnesium levels rapidly decline upon withdrawal from alcohol.[54,55] Hypomagnesemia occurs independently of liver dysfunction or deficiencies in serum protein or thiamine. It appears to be due to an increase in urinary excretion of the cation and occurs even when serum magnesium levels are low. The enhanced excretion of magnesium during withdrawal may be related to the naturesis and diuresis observed during this period. Serum magnesium levels return to normal in 40 to 60 hours following withdrawal.[53,56]

Thirty percent of withdrawing alcoholics have been reported to exhibit low serum magnesium levels.[54] The time course of hypomagnesemia correlates well with the period of neuromuscular hyperexcitability, e.g. tremulousness and seizures, seen during withdrawal.[51]

Another sign of neuromuscular irritability, that shows the same temporal relationship to cessation of drinking as does the incidence of spontaneous seizures, is sensitivity to photically-induced convulsions. Stroboscopic stimulation elicits in about 50% of withdrawing alcoholics, either tonic-clonic convulsions with loss of consciousness or coarse myoclonic movements. This photic sensitivity is never seen in the normal, and only rarely in the epileptic, individual. In one reported study, positive stroboscopic sensitivity was correlated with significantly reduced serum magnesium levels in ten alcoholics, compared to eight alcoholics exhibiting no photosensitivity.[56] The latter group had serum magnesium concentrations which were not different from those of control nonalcoholic subjects.

Hypokalemia, due to hyperventilation which commonly occurs during withdrawal from alcohol, has been observed to follow the same time course as neuromuscular hypersensitivity and hypomagnesemia during ethanol abstinence.[47,56] Both factors may be involved in the etiology of the neuromuscular symptoms of alcohol abstinence.

It appears, therefore, that a rapidly occurring, though transient, hypomagnesemia and alkalosis observed during early alcohol withdrawal may be responsible for many of the symptoms of the withdrawal phase, especially the early signs of tremulousness and seizures. The period of delirium tremens displays a less satisfactory correlation with serum magnesium levels but may, nevertheless, be related to obscured reductions in total body magnesium.[51,56]

The duration of withdrawal varies, but studies of free recall, i.e., how many words in a spoken series of twelve can immediately be remembered, and of the return to normal of REM sleep (as a percentage of total sleep) indicate that two weeks are necessary for recovery from the withdrawal phase.[57]

NONBARBITURATE HYPNOSEDATIVE DEPENDENCE

For the purposes of this presentation, both drugs accepted as hypnosedative agents, and those promoted as minor tranquilizers, will be included. Dependence on this group of drugs has been discussed, in relation to general drug abuse, by several authorities in the field.[2,3,7,58] In addition, Essig has presented two reviews exclusively devoted to a consideration of intoxication and dependence in relation to nonbarbiturate sedative and tranquilizing agents.[59,60]

In this section, the drugs under consideration will be categorized according to general chemical relationships, into derivatives of acetaldehyde (chloral hydrate, paraldehyde), propanediol (meprobamate, tybamate), piperidinedione (glutethimide, methyprylon), pentynol (ethchlorvynol, ethinamate), and benzodiazepine (chlordiazepoxide, diazepam).

All of the drugs in these classes produce signs of intoxication which are similar to one another, and to both barbiturates and ethanol. These symptoms include drowsiness, confusion, motor incoordination with staggering gait, memory impairment, diplopia, blunting of intellectual function, rage reactions, and, in excessive doses, a comatose state which may terminate fatally. Such deaths have been attributed to meprobamate, glutethimide, methyprylon, ethchlorvynol, and ethinamate.[7]

The compounds in this general group present an abstinence syndrome which is common to all, and similar to that of alcohol and barbiturates. Minor withdrawal symptoms of anxiety, tremulousness, insomnia, gastrointestinal upset, and heightened sympathetic tone predominate. Major abstinence symptoms of convulsive seizures, delirium, or both have been reported. Such withdrawal may be life-threatening, and death has been reported during abstinence from meprobamate and methyprylon.[7]

Acetaldehyde Group

Chloral Hydrate (Noctec®, Somnos®)

Abuse of this agent seems to have been fairly common following its introduction into medicine in 1869. More recently chloral hydrate dependence has become rare, with only three cases reported in the English-language literature since 1907, the latest in 1966.[61] The most complete description of chloral intoxication and withdrawal in the recent literature is that by Margetts written in 1950.[62]

Mental manifestations of chronic chloral intoxication may include apathy, depression, drowsiness, impaired memory and judgment, apprehension, restlessness, euphoria, hallucinations, impaired libido, and, commonly, paranoia. Physical symptoms of chronic chloralism include some which appear to be characteristic of the drug, such as suffusion of the conjunctivae, lacrimation, scaling of the eyelids and scalp, cutaneous vasodilatation, the tell-tale odor of the drug on the breath, and arthralgia and myalgia which may mimic arthritis. Other somatic symptoms are similar to those observed in chronic alcoholism. Loss of weight, hypovitaminosis, ataxia, incoordination, slurred speech, gastric irritation, skin eruptions, and grand mal seizures occur. A number of parenchymatous pathologies have been attributed to chloral hydrate including fatty degeneration of the heart, congestion of lungs and liver, and renal damage.

Chloral dependence and withdrawal develop in individuals taking 4.5 to 7.0 g/day, although a recent report describes an habitué who took approximately 22 g/night for ten months prior to withdrawal.[61]

Abrupt withdrawal from chloral hydrate results, within a few hours, in agitation, restlessness, and disorientation. After 48 to 72 hours the symptoms of acute chloral delirium appear. Auditory and visual hallucinations occur, as well as delusions and illusions. Fear and acute paranoid reactions appear to be common. In addition, feelings of unreality, impaired insight, euphoria, agitation, impaired memory, and dream states may be seen. Suicide may be attempted because of depression, paranoia, or confusion. The symptoms of chloral withdrawal are largely mental (although any of the physical manifestations may occur during acute abstinence) and the state is often referred to as "chloral delirium". The duration of the withdrawal syndrome varies from one to three weeks. No cases of death attributable to chloral hydrate withdrawal appear to have been reported.

Paraldehyde

Mendelson et al.[63] report that alcoholics may

develop a preference for paraldehyde over alcohol, after being given the former drug in hospital to treat alcoholic delirium tremens. Chronic paraldehyde intoxication produces symptoms similar to those of alcohol, with pronounced gastrointestinal disturbances, headache, and dizziness. Withdrawal appears to be characterized by a syndrome similar to that of alcohol, including tremor, confusion, hallucinosis, and delirium tremens.

Propanediol Group

Meprobamate (Miltown®, Equanil®)

Physical dependence to meprobamate and an alcohol-barbiturate type withdrawal syndrome have been well documented.[59,60] Grand mal seizures following abrupt drug withdrawal occur when doses as small as 2.4 g/day are taken for less than one month. Withdrawal from larger doses of the drug results in the development of an abstinence syndrome in from ten hours to four days. Abstinence is characterized by extreme nervousness and excitability, incoherence, irrationality, hostility, paranoia, and hallucinations. One or more of the following physical symptoms are often present: tremor, grand mal seizures, hyperhidrosis, hypotension or hypertension, and high fever.

In one report of 47 patients receiving 3.2 or 7.4 g of meprobamate for 40 days, 30 developed a withdrawal syndrome, following abrupt discontinuance of the drug, consisting of insomnia anxiety, headache, tremulousness, and vomiting. Three of the patients had seizures and eight developed psychotic behavior which terminated spontaneously within three days.[64] Death during withdrawal from daily doses of 10 g of meprobamate has been reported.[65]

Tybamate (Solacen®, Tybatran®)

Other agents structurally related to meprobamate presumably will produce a similar pattern of abuse and dependence. One such congener, tybamate, has been found to be devoid of dependence in volunteers receiving up to nine g/day for periods of up to 12 days.[66] These individuals received the drug in divided doses four times a day. In another study,[67] the drug was given, on the same dosage schedule, in doses up to 14 g/day for 15 weeks without signs of physical dependence. In explaining this result, Hollister points out the short plasma halflife (about four hours) of tybamate and suggests that administration of the drug four times a day does not allow the accumulation of sufficiently high plasma levels to produce physical dependence. On the other hand, dependence will likely occur in a prone individual, since he will take the drug as often as is necessary to maintain a state of chronic intoxication, though the necessity of frequent doses of tybamate tends to reduce its dependence liability compared to meprobamate.

Piperidinedione Group

Glutethimide (Doriden®)

Glutethimide abuse has been reviewed by Essig.[59,60] Signs of intoxication occur at daily doses of greater than 2.5 g, and closely parallel symptoms of typical hypnosedative overdosage. These include drowsiness, staggering gait, slurred speech, disorientation, loss of memory, and deterioration of intellectual functions. Coma is produced with as little as 5 g of the drug, and death has been reported due to 12 g.

Glutethimide dependence may occur when the drug is taken in doses of 2.5 g over a period of three months. Symptoms of the glutethimide abstinence syndrome are similar to those produced by barbiturate or meprobamate withdrawal. They include vomiting, abdominal cramps, agitation, tremor, sweating, hyperpyrexia, and tachycardia. The major withdrawal manifestations are seizures and a delirium consisting of disorientation, confusion, and hallucinations. Multiple seizures have been precipitated 16 hours after withdrawal of the drug, though the onset of convulsions may be delayed until the sixth day of abstinence.

Methyprylon (Noludar®)

Methyprylon intoxication,[59] like that due to barbiturates, is marked by confusion, unsteady gait, and thick speech. Acute toxicity appears to be low with recovery recorded following doses of up to 20 g of the drug. However, delayed death has occurred following a single dose of 6 g.

Abrupt abstinence from methyprylon precipitates a syndrome characterized by confusion, restlessness, agitation, sweating, and polyuria. Grand mal-like seizures, and a schizophreniform delirium with auditory and visual hallucinations may also occur. Death has been reported in a case involving withdrawal from daily doses of 7.5 to 12 g of the drug taken for about 18 months.[59]

Pentynol Group

Ethchlorvynol (Placidyl®)

Ethchlorvynol was introduced as a nonbarbiturate hypnosedative in 1955. The most common symptoms of intoxication with this agent are weakness, ataxia, slurred speech, and drowsiness. With larger chronic doses, tremor, nystagmus, and decreased or absent tendon reflexes are seen. Early reports on the drug indicated that it was nonaddicting, but in 1961 a case was reported of withdrawal from ethchlorvynol involving a schizophreniform reaction with epileptiform seizures occurring about ten days after the drug was discontinued.[68] In two instances, doses of 500 to 2000 mg/day were taken over a period of one to two years.[69] Six to ten days following discontinuance of the drug a sudden schizophrenia-like delirium occurred, characterized by auditory hallucinations, delusions, thought disorder, and affective symptoms. Other withdrawal symptoms included restlessness, confusion, tremulousness, and disorientation. One of these two cases suffered an initial grand mal seizure prior to the onset of delusional symptoms. Both cases were treated with chlorpromazine and diphenylhydantoin and were free of withdrawal symptoms after about one week. In another instance in which the dose of ethchlorvynol varied over a period of several months, but rose to 5000 to 7500 mg/day prior to hospital admission, the patient exhibited multiple seizures on days four and five of withdrawal, together with auditory and visual hallucinations.[70]

Ethinamate (Valmid®)

A characteristic general depressant-type abstinence syndrome has been described following chronic use of this drug.[59,60] Convulsions and delirium have followed withdrawal from daily doses of 2 to 2.5 g taken for a period of ten months. Daily doses of up to 15 g have been reported during chronic abuse, with confusion, agitation, disorientation, and ataxia as prominent signs of intoxication.

Sudden abstinence from ethinamate precipitates a syndrome characterized by agitation, hyperreflexia, fainting, and tremor. A psychotic delirium, with disorientation, delusions and hallucinations, and multiple generalized seizures, occurs 12 to 24 hours after withdrawal of the drug. Calmness and rationality are evident after about two weeks.

Benzodiazepine Group

Chlordiazepoxide (Librium®)

Chlordiazepoxide can produce drowsiness, delayed reaction times, ataxia, rage reactions, and, in acute overdosage, coma may develop.[59]

Abuse of and dependence on chlordiazepoxide has been reported to occur in 3.6% of 111 alcoholic patients treated with this drug, as compared to 7.7% of 78 such patients treated with meprobamate.[71] Chlordiazepoxide withdrawal, following five to six months' administration of increasing doses culminating in a daily dose of 300 to 600 mg, has produced insomnia, anorexia, nausea, agitation, depression, hyperhidrosis, and muscle twitching in nine of ten patients.[60] Two of the patients had convulsions. Convulsions also occurred in one patient whose final daily dose was 300 mg after three months.

Diazepam (Valium®)

Diazepam dependence developed in 2.3% of 302 alcoholics treated with this drug.[71] Dependence upon diazepam may develop with daily doses of 40 to 60 mg taken over periods of three or more months. In one such case the period of intoxication was characterized by drowsiness, unsteadiness, slurred speech, restlessness, and hostility.[72] Upon withdrawal, a single grand-mal type seizure at 72 hours after cessation of drug ingestion heralded the onset, one day later, of confusion, incoherent speech and a delirium manifesting paranoid delusions, disorientation with respect to time, agitation, hostility, and hallucinations. The latter were of an auditory, visual, olfactory, and gustatory nature. On the ninth withdrawal day a Korsakoff-like syndrome appeared with loss of recent memory and confabulation. By the eleventh day of abstinence clinical symptoms of withdrawal had disappeared. Recovery was complete. In most other reported studies, dose levels of 100 to 150 mg/day are associated with withdrawal seizures.

A fatal withdrawal following administration of 40 to 60 mg diazepam for eleven days has been reported.[73] In this case, tremor, diaphoresis, mydriasis, hyperpyrexia, and tachycardia occurred 36 hours after cessation of drug treatment, and death occurred at 72 hours. The interpretation of this fatality as specifically diazepam-related is, however, speculative, since the patient was suffering from a disease of the basal ganglia associated with neuronal lipidosis throughout the whole of the cerebrum and cerebellum.

Benzodiazepines, therefore, even in doses which may be considered therapeutic, may produce dependence which is manifested, during withdrawal, by symptoms similar to those elicited by abstinence from other nonselective central nervous system depressants. However, the dependence liability of this class of drugs appears to be significantly less than that of meprobamate.

SUMMARY

Barbiturates, ethyl alcohol, nonbarbiturate hypnosedatives, and the so-called minor tranquilizers appear to represent a homogeneous class of compounds in terms of the characteristics of abuse and dependence which they display. In this regard, the use of a term such as "dependence of the nonselective depressant type" might be more meaningful than the more restrictive nomenclature, "dependence of the alcohol-barbiturate type".

Intoxication with this category of drugs commonly causes drowsiness, ataxia, mental confusion, and loss of mood control. In excessive doses, coma, which may terminate fatally, is induced. Chronic intoxication induces a low-grade tolerance, with evidence of cross-tolerance existing to some degree between the various members of the group. Characteristically, tolerance is associated with an enhanced rate of hepatic metabolism of the abused agent, although a central adaptive process cannot be ruled out as contributory to the development of the tolerant state. The characteristics of tolerance to nonopiate dependence-producing agents have been reviewed recently by Kalant el al.[74]

Abrupt abstinence following chronic administration of increasing doses of the nonselective central depressants precipitates a withdrawal syndrome which is qualitatively similar for all members of this category of drugs. Minor symptoms of anxiety, tremor, gastrointestinal upset, and enhanced sympathetic activity are common. These are followed, after a variable period of time, by the major symptoms of abstinence: a state of delirium with hallucinations, delusions, disorientation and paranoid or schizoid behavior, and grand mal-type convulsive seizures. The incidence of major symptoms appears to depend upon the duration of drug abuse as well as upon the ultimate dose achieved by the abuser.

The use of terms such as "nonbarbiturate hypnosedative" and "minor tranquilizer" has done much to dispel well-founded fears of dependence liability in regard to many of these drugs. It should be emphasized that none of the newer nonselective central depressants has been found to be devoid of this insidious complication, and, as far as it is possible to predict, it is unlikely that any will be forthcoming.

REFERENCES

1. Domino, E. F., Human pharmacology of tranquilizing drugs, *Clin. Pharmacol. & Ther.*, 3, 599, 1962.

2. Deneau, J. and Seevers, M. H., Drug dependence, in, *Evaluation of Drug Activities*, 1st ed., Laurence, D. R. and Bacharach, A. L., Eds., Academic Press, New York, 1964, 176.

3. Eddy, N. B., Halbach, H., Isbell, H., and Seevers, M. H., Drug dependence: its significance and characteristics, *Bull. W.H.O.*, 32, 721, 1965.

4. Isbell, H., Altschul, S., Kornetsky, C. H., Eisenman, A. J., Flanary, H. G., and Fraser, H. F., Chronic barbiturate intoxication, *Arch. Neurol. Psychiat.*, 64, 1, 1950.

5. Fraser, H. F., Isbell, H., Eisenman, A. J., Wikler, A., and Pescor, F. T., Chronic barbiturate intoxication: further studies, *Arch. Intern. Med.*, 94, 34, 1954.

6. Devenyi, P. and Wilson, M., Barbiturate abuse and addiction and their relationship to alcohol and alcoholism, *Canad. Med. Ass. J.*, 104, 215, 1971.

7. Essig, C. F., Addiction to barbiturate and nonbarbiturate sedative drugs, *Ass. Res. Nerv. Dis.* (Res. Publ.), 68, 188, 1968.

8. Wikler, A., Diagnosis and treatment of drug dependence of the barbiturate type, *Amer. J. Psychiat.*, 125, 6, 1968.

9. Fraser, H. F., Wikler, A., Essig, C. F., and Isbell, H., Degree of physical dependence induced by secobarbital or pentobarbital, *J. A. M. A.*, 166, 126, 1958.

10. Evans, J. I., Lewis, S. A., Gibb, I. A. M., and Cheetham, M., Sleep and barbiturates: some experiments and observations, *Brit. Med. J.*, 4, 291, 1968.

11. Evans, J. I. and Lewis, S. A., Drug withdrawal state: an EEG sleep study, *Arch. Gen. Psychiat.*, 19, 631, 1968.

12. Oswald, I., Human brain protein, drugs and dreams, *Nature*, 223, 893, 1969.

13. American Medical Association, Committee on Medicolegal Problems, *Alcohol and the Impaired Driver*, AMA, Chicago, 1968.

14. Gaddum, J. H., *Pharmacology*, 5th ed., Oxford University Press, New York, 1968.

15. Carson, D. J. L., Pathologic findings following alcohol, *Anesth. Analg.*, 48, 670, 1969.

16. Malerstein, A. J., Korsakoff's syndrome in the alcoholic, *Med. Trial Tech. Quart.*, 17, 59, 1970.

17. Boeke, P. E., Some remarks about alcohol-dementia in clinically-treated alcoholics, *Brit. J. Addict.*, 65, 173, 1970.

18. Walsh, J. C. and McLeod, J. G., Alcoholic neuropathy: an electrophysiological and histological study, *J. Neurol. Sci.*, 10, 157, 1970.

19. Schneider, R., Acute alcoholic myopathy with myoglobinuria, *Southern Med. J.*, 63, 485, 1970.

20. Muller, P., Regli, F., and Meyer, M., Alcoholic myopathy, *German Med. Monthly*, 13, 511, 1968.

21. O'Brien, E. T. and Goldstraw, P., Alcoholic myopathy, *Brit. Med. J.*, 4, 785, 1969.

22. Seelig, M. S., Electrographic patterns of magnesium depletion appearing in alcoholic heart disease, *Ann. N. Y. Acad. Sci.*, 162, 906, 1969.

23. Sanders, M. G., Alcoholic cardiomyopathy: a critical review, *Quart. J. Stud. Alcohol*, 31, 324, 1970.

24. Gould, L. and Gomprecht, R. F., Alcoholic heart disease, *Geriatrics*, 25, 130, 1970.

25. Helman, R. A., Temko, M. H., Nye, S. W., and Fallon, H. J., Alcoholic hepatitis: natural history and evaluation of prednisolone therapy, *Ann. Intern. Med.*, 74, 311, 1971.

26. Leevy, C. M., Cirrhosis in alcoholics, *Med. Clin. N. Amer.*, 52, 1445, 1968.

27. Kallio, V., Saarimaa, H., and Saarimaa, A., Serum lipids and postprandial lipemia in alcoholics after a drinking bout, *Quart. J. Stud. Alcohol*, 30, 565, 1969.

28. Kudzma, D. J. and Schonfeld, G., Alcoholic hyperlipidemia: induction by alcohol but not by carbohydrate, *J. Lab. Clin. Med.*, 77, 384, 1971.

29. Ogata, M., Mendelson, J. H., Mello, N. K., and Majchrowicz, E., Adrenal function and alcoholism, II. catecholamines, *Psychosomat. Med.*, 33, 159, 1971.

30. Rubin, E. and Lieber, C. S., Alcohol-induced hepatic injury in non-alcoholic volunteers, *New Eng. J. Med.*, 278, 869, 1968.

31. Douglass, C. C. and Twomey, J. J., Transient stomatocytosis with hemolysis: a previously unrecognized complication of alcoholism, *Ann. Intern. Med.*, 72, 159, 1970.

32. Anonymous, Alcohol and the blood, *Lancet*, 2, 675, 1969.

33. Hines, J. D. and Cowan, D. H., Studies on the pathogenesis of alcohol-induced sideroblastic bone-marrow abnormalities, *New Eng. J. Med.*, 283, 441, 1970.

34. Cowan, D. H. and Hines, J. D., Thrombocytopenia of severe alcoholism, *Ann. Intern. Med.*, 74, 37, 1971.

35. Hourihane, D. O'B., Suppression of erythropoiesis by alcohol, *Brit. Med. J.*, 1, 86, 1970.

36. Hed, R. and Nygren, A., Alcohol-induced hypoglycaemia in chronic alcoholics with liver disease, *Acta Med. Scand.*, 183, 507, 1968.

37. Leevy, C. M. and Baker, H., Vitamins and alcoholism: introduction, *Amer. J. Clin. Nutr.*, 21, 1325, 1968.

38. Thomson, A. D., Baker, H., and Leevy, C. M., Patterns of ^{35}S-thiamine hydrochloride absorption in the malnourished alcoholic patient, *J. Lab. Clin. Med.*, 76, 34, 1970.

39. Carney, M. W. P., Serum folate and cyancobalamin in alcoholics, *Quart. J. Stud. Alcohol*, 31, 816, 1970.

40. Roggin, G. M., Iber, F. L., Kater, R. M. H., and Tabon, F., Malabsorption in the chronic alcoholic, *Hopkins Med. J.*, 125, 321, 1969.

41. Williams, I. R. and Girdwood, R. H., The folate status of alcoholics, *Scot. Med. J.*, 15, 285, 1970.

42. Mezey, E., Jow, E., Slavin, R. E., and Tobon, F., Pancreatic function and intestinal absorption in chronic alcoholism, *Gastroenterology*, 59, 657, 1970.

43. Smith, J. W. and Brinton, G. A., Color-vision defects in alcoholism, *Quart. J. Stud. Alcohol*, 32, 41, 1971.

44. Ugarte, G., Cruz-Coke, R., Rivera, L., Altschiller, H., and Mardones, J., Relationship of color blindness to alcoholic liver damage, *Pharmacology*, 4, 297, 1970.

45. Marjot, D. H., The length of the drinking bout preceding alcohol withdrawal states, *Brit. J. Addict.*, 74, 307-313, 1970.

46. Marvin, T. R., Acute alcoholic withdrawal syndrome, *Minn. Med.*, 53, 999-1003, 1970.

47. Knott, D. H. and Beard, J. D., Diagnosis and therapy of acute withdrawal from alcohol, *Curr. Psychiat. Ther.*, 10, 145-153, 1970.

48. Johnson, L. C., Burdick, J. A., and Smith, J., Sleep during alcohol intake and withdrawal in the chronic alcoholic, *Arch. Gen. Psychiat.*, 22, 406, 1970.

49. Mello, N. K. and Mendelson, J. H., Behavioral studies of sleep patterns in alcoholics during intoxication and withdrawal, *J. Pharmacol. Exp. Ther.*, 175, 94, 1970.

50. Oswald, I., Sleep, dreaming and drugs, *Proc. Roy. Soc. Med.*, 62, 151, 1969.

51. Mendelson, J. H., Ogata, M., and Mello, N. K., Effects of alcohol ingestion and withdrawal on magnesium states of alcoholics: clinical experimental findings, *Ann. N. Y. Acad. Sci.*, 162, 918, 1969.

52. Victor, M., The alcohol withdrawal syndrome, *Postgrad. Med.*, 47, 68-72, 1970.

53. Ogata, M., Mendelson, J. H., and Mello, N. K., Electrolytes and osmolality in alcoholics during experimentally induced intoxication, *Psychosom. Med.*, 30, 463, 1968.

54. Sullivan, J. F., Wolpert, P. W., Williams, R., and Egan, J. D., Serum magnesium in chronic alcoholism, *Ann. N. Y. Acad. Sci.*, 162, 947, 1969.

55. Beard, J. D., Fluid and electrolyte abnormalities in alcoholism, *Psychosom. Med.*, 11, 502, 1970.

56. Wolfe, S. M. and Victor, M., The relationship of hypomagnesemia and alkalosis to alcohol withdrawal symptoms, *Ann. N. Y. Acad. Sci.*, 162, 973, 1969.

57. Allen, R. P., Faillace, L. A., and Wagman, A., Recovery time for alcoholics after prolonged alcohol intoxication, *Johns Hopkins Med. J.*, 128, 158-164, 1971.

58. Seevers, M. H., Psychopharmacological elements of drug dependence, *J. A. M. A.*, 206, 1263, 1968.

59. Essig, C. F., Addiction to nonbarbiturate sedative and tranquilizing drugs, *Clin. Pharmacol. Ther.*, 5, 334, 1964.

60. Essig, C. F., Newer sedative drugs that can cause states of intoxication and dependence of barbiturate type, *J. A. M. A.*, 196, 714, 1966.

61. Robinson, J. T., A case of chloral hydrate addiction, *Int. J. Soc. Psychiat.*, 12, 66, 1966.

62. Margetts, E. L., Chloral delirium, *Psychiat, Quart.*, 24, 278, 1950.

63. Mendelson, J., Wexler, D., Leiderman, P. H., and Solomon, P., A study of addiction to nonethyl alcohols and other poisonous compounds, *Quart. J. Stud. Alcohol*, 18, 561, 1957.

64. Haizlip, T. M. and Ewing, J. A., Meprobamate habituation: a controlled clinical study, *New Eng. J. Med.*, 258, 1181, 1959.

65. Swanson, L. A. and Okada, T., Death after withdrawal of meprobamate, *J. A. M. A.*, 184, 780, 1968.

66. Colmore, J. P. and Moore, J. D., Lack of dependence and withdrawal symptoms in healthy volunteers given high doses of tybamate, *J. Clin. Pharmacol.*, 7, 319, 1967.

67. Shelton, J. and Hollister, L. E., Simulated abuse of tybamate in man, *J. A. M. A.*, 199, 116, 1967.

68. Hudson, H. S. and Walker, H. I., Withdrawal symptoms following ethchlorvynol dependence, *Amer. J. Psychiat.*, 118, 361, 1961.

69. Aycrigg, J. B., Two cases of withdrawal from ethchlorvynol, *Amer. J. Psychiat.*, 120, 1201, 1964.

70. Magness, J. L., Ethchlorvynol intoxication and severe abstinence reaction, *Lancet*, 85, 80, 1965.

71. Glatt, M. M., Benzodiazepines, *Brit. Med. J.*, 2, 444, 1967.

72. Barten, H. H., Toxic psychosis with transient dysmnestic syndrome following withdrawal from Valium, *Amer. J. Psychiat.*, 121, 1210, 1965.

73. Relkin, R., Death following withdrawal of diazepam, *N. Y. State J. Med.*, 66, 1770, 1966.

74. Kalant, H., LeBlanc, A. E., and Gibbins, R. J., Tolerance to, and dependence on, some non-opiate psychotropic drugs, *Pharmacol. Rev.*, 23, 135, 1971.

CNS STIMULANTS AND HALLUCINOGENS

S. H. Snyder

TABLE OF CONTENTS

INTRODUCTION

Both the terms, "stimulant" and "hallucinogen" are ambiguous words. They encompass many drugs, some of which are highly susceptible to abuse and others which are rarely associated with excess usage. Of course, some persons will ingest anything that can alter mental function in any way, seemingly in an attempt to almost literally "blow" their minds. Such individuals are known to "abuse" close-to-fatal doses of digitalis, large amounts of reserpine, or other available drugs. In discussing drugs of dependence, however, we will focus on those agents which reliably induce a dependent state, often demonstrable in animals, as well as man.

CNS STIMULANTS

A straightforward definition of a "stimulant" is "a drug which stimulates some bodily function." But, defined this way, it includes fully half of all existing pharmaceutical agents, ranging from cathartics and insulin to psychedelic drugs. Popular usage refers to agents which are central stimulants in the sense that they elicit a state associated with *heightened alertness and/or elevation of mood*.

Among the stimulants, some are liable to abuse because of induced dependent states, while others are virtually "abuse-free." The most widely used central stimulants are the methylxanthines, caffeine, theophylline, and theobromine; the active ingredients of coffee, tea, cocoa, and cola drinks. Since more than two billion pounds of coffee are consumed each year in the United States, as well as comparably large quantities of tea, cocoa, and cola, these are probably the most widely used of all "drugs." Despite the extensive use of these beverages and the well-known dependence of many individuals on their "morning cup of coffee," these drugs, unlike the amphetamines, are not usually thought of as eliciting "dependence." This is so despite the repeated demonstrations that, in many ways, the stimulant effects of amphetamine and caffeine are similar. Several experimental studies have shown that caffeine, like amphetamine, produces a more rapid and clearer flow of thought and allays drowsiness and fatigue. Besides evoking sustained intellectual effort and better association of ideas, caffeine shares with amphetamine the capacity to enhance discrimination of sensory stimuli and to quicken reaction time.[1] The reasons for the difference in dependence liability between the two drugs are not clear. The two central stimulants most associated with serious dependence problems are cocaine and amphetamine.

Cocaine

One of the first central stimulants to be widely abused in Western culture was cocaine. Characteristics of dependence to cocaine are very much like those of amphetamine. Indeed, the neuropharmacological mechanism of action of the two types of drug appears to be quite similar. Since the phenomenon of cocaine dependence has been well documented in Western European and American medical literature since the late nineteenth century and its clinical characteristics more fully described than amphetamine, we will begin with a consideration of cocaine dependence.*

Many people are not aware that the psychic actions of synthetic cocaine were first widely advocated by Sigmund Freud.[2] Shortly after cocaine was extracted in pure form from Peruvian coca leaves, the Merck Company provided Freud with samples of the alkaloid to evaluate its pharmacological properties. Besides performing a series of animal experiments, he ingested some of the drug himself and described the effects in this way, "If one takes a minimally active dose (0.05 to 0.10 g) while in excellent health and does not expect any special exertion thereafter, one can hardly perceive any surprising effect. It is different, however, if this dose of cocaine hydrochloride is taken by a subject whose general health is impaired by fatigue or hunger. After a short time (10 to 20 minutes) he feels as though he had been raised to the full height of intellectual and bodily vigor, in a state of euphoria, which is distinguished from the euphoria after consumption of alcohol by the absence of any feeling of alteration. However astonishing this effect of ingestion of coca may be, the absence of signs that could distinguish the state from the normal euphoria of good health makes it even more likely that we will underestimate it. As soon as the contrast between the present state and the state before the ingestion of cocaine is forgotten, it is difficult to believe that one is under the influence of a foreign agent, and yet one is very profoundly altered for four to five hours, since so long as the effects of the drug persist, one can perform mental and physical work with great endurance, and the otherwise urgent needs of rest, food, and sleep are thrust aside, as it were. During the first hours after cocaine, it is even impossible to fall asleep."[2]

As is evident from this description, the subjective effects of cocaine are very much like those of amphetamine. An interesting facet of amphetamine action which is not well recognized is its lack of stimulant effects upon an individual remaining at rest. Subjects maintained in bed after receiving 10 mg of *d*-amphetamine sulfate may even seem sedated.[3] According to Freud's description cocaine shares this property. Freud's publications describing cocaine as a miraculous "psychic energizer" gained wide currency throughout Europe and may have been a factor in the subsequent epidemic of cocaine abuse toward the end of the nineteenth century.

Because of medical reports that cocaine eased withdrawal symptoms from morphine, many patients in the early twentieth century became cocaine addicts via this iatrogenic route. To the morphine addict, cocaine brought a welcome change by temporarily enabling him to surmount his passivity and lethargy. Accordingly, combined dependence to both drugs has been much commoner than cocaine addiction alone.

Although cocaine can be administered orally, one of the most common techniques among cocaine addicts is to snuff the drug. Presumably, this affords a more rapid absorption. As described in the quotation from Freud, the *primary effects are an immediate elation with a subjective feeling of greater mental agility, greater precision of thought and action, immunity to fatigue and greater muscular power.* All of these effects also can be objectively demonstrated. Indeed, it has been speculated that the capacity of the drug to induce resistance to fatigue facilitated legendary physical exploits of Peruvian mountain climbers.[4] As already mentioned, these effects are virtually identical to those of amphetamine.

After being high on cocaine and stopping the drug, there ensues a profound depression whose duration is related to the length of period during which the subject has been intoxicated by the drug. If the individual has been taking the drug for several days consecutively with little sleep, he will then sleep for 1 to 2 days.

Cocaine addicts develop a number of interesting behavioral characteristics. Sexual alterations become prominent. Most frequently, hypersexuality is evident, especially in women. Men may gravitate to a wide variety of sexual aberrations. Another striking characteristic is the presence of stereotyped compulsive behavior which can be experimentally demonstrated in animals. Chronic cocaine users will pursue a single, seemingly meaningless activity in a strange repetitious manner. For instance, women will compulsively clean their apartments over and over again.

The stereotyped, compulsive behavior often merges into cocaine psychosis. This condition is a paranoid psychosis which is almost indistinguishable from acute paranoid schizophrenia.[5] Patients invariably have vague or systematic delusions of

* Although the terms dependence and addiction are used interchangeably, it is understood to mean with reference to the CNS stimulants only "psychogenic dependence."

persecution. Both auditory and visual hallucinations occur. Despite the presence of psychotic thinking processes, most psychiatrists feel that these patients lack a typically schizophrenic thought disorder, with looseness of associations and concrete rather than abstract conceptualization.

As with the single dose effects, chronic actions of cocaine in addicts and the symptoms of cocaine psychosis are all the same as comparable effects of amphetamine. The general pharmacological features of these two drugs in man and in animals are also similar. Tolerance builds up rapidly to the stimulant actions. Cocaine and amphetamine addicts often consume 10 to 50 times as much drug as would be indicated for novice. Also, for both agents there are no prominent physical withdrawal symptoms, except for depression. Accordingly, in patients with amphetamine or cocaine psychosis, the drug may be stopped abruptly. The interactions of these agents with brain catecholamines, whereby the clinical effects appear to be mediated, will be described in the subsequent discussion of the amphetamines.

Amphetamines

Amphetamines have enjoyed widespread use for over 30 years, but have been notoriously abused, at least as far as public awareness is concerned, only in the past five years. Although addiction to massive doses of intravenously injected amphetamine is a fairly recent phenomenon, it is quite conceivable that millions of dieting housewives have for many years been more or less secret addicts.

The central stimulant properties of amphetamine were described in the early 1930's.[6] Amphetamine had been synthesized as a sympathomimetic agent for use in asthma and shock. It differed from the many sympathomimetics available at the time, the best known of which was ephedrine, in being more lipid soluble. Hence, it entered the brain with great facility and could produce central actions in low doses which had few peripheral autonomic effects. Its central stimulant properties were put to clinical use by Printzmetal and Bloomberg in the treatment of narcolepsy, for which it is still the drug of choice.[7]

In the early 1940's the anorexic activity of amphetamine became well established, and extensive use of this class of drugs in dieting began. In 1947, Bradley made the key observation that amphetamine, paradoxically, calmed hyperactive children; a clinical use which is becoming generally accepted only quite recently.[8] Finally, though frowned upon by most pharmacologists and the Food and Drug Administration, some analogues have been extensively prescribed for the relief of mild depression.

How does amphetamine do all these things? The mechanisms of action of amphetamine and cocaine are probably similar. Most pharmacologists feel that all the central effects of these drugs can be ascribed to an interaction with the catecholamines in the brain, norepinephrine, and/or dopamine. Histochemical fluorescent studies have revealed that cell bodies for the norepinephrine neurons in the brain are distributed diffusely in the brain stem (Figure 1).[9] Axons of the norepinephrine neurons ascend in the medial forebrain bundle and give off terminals throughout the brain, with the highest density in the hypothalamus. There is fairly sound evidence for the generalization that synaptic release of norepinephrine from many of its terminals in the brain is associated with central stimulation and euphoria. The tricyclic antidepressants, such as imipramine (Tofranil) and amitriptyline (Elavil), appear to exert their clinical actions by inhibiting the reuptake inactivation of norepinephrine, hence potentiating its synaptic effects.[10]

Dopamine, the other major catecholamine in the brain, is localized to several circumscribed neuronal tracts. The largest and best known has cell bodies in the substantia nigra and terminals in the caudate nucleus and putamen, collectively called the corpus striatum. It is this tract which is degenerated in patients with Parkinson's disease with an attendant depletion of dopamine.

Besides the nigrostriatal tract, there are several other prominent dopamine tracts (Figure 1).[9] Dopamine neurons exist in the retina. A dopamine tract with cell bodies in the arcuate nucleus of the hypothalamus and terminals surrounding the capillary plexus to the anterior pituitary gland may play a role in regulating the release of pituitary trophic hormones. Of perhaps even greater interest are tracts with cell bodies near the interpeduncular nucleus of the midbrain with terminals in the nucleus accumbens in the septal area or the olfactory tubercle. The latter two neuronal systems are in parts of the brain that are implicated in the regulation of emotions.

A differential neurochemical mediation of

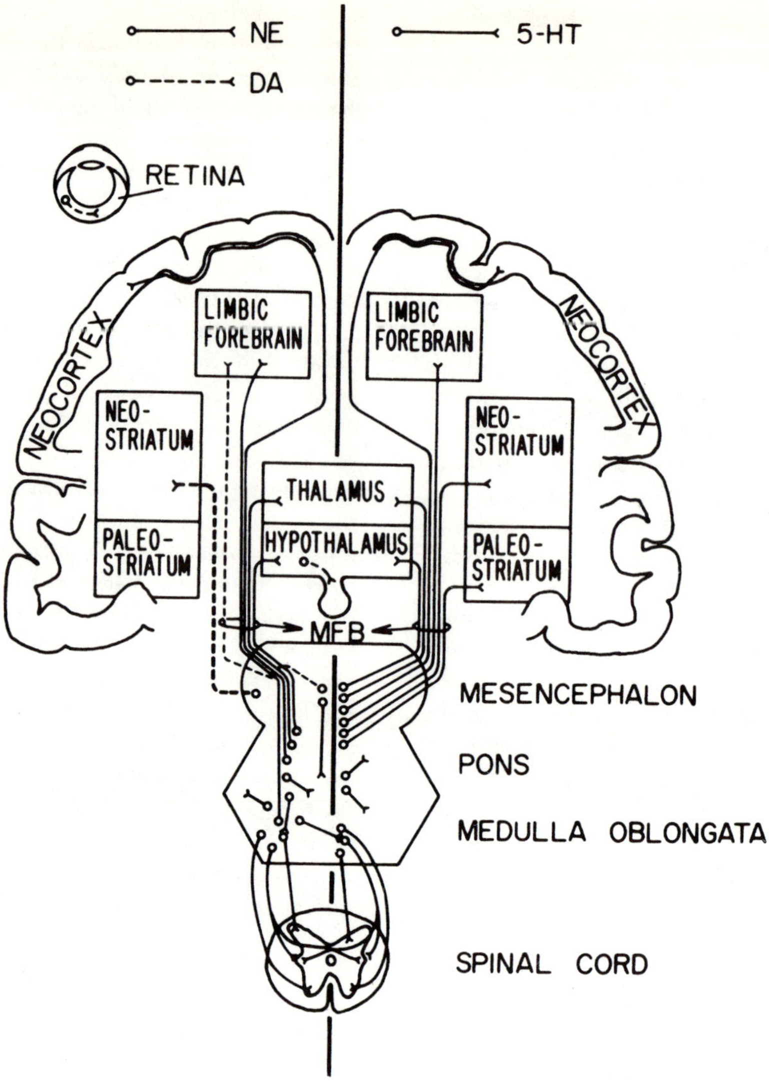

FIGURE 1. Diagrammatic representation of norepinephrine (NE), dopamine (DA), and serotonin (5-HT) tracts in the rat brain. Adapted from Anden et al.[9]

euphoria and the psychotic effects of amphetamine and cocaine is hinted at by differences in the clinical features of the two phenomena. Low doses of amphetamine produce moderate euphoria and increased alertness in adults. Since tolerance can develop to these actions, dieting patients using amphetamine may, in the absence of close medical supervision, gradually increase their intake to as much as ten times the recommended dose. Some of these patients may become psychotic. However, amphetamine or cocaine psychosis usually occurs among more bonafide addicts. Methamphetamine, whose subjective effects are essentially the same as those of amphetamine and other amphetamine analogues such as methylphenidate (Ritalin), are injected intravenously by addicts in rapidly escalating amounts. They seek an immediate "rush", a massive whole body euphoria much like an orgasm that takes place as soon as the drug enters the bloodstream. While amphetamine is consistently a euphoriant in low doses, addicts, surprisingly, experience negligible euphoria after the initial rush. They spend most of their time depressed, possibly as a rebound phenomenon. They take the drug in "runs" of four consecutive days when they hardly sleep or eat at all, followed by three days of rest with no drug and almost constant sleep to recuperate.

Almost all addicts become psychotic on one or more occasions. The psychosis is very similar for amphetamine and cocaine, and difficult to distinguish from paranoid schizophrenia. Indeed, many misdiagnoses have been made by psychiatrists not provided with the history of drug use. One of the hallmarks of amphetamine psychosis or the prepsychotic state is stereotyped, compulsive behavior.[11] Some amphetamine psychotics will compulsively search for bugs under their skin. Others will go back and forth to the refrigerator opening and closing it, seeming to search for something which is not present. Still others have been reported to take apart and attempt to reassemble every radio, television, or other appliance in sight.

Thus, there are two different types of behavioral actions of amphetamine in adult humans, central stimulation at low doses and amphetamine psychosis at high, prolonged doses. These two states have their animal counterparts. At low doses amphetamine elicits central stimulation in animals, an effect which can be readily measured in rodents as enhancement of locomotor activity. At higher and more chronic doses, animals evince a stereotyped compulsive behavior[12] which, in monkeys, bears certain resemblances to the behavior of human amphetamine psychotics.[13]

Recent research has suggested that the central stimulant effect of amphetamine in animals and presumably in humans, may be mediated by brain norepinephrine, while the stereotyped behavior involves brain dopamine.[14-16] Experiments in our laboratory with the two isomers of amphetamine have supported this notion.

It is likely that similar interactions with brain catecholamines underlie the behavioral effects of cocaine. Both drugs block the reuptake inactivation of catecholamines.[10] Amphetamines, in addition, can elicit a direct release of catecholamines into the synaptic cleft. *d*-Amphetamine is about 10 times as potent in inhibiting catecholamine reuptake at norepinephrine synapses, while the two isomers show similar potencies in facilitating events at dopamine synapses.[17]

Behavioral observations strikingly parallel the neurochemical results. *d*-Amphetamine is ten times as potent as its *l*-isomer in enhancing locomotor activity in rats, strongly suggesting that this effect, and hence central stimulation in man, is mediated by brain norepinephrine.[16] The two amphetamine isomers, however, have only a twofold difference in potency in eliciting stereotyped compulsive behavior in rats. Angrist and Gershon[18] have obtained support for a dopaminergic basis of amphetamine psychosis by showing that *d*- and *l*-amphetamine have similar milligram potencies in eliciting amphetamine psychosis in human volunteers.

It is quite impressive that a behavioral effect of a drug can be attributed to a single neurochemical system in the brain. Perhaps there are even broader implications. Since amphetamine psychosis so closely resembles paranoid schizophrenia, many investigators have suggested that it is an experimental model for schizophrenia. Thus, new knowledge of the neuronal basis of amphetamine psychosis may have implications for understanding brain mechanisms operative in schizophrenia. In this connection, it is important to bear in mind the fact that the potency of antischizophrenic phenothiazines and butyrophenones is closely paralleled by their ability to block dopamine receptors in the brain.[19,20] Moreover, phenothiazines are extraordinarily effective in the treatment of amphetamine psychosis, producing dramatic and rapid amelioration of symptoms (B. Angrist, personal communication).

HALLUCINOGENS

These agents have had many labels, including hallucinogenic, psychotomimetic, psychodysleptic, and psychosomimetic, but most of these are somewhat misleading. For instance, "hallucinogenic" suggests that the drug gives rise to formed hallucinations in the sense that the user will see things that "aren't there." The term "psychedelic" is tinged with disrepute since it connotes the fascinating effects of these drugs and thus suggests a tacit approval of their use. Actually, although hallucinogens generally elicit perceptual distortions, they rarely produce true hallucinations. "Psychotomimetic" is a poor term, since drugs that give rise to toxic mental effects, agents as diverse as atropine, gasoline and alcohol, also produce psychosis. Yet the toxic delirium of gasoline intoxication is surely very different from the transcendental state elicited by LSD.

"Psychedelic" is a term coined by Humphrey

Osmond in 1957[21] from the Greek meaning "mind manifesting." Osmond was referring to the capacity whereby these drugs seem to enhance awareness of the self and of nuances of the environment. Subsequent research with a large number of psychedelic drugs has demonstrated that changes in internal and external perception are indeed the *sine qua non* of the psychedelic experience shared by all drugs of this class though they may differ in other respects. A brief description of the remarkable state of consciousness that occurs during a "trip" on one of these drugs provides valuable insight into the attraction they hold for young people.

After a moderate dose of LSD (about 100 to 150 μg) taken by mouth the first effect, noted about 30 to 45 min after drug ingestion, is slight nausea, after which perceptual changes commence. At first objects may look different, though the viewer cannot pinpoint what has changed. Then, he may begin to feel that he is perceiving things more intensely than ever before. For instance, he may find himself visualizing pores in people's skin. Objects become distorted, and the distortions are determined in part by the viewer's wishes. If he focuses on his thumb, it may grow and undulate. One remarkable effect is synesthesia, a transmutation of the senses. When someone claps his hands, the drug user may visualize the sound waves moving across the room.

Changes in sensory perception are often followed by alterations in mental or emotional perception. The individual feels that he can "see" what those about him are feeling. He may then groove on the perception of his own mind, sensing it to be at one with the universe. Leaders of the LSD drug cult maintain that this is the essence of the "psychedelic experience." Boundaries between self and nonself dissolve. The ego evaporates and merges with the totality of all "being." Such an experience is ineffable and strongly reminiscent of mystical states attained by practitioners of profound meditation whether of Christian, Buddhist, or Hindu persuasion.

But the same mental state that affords the possibility of a profound "religious" experience also provides the greatest danger of hallucinogen use. For many people cannot tolerate a loss of the sense of self. Together with ego dissolution may come overwhelming terror. When the individual feels that he does not know who he is, or what or where the world is, he may become panic-stricken. It is in such states of panic that LSD users have jumped to their death from the windows of high buildings. These "bad trips" are the most serious adverse effect from hallucinogens and are the most frequent complication of psychedelic drug taking. Dealing with them is fairly easy, if one understands the nature of the reaction and the pharmacology of hallucinogens.

First, bear in mind the enormous suggestability of the subject under the influence of these drugs. This has already been alluded to in describing how perceptual distortions are largely determined by the patient's volition. Since much of the psychedelic experience has been brought on by suggestion, this is the best tool in alleviating the panic reaction. More important than any drug antidotes is the calm "talking down" of the patient. Since panic has resulted from the patient's rigid refusal to tolerate the riotous changes in his sense of self, the patient should be urged to relax and accept calmly the changes in mental function, to "ride with the drug experience." He should be reassured that he is not going crazy but only experiencing a self-limited drug induced state.

What about chemical antidotes? Phenothiazines have been used commonly to bring patients down from bad trips. Probably, the rationale for the use of these drugs derived from the pioneering neurophysiological studies of Bradley and Elkes[22] and Bradley and Key.[23] Using the *encephalè isoleé* preparation of the cat, they were able to distinguish between the exciting effects of LSD and amphetamine and between the sedating effects of phenobarbital and chlorpromazine. Small doses of amphetamine facilitated behavioral arousal whether induced by direct stimulation of the reticular activating system or by a sensory stimulus such as an auditory click. LSD, however, had no effect on the threshhold of arousal to electrical stimulation of the reticular activating system but, in very small doses, greatly enhanced arousal elicited by sensory stimulation. They concluded that a primary mode of action of LSD was to augment sensitivity to sensory perception. An analogous, but inverse, situation occurred in comparing phenobarbital and chlorpromazine. Phenobarbital attenuated arousal whether elicited by brain stem stimulation or sensory stimuli, while chlorpromazine attenuated arousal only to sensory stimuli for which it was effective in very small doses. Not only did these experiments suggest a neurophysiologic explanation of the actions of

LSD, but they suggested an antagonist. Chlorpromazine would be predicted to be a specific and potent antidote to bad trips.

In recent years clinicians who deal with large numbers of patients having adverse reactions to hallucinogens have come to feel that sedatives, particularly the minor tranquilizers chlordiazepoxide (Librium®) and diazepam (Valium®), are at least as effective. Since some LSD is spiked with strychnine, and since phenothiazines potentiate the convulsive effects of strychnine, many doctors are reluctant to administer phenothiazines to trippers so that Librium and Valium become the drugs of choice. Also, because of the growing realization that much of the hallucinogen syndrome is the product of suggestion, it is widely felt that for most bad trips patients can be "talked down" and drugs should be employed only when reassurance fails.

Ways of dealing with these drugs in the future may be determined by current research demonstrating a highly selective specific interaction between these agents and serotonin neurons in the brain. Aghajanian et al.[24] found that miniscule doses of LSD, too low to produce overt behavioral effects, stopped or markedly slowed the firing of the serotonin-containing raphe neurons in the brain stem.

Histochemical fluorescent studies have revealed that all the serotonin in the brain is contained in a system of neurons whose cell bodies constitute the raphe nuclei in the midbrain and upper pons (Figure 1). Axons ascend in the medial forebrain bundle to give terminals in all parts of the brain, but with highest incidence in the hypothalamus and the limbic forebrain.

Aghajanian found that raphe cells were the only neurons in the brain that responded to LSD in this way. Moreover, this effect was shared by all hallucinogens even though of markedly different chemical structure, such as mescaline and DOM (STP), while chemically similar agents which are not psychedelic drugs, such as amphetamine, lacked this effect. A variety of evidence has led Aghajanian to postulate that the LSD slowing of raphe neuronal firing is an indirect effect.[24] LSD mimicks the effects of serotonin at its postsynaptic receptors. The postsynaptic cells, via a hypothetical interneuron, send back to the raphe cells the message to stop firing.

What are the implications of these findings? A great deal of other research has linked the serotonin neuronal system to sleep-wakefulness and arousability.[25] It is quite possible that the serotonin neurons regulate the influence of sensory stimuli on attention and feelings, providing a link to the earlier neurophysiological studies.[22,23] Certainly, the ideal antidote to LSD would be an antagonist of serotonin and its receptors in the brain.

What psychedelic drugs exist besides LSD? There are the tryptamine derivatives; psilocybin, psilocin, dimethyltryptamine (DMT), diethyltryptamine, and dipropyltryptamine, as well as the phenethylamine, mescaline. Quite recently a large number of agents chemically related both to mescaline and amphetamine, most of which were first synthesized by Shulgin,[26] have come into widespread use. Shulgin systematically varied substituents of the amphetamine analogue of mescaline and was able to greatly enhance potency on a milligram basis. Thus, DOM (STP) differs from the mescaline analogues only in the location of the methoxy group, yet is 50 times as potent as mescaline.

Despite their chemical diversity, all of these drugs produce essentially the same effects. Effects of mescaline and DOM last somewhat longer than those of LSD. With the bromine and ethyl derivatives of DOM, enhanced self-awareness can occur over a wide range of doses without any perceptual distortions or psychotomimetic effects (Shulgin, personal communications, Reference 27). These results suggest that their action may indeed be "psychedelic," i.e., to enhance self-awareness, while the hallucinogenic and psychotomimetic effects may only be secondary phenomena, which conceivably may be eliminated by appropriate chemical modification of the drug.

REFERENCES

1. Foltz, E., Ivy, A. C., and Barborka, C. J., The use of double work periods in the study of fatigue and the influence of caffeine on recovery, *Amer. J. Physiol.*, 136, 79, 1942.

2. Freud, S., On the general effects of cocaine, *Drug Dependence*, 5, 15, 1970.

3. Snyder, S. H., Faillace, L. A., and Weingartner, H., A new psychotropic agent: psychological and physiological effects of 2,5-dimethoxy-4-ethylamphetamine (DOET) in man, *Arch. Gen. Psychiat.*, 21, 95, 1969.

4. Taylor, N., *Narcotics, Nature's Dangerous Gifts*, Dell, New York, 1970, 59.

5. Mayer-Gross, W., Slater, E., and Roth, M., *Clinical Psychiatry*, Cassell, London, 1961, 378.

6. Alles, G. A., The comparative physiological actions of dl-β-phenylisopropylamines. I. Pressor effect and toxicity, *J. Pharmacol. Exp. Ther.*, 47, 339, 1933.

7. Printzmetal, M. and Bloomberg, W., The use of Benzedrine for the treatment of narcolepsy, *J.A.M.A.*, 105, 2051, 1935.

8. Bradley, C. B., Treatment of the convulsive child in a children's psychiatric hospital, *Nerv. Child*, 6, 76, 1947.

9. Anden, N. E., Dahlstrom, A., Fuxe, K., Larsson, K., Olson, L., and Ungerstedt, U., Ascending monoamine neurons to the telencephalon and diencephalon, *Acta Physiol. Scand.*, 67, 313, 1966.

10. Snyder, S. H., Catecholamines, brain function and how psychotropic drugs act, in *Principles of Psychopharmacology*, Clark, W. G. and del Giudice, J., Eds., Academic Press, New York, 1970, 115.

11. Ellinwood, E. H., Jr., Amphetamine psychosis: I. description of the individuals and process, *J. Nerv. Ment. Dis.*, 144, 273, 1967.

12. Randrup, A. and Munkvad, I., Stereotyped activities produced by amphetamine in several animal species and man, *Psychopharmacologia*, 11, 300, 1967.

13. Ellinwood, E. H., Jr., Chronic methamphetamine intoxication in three experimental animals, in *Amphetamine Abuse*, Ellinwood, E. H. and Cohen, S., Eds., 1972, in press.

14. Ernst, A. M., Modes of action of apomorphine and dexamphetamine on gnawing compulsion in rats, *Psychopharmacologia*, 10, 316, 1967.

15. Fog, R. L., Randrup, A., and Pakkenberg, H., Aminergic mechanisms in corpus striatum and amphetamine-induced stereotyped behavior, *Psychopharmacologia*, 11, 179, 1967.

16. Taylor, K. M. and Snyder, S. H., Differential effects of *d*- and *l*-amphetamine on behavior and on catecholamine disposition in dopamine and norepinephrine containing neurons of rat brain, *Brain Res.*, 28, 295, 1971.

17. Snyder, S. H., Taylor, K. M., Coyle, J. T., and Meyerhoff, J. L., The role of brain dopamine in behavioral regulation and the actions of psychotropic drugs, *Amer. J. Psychiat.*, 127, 199, 1970.

18. Angrist, B. M., Shopsin, B., and Gershon, S., The comparative psychotomimetic effects of stereoisomers of amphetamine, *Nature*, 234, 152, 1971.

19. Jannsen, A. J., The evolution of the butyrophenones haloperidol and trifluperidol from meperidine-like 4-phenylpiperidines, *Int. Rev. Neurobiol.*, 8, 221, 1965.

20. Horn, A. S. and Snyder, S. H., Chlorpromazine and dopamine: conformational similarities that correlate with the antischizophrenic activity of phenothiazine drugs, *Proc. Natl. Acad. Sci. U.S.A.*, 68, 2325, 1971.

21. Osmond, H., A review of the effects of psychotomimetic agents, *Ann. N.Y. Acad. Sci.*, 66, 429, 1957.

22. Bradley, P. B. and Elkes, J., The effects of some drugs on the electrical activity of the brain, *Brain,* 80, 77, 1957.

23. Bradley, P. B. and Key, B. J., The effect of drugs on arousal responses produced by electrical stimulation of the reticular formation of the brain, *Electroenceph. Clin. Neurophysiol.*, 10, 97, 1958.

24. Aghajanian, G. K., Foote, W. E., and Sheard, M. H., Action of psychotogenic drugs on single midbrain raphe neurons, *J. Pharmacol. Exp. Ther.*, 171, 178, 1970.

25. Jouvet, M., Biogenic amines and the states of sleep, *Science*, 163, 32, 1969.

26. Shulgin, A. T., Sargent, T., and Naranjo, C., Structure-activity relationships of one-ring psychotomimetics, *Nature*, 221, 537, 1969.

27. Snyder, S. H., Weingartner, H., and Faillace, L. A., DOET (2,5-dimethoxy-4-ethylamphetamine), a new psychotropic drug: effects of varying doses in man, *Arch. Gen. Psychiat.*, 24, 50, 1971.

CANNABIS

R. T. Jones

TABLE OF CONTENTS

INTRODUCTION

During the past five years cannabis has become a fashionable drug to use and to research. A number of factors stimulated renewed scientific interest in *cannabis sativa* after many years of relative neglect. Certainly a concern over the increase in the use of cannabis by young people in most Western countries is important. Advances in the understanding of cannabis chemistry and the availability of government research funds earmarked for cannabis research are significant. A complete review of the extensive and rapidly growing literature on cannabis is not practical in a short chapter. Besides, any review of cannabis dependence will soon be dated. This is a selective review with an emphasis on references and topics that have received insufficient attention elsewhere. A number of recent comprehensive reviews and books concerned with cannabis effects are available.[1-6]

BOTANY AND CHEMISTRY

Cannabis sativa is one of man's oldest cultivated plants.[7] World-wide dissemination is largely a result of the plant's value as a source of fiber. Grown as hemp, it was mainly used to make rope, but biologically active constituents in some varieties of plant were recognized thousands of years ago and used for both medical purposes and as a social intoxicant.[4] The general term, cannabis, refers to a variety of preparations derived from the herbaceous plant *cannabis sativa*. Marijuana or marihuana (grass, pot, weed in North America) usually consists of variable proportions of crushed *cannabis sativa* leaves, flowers, and stems. Similar preparations are known as *bhang* in India. The relatively pure resin from the plants is called *hashish* or *charas* and is about five times as potent by weight as marijuana. *Ganja* is somewhere between bhang and charas in potency and consists of resinous masses of small leaves.

Failure to properly consider and appreciate the tremendous variation in composition and biological potency of cannabis[7] has contributed to unnecessary confusion concerning much of its psychopharmacology. Most plants cultivated for their biological products vary in potency due to genetic, environmental, and processing factors. Unfortunately for the cannabis user and the scientist, *cannabis sativa* may vary more than most plants. It is an extremely adaptable plant, showing great genetic plasticity and susceptibility to environmentally induced changes.[7] As with any other biologically active plant, the methods used for preparing crude plant material and conditions of storage are important in determining its chemistry.[8,9] In the illicit market, these factors are completely uncontrolled.

Cannabis contains a great array of organic chemicals. Current interest has centered on its unique constituents called cannabinoids. Cannabinoids are not known to occur in any other plant material. Although numerous cannabinoids have been considered as active principles of cannabis, it now appears that certain isomers of tetrahydrocannabinol are the most potent psychoactive constituents.[2,3,10] The major tetrahydrocannabinol believed to account for the sought after psychoactive properties of cannabis is referred to as delta-9-tetrahydrocannabinol or delta-1-THC in the monoterpinoid numbering system.[10] In this chapter, unless otherwise qualified, the abbreviation THC will refer to delta-9-tetrahydrocannabinol. Delta-8-THC is also biologically active but occurs in only small amounts in cannabis. Cannabidiol and cannabinol are present in substantial amounts but, on the basis of animal studies, are not thought to be psychoactive.[3,10] However, before it is correct to say that *the* active ingredient has been established, much more basic psychopharmacologic work needs to be done, particularly with human subjects judging psychoactivity. As with other drugs, there are marked species differences in response to cannabis.[11] Animal assays are not always accurate predictors of psychoactivity in man.

PATTERNS OF USE

Because of the variability of the substance ingested, any answer to the question, what are the characteristics of cannabis dependence, becomes exceedingly complex. Both the short and long-term health consequences of any drug use are determined by the dose the frequency of use, the form in which the drug is used, and the route of administration. The variable chemical composition of cannabis presents a serious problem in making general statements about many of the characteristics of cannabis dependence. For example, reliable data concerning the usual dose of cannabis consumed are not yet available. One can make only educated guesses about this basic variable. Information on the dose used by people in the real world is as important in designing appropriate laboratory experiments as it is in gathering meaningful epidemiological data on the consequences of cannabis use.

There is much to suggest that most American experience is based on the widespread but relatively infrequent use of an exceedingly weak form of cannabis. Much of the cannabis consumed in the U.S. is the fiber genotype containing little THC. Wild growth gathered in the midwestern U.S. contained only 0.1 to 0.5% THC.[9] Cannabis of Mexican origin ranged from 0.8 to 1.4% with an average of 1.2%.[12] Numerous specimens given to me by San Francisco users and described as better than average marijuana contained from 0 to 1.6% THC. A survey in Ontario, Canada found that of 36 samples obtained from users and alleged to be marijuana with high cannabinoid content, 34% contained no marijuana at all and much of the remainder was diluted with other plant substances.[13] It is possible to obtain far more potent marijuana. Plants grown in Mississippi from Mexican drug type plant seeds contained 1 to 4% THC[14] and a sample of Thailand marijuana contained 5% THC.[9] Such potent material is probably rare in most areas of the U.S. A fair assumption is that the cleaned marijuana generally available in this country averages about 1% THC. This estimate is in keeping with potency ratings made by users serving as experimental subjects in laboratory studies. They judged marijuana containing 0.9% THC to be of average quality.[15,16] Subjects who smoked marijuana containing 2.8% THC described it as potent as anything encountered in their years of cannabis use.

Although fresh hashish is generally reported to be about five times as potent as marijuana or bhang, it too is subject to great variation.[17] Lebanese hashish averaged 4 to 5% THC.[10] Specimens available in this country contain as little as 1 or 2%.[12,14] The average THC content of ganja is about 3% but this is an inference based on its preparation and comparisons to charas.[18]

Appropriate large-scale surveys and chemical analyses will ultimately provide better data on average potency. However the fact that most cannabis is smoked presents further complications in determining just what dose people are using.[19] Less than 10% of cannabis is smoked in pipes and a negligible amount is taken in the form of oral preparations in the U.S.[19] India is the only country where a significant amount of cannabis is taken orally, usually in the form of bhang drinks or as a constituent of sweet cakes. A distinction concerning route of administration must be made because of differences in rate and degree of absorption and differences in onset and duration of action between smoked and eaten cannabis.[18,20]

In studies with tobacco cigarettes, measures of cigarettes per day are not a good index of tobacco consumption because of wide variations in patterns of inhalation, length of butt, varying chemical characteristics of tobacco, etc.[21] The quality of marijuana smoked by American users will be an equally difficult figure to obtain. As with alcohol or tobacco dependence, it is necessary to consider amount and frequency of use in understanding cannabis dependence. Few of the numerous surveys of characteristics of users considered these variables.[19] Cigarettes in the eastern U.S. are generally smaller than those rolled in the West.[19] Experienced cannabis users judged 1 g cigarettes to be consistent with their usual experience.[16] When 20 highly experienced smokers were asked to roll cigarettes similar in size to what they usually smoked, the weights ranged from 0.49 to 2.1 g with a mean of 1.2 g.[16] They reported smoking one or two such cigarettes during an evening of smoking.[19,22] These quantities are consistent with the amount of marijuana smoked in ad libitum experimental sessions.[23]

Estimates based on a variety of sources suggest that 8 to 20 million Americans have tried cannabis.[4-6] However, far more people have *tried* cannabis than use it regularly. Whether the focus is on the individual user or on the significance of groups of users to society, it is necessary to make a distinction between the occasional experimenter and the person who smokes five to ten cannabis cigarettes daily. This is an obvious consideration but often overlooked in attempts to find, for example, drug induced changes in "marijuana users."[24]

The task of describing the scope of cannabis use is an enormous one. All the data currently available have questionable validity and reliability. The reluctance of some users to admit to illegal activity and the eagerness of some nonusers, particularly younger students, to pretend use may seriously distort prevalent data. Drug use has been surveyed in numerous high schools and colleges.[25] There is a suggestion of a leveling off or even a decrease in numbers of users in a recent West Coast junior and senior high school population.[26] In surveys where frequency of use has been considered, 46% of 8 to 20 million "users" in the U.S. have used cannabis less than 10 times or have stopped completely.[27] Young adults who consider themselves as regular and enthusiastic cannabis users often report using the drug once weekly or less.[16,23,27,28] Such infrequent, albeit regular use is a pattern that must be considered in any discussion of the presence or absence of chronic effects in drug-using populations.

If possible differences in patterns of use, dose, and potency of material used are kept in mind, then the disparity between the "American experience" with cannabis and reports of adverse acute and chronic effects from abroad becomes more understandable.[5,6,15] High dose level, continuous use of potent cannabis is commonly reported in India, the Middle East, and North Africa. For example, Indian reports define moderate use of cannabis as equivalent to 30 to 60 mg of THC *daily* or about 5 to 10 average U.S. cigarettes.[18] Cultural forces are important determinants of drug use patterns, but simply the availability of potent material may be a factor in frequency of cannabis use. Tennant et al. described a group of American soldiers stationed in Germany where hashish was plentiful and cheap, who consumed 100 g or more of hashish monthly (perhaps equivalent to 500 domestic American marijuana cigarettes).[29] It would be surprising if there were no differences between that group of hashish smokers and a group of U.S. college freshmen who smoked a total of 20 marijuana cigarettes over a one-year period. In fact, there are very significant differences between frequent and infrequent users.[16,23,28] However, only prospective studies will clarify the role of cannabis in producing the differences.

EFFECTS ON HUMANS

We know more about the effects of cannabis in man than the effects of many other drugs of abuse. As Hollister points out in an excellent review of human effects, "Much of the newer work with marihuana involves the rediscovery of phenomena known for a long time, sometimes camouflaged by coining new names for old phenomena or by elegantly proving the obvious."[1] Much of the older literature presents a consistent and valid description of the psychological and behavioral effects of cannabis if the reader keeps in mind the varied effects of dose, route of administration and the nondrug factors of personality, set, setting, and prior drug experience.

The results of current research add little to the elegant accounts of Baudelaire, Dumas, and Gautier, and other writers active in the mid-19th century French hashish cult.[30] They described cannabis induced feelings of euphoria, excitement, disturbed associations, changes in the perception of time and space, enhanced auditory and tactile sensitivity, paresthesia and weakness, perseveration, rapidly changing mood, mental disorganization, delusions, illusions, and hallucinations. All these phenomena have been observed in recent laboratory experiments, although reported far less poetically. Even after a century, it is difficult to improve on Moreau de Tours' clinical studies with hashish except that we can now more reliably specify the dose administered.[31] A psychiatrist, he encouraged his students to experience cannabis intoxication so that by their experiences they could gain insights into schizophrenia and other mental disturbances. The use of cannabis to induce a model psychosis may seem inconsistent with the experience of cannabis users in this country and statements concerning the undramatic effects produced in recent laboratory studies.[5,6,15] We should remember that Moreau de Tours was probably talking about doses of hashish containing 50 to 100 mg or more of THC, while most American users are reporting on the effects of 1 to 10 mg of THC.

Public concern over the use of cannabis in the U.S. led to extensive investigations in the early 1940's under the direction of the LaGuardia Committee on Marihuana.[32] Cannabis users and nonusers were given orally administered and smoked marijuana. Measures of dose were in terms of quantity of raw material but probably were in the range of 30 to 50 mg THC orally (with up to 300 mg in a few subjects) and 8 to 30 mg THC smoked. Clinical effects were consistent with those previously described. Euphoria and difficulty in concentrating or controlling attention were prominent. Feeling of lightness or heaviness, dry mouth, blurred vision, tachycardia and palpitation, and increased appetite were commonly reported. Clinical biochemical studies were within normal limits. Electroencephalographic studies showed increased alpha after the drug but without proper control groups, it is impossible to say whether this and other changes were simply due to the passage of time, boredom, fatigue, etc. Simple psychomotor functions were only slightly altered. More complex functions were impaired at all doses. Generally, nonusers were more affected by marijuana than those with previous experience. There were nine cases of psychotic reactions in the group of 72 prisoners studied. None of the individuals so affected was a regular user of cannabis.

The conclusions of the LaGuardia report, like other significant earlier contributions to the cannabis literature, must be qualified because of the many weaknesses in experimental methodology. Double blind and placebo controls were lacking, statistical analyses of changes were rarely used, the reporting tended to be biased if the data were ambiguous, and the use of subject populations like prison inmates or writers limited the generalizations that could be made from the data. However, more recent controlled studies have added little new information.

Since the 1940's, it was suspected that the tetrahydrocannabinols were mainly responsible for the activity of cannabis.[11] The availability of pure THC, and improved chemical techniques for its quantification, has led to a rapidly increasing series of pharmacological studies where, for the first time, there is some precision in dose. Isbell et al. first reported the effects of pure synthetic THC in man and confirmed it was similar to cannabis.[33]

Soon after, Hollister[34] and Waskow[35] and their colleagues reported on studies of THC in man. A number of clinical studies using smoked or oral doses of plant material extracts assayed for THC content have followed during the past three years.[15,16,20,23,36-51] Not surprisingly, it appears the effects are closely related to the dose consumed. At levels of THC below 2 to 20 mg THC administered in a single smoked dose or 5 to 40 mg THC given orally, typical subjective reports include euphoria and silliness, subjective slowing of time, difficulty in thinking, loss of attention, sleepiness, floating sensations, depersonalization, weakness, relaxation, impairment of immediate memory, and perceptual changes (auditory, visual, tactile). It is important to note that experience in the laboratory setting is consistent with descriptions from users' experience in a social situation obtained by questionnaire or interview techniques.[52,53]

In the laboratory oral administration of doses above 40 mg THC and smoked doses above 20 mg THC produces a generally dysphoric state with unpleasant somatic symptoms (nausea, vomiting, headache, sedation) and on occasion, anxiety, delusions, illusions, and hallucinations.[20,33,34]

The dose of cannabis is only one determinant of the resulting subjective experience. The importance of set and setting and the subject's past experience in determining subjective effects is illustrated by differences in the reactions to THC given to Isbell's addicts[33] who were familiar with and who knew they were receiving a cannabis-like drug and Waskow's subjects who were "marihuana naïve" state hospital patients, and unaware of the type of drug they were to ingest.[35] The former developed the expected euphoria, perceptual and time sense changes, delusions, and hallucinations. The latter group mainly experienced a feeling of sedation, slight euphoria, mildly unpleasant and nonspecific somatic effects, and few mental changes. Similar differences in subjective reactions to smoked cannabis determined by set, setting, and past experiences have been reported.[15,16,23]

Physiologic Effects

Pulse rate increase is perhaps the most consistent physiologic correlate of cannabis intoxication. It is sufficiently dose-related and reproducible for use in quantitative assays.[33,51,54-56] The tachycardia may be mediated through a beta-adrenergic mechanism and is blocked by propranolol.[55] Cannabis may suppress the normal sinus arrhythmia.[51] Other than a slight flattening of T waves and occasional premature ventricular contractions in 2 of 15 subjects, no electrocardiographic changes have been reported.[54] Blood pressure tends to fall slightly or remain unchanged.[34,54] Orthostatic hypotension can occur at higher doses.[1]

Conjuctival vascular congestion is dose-related and occurs after oral or smoked administration.[15,16,34,55,56] Both the pulse and conjunctival vessel changes correlate well with time of appearance, duration, and intensity of psychological effects.[33,55] Dilated pupils and a sluggish reaction to light have been reported consistently in other studies,[32,57] but recent experiments have noted no dilation.[15,16,33,34] Ptosis and edema of eyelids have been reported along with photophobia and nystagmus.[58,59]

Salivary flow is decreased after cannabis.[16] Body temperature is generally unchanged[34] or slightly decreased.[35] Neurological effects include fine tremors,[32,58] muscle weakness,[32,34] and decrements in static body equilibrium.[34,45] There are decrements in auditory and visual acuity.[32,36,38,60]

Relatively few studies have included biochemical measures. Most recent studies have found no changes in blood glucose levels attributable to cannabis.[33,34,41,42] An increase in food intake after cannabis has been reported but with great between-subject variability.[42,61] Hollister et al. found total leukocytes increased and phosphorous and creatinine clearance decreased slightly by THC and synhexyl. No changes were noted in free fatty acid levels, platelet serotonin content, plasma cortisol, or urinary catecholamine excretion.[34,62,63] There is a great need for precise biochemical studies with proper dietary and other appropriate controls.

Studies of acute cannabis effects on the electroencephalograph have shown inconsistent and minimal changes. A decrease in percent alpha time,[57,58,64] together with increased fast activity[9] has been reported. A recent study reports more alpha and less fast activity after smoking marijuana.[66] The published studies often do not include a placebo control group, so it is difficult to determine if the background EEG changes are drug related or more a function of nonspecific drowsiness, boredom, or fatigue. Rodin et al. found no changes in auditory or visual EEG evoked responses.[48] However, Tinklenberg reports increased amplitudes of visual EEG evoked responses.[67]

Effects on Intellectual and Motor Performance

Simple and well-practiced tasks are least affected by cannabis. As tasks become more complicated, decrements in performance are usually noted. Experimental confirmation is evident from a wide range of studies.[15,16,23,32,36,37,41,43,46,47,61] Experienced users demonstrate less impairment than novices or infrequent users, at least at lower dose levels.[15,16,20,23,36,37,40] Doses of THC as low as 6 μg/kg have produced decrements in psychomotor performance.[55] As with other psychoactive agents, there were marked individual differences in cannabis effects on performance.[36,37,45] A problem in interpreting the relevance of many laboratory studies is a tendency for investigators to infer too much concerning the face validity of some of the measures. For example, much has been made of the memory deficit produced by cannabis.[46,47,50] The tasks used to measure this memory deficit in fact tap a complex array of mental functions – concentration, attention, and set and are subject to effects of motivation, cooperation, etc. A deficit in performance after cannabis may be secondary to a memory defect, but could be a result of changes in the other variables. The specificity of many of the cannabis effects is still open to question. When cannabis is compared to modest doses of ethanol, a similar "memory defect" and other performance deficits are seen.[20,43,67-69]

The frequent use of cannabis while driving[19] aroused interest in its effects on driving skills. One study compared the effects of alcohol (1.2 g/kg body weight) and smoked marijuana (22 mg of THC in 2 cigarettes) on a driving simulator task. The alcohol impaired simulator scores, while the marijuana produced only minimal decrements.[40] This well-publicized study has been criticized as an inappropriate comparison of single doses of drugs rather than obtaining dose effect data.[70] The validity of simulator data as a predictor of real life driving is also open to question.

Route of Administration and Metabolism

Smoking cannabis produces quantitative and probably qualitative differences in a subjective state when compared to the effects of oral consumption, even when roughly equivalent doses are compared.[1,15,16,19,32] However, there are more similarities than differences between the different routes of administration, particularly on behavioral measures.[1] When smoked, there is a rapid onset of effects within seconds. Effects may be subtle and brief or last 2 or 3 hours after a single cigarette containing 5 to 20 mg of THC. At about 1 hour after smoking, most individuals are rapidly becoming less intoxicated. About 50% of the THC originally in the cigarette is delivered to the mouth if the butt is totally consumed.[16,45,71] Relatively little THC is lost by pyrolysis, but it is progressively concentrated in the cigarette butt.[45,71,72]

Symptoms develop about 30 to 120 minutes after ingestion of THC or cannabis extract.[1] Although oral administration gives the illusion of more precision and control of dose, as little is known about absorption of THC from the gut as from the lungs.[1] The amount inactivated or altered during passage through the liver is unknown. Until a suitable quantitative estimation of THC concentration in tissue, plasma, or urine is available, arguments over what provides most control over dose are moot. It is possible to get reliable data in humans with both smoked[33,51,54,56] and oral routes.[46,49] Both deserve study. The intraperitoneal route has been widely used in animal studies. Because of the irritating qualities of THC and cannabis extracts and their poor solubility, caution is warranted until tissue levels can be assayed.

The metabolism of cannabis in animal and man is poorly understood. Research with radioactive THC indicates that breakdown products remain in the body for some time after the acute intoxication is over.[73,74] In rats the halflife of radioactive THC may be a week or more.[75] Recently a pharmacologically active 11-hydroxy metabolite of THC was reported.[10] When injected intercerebrally into mice, it is 15 times more active than THC.[76] Metabolites of THC appear in plasma within 10 minutes after intravenous administration, but only small quantities of THC appear in the urine.[73] When a tracer (0.6 mg) dose of THC was injected into three humans who had never smoked marijuana, the halflife of blood THC was 56 hours.[73] Metabolites appeared in plasma within 10 minutes. The 11-hydroxy metabolite was only a small fraction of material in plasma. The THC disappeared twice as rapidly from the blood of experienced users and excretion in the urine was more rapid.[74]

Some experienced users of cannabis report that instead of becoming tolerant to its effects, they become more sensitive to cannabis after the first few trials.[15] There has been a fair amount of speculation as to biochemical mechanisms for this so-called "reverse tolerance" phenomenon.[10,73,74] Mechoulam suggested enzyme induction may result in more effective metabolism with repeated exposure.[10] This would be consistent with the shorter halflife of THC in the blood of users particularly if cannabis psychoactivity is associated primarily with a metabolite. There is, however, some suggestion that the often cited decreased sensitivity to cannabis on the first few exposures may be folklore with little basis in fact.[19,20] If it is a common phenomenon, it can be explained readily on the basis of repeated exposure to low potency marijuana where psychological factors are the primary determinants of the subjective state.[16] Shared cultural values and learning are thought to play an important role in determining the interpretation and labeling of the state resulting from smoking cannabis.[77] If the "reverse tolerance" is chemically determined, it is remarkable that only sensitivity to psychic effects appears and more traditional tolerance is seen with behavioral and physiologic measures.[16,23,78-80]

Animal Pharmacology

A large number of animal investigations have looked into the neurological, biochemical, and behavioral effects of cannabis.[2,3] The relevance of many animal studies to the human use of cannabis and to the drug's psychotropic actions in man remains uncertain. The reasons for this stem from the tendency for animal investigators to use high dose levels and methods of administration unlike those used by humans. This is not to say that animal studies are unwarranted. To gain an understanding of mechanisms of drug action, to obtain certain chronic and acute toxicity data, and to provide clues for human studies, demands animal experiments. However, one should be cautious in attempts to explain human behavior on the basis of data derived from animals. The caution which holds for all psychoactive drugs is even more appropriate for cannabis studies since there are enormous species differences in cannabis activity.[11] For example, cannabichromene produces ataxia and sedation in the dog[81] but is without activity in man and monkey.[33,82] Cannabidiol produces marked motor deficits in rabbits, but is without activity in dog and man.[83,10] Tachycardia is one of the more predictable cannabis effects in man, but cannabis produces bradycardia in the dog.[11]

The single dose toxicity of THC in animals is low. The LD_{50} is between 800 and 1400 mg/kg orally and 20 to 40 mg/kg by intravenous injection depending on species.[3] Death occurs by respiratory arrest. This low lethal toxicity reflects the experience in humans where there is no convincing report of death by simple overdosage of cannabis.

A frequently used measure of cannabis effects in animals is analgesia. The spectrum of analgesia is different from that of morphine.[80,84] Cannabis has been used clinically for its analgesic effects but it is not established if these are primary or secondary to the hypnotic effects.[85] Both THC and synhexyl potentiate barbiturate sleeping time.[86,87] It is not yet established whether this is a result of enzyme induction. Paradoxically, cannabis prolongs the stimulant action of amphetamine.[86] Electroencephalographic changes produced by cannabinoids are not similar to those reported in humans.[88-90]

Behaviorally, cannabis decreases aggression in mice,[91] but increases fighting in starved rats.[92] Boyd et al.[?] found that synthetic tetrahydrocannabinols generally depress rat operant behavior and have effects similar to pentobarbital.[93] Monkeys become stimulated or depressed depending on dose of THC. They lose the ability to perform complex tasks.[94]

TOLERANCE AND DEPENDENCE

Although marked tolerance to the major effects of cannabis is not commonly observed among users in this country, there is increasing evidence that it can develop in both man[16,57] and animal.[79,80,95] As with most cannabis effects, the development of tolerance is related to dose and frequency of use. The cannabis user consuming 5 or 10 mg of THC two or three times weekly is no more likely to demonstrate measurable tolerance to cannabis than would someone drinking two or three beers weekly demonstrate tolerance to alcohol. There is little tendency for most intermittent users of cannabis to increase dose.[27] However, a survey by Chopra in India found dose to be gradually increased by certain users.[64] There are other reports of chronic frequent users in the Middle East who consume what would be large quantities of cannabis by Western standards.[96,97] Doses of THC over 60 to 70 mg given in experimental settings in this country produce generally unpleasant states in cannabis-using subjects.[20,27] In contrast, smokers in Chopra's survey consumed approximately 700 mg of THC daily. Tennant reported some U.S. military personnel to be consuming between 150 and 700 mg of THC daily (in hashish), a dose equivalent to well over 10 marijuana cigarettes.[29] Such clinical reports certainly suggest the development of tolerance.

In laboratory studies, frequent (daily) marijuana users showed fewer heart rate increases[16,23] and salivary flow decreases[16] after smoking marijuana when compared to infrequent users. The frequent users demonstrated less impairment on psychomotor tasks in both studies. Studies comparing heart rate increases in naïve and experienced but less frequent cannabis smokers (smoking marijuana at least once a week) found both groups to show a similar change.[51,54] This suggests that daily use may be required to demonstrate measurable tolerance on this measure.

Recent animal experiments demonstrated marked tolerance to the behavioral effects of THC in the pigeon,[79,84] rat,[84] and dog.[80] The pigeons developed tolerance to increases of 100 times the dose of THC that initially depressed the pecking response in an operant task. Carlini found that rats develop tolerance to the inhibitory effects of cannabis extracts on rope climbing, bar pressing and isolation induced aggressiveness.[95] Tolerance to the hypothermic effects produced by THC in rats occurred after only 15 days of repeated doses.[78] Tolerance has not been observed in all chronic animal studies.[98] The reasons for this are not entirely clear.

The ideal way to investigate the development of tolerance and dependence in man is to administer high doses of the drug over a prolonged length of time under controlled conditions. Only one major experiment with cannabis approximated these conditions.[57] Williams and co-workers gave synhexyl (a synthetic marijuana analogue) for 26 days followed by marijuana cigarettes for 39 days to prisoners who had prior experience with marijuana. The daily dose was determined by the subjects. The average amount of synhexyl was increased from 200 mg the first day to 1600 mg daily with decreasing physiologic effects. Restlessness, insomnia, decreased appetite, and perspiration developed three days after the synhexyl administration stopped. One subject had a hypomanic reaction and a second suffered from disorientation and severe mood swings. The number of marijuana cigarettes consumed increased only slightly during the chronic marijuana administration. The range was 9 to 26 cigarettes with a mean of 17 daily. By three weeks, the elevated pulse rate returned to normal. After termination of the smoking portion of the experiment no withdrawal symptoms were noted other than subjective reports of feeling "jittery." Thus, although tolerance clearly developed to the synhexyl and marijuana, the evidence of physical dependence was equivocal for the synhexyl and lacking for marijuana.

Although the distinction between physical and psychological dependence implies a dichotomy between body and mind that is becoming increasingly untenable; it is traditional to consider the two types of dependence separately. There is clinical evidence for considerable difficulty in discontinuing regular use of high doses of cannabis without external restraint.[17,18] Studies from the U.S. considering the effects of lower doses used for shorter time periods concluded there was no evidence of marked psychological dependence.[134] In order to produce significant physical dependence to cannabis, it may be necessary to take enough to maintain a state of chronic intoxication during a major portion of each day. Such a sustained level of intoxication is necessary to demonstrate physical dependence to barbiturates.[99] A single large daily dose or even two or three doses daily will not usually result in an abstinence syndrome. It is rare for a cannabis user in the U.S. to maintain a chronic intoxicated state.

PHARMACOLOGIC CLASSIFICATION

Cannabis cannot be properly classified unless dose level is specified. It has some similarities to stimulant, sedative, analgesic, and psychotomimetic drugs.[84] In man, it produces a mild feeling of stimulation, followed by sedation; and in large doses, by psychotomimetic effects. Alcohol and cannabis have similar effects on mood and mental function under certain conditions.[20,43,67-69] There is suggestive evidence of cross tolerance between alcohol and cannabis.[20,100,101] However, the complete dose effect pattern of the two drugs is quite different. At high doses cannabis can produce marked distortion of auditory and visual perception, hallucinations, delusions with a relatively clear sensorium and depersonalization, synesthesia, and deeper awareness of meanings; phenomena rarely reported after alcohol.[33,102] However, in contrast to most psychotomimetics, cannabis produces a generally sedated rather than stimulated picture. Cannabis does not increase body temperature and blood pressure, lower knee jerk threshold, or dilate pupils.[33] Experienced users can easily distinguish the effects of the two drugs.[44] In man there is no cross tolerance between LSD and THC.[44]

When given to animals, cannabis drugs potentiate amphetamine excitement in mice,[86] but prolong barbiturate sleeping time[2,103] and exhibit anticonvulsant activity.[104] There is no cross tolerance between LSD and cannabis in rats.[105] Probably the only certain thing concerning classification is that cannabis is not a narcotic. At doses used by most people in this country, it has the characteristics of a sedative-hypnotic. However, those who prefer to put it in a class by itself[106] may ultimately be found to be correct.

MEDICAL USES

Cannabis was used medically for a long time, resulting in an extensive literature on its therapeutic applications. The indications for its use are described in a number of reviews.[4,6,17,85] It gradually disappeared because of difficulty in standardizing potency, great variability of individual responses to a given dose, and the introduction of synthetic drugs easier to administer. Sedative, antispasmodic, and analgesic properties accounted for much of its popularity. Trial as a diuretic[58] and anticonvulsant[107] has been suggested but not tested clinically to any great extent.

The availability of a semi-synthetic THC analog, synhexyl, led to a number of clinical studies. Synhexyl was initially reported to be an effective antidepressant[108] but subsequent studies failed to confirm this.[109,110] Synhexyl may help relieve alcohol and barbiturate abstinence symptoms[101] but is not effective in opiate withdrawal.[111] It was reported to be a substitute for alcohol in a single patient with alcohol dependence.[100] Recent controlled studies with synhexyl in normal human subjects have confirmed its cannabis-like activity.[34] The rapid progress in cannabinoid chemistry may result in some potentially useful derivatives. At this point, the natural material or THC appears to offer little advantage over currently used medications used as sedatives, analgesics, antidepressants and antihypertensive drugs.[1]

ADVERSE EFFECTS

In discussing the adverse effects of cannabis or for that matter any psychoactive drug, it is useful to distinguish somatic or "organ" toxicity and behavioral toxicity. In assessment of the consequences of cannabis dependence there has been too much attention paid to the former and too little consideration of behavioral toxicity.[16,112]

None of the reports concerning the presence of, or the absence of somatic effects resulting from cannabis use meet modern epidemiological research standards. Frequent use of smoked material may produce bronchitis[18] and sinusitis[29] and chronic conjunctival congestion.[17,58] The tendency of cannabis smokers to also use tobacco may contribute to such findings. Kew reported mild hepatic dysfunction in frequent cannabis smokers.[113] This was not confirmed in a group of U.S. Army hashish users.[29] The LaGuardia report and the Indian Hemp Drugs Commission concluded that moderate use of cannabis produced no mental or physical deterioration.[18,32] Of course, a similar statement could be made about alcohol, heroin, or barbiturates.

No adverse effects of cannabis on fetal mortality or fetal development have been observed in humans. After injecting large quantities of cannabis extracts preliminary studies found fetal abnormalities in rats, hamsters, and rabbits,[114-116] but other researchers administering pure THC have not been able to duplicate such findings in rats and hamsters.[117,118] THC does pass the placental barrier.[119] Thus far, no cannabis related chromosomal changes have been found.[120,121] Great species differences and the tendency of researchers to use unrealistic doses make it difficult to apply animal findings concerning teratogenesis to the human situation.

Careful, properly controlled, longitudinal studies of chronic cannabis users are indicated. Experience with attempts to clarify the significance of somatic changes in alcoholics or tobacco addicts suggests any definitive and generally acceptable findings may be a long way off.

The major adverse effect of cannabis may well be behavioral toxicity. Behavioral toxicity is a relatively new term referring to the adverse effects of drugs on behavior or psychological functioning. It has been defined as "the alterations in perceptual and cognitive functions, psycho-motor performance, motivation, mood, interpersonal relationships or intrapsychic processes of an individual to the degree that they limit the capacity of the individual to function within his setting or constitute a hazard to his physical well being."[122] It is a relative term and has to be considered in the context of the purposes for which the drug is taken and the desired effects. When applied to the effects of a self-selected and self-administered drug, behavioral toxicity, like beauty, often is chiefly in the eye of the observer. The purpose for which a drug is self-administered might be defined as a sought after and desirable consequence by the user, but termed behavioral toxicity by a physician or society.[122]

Many of the acute effects of cannabis are clearly associated with decrements in the ability to think and perform in a laboratory situation. There are unfortunately serious problems in generalizing from the psychopharmacology laboratory to the real world. Does impaired reaction time or impaired performance on a serial subtraction task have any implications concerning the use of cannabis while driving or studying? It probably does. Many of the regularly occurring acute behavioral effects of cannabis when sufficiently intense could be expected to impair driving skills, ability to study, and optimum performance in an interpersonal situation.

There is abundant evidence that cannabis can precipitate sudden psychotic or anxiety reactions. Nonpharmacological factors play an important role in the etiology of such reactions.[123,124] The complex interaction of specific drug effects with personality, mood and prior drug experience of the recipient and the setting in which the drug is ingested makes precise analysis of published reports difficult.

Brief psychotic or psychotic-like episodes have occurred during a number of experimental trials of cannabis or THC.[32,33,45,57,58] In the mildest form, the reactions appear to be an acute brain syndrome with excitement, restless delirium, and anxiety. In more extreme cases, the symptoms progress to thought disorganization, paranoid delusions, depersonalization, and hallucinations. The time course is variable; ranging from only a few hours with smoked material or low oral doses, to days, weeks, or months. The longer-lasting psychoses (longer than 24 to 72 hours) resulting from a single dose of cannabis are poorly understood. Their clinical courses are similar to those of spontaneously occurring schizophrenia. Experimental[31,125] and clinical evidence[24] suggests that schizophrenics may be unusually sensitive to the disrupting effects of cannabis. Perhaps an individual with the genotype for schizophrenia is more likely to develop a long-lasting psychotic episode to a given dose of cannabis. The preliminary evidence for slow excretion of THC from the body suggests these longer-lasting episodes may be true toxic psychoses.[73]

Talbott and Teague described 12 cases of cannabis-related psychosis in U.S. soldiers serving in Vietnam.[102] All occurred during the first admitted exposure to cannabis. A majority recovered within three days. A number of similar cases have been reported in both inexperienced and experienced users.[24,123,126,127] Experiences in our laboratory suggest high doses and environmental stress may be important factors, and capable of contributing to an acute, three to six hours long "cannabis psychosis" even in well-integrated, stable individuals.

The incidence of adverse reactions to cannabis is difficult to estimate. On one hand, Smith in San Francisco reports he has never observed "cannabis psychosis" in over 35,000 marijuana users seen in the Haight-Ashbury Clinic.[124] Pillard estimates "5 to 7 marijuana associated anxiety reactions" are seen yearly in a college student health service caring for a student population of 20,000.[106] In contrast, "freaking out" one or more times was reported by 21% of the experienced users responding to Tart's survey of common marijuana experiences.[52] "Freaking out" was defined as an intense, transient emotional upset. Twenty percent of his respondents report that on at least one occasion after using cannabis, they lost control and were "taken over" by an outside "force or will" which was hostile or evil in intent. Tart believes this population of cannabis enthusiasts probably under reported such negative effects. Apparently many adverse reactions are not reported to physicians.

Mental deterioration resulting from chronic heavy use of cannabis has been reported by a number of Far and Middle Eastern clinicians.[17,18,96,128,129] A majority of the cases are acute psychoses probably from toxic overdoses and clear much more rapidly than is usual in acute schizophrenia. The existence of a characteristic mental deterioration in cannabis habitues after many years' use is reported.[18,64] The etiologic role of cannabis in these cases is not established.

Of more current concern in this country are questions of subtle personality and behavior changes resulting from frequent use of cannabis. The "amotivational syndrome" referring to loss of interest in school, work, achievement, and other traditional long-term goals has been described in cannabis users.[124] The question of whether there exists a causal relationship between cannabis use and this syndrome or simply a correlation between these traits and cannabis use is yet to be answered. Recent reports suggest that many regular but infrequent cannabis users in this country do not demonstrate these traits, but that frequent (once daily or more) users do.[130,131] Consideration of differences in pattern of use and age of the user is essential in any attempt to answer such questions. Many of the issues concerning the behavioral toxicity of cannabis are precisely those that have not been adequately answered with respect to LSD or alcohol; thus progress may be slow.

Despite much speculation and claims to the contrary most research data indicate cannabis use does not lead directly to the use of heroin or other drugs.[17,18,132] It is true that a majority of heroin users in this country used cannabis before heroin. However, it appears most cannabis users do not go on to use heroin. The more frequently a person uses cannabis, the more likely other drugs will be used. This is likely a result of a disposition toward psychoactive drug use in general.[5,52] Knowing a person uses cannabis is not as good a predictor of other drug use as knowing he uses a great deal of cannabis. A related belief is that cannabis may substitute for alcohol as a social intoxicant. Recent surveys do not always show this to be true.[132,133] Cannabis users use alcohol roughly in proportion to the degree that they use cannabis. The more often they use cannabis, the more alcohol they drink. Longitudinal prospective studies of patterns of drug use should clarify this issue.

The interest in the relationship between cannabis use, crime, and violence goes back many years. It was one of the issues considered by the Indian Hemp Commission.[18] That group concluded that taking cannabis is not a direct cause of serious crime or violence. Every major review group since has made a similar decision.[32] A recent review of the interaction between drugs and violence arrived at a similar conclusion.[134]

It is impressive how many of the popular beliefs about cannabis and its effects are based on spurious correlations between traits and behaviors and drug use, intermixed with much anecdotal evidence.

REFERENCES

1. Hollister, L. E., Marihuana in man: three years later, *Science*, 172, 21, 1971.

2. Gershon, S., On the pharmacology of marijuana, *Behav. Neuropsychiat.*, 1, 9, 1970.

3. Neumeyer, J. L. and Shagoury, R. A., Chemistry and pharmacology of marijuana, *J. Pharm. Sci.*, 60, 1433, 1971.

4. Snyder, S., *Uses of Marijuana*, Oxford University Press, New York, 1971.

5. Goode, E., *The Marijuana Smokers*, Basic Books, New York, 1970.

6. Grinspoon, L., *Marihuana Reconsidered*, Harvard University Press, Cambridge, 1971.

7. Schultes, R. E., Random thoughts and queries on the botany of cannabis, in *The Botany and Chemistry of Cannabis*, Joyce, C. R. B. and Curry, S. H., J. and A. Churchill, London, 1970, 11.

8. Lerner, P., The precise determination of tetrahydrocannabinol in marihuana and hashish, *U.N. Bull. Narc.*, 21, 39, 1969.

9. Phillips, R., Turk, R., Manno, J., Jain, N., and Forney, R. B., Seasonal variation in cannabinolic content of Indiana marihuana, *J. Forensic Sci.*, 15, 191, 1970.

10. Mechoulam, R., Marihuana chemistry, *Science*, 168, 1159, 1970.

11. Loewe, S., Studies of the pharmacology and acute toxicity of compounds with marihuana activity, *J. Pharmacol. Exp. Ther.*, 88, 154, 1946.

12. Lerner, M. and Zeffert, J. T., Determination of tetrahydrocannabinol isomers in marijuana and hashish, *U.N. Bull. Narc.*, 20, 53, 1968.

13. Marshman, J. A. and Gibbins, R. J., A note on the composition of illicit drugs, *Ontario Med. Rev.*, 1, 3, 1970.

14. Fetterman, P. S., Keith, E. S., Waller, C. W., Guerrero, O., Doorenbos, N. J., and Quimby, M. W., Mississippi grown Cannabis sativa L. A preliminary observation on the chemical definition of genotype and variations in THC content versus age, sex, and plant part, *J. Pharm. Sci.*, in press.

15. Weil, A. T., Zinberg, N. E., and Nelsen, J. M., Clinical and psychological effects of marihuana in man, *Science*, 162, 1234, 1968.

16. Jones, R. T., Tetrahydrocannabinol and the marijuana induced social "high" or the effects of the mind on marijuana, *Ann. N.Y. Acad. Sci.*, in press.

17. Chopra, I. C. and Chopra, R. N., The use of the cannabis drugs in India, *U.N. Bull. Narc.*, 9, 4, 1957.

18. *Indian Hemp Drugs Commission Report, 1893-1894, Marijuana*, Introduction by Kaplan, J., Thomas Jefferson Publishing Co., Silver Spring, Md., 1969.

19. Haines, L. and Green, W., Marijuana use patterns, *Brit. J. Addict.*, 65, 347, 1970.

20. Jones, R. T. and Stone, G. C., Psychological studies of marijuana and alcohol in man, *Psychopharmacologia*, 18, 108, 1970.

21. Hilding, A. C., On cigarette smoking, bronchial carcinoma and ciliary action. I. Smoking habits and measurement of smoke intake, *New Eng. J. Med.*, 254, 775, 1956.

22. Shean, G. D. and Fechtmann, F., Purpose in life scores of student marijuana users, *J. Clin. Psychol.*, 27, 112, 1971.

23. Meyer, R. E., Pillard, R. C., Shapiro, L. M., and Mirin, S. M., Administration of marijuana to heavy and casual marijuana users, *Amer. J. Psychiat.*, 128, 198, 1971.

24. Kolansky, H. and Moore, W. T., Effects of marihuana on adolescents and young adults, *J.A.M.A.*, 216, 486, 1971.

25. Berg, D. F., The non-medical use of dangerous drugs in the United States: A comprehensive view, *Int. J. Addict.*, 5, 777, 1970.

26. San Mateo, California Dept. of Public Health and Welfare, Research and Statistics Section. The use of alcoholic beverages, amphetamines, LSD, marijuana, and tobacco reported by high school and junior high school students. San Mateo, Cal. 94403, 1968-1969; and preliminary release of 1970.

27. McGlothlin, W. H., The use and effects of cannabis. Report prepared for the National Commission on Marihuana and Dangerous Drugs, Washington, D.C., 1971.

28. Mirin, S. M., Shapiro, L. M., Meyer, R. E., Pillard, R. C., and Fisher, S., Casual versus heavy use of marijuana: A redefinition of the marijuana problem, *Amer. J. Psychiat.*, 127, 1134, 1971.

29. Tennant, F. S., Preble, M., Pendergast, T. J., and Ventry, P., Medical manifestations associated with hashish, *J.A.M.A.*, 216, 1965, 1971.

30. Ebin, D., *The Drug Experience. First Person Accounts of Addicts, Writers, Scientists, and Others*, Orion, New York, 1961.

31. Moreau de Tours, J., *Du Hachich et de l'Alienation Mentale - Etudes Psychologiques*, Paris, Masson, 1845. Translation, *Hashish and Mental Illness*, translated by Barnett, G. J., Raven Press, New York, 1971.

32. Mayor's Committee on Marihuana Report, *The Marihuana Problem in the City of New York*, Cattell Press, Lancaster, 1944.

33. Isbell, H., Gorodetzsky, C. W., Jasinki, D. R., Claussen, U., Von Spulek, F., and Korte, F., Effects of (-)-delta-9-trans-tetrahydrocannabinol in man, *Psychopharmacologia,* 11, 184, 1967.

34. Hollister, L. E., Richards, R. K., and Gillespie, H. K., Comparison of tetrahydrocannabinol and synhexyl in man, *Clin. Pharmacol. Ther.*, 9, 783, 1968.

35. Waskow, I. E., Olsson, J. E., Salzman, C., and Katz, M. M., Psychological effects of tetrahydrocannabinol, *Arch. Gen. Psychiat.*, 22, 97, 1970.

36. Clark, L. D. and Nakashima, E. N., Experimental studies of marihuana, *Amer. J. Psychiat.*, 125, 379, 1968.

37. Clark, L. D., Hughes, R., and Nakashima, E. N., Behavioral effects of marihuana; experimental studies, *Arch. Gen. Psychiat.*, 23, 193, 1970.

38. Caldwell, D. F., Myers, S. A., Domino, E. F., and Merriam, P. E., Auditory and visual threshold effects of marihuana in man, *Percept. Mot. Skills*, 29, 755, 1969.

39. Caldwell, D. F., Myers, S. A., Domino, E. F., and Merriam, P. E., Auditory and visual threshold effects of marihuana in man: Addendum, *Percept. Mot. Skills*, 29, 922, 1969.

40. Crancer, A., Dille, J. M., Delay, J. C., Wallace, J. E., and Haykin, M. D., Comparison of the effects of marihuana and alcohol on simulated driving performance, *Science*, 164, 851, 1969.

41. Dornbush, R. L., Fink, M., and Freedman, A. M., Marijuana, memory, and perception, *Amer. J. Psychiat.*, 128, 194, 1971.

42. Hollister, L. E., Hunger and appetite after single doses of marihuana, ethanol and dextroamphetamine, *Clin. Pharmacol. Ther.*, 12, 44, 1971.

43. Hollister, L. E. and Gillespie, H. K., Marihuana, ethanol, and dextroamphetamine: Mood and mental function alterations, *Arch. Gen. Psychiat.*, 23, 199, 1970.

44. Isbell, H. and Jankinski, D. R., A comparison of LSD-25 with (–)-delta- 9-trans-tetrahydrocannabinol (THC) and attempted cross tolerance between LSD and THC, *Psychopharmacologia*, 14, 115, 1969.

45. Manno, J., Kiplinger, G. R., Bennett, I. F., Hayne, S., and Forney, R. B., Comparative effects of smoking marihuana on motor and mental performance in humans, *Clin. Pharmacol. Ther.*, 11, 808, 1970.

46. Melges, F. T., Tinklenberg, J. R., Hollister, L. E., and Gillespie, H. K., Marihuana and temporal disintegration, *Science*, 168, 1118, 1970.

47. Melges, F. T., Tinklenberg, J. R., Hollister, L. E., and Gillespie, H. K., Temporal disintegration and depersonalization during marijuana intoxication, *Arch. Gen. Psychiat.*, 23, 204, 1970.

48. Rodin, E., Domino, E. F., and Porzak, J. P., The marijuana-induced "social high" – Neurological and electroencephalographic concomitants, *J.A.M.A.*, 213, 1300, 1970.

49. Tinklenberg, J. R., Melges, F. T., Hollister, L. E., and Gillespie, H. K., Marihuana and immediate memory, *Nature*, 226, 1171, 1970.

50. Weil, A. T. and Zinberg, N. E., Acute effects of marihuana on speech, *Nature*, 222, 434, 1969.

51. Renault, P. F., Schuster, C. R., Heinrich, R., and Freedman, D. X., Marihuana: standardized smoke administration and dose effect curves on heart rate in humans, *Science*, 174, 589, 1971.

52. Tart, C. T., Marihuana intoxication: common experiences, *Nature*, 226, 701, 1970.

53. Halikas, J. A., Goodwin, D. W., Guze, S. B., Marijuana effects, *J.A.M.A.*, 217, 692, 1971.

54. Johnson, S. and Domino, E. F., Some cardiovascular effects of marihuana smoking in normal volunteers, *Clin. Pharmacol. Ther.*, 12, 762, 1971.

55. Kiplinger, G. F., Human motor and mental performance as influenced by cannabis, *Psychopharmacol. Bull.*, 8, 16, 1971.

56. Kiplinger, G. F., Manno, J. E., Rodda, B. E., and Forney, R. B., Dose-response analysis of the effects of tetrahydrocannabinol in man, *Clin. Pharmacol. Ther.*, 12, 650, 1971.

57. Williams, E. G., Himmelsbach, C. K., Wikler, A., Ruble, D. C., and Lloyd, B. N., Studies on marihuana and pyrahexl compound, *Public Health Rep.*, 61, 1059, 1946.

58. Ames, F., A clinical and metabolic study of acute intoxication with *Cannabis sativa* and its role in the model psychoses, *J. Mental Sci.*, 104, 972, 1958.

59. Allentuck, S. and Bowman, K. M., The psychiatric aspects of marihuana intoxication, *Amer. J. Psychiat.*, 99, 248, 1942.

60. Aldrich, C. K., The effect of a synthetic marihuana-like compound on musical talent as measured by the Seashore test, *Public Health Rep.*, 59, 431, 1944.

61. Abel, E. L., Effects of marihuana on the solution of anagrams, memory and appetite, *Nature*, 231, 260, 1971.

62. Hollister, L. E., Steroids and moods: Correlations in schizophrenics and subjects treated with lysergic acid diethylamide (LSD), mescaline, tetrahydrocannabinol, and synhexyl, *J. Clin. Pharmacol.*, 9, 24, 1969.

63. Hollister, L. E., Moore, F., Kanter, S., and Noble, E., Delta-1-tetrahydrocannabinol, synhexyl and marijuana extract administered orally in man: catecholamine excretion, plasma cortisol levels and platelet serotonin content, *Psychopharmacologia*, 17, 354, 1970.

64. Wikler, A. and Lloyd, B. J., Effect of smoking marihuana cigarettes on cortical electrical activity, *Fed. Proc.*, 4, 141, 1945.

65. Hollister, L. E., Sherwood, S. L., and Cavasino, A., Marihuana and the human electroencephalogram, *Pharmacol. Res. Commun.*, in press.

66. Volavka, J., Dornbush, R., Feldstein, S., Clare, G., Zaks, A., Fink, M., and Freedman, A. M., Marijuana, EEG and behavior, *Ann. N.Y. Acad. Sci.*, in press.

67. Tinklenberg, J. R., Marihuana and alcohol, *Psychopharmacol. Bull.*, 8, 9, 1971.

68. Jones, R., The marijuana induced "social high" – a note of caution regarding specificity, *Psychopharmacol. Bull.*, 8, 13, 1971.

69. Manno, J. E., Kiplinger, G. F., Scholz, N., and Forney, R. B., The influence of alcohol and marihuana on motor and mental performance, *Clin. Pharmacol. Ther.*, 12, 202, 1971.

70. Kalant, H., Marihuana and simulated driving, *Science*, 166, 640, 1969.

71. Foltz, R. L., Kinzer, G. W., Mitchell, R. I., and Truitt, E. B., Jr., The fate of cannabinoid components of marijuana during smoking, *J. Anal. Chem.*, in press.

72. Miras, C., Simon, S., and Kiburis, J., Comparative assay of the constituents from the sublimate of smoked cannabis with that from ordinary cannabis, *U.N. Bull. Narc.*, 16, 13, 1964.

73. Lemberger, L., Delta-9-tetrahydrocannabinol; metabolism and disposition in long-term marihuana smoking, *Science*, 173, 72, 1971.

74. Lemberger, L., Silberstein, S. D., Axelrod, J., and Kopin, I. J., Marihuana: studies on the disposition and metabolism of delta-9-tetrahydrocannabinol in man, *Science*, 170, 1320, 1970.

75. Agurell, S., Nilsson, I. M., Ohlsson, A., and Sandberg, F., On the metabolism of tritium-labelled delta-1-tetrahydrocannabinol in the rabbit, *Biochem. Pharmacol.*, 19, 1333, 1970.

76. Christensen, H. D., Freudenthal, R. I., Boegli, G., Testing, L., Brine, D. R., Pitt, C. G., and Wall, M. E., Activity of delta-8 and delta-9-tetrahydrocannabinol and related compounds in the mouse, *Science*, 172, 165, 1971.

77. Becker, H. S., History, culture and subjective experience: an exploration of the social bases of drug-induced experiences, *J. Health Soc. Behav.*, 8, 163, 1967.

78. Lomax, P., Animal pharmacology of marihuana, *Proc. West. Pharmacol. Soc.*, 14, 10, 1971.

79. McMillan, D. E., Harris, L. S., Frankenheim, J. M., and Kennedy, J. S., 1-delta-9-trans-tetrahydrocannabinol in pigeons, tolerance to the behavioral effects, *Science*, 169, 501, 1970.

80. McMillan, D. E., Dewey, W. L., and Harris, L. S., Pharmacological and behavioral effects of delta-8 and delta-9-tetrahydrocannabinols, Paper presented at New York Academy of Sciences Conference on Marijuana; Chemistry, Pharmacology and Patterns of Social Usage, May 21, 1971, New York, New York.

81. Gaoni, Y. and Mechoulam, R., Cannabichromene, a new active principle in hashish, *Chem. Comm.*, 1, 20, 1966.

82. Grunfeld, Y. and Edery, H., Psychopharmacological activity of the active constituents of hashish and some related cannabinoids, *Psychopharmacologia*, 14, 200, 1969.

83. Lipparini, F., DeCarolis, A., and Longo, V. A., Neuropharmacological investigation of some trans-tetrahydrocannabinol derivatives, *Physiol. Behav.*, 4, 527, 1969.

84. Harris, L. S., Pharmacology of marihuana and constituents, *Psychopharmacol. Bull.*, 8, 10, 1971.

85. Kabelik, J., Krejci, Z., and Santavy, F., Cannabis as a medicament, *U.N. Bull. Narc.*, 12, 5, 1960.

86. Garriott, J. C., King, L. J., Forney, R. B., and Hughes, F. W., Effects of some tetrahydrocannabinols on hexobarbital sleeping time and amphetamine induced hyperactivity in mice, *Life Sci.*, 6, 2119, 1967.

87. Kubena, R. K. and Barry, H., Interactions of delta-1-tetrahydrocannabinol with barbiturates and methamphetamine, *J. Pharmacol. Exp. Ther.*, in press.

88. Bose, B. C., Saifi, A. Q., and Bhagwat, A. W., Observations on the pharmacological actions of Cannabis indica. Part II, *Arch. Int. Pharmacodyn. Ther.*, 147, 285, 1964.

89. Boyd, E. S. and Meritt, D. A., Effects of thiopental and a tetrahydrocannabinol derivative on arousal and recruiting in the cat, *J. Pharmacol. Exp. Ther.*, 149, 138, 1965.

90. Bicher, H. I. and Mechoulam, R., Pharmacological effects of two active constituents of marihuana, *Arch. Int. Pharmacodyn. Ther.*, 172, 24, 1968.

91. Santos, M., Sampaio, M. R., Fernandes, N. S., and Carlini, E. A., Effects of cannabis sativa on fighting behavior of mice, *Psychopharmacologia*, 8, 437, 1966.

92. Carlini, E. A. and Masur, J., Development of aggressive behavior in rats by chronic administration of cannabis sativa (marihuana), *Life Sci.*, 8, 607, 1969.

93. Boyd, E. S., Hutchinson, E. D., Gardner, L. C., and Merritt, D., Effects of tetra-hydrocannabinols and other drugs on operant behavior in rats, *Arch. Int. Pharmacodyn. Ther.*, 144, 533, 1963.

94. Scheckel, C. L., Boff, E., Dahlen, P., and Smart, T., Behavioral effects in monkeys of racemates of two biologically active marihuana constituents, *Science*, 160, 1467, 1968.

95. Carlini, E. A., Tolerance to chronic administration of Cannabis sativa (marihuana) in rats, *Pharmacology*, 1, 135, 1968.

96. Bouquet, J., Cannabis, *U.N. Bull. Narc.*, 3, 22, 1951.

97. Benabud, A., Psycho-pathological aspects of the cannabis situation in Morocco: statistical data for 1956, *U.N. Bull. Narc.*, 9, 1, 1957.

98. Forney, R. B., Toxicology and pharmacology of marijuana, *Ann. N.Y. Acad. Sci.*, in press.

99. Fraser, H. F., Wikler, A., Essig, C. F., and Isbell, H., Degree of physical dependence induced by secobarbital or pentobarbital, *J.A.M.A.*, 166, 126, 1953.

100. Mikuriya, T. H., Cannabis substitution, an adjunctive therapeutic tool in the treatment of alcoholism, *Med. Times*, 98, 187, 1970.

101. Thompson, L. J. and Proctor, R. C., The use of pyrahexyl in the treatment of alcoholic and drug withdrawal conditions, *N.C. Med. J.*, 14, 520, 1953.

102. Talbott, J. A. and Teague, J. W., Marihuana psychosis, acute toxic psychosis associated with the *Cannabis* derivatives, *J.A.M.A.*, 210, 299, 1969.

103. Bose, B. C., Saifi, A. Q., and Bhagwat, A. W., Effect of Cannabis indica on hexobarbital sleeping time and tissue respiration of rat brain, *Arch. Int. Pharmacodyn. Ther.*, 141, 520, 1963.

104. Garriott, J. C., Forney, R. B., Hughes, F. W., and Richards, A. B., Pharmacologic properties of some cannabis related compounds, *Arch. Int. Pharmacodyn. Ther.*, 171, 425, 1968.

105. Silva, M. T. A. and Carlini, E. A., Lack of cross-tolerance in rats among (-)-delta-9-trans-tetrahydrocannabinol (delta-9-THC), cannabis extract, mescaline and lysergic acid diethylamide (LSD-25), *Psychopharmacologia*, 13, 332, 1968.

106. Pillard, R. C., Marihuana, *New Eng. J. Med.*, 283, 294, 1970.

107. Davis, J. P. and Ramsey, H. H., Antiepileptic action of marihuana-active substances, *Fed. Proc.*, 8, 284, 1949

108. Stockings, G. T., A new euphoriant for depressive mental states, *Brit. Med. J.*, 918, 1947.

109. Parker, C. S. and Wrigley, F., Synthetic cannabis preparations in psychiatry: (1) synhexyl, *J. Mental Sci.*, 96, 276, 1950.

110. Pond, D. A., Psychological effects in depressive patients of the marihuana homologue synhexyl, *J. Neurol. Neurosurg. Psychiat.*, 11, 271, 1948.

111. Himmelsbach, C. K., Treatment of the morphine abstinence syndrome with a synthetic cannabis-like compound, *South. Med. J.*, 37, 26, 1944.

112. Seevers, M. H., Drug dependence and drug abuse, a world problem, *Pharmacologist*, 12, 172, 1970.

113. Kew, M. C., Bersohn, L., and Siew, S., Possible hepatotoxicity of cannabis, *Lancet*, 1, 578, 1969.

114. Geber, W. F. and Schramm, L. C., Effect of marihuana extract on fetal hamsters and rabbits, *Toxicol. Appl. Pharmacol.*, 14, 276, 1969.

115. Geber, W. F. and Schramm, L. C., Teratogenicity of marihuana extract as influenced by plant origin and seasonal variation, *Arch. Int. Pharmacodyn. Ther.*, 177, 224, 1969.

116. Persaud, T. V. N. and Ellington, A. C., The effects of Cannabis sativa L. (ganja) on developing rat embryos – preliminary observations, *West Indian Med. J.*, 17, 232, 1968.

117. Pace, H. B., Davis, W. M., and Borgen, L. A., Teratogenesis and marijuana, *Ann. N.Y. Acad. Sci.*, in press.

118. Borgen, L. A. and Davis, W. M., Effects of synthetic delta-9-tetrahydrocannabinol on pregnancy and offspring in the rat, *Toxicol. Appl. Pharmacol.*, in press.

119. Idanpaan-Heikkila, J., Fritchie, G. E., Englert, L. F., Ho, B. T., and McIsaac, W. M., Placental transfer of tritiated-1-delta-9-tetrahydrocannabinol, *New Eng. J. Med.*, 281, 330, 1969.

120. Martin, P. A., Cannabis and chromosomes, *Lancet*, 1, 370, 1969.

121. Neu, R. L., Powers, H., King, S., and Gardner, L. I., Cannabis and chromosomes, *Lancet*, 1, 675, 1969.

122. Shader, R. I. and DiMascio, A., *Psychotropic Drug Side Effects, Clinical and Theoretical Perspectives*, Williams and Wilkins, Baltimore, 1970, 127.

123. Weil, A. T., Adverse reactions to marijuana, *New Eng. J. Med.*, 282, 997, 1970.

124. Smith, D. E., Acute and chronic toxicity of marijuana, *J. Psyched. Drugs*, 2, 37, 1968.

125. Lindemann, E. and Malamud, W., Experimental analysis of the psychopathological effects of intoxicating drugs, *Amer. J. Psychiat.*, 90, 853, 1934.

126. Baker, A. A. and Lucas, E. G., Some hospital admissions associated with cannabis, *Lancet*, 1, 148, 1969.

127. Grossman, W., Adverse reactions associated with cannabis products in India, *Ann. Intern. Med.*, 70, 529, 1969.

128. Asuni, T., Socio-psychiatric problems of cannabis in Nigeria, *U.N. Bull. Narc.*, 16, 17, 1964.

129. Watt, J. M., Dagga in South Africa, *U.N. Bull. Narc.*, 13, 9, 1961.

130. Goode, E., Drug use and grades in college, *Nature*, 234, 225, 1971.

131. Beill, N. Q., Crumptom, E., and Grayson, H. M., Personality factors in marihuana use, *Arch. Gen Psychiat.*, 24, 163, 1971.

132. Robins, L. N. and Murphy, G. E., Drug use in a normal population of young Negro men, *Amer. J. Public Health*, 57, 1580, 1967.

133. Blum, R. H. and associates, *Drugs II, Students and Drugs*, Jossey-Bass, San Francisco, 1969.

134. Tinklenberg, J. R. and Stillman, R. S., Drug use and violence, in *Violence and Man's Struggle for Existence*, Daniels, D. N., Gilula, M. F., and Ochberg, F. M., Eds., Little, Brown and Co., Boston, 1970, 327.

CRITERIA FOR EVALUATING DRUG DEPENDENCE

CRITERIA FOR EVALUATING PHYSICAL AND PSYCHIC DEPENDENCE AND OVERALL ABUSE POTENTIAL OF DRUGS IN MAN

H. F. Fraser

TABLE OF CONTENTS

DEFINITION OF DEPENDENCE AND ABUSE AND SCOPE OF THIS REVIEW

In 1964, the World Health Organization (WHO) Expert Committee on Addiction-Producing Drugs recommended substitution of the term "drug dependence" for the terms "drug addiction" and "drug habituation." The WHO Scientific Group (1964) endorsed this recommendation.

Drug dependence is defined as a state arising from the repeated administration of a drug on a periodic or continuous basis. It includes the attributes "physical" and/or "psychic" dependence. Although the characteristics of dependence vary with the agent involved, it carries no connotation in regard to degree of risk to the public or need for a particular type of control.

Drug abuse takes into account not only the concept of dependence, but also the degree of risk to the public. It is defined as follows: abuse of a drug exists if its use so harmfully affects the individual and/or society as to require its control.[1] Risks to the public are often reflected in the type and extent of controls promulgated. To a considerable extent, however, the degree of control of a drug or substance depends upon whether the "addiction" is socially accepted. In the case of alcohol and tobacco, for example, the controls are quite lenient, since these are socially accepted forms of addiction. Heroin abuse, on the other hand, is not socially accepted, and controls are strict.

It would be preferable to have screening procedures and tests in animals and man which would predict not only "drug dependence" but also, if possible, the extent to which drugs might be abused by society. This review will point out that, in the case of narcotic drugs (both agonistic and antagonistic), considerable sophistication has been attained in developing a multiplicity of tests in man that are satisfactorily predictive of abuse liability.

The classes of drugs covered in this review include narcotics and narcotic antagonists, central nervous system depressants of the barbiturate and alcohol types, major and minor tranquilizers, amphetamines, and hallucinogens.

EVALUATION OF NARCOTICS

The methods described below for evaluating abuse liability of narcotic-like drugs are those employed at the Addiction Research Center in Lexington, Kentucky. The subjects are male prisoner volunteers in good physical condition with a long history of asocial behavior, including abuse of opiate-like drugs, and with a poor prognosis for recovery.

Tests for Physical Dependence of Morphine-like Drugs

Substitution of Test Drug for Morphine in Subjects Physically Dependent on Daily High Doses of Morphine[2,3]

This test, utilizing the principle developed by Himmelsbach,[3] is conducted as follows: a group of 5 to 12 nontolerant opiate addicts is given morphine sulfate subcutaneously four times daily; the dose is rapidly increased as tolerance and safety permit until each patient is receiving 240 mg of morphine daily. Morphine is discontinued, and coded substances are then substituted for the morphine for 24 hours. Fourteen hours after the last regular dose of morphine, observations for intensity of abstinence (withdrawal) are made for 10 hours. The substitution procedure is repeated at weekly intervals until each subject has received, in random double-blind order, the experimental drug, injections of saline (placebo), the regular stabilization dose of morphine, and, usually, one or more other agents. Substitution of test drugs may also be made for 14 days; then the substituted drug is abruptly withdrawn and observations for intensity of abstinence are made for 10 days.

If the drug substituted for morphine completely suppresses signs of abstinence (withdrawal illness), it will induce physical dependence when given chronically to nonaddicted persons.

Scores for accurately measurable signs of abstinence include:

- Fever: one point for each 0.1° C (rectal) rise.
- Hyperpnea: one point for each respiration/minute increase.
- Systolic blood pressure: one point for each 2 mm Hg rise (up to 30 mm).
- Weight: one point for each pound loss.

Scores for signs of abstinence not accurately measurable include:

Yawning Lacrimation Rhinorrhea Perspiration	one point only for any of these signs observed on any one day
Anorexia Goose flesh Dilated pupils Tremor	three points only for any of these signs observed on any one day
Restlessness	five points only in one day
Emesis	five points for each emesis observed

The score for any 24-hour day is the sum of these points.

Direct Addiction Test[2-4]

With this technique, the experimenter attempts to duplicate the abuse pattern which an addict might employ if he had free access to an addictive agent. In the comparison of a drug with morphine for its relative abuse liability by the direct addiction technique, administration of the test drug is started in the therapeutic dosage range and rapidly increased, as safety and tolerance permit, for 18 days or more. The drug is then abruptly withdrawn and the subject observed for the intensity of abstinence. In addition, the patient is challenged with 3 or 5 mg of nalorphine during maintained addiction to the new drug to ascertain whether an abstinence syndome can be precipitated by nalorphine.

Throughout the period of chronic intoxication, rectal temperature, pulse and respiratory rates, and systolic and diastolic blood pressures are noted three times daily. Body weight and caloric intake are recorded daily, and urine and blood tests are made at intervals of one or two weeks to detect any abnormalities. By means of questionnaires completed daily by the patient and independently by the observer, an attempt is made to analyze the patient's attitude concerning the drug.

Drugs are withdrawn abruptly after 10, 20, 30, or 60 days. The intensity of the abstinence syndrome is then observed over a period of 10 days and is compared with that for standard and unknown drugs. The general plan is to match the unknown with a standard of corresponding dependence characteristics. For example, the currently used standards include morphine, codeine, and propoxyphene.

Tests for Psychic Dependence of Morphine-like Drugs

Until about 15 years ago, the emphasis at the Addiction Research Center in evaluating the abuse liability of opiate-like drugs had been on the physical dependence aspects. This approach was satisfactory as long as the compounds presented for evaluation possessed typical morphine-like patterns; however, many compounds with atypical morphine-like patterns have been discovered; these might even antagonize the effects of morphine (for example, a morphine antagonist), and yet they possess valuable analgesic characteristics. In addition, these antagonists induce tolerance and a moderate degree of physical dependence, as indicated by definite abstinence syndromes when the drugs are withdrawn, although after withdrawal the subjects exhibit no drug-seeking behavior.

These observations, as well as others, have necessitated a broader evaluation of compounds with atypical morphine-like patterns. The new approach has been to carry out not only the physical-dependence type of experiment, but also a systematic evaluation of the addict's attitude toward the new drug. One useful procedure for evaluating psychic (as distinguished from physical) dependence on morphine-like drugs involves the use of tests with a questionnaire that provides for subjective ratings by the patient and parallel ratings on the part of the observer, the latter being based on the behavior of the subject.

The single-dose questionnaire for rating the effects of a drug includes the following questions:

1. Do you feel the medicine?
2. This drug is most like what drug listed below (check one); a blank, dope (opiates), cocaine, marihuana, goof balls (barbiturates), benzedrine ("Benny"), other.
3. Check each sensation which you feel: Normal, "turning of stomach," skin itchy, relaxed, "coasting," "soap-box," pleasant "sick," "drive," sleepy, drunken, nervous, other.
4. My liking for this drug is most nearly described by which of the following: not at all, slight, moderate, a lot, an awful lot, other.
5. Comments.

For typical morphine-like drugs for many of these parameters, such as "turning of the stomach, skin itchy, relaxed, coasting, soap-box, pleasant sick, and drive," very satisfactory dose-response curves can be obtained. Using as few as 8 to 12 subjects, the single dose questionnaire is generally administered at weekly intervals on a double-blind basis with a base line observation prior to drug and then at hourly intervals for 7 observations post-drug. The results are compared with an observation prior to administration of the drug and with observations subsequent to drug administration. The studies are conducted with a positive control, such as codeine, morphine, or propoxyphene, depending upon the characteristics of the unknown. A placebo is also used in these double-blind set-ups.

The subjective ratings reported by the patient are compared with objective findings, such as photographs of the pupils made at parallel time intervals and with another questionnaire completed by the observer (aide). With the single dose questionnaire, it has been possible to identify the type of drug being administered, its potency, and its abuse potential as related to the standard drug.

In recent years, the Addiction Research Center has employed three additional subjective ratings that have proved valuable.[5] These include 40 items from the morphine-benzedrine group scale (MBG) which measures euphoria, the LSD-specific scale

(LSD) which measures psychotomimetic effects, and the pentobarbital-chlorpromazine-alcohol group scale (PCAG) which measures sedation, lethargy, etc. These scales are not specific except in the case of the LSD scale; nevertheless, very satisfactory dose-response curves can be obtained for drugs in any of the categories above mentioned.

In the case of the potent morphine-like drugs, a subjective report of former addicts and interpretation of their behavior by observers are in good agreement; however, in the case of drugs with weak or atypical morphine-like characteristics, particularly those administered orally, a discrepancy frequently develops between the subjective report of the former addict and the objective interpretation. In such instances, it is nearly always necessary to use direct addiction tests. These chronic studies accentuate the difference between the subjective interpretations of the former addicts and the behavioral interpretations of the observers with respect to the abuse potential of drugs.

These points are illustrated by studies of Fraser[6] on the addictiveness of 1,2-dimethyl-3-phenyl-3-propionoxy pyrrolidine hydrochloride (The Addiction Research Center code is I-O-1). This agent was administered in progressively increasing doses as tolerated by 5 subjects with the following overall results. Three subjects elected to discontinue the test after 17 days, and 2 subjects after 39 days. During the test the specific effects reported and observed included nausea (which in some patients is continuous), constipation, a moderate degree of respiratory depression, miosis, difficult micturition, a "sleepy and/or dull-headed" feeling, and a gradual progressive loss of weight in 4 of the 5 subjects. The incidence of vomiting was outstanding (for example, subject one had 21 such episodes), and tolerance to this effect did not develop in any of the subjects. During this study, the discrepancy between evaluation by patients and by aides (observers) is presented in Figure 1, a and b. This discrepancy is especially noteworthy in the responses to the items "would like to take

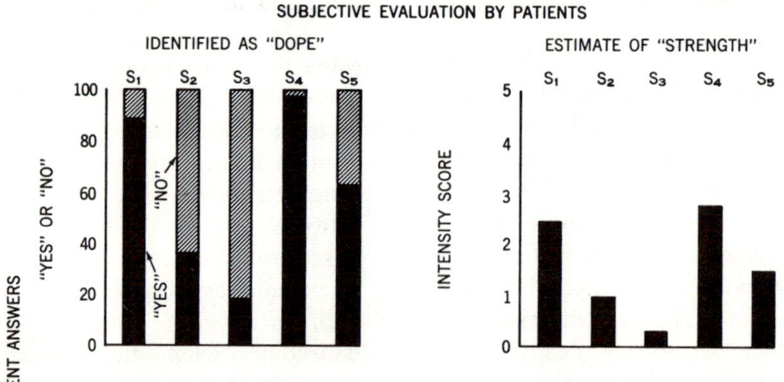

FIGURE 1a. Summary of "subjective" evaluations of individual patients (S1, S2, S3, S4, and S5) tabulated from questionnaires while each patient was receiving I-O-1 in direct addiction test. Note the excellent correlation for all subjects between the items "identified as 'dope' ", and "estimate of 'strength' ", also the high incidence of reports that "drug makes me feel bad" particularly for subjects S1 and S2. (Reprinted by permission, *Bull. Narc.* (U. N.), 16, (1), 37, 1964.)

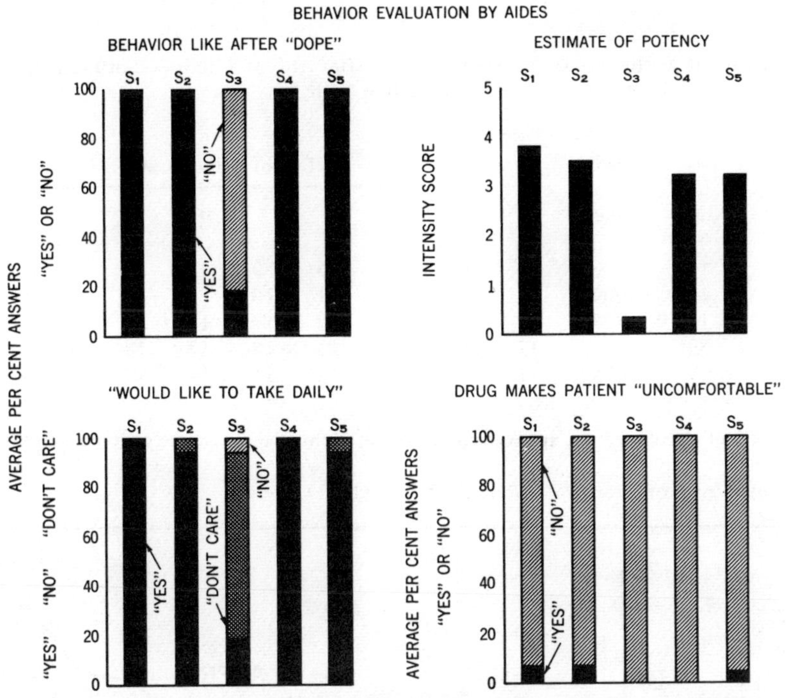

FIGURE 1b. Summary of results of questionnaires prepared by observers when they evaluated the effects induced in individual patients while receiving I-O-1 in the direct addiciton test. The observers interpreted (1) the behavior of four of the five patients as being similar to that observed after "dope" (opiate); (2) that the drug was quite potent; (3) that four of these patients "would like to take I-O-1 daily;" and (4) the incidence of reporting that drug makes patient "uncomfortable" was very low. Note that marked discrepancy between the evaluation of the patients (Figure 1a,) and that of the observers respecting the items "would like to take daily" and "the drug makes the patient feel 'bad' or 'uncomfortable' ". (Reprinted by permission, *Bull. Narc.* (U. N.), 16 (1), 37, 1964.)

daily" and "drug makes me feel bad" or "uncomfortable."

When I-O-1 was discontinued abruptly, all patients exhibited mild to moderate signs of abstinence. The daily point scores are shown in Table 1. In addition I-O-1 was partially substituted for morphine in morphine-dependent patients (Figure 2).

Despite the substitution test and the direct addiction test, both of which showed definite evidence of physical dependence, it was concluded that I-O-l had substantially less addictiveness than codeine and probably less addictiveness than propoxyphene. In the overall evaluation, emphasis was placed on the negative attitude of addicts; for example, one said, "I wouldn't buy it; in fact, I wouldn't take it for free, even if I were kicking the habit."

EVALUATION OF NARCOTIC ANTAGONISTS (SPECIAL FEATURES)

Many morphine antagonists, such as nalorphine, are capable of producing physical dependence in animals and man, since many of them contain a significant amount of agonistic properties, which account for their analgesic activity as well as their capacity to produce drug-seeking behavior. One member of the morphine antagonist group, however, which possesses no morphine-like agonistic properties, only antagonistic characteristics, is naloxone. The abstinence syndromes for the antagonists nalorphine, cyclazocine, and pentazocine are much milder than that of morphine, and in addition, are qualitatively different.[7,8] For example, in the case of morphine, the percentages of abstinence points

TABLE 1

Intensity of Abstinence (Daily Point Scores) After Abrupt Withdrawal of I-O-1 in Direct Addiction Test*

Subject	Days on drug	Daily dose (mg)	Day of withdrawal 1	2	3	4	5	6	7	8	9	10
1	17	600	3	16	13	15	5	11	9	9	9	6
2	17	600	6	10	13	11	10	8	7	3	5	9
3	17	825	1	13	9	9	10	12	3	8	4	5
4	39	675	17	24	18	13	15	12	14	16	12	8
5	39	675	11	19	12	12	11	14	12	14	a	a

[a]This patient developed an upper respiratory infection, hence scores on these days were not calculated.

*Reprinted by permission, *Bull. Narc.* (U. N., 16 (1), 37, 1964.

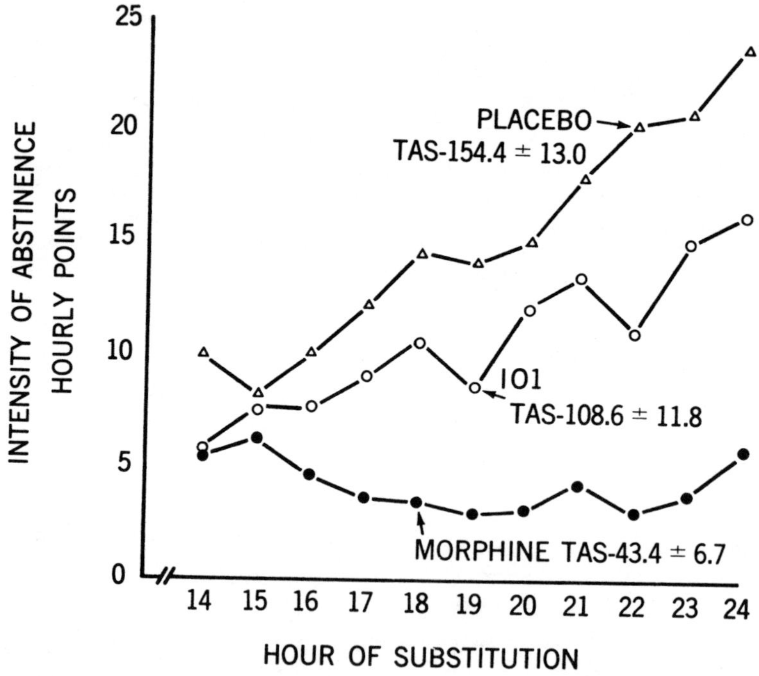

FIGURE 2. This figure compares in a cross-over experiment the average intensity of abstinence in 11 subjects when I-O-1 and a placebo were substituted for morphine, and when the customary dosage of morphine was continued in these subjects. (Reprinted by permission, *Bull. Narc.* (U. N.), 16 (1), 37, 1964.)

derived from fever, hyperpnea and systolic blood pressure are 12.3, 31.1, and 25.5, respectively, whereas for nalorphine the percentages are 35.8, 10.8, and 9.9, respectively, for these parameters. In addition, there is very little drug-seeking behavior following withdrawal of the antagonists, as distinguished from very marked drug-seeking behavior when morphine is withdrawn.

In general, the same battery of physical and psychic dependence tests is conducted on the antagonists that has been outlined above for agonists such as morphine. The antagonists are evaluated for their potency by comparing them with a standard drug, such as nalorphine, and with a placebo. In addition, the unknown is quantitatively compared with nalorphine or naloxone for its potency in precipitating an abstinence syndrome in morphine-dependent persons; however, some partial agonists of the morphine type (weak narcotic antagonists) have the capacity to precipitate abstinence syndromes in subjects with a high level of morphine dependence, but will suppress such symptoms in subjects with a lower level of dependence.[9]

OVERALL ABUSE POTENTIALS OF NARCOTICS AND NARCOTIC ANTAGONISTS, AS PREDICTED EXPERIMENTALLY, AND THEIR RELIABILITY

The abuse potential of a drug often is influenced significantly by subtle characteristics other than physical and psychic dependence. Questions which may play a part, for instance, are whether the compound is soluble in water, so that it may be readily injected intravenously, and whether the quality of the subjective effects upon injection resembles that of morphine or heroin. For example, codeine has a pattern typical of morphine when injected intravenously, with the exception that it releases considerably more histamine. While a moderate amount of histamine release is desired by the addict (that is, the induction of a flush), an excessive release is disliked. Furthermore, when injected rapidly or in doses that are sufficient to produce the desired subjective effect, codeine has the capacity for inducing postural hypotension and even fainting, a characteristic not observed when either morphine or heroin is injected intravenously. In addition, since codeine phosphate is relatively insoluble, the addict has difficulty getting a large enough dose in his 2 or 5 cc syringe. The precipitate frequently blocks a small needle.

Another characteristic that the addict demands is the rapid development of morphine- or heroin-like effects when the drug is injected intravenously. Failure of a morphine-like drug to induce such an effect promptly is illustrated by diphenoxylate (Lomotil®). This compound is so insoluble in water that it must be dissolved in pure propylene glycol, and if even a drop of water is present in the syringe, the diphenoxylate will be precipitated out of the solution. Apparently, when diphenoxylate is injected into the vein, it precipitates in the bloodstream and is absorbed by the central nervous system at such a slow rate that the addict does not recognize significant effect for at least 20 minutes. Such a drug would have relatively low abuse potential on two grounds: (1) for practical purposes, the addict is precluded from injecting it, since water is his only readily available solvent, and (2) he would be dismayed by the lack of effect when it is injected intravenously, even though quite good morphine effects are obtained after 30 to 45 minutes.

The Addiction Research Center at Lexington has evaluated some 30 compounds in the opiate agonist or antagonist series that have been made clinically available to physicians. In every instance, the overall abuse potential as evaluated in post-narcotic addicts has subsequently been confirmed by the clinical experience with these compounds.[10] Although the studies at Lexington have been highly predictive, the final court for determining the abuse potential of any drug is the experience observed with its extensive clinical use.

EVALUATION OF THE BARBITURATE–ALCOHOL TYPE OF DRUG

Tests for Physical Dependence

Dependence can be induced readily in man with several different barbiturates[11,12] and it has been observed in experimental alcoholic intoxication.[13,14] The signs of intoxication with barbiturates are similar to those provoked by alcohol.

The abstinence syndrome of abrupt withdrawal of alcohol[13] and barbiturates[11] differs considerably from that observed following abrupt withdrawal of opiates and may be described as follows. There is a progressive decrease in signs of intoxication over a period of 6 to 15 hours, depending upon the length of action of the barbiturate or alcohol and the degree of intoxication. When signs of intoxication disappear, the patient begins to show anxiety, nervousness, coarse tremor of the hands and face, progressive weakness, loss of appetite, nausea and even vomiting, and acute loss of weight. These symptoms may be followed after 24 hours or more by grand mal convulsions, auditory or visual hallucinations, and by a frank delirium in some patients. Hyperpyrexia and death may ensue for certain patients withdrawn abruptly from barbiturates.[15] In the case of alcoholic delirium, as many as 15% of the patients may die if inadequately treated.[14]

It should be pointed out that in order to induce experimental dependence with alcohol and barbiturates, it is necessary to intoxicate such patients around the clock for approximately 45 days. Such a procedure is hazardous to the individual and should not be undertaken, certainly, as a routine test procedure. Acute withdrawal also is hazardous, since such serious complications as grand mal convulsions and delirium may ensue.

However, a panel of experts (Workshop on Sedatives-Hypnotics, jointly sponsored by the Bureau of Narcotics and Dangerous Drugs and the Food and Drug Administration, Washington, D.C., 1966)[16] agreed that short-term, direct addiction preference tests might be made comparing an unknown drug with a known agent that is abused, such as secobarbital.

Tests for Psychic Dependence

These tests should be conducted preferably in sophisticated drug addicts and could utilize single doses capable of inducing definite effects. Comparisons would then be made with a standard drug such as secobarbital or pentobarbital. The pentobarbital-chlorpromazine-alcohol group scale of the Addiction Research Center Inventory could be employed, as well as the degree-of-liking scale. The unknown drug would be compared with the standard at two or more dose levels and with a placebo. The questions from the single dose opiate questionnaire, which involve relating the characteristics of the drug to other agents with which the patient is familiar and the degree of liking, could also be utilized.[4]

RELIABILITY OF THE TESTS ON BARBITURATE–LIKE DRUGS FOR PREDICTING ABUSE LIABILITY IN MAN

Although effective techniques have been developed for assessing the abuse potential of drugs in the barbiturate-alcohol group, nevertheless, the quantification of abuse has not been developed to the same degree as that attained for opiate-like drugs. Caution is necessary in extrapolating from animals to man in this class of drugs in respect to substitution studies. For example, carisoprodol and tybamate are effective substitutes for barbital, but these drugs do not demonstrate dependence in a direct addiction test in animals,[16] and carisoprodol has not shown physical dependence in human studies.[17] Not all drugs that satisfactorily substitute for barbital can be considered dependence-inducing agents, nor will any one procedure predict dependency.

Again, phenobarbital is capable of producing physical dependence in a manner similar to that of the other barbiturates, but dependence on phenobarbital is rarely voluntarily undertaken by man. A partial explanation of this fact is that the onset of signs of intoxication following phenobarbital administration is gradual, whereas signs of intoxication following administration of secobarbital, pentobarbital, and amobarbital are rapid and, in many respects, similar to those of alcohol in their onset.

EVALUATION OF TRANQUILIZERS

Tranquilizers may be divided roughly into two classes: major and minor. Drugs in the major classification include the phenothiazines, the reserpine alkaloids, and butyrophenones. These agents have in common an ability to decrease response. They apparently do not elicit self-administration in animals. It has been agreed that drugs in this category which have thus far been used in medicine do not possess any significant abuse potential. Whether new compounds of the major tranquilizer class will produce addiction liability is unknown. Each new drug should be evaluated in animals and man by means of techniques applicable to the barbiturate-alcohol group.

Physical and Psychic Dependence Tests for the Minor Tranquilizers

The most commonly used clinical drugs in this

category include chlordiazepoxide, diazepam, and meprobamate. In general, substances belonging to this class are somewhere between barbiturates and the major tranquilizers in their abuse potential. The test for physical dependence in man should be patterned after those tests described for the barbiturate-alcohol group. Again, it is necessary to administer these drugs chronically in very high doses over a considerable interval in order to ascertain whether or not physical dependence may be induced. The syndrome of abrupt withdrawal is analogous to that observed with the barbiturate group, the major complications being convulsions and/or psychosis.

As yet, no satisfactory procedures using only psychic dependence parameters have been published for discriminating the various members of this group for abuse potential.

The Workshop on Sedatives-Hypnotics concluded that methods suitable for evaluating the abuse potential of minor tranquilizers were unsophisticated and that it was not advisable to recommend a specific set of tests.[16]

EVALUATION OF STIMULANTS

Cocaine and the amphetamines are prototypes of stimulant drugs which have been subject to abuse by man. These compounds demonstrate the following properties in man:

1. Increased wakefulness and activity.
2. Tolerance, a common but not an invariable attribute: i.e., cocaine lacks this property.
3. No readily identifiable physical withdrawal syndrome.
4. A euphoric effect in man of relatively rapid onset and characterized by a feeling of relaxation rather than stimulation, unless the dosage is excessive.
5. Appetite suppression, at least on initial administration.

In animals, particularly in monkeys, self-administration tests have demonstrated that all of the compounds known to be abused by man are taken excessively and even in fatal doses by animals; however, there has been no systematic evaluation of these compounds for their relative abuse liability: that is, how reinforcing the injection of any given effective dose of one compound would be in comparison with the reinforcement capacity of another.

Martin et al.[17] have compared the pharmacological effects of single subcutaneous doses of ephedrine, *l*-ephedrine, amphetamine, *d*-methamphetamine, phenmetrazine, and methylphenidate in man. Ephedrine was selected for the study by these authors "because it is a widely used sympathomimetic amine which, we thought, had not been abused and could therefore serve as a negative control in validating a method." A review of the literature revealed several case reports of abuse of ephedrine; however, even though ephedrine has been widely used in medicine and its salts are quite water soluble, the incidence of abuse is minute compared to that of amphetamine and methamphetamine. The experiments of Martin et al. demonstrated that the subjective effects of ephedrine in appropriate dosages were similar to those of the other amphetamines and relatively similar in all of the physiological tests.

In view of the limited number of controlled studies in man, it is thought that we do not have satisfactory methods for predicting the relative abuse potential of central nervous system stimulants in man.

EVALUATION OF HALLUCINOGENIC DRUGS

It is generally agreed that man is the best experimental animal for studies of hallucinogens. The use of these drugs in normal volunteer subjects raises certain ethical questions, especially in regard to creating drug-dependent individuals. The workshop on methods for evaluating the abuse potential of drugs mentioned above,[16] however, agreed that there is no evidence of significant psychological risk nor is there evidence that administering such drugs to nonaddictive normal persons has been followed by subsequent abuse.

The hallucinogenic effects can be readily detected by a variety of psychological tests, which may be supervised by physiological measures to detect impairment. There are no specific biochemical changes due to the administration of hallucinogenic drugs. None of these agents produces physical dependence or compulsive psychic dependence. There has been no evidence that a drug, simply by being a hallucinogen, is, therefore, subject to abuse. The choice of such agents will depend on certain pharmacological properties of the drug which the potential addict considers beneficial. In general, drugs which will be abused are those that are quickly effective and have a relatively brief span of action, usually measured in hours.

There have been no adequate studies to establish methods that would predict the relative abuse of a new agent in this category.

SUMMARY

Drug dependence is defined as a state arising from the repeated administration of a drug on a periodic or continuous basis. It includes the attributes "physical" and/or "psychic."

Drug abuse takes into account the concept of dependence, but also the degree of risk to the public. It is defined as follows: abuse of a drug exists if its use so harmfully affects the individual and/or society as to require its control. Risks to the public are often reflected in the type and extent of controls promulgated. However, socially accepted drugs of "addiction" such as alcohol and tobacco have lenient controls; whereas, heroin addiction, which is socially taboo, has strict controls.

Methods have been described for man which are highly predictive of the abuse potential of narcotics on an experimental basis and narcotic anatagonists, since subsequent clinical use of such agents has confirmed the experimental studies.

In the case of central nervous system depressants of the barbiturate-alcohol type, experimental procedures have been developed in man that are positive for known highly abused agents, but the relative abuse capacity of such agents cannot be readily assessed as yet. A part of this difficulty is due to the fact that acute and chronic intoxication and abrupt withdrawal of chronically administered drugs of this class of compounds are hazardous for man.

The major tranquilizers (such as the phenothiazines, the reserpine alkaloids, and the butyrophenones) do not exhibit any significant abuse potential.

The minor tranquilizers, such as chlordiazepoxide, diazepam, and meprobamate, and particularly the latter, have shown some abuse, but methods have not been developed in man for prediciting their *relative* abuse.

Similarly, in the case of the amphetamines and the hallucinogens, methods have not been developed in man to determine their *relative* abuse potential on an experimental basis.

In the assessment of overall abuse potential of a drug, in addition to its potential for inducing physical and psychic dependence under arbitrary conditions of administration, there are several adjuvant phenomena that must be considered. These include the quality of the subjective effects by several routes of administration, its water solubility (low solubility practically precludes intravenous injection), the rapidity of the onset of subjective effects, and its tissue irritant capacity since highly irritating drugs will progressively occlude veins and interfere with intravenous use.

REFERENCES

1. Fraser, H. F., Methods for testing for narcotic addiction in animals and man and their efficacy for predicting human abuse, in *Methods in Drug Evaluation,* North Holland Publishing Company, Amsterdam, 1966, 297.

2. Kolb, L. and Himmelsbach, C. K., Clinical studies of drug addiction. III. A critical review of the withdrawal treatments with method of evaluating abstinence syndromes, *Amer. J. Psychiat.*, 94, 759, 1938.

3. Himmelsbach, C. K., Studies of certain addiction characteristics of (a) dihydromorphine ("paramorphan"), (b) dihydrodesoxymorphine-D ("Desomorphine), (c) dihydrodesoxycodeine-D ("Desocodeine) and (d) methyldihydromorphinone ("Metopon"), *J. Pharmacol. Exp. Ther.*, 67, 239, 1939.

4. Fraser, H. F., Van Horn, G. D., Martin, W. R., Wolbach, A. B., and Isbell, H., Methods for evaluating addiction liability, (A) "Attitude" of opiate addicts toward opiate like drugs, (B) A short-term "direct" addiction test, *J. Pharmacol. Exp. Ther.*, 133, 371, 1961.

5. Jasinski, D. R., Martin, W. R., and Sapira, J. D., Antagonism of the subjective, behavioral, pupillary, and respiratory depressant effects of cyclazocine by naloxone, *Clin. Pharmacol. Ther.*, 9, 215, 1968.

6. Fraser, H. F., Addictiveness of 1,2-dimethyl-3-phenyl-3-propionoxy pyrrolidine hydrochloride (ARC I-O-1), *Bull. Nar.*, 16 (1), 37, 1964.

7. Fraser, H. F. and Rosenberg, D. E., Studies on the human addiction liability of 2′-hydroxy-5,9-dimethyl-2-(3,3-dimethylallyl)-6,7-benzomorphan (WIN 20,228), a weak narcotic antagonist, *J. Pharmacol. Exp. Ther.*, 143, 149, 1964.

8. Martin, W. R. and Gorodetzky, C. W., Demonstration of tolerance to and physical dependence on N-allylnormorphine (nalorphin), *J. Pharmacol. Exp. Ther.*, 150, 437, 1965.

9. Martin, W. R., Pharmacological redundancy as an adaptive mechanism in the central nervous system, *Fed. Proc.*, 29, 13, 1970.

10. Halbach, H. and Eddy, N. B., Tests for addiction (chronic intoxication) of morphine type, *Bull. W.H.O.*, 28, 139, 1963.

11. Isbell, H., Altschul, S., Kornetsky, C. H., Eisenman, A. J., Flanary, H. G., and Fraser, H. F., Chronic barbiturate intoxication: An experimental study, *Arch. Neurol. Psychiat.*, 64, 1, 1950.

12. Fraser, H. F., Isbell, H., Eisenman, A. J., Wikler, A., and Pescor, F. T., Chronic barbiturate intoxication: Further studies, *A.M.A. Arch. Intern. Med.*, 94, 34, 1954.

13. Isbell, H., Fraser, H. F., Wikler, A., Belleville, R. E., and Eisenman, A. J., An experimental study of the etiology of "rum fits" and delirium tremens, *Quart. J. Stud. Alcohol,* 16, 1, 1955.

14. Victor, M., Alcohol and nutritional diseases of the nervous system, *J.A.M.A.*, 167, 65, 1958.

15. Fraser, H. F., Shaver, M. R., Maxwell, E. S., and Isbell, H., Death due to withdrawal of barbiturates, *Ann. Intern. Med.*, 38, 1319, 1953.

16. Harwood, T., personal communication.

17. Martin, W. R., Sloan, J. W., Sapira, J. D., and Jasinski, D. R., Physiologic, subjective and behavioral effects of amphetamine, methamphetamine, ephedrine, phenmetrazine, and methylphenidate in man, *Clin. Pharmacol. Ther.*, 12, 245, 1971.

CHEMICAL ASPECTS OF DRUG DEPENDENCE

CHEMICAL ASPECTS OF DRUG DEPENDENCE

Chemical Characteristics of Drugs Inducing Physical and/or Psychic Dependence to:

NARCOTIC ANALGESICS AND ANTAGONISTS

A. E. Jacobson

TABLE OF CONTENTS

INTRODUCTION

Opium has been known and used since antiquity; the alkaloid morphine was isolated from this plant almost two centuries ago. The use of opium or alkaloids derived from it, for the purpose of alleviating pain, is about as old as medicine itself. Yet, for the past 50 years scores of chemists have worked to synthesize analgesics. This anomaly is due to three unfortunate features of morphine. It is a respiratory depressant, it can produce drug dependence, and tolerance is developed to it.

Until 1939 synthetic work on analgesics was mostly limited to derivatives of the opium alkaloids. One such derivative, the diacetyl analog of morphine, was proclaimed as the perfect analgesic in 1899. Subsequent work on that compound, heroin, proved otherwise. Odd errors of this sort have occurred occasionally, probably because the biological tests for analgesia and dependence liability of the opiate type were inadequate. Until rather recently compounds showing strong analgesic activity in the available animal tests were invariably found to be drugs having physical dependence liability of the opiate-type in man. Even today, using the newer analgesic test procedures, some synthetic compounds which seem to be excellent analgesics, appearing free from the liability of dependence in animal species and causing much less respiratory depression than morphine, have been shown to have drug dependence liability in man. Man is an expensive and time-consuming test animal. It is not surprising, therefore, that new improved analgesics appear infrequently in medical practice. It has been said that, at present, all compounds which have the chemical characteristics of strong analgesics induce some type of physical dependence in man, in varying degree; however, the agonist-antagonists have a quantitatively and qualitatively different type of physical dependence liability.

Thousands of synthetic analgesics have been prepared. It is impossible to list all of them in this short chapter, excellent compilations can be found in the more complete texts.[1-3] This chapter will be restricted mostly to analgesics which have morphine-like analgesic activity, and are commercially available. Some very active analgesics, not in clinical use but having found utility in other areas, will be discussed; as will the relatively new and fascinating agonist-antagonists. The innumerable codeine-like compounds will not be included.

There are five main classes of clinically useful analgesics for man. These are, in order of their historical rise: 1) the opium alkaloids and their derivatives; 2) pethidine and its congeners, originated by Eisleb and Schaumann; 3) methadone and its cognates, due to Bockmühl and Ehrhart; 4) the morphinans and relatives, discovered by Grewe; and the last and very important class, 5) the 6,7-benzomorphans, originated by E. L. May.

Almost all of the strong narcotic analgesics in these five classes of drugs have three or four structurally similar characteristics. They have: 1) a quaternary carbon atom, 2) an aromatic nucleus linked to this carbon; 3) a tertiary amino group two saturated carbon atoms away from the quaternary carbon atom; and, 4) a phenolic hydroxyl group situated *meta* to the quaternary carbon – if the tertiary nitrogen is a part of a fused piperidine ring system. These structure-activity correlations for narcotic analgesics are illustrated in Figure 1.

With only one exception, all clinically accepted strong narcotic analgesics have these features. A fifth structural feature in all but the pethidine and methadone class of analgesic has produced the agonist-antagonist. This involves a change in the nitrogen substituent. When an *N*-methyl is replaced by an *N*-allyl, *N*-3,3-dimethylallyl or an *N*-cyclopropylmethyl, among other possibilities, then certain of the compounds in these classes of analgesics are transformed into agonist-antagonists. That is, they become capable of cancelling or reversing most of the pharmacologic effects of morphine-like compounds and yet are, themselves, analgesics of varying effectiveness. Some other moieties known to confer agonist-antagonist properties to the nor derivative (*N*-desmethyl) of some of the narcotic analgesics, when substituted on the nitrogen atom, are propargyl, 2-methylallyl, cyclobutylmethyl, 3-chloroallyl (*cis* and *trans*), 2-chloro and 2-bromoallyl, *n*-propyl, cyclopentylmethyl, cyclopropylethyl, 3,3-dichloroallyl and, possibly, cyclohexylmethyl.

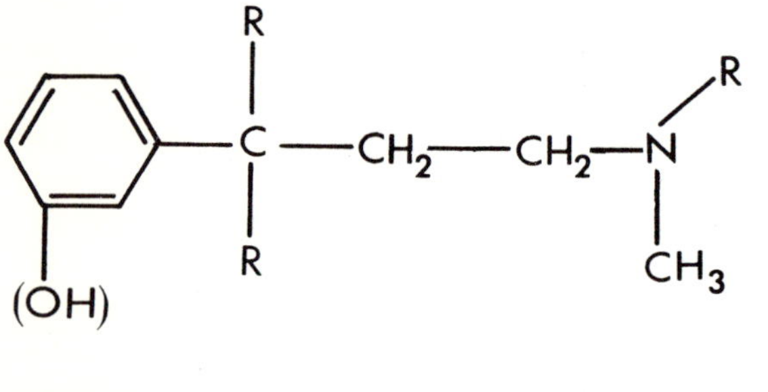

FIGURE 1. Minimal structural features usually associated with narcotic analgesic activity.

The four criteria for structure-activity correlation of narcotic analgesics, and the fifth (*N*-substitution) for antagonist activity have recently been joined by a sixth factor – optical resolution of some of the *N*-methyl-6,7-benzomorphans.[3] The latter produces agonist-antagonists (at least in animal species) which have the added feature of being difficult, if not impossible, to reconvert chemically to the racemic parent narcotic analgesic; a property which may become rather important in the future.

These structure-activity correlations, although interesting as an ex post facto analysis, are lacking in their predictive capacity. Their limited usefulness will be discussed at the conclusion of this chapter.

THE OPIUM ALKALOIDS AND THEIR DERIVATIVES

Out of all of the opium alkaloids, and all of their chemical modifications, morphine remains the most widely used analgesic.[4] Morphine (Formula 1) meets all of the narcotic analgesic structure-activity criteria listed in the Introduction.

There are several variants of the morphine structure which have attained some clinical utility. If the 6-hydroxy group of morphine is oxidized to a ketone, the 7,8-double-bond saturated, and a 14-hydroxyl group introduced, the compound oxymorphone (7,8-dihydro-14-hydroxymorphinone. Formula 2) is produced. Although

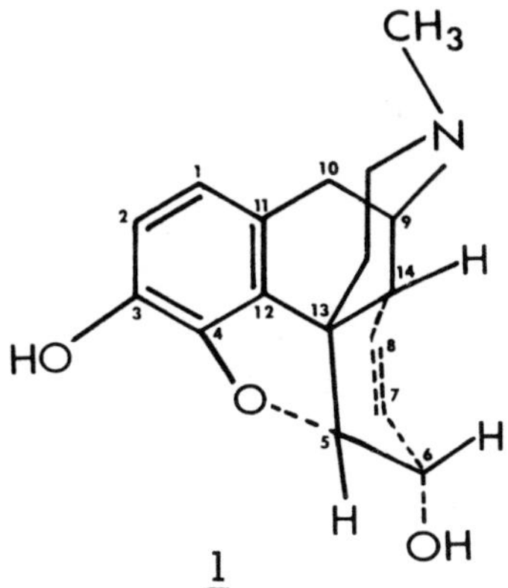

1

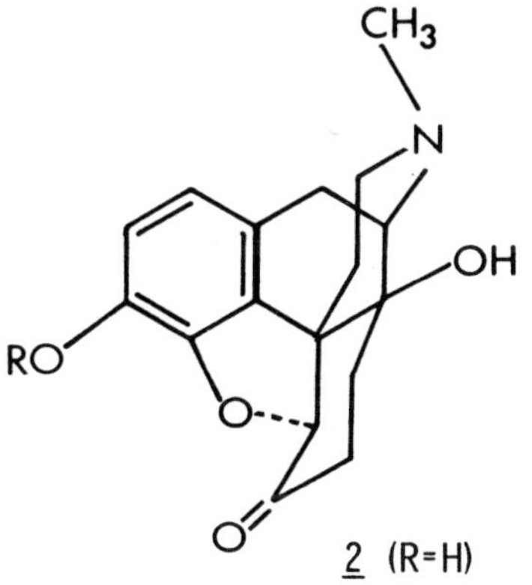

2 (R=H)
3 (R=CH_3)

oxymorphone, originally synthesized by Weiss,[5] is much more active than morphine as an analgesic (Table 1) it offers little clinical advantage, retaining the adverse effects of the morphine.[6] Oxycodone (7,8-dihydro-14-hydroxycodeinone. Formula 3), more widely used than oxymorphone, is a similarly modified compound (from codeine).[7,8] Identical to oxymorphone in all but the 3-hydroxy group, oxycodone is illustrative of the reduction in analgesic potency which occurs by etherification of the phenolic group in almost all classes of analgesics. However, etherification of the phenolic oxygen may result in orally effective drugs. Almost all analgesics are much less effective by the oral route of administration than they are by injection; thus oxycodone, utilized orally as an analgesic or antitussive, acts more like codeine than morphine. However, oxycodone retains the respiratory depressant effect and addiction liability of morphine, and these are rather undesirable properties for antitussives. Hydrocodone (7,8-dihydrocodeinone, Formula 4) can be looked at as a compound in which the 14-hydroxyl group of oxycodone has been replaced by hydrogen.[8,9] Again, like oxycodone, it is used orally as an antitussive. Used orally, it is a rather ineffective analgesic and is more addictive than codeine. Hydromorphone (7,8-dihydromorphinone, Formula 5),[8,10] the 3-hydroxy relative of hydrocodone, is used orally and parenterally. As used parenterally, it is at least five times as active as morphine. All of them are equal to, or worse than morphine in their physical dependence producing properties, respiratory depression, and other toxic effects.

The morphine variants offer slight, if any, advantage over morphine parenterally except,

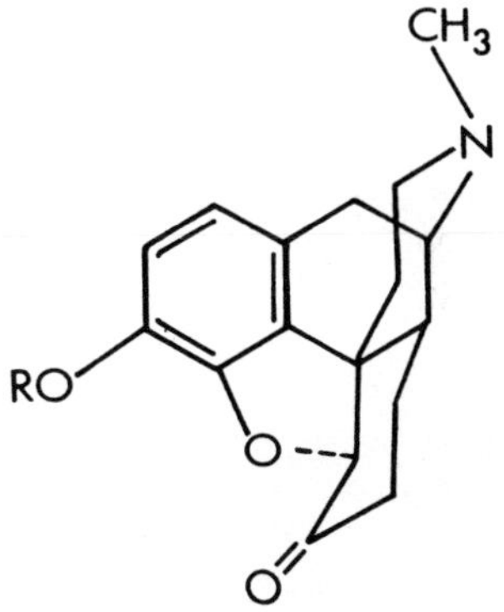

4 (R=CH_3)
5 (R=H)

perhaps, oxymorphone which might be preferable in those instances where depression of the cough reflex is contraindicated.

These are the only narcotic analgesics derived from the opium alkaloids which are used in the United States. Heroin (Formula 6), the 3,6-diacetyl

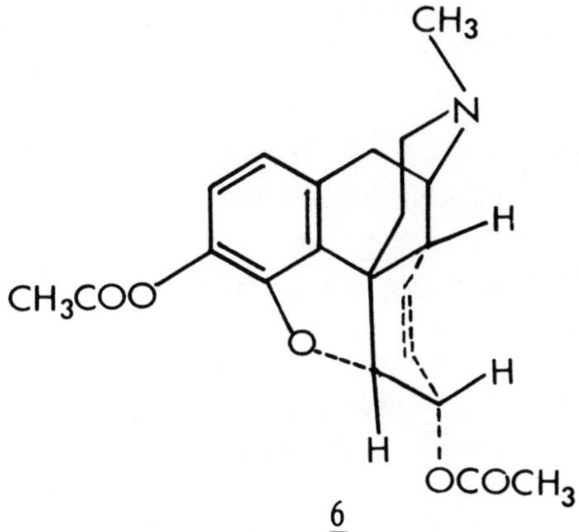

6

TABLE 1

Activity of Narcotic Analgesics and Agonist-Antagonists in Mice and Man.

Formula no.	International nonproprietary name[a]	Some trade and common names	Mice ED_{50} (mg/kg)[b]	Man[c] (mg)	Dependence liability[d] (man)
1	Morphine		1.2	10	High[e]
2	Oxymorphone	Numorphan®	0.08	1.12-1.15	High
3	Oxycodone	Nucodan®, Eucodal. Eumorphal, Eucosan, Percodan®	0.3	10-15	High
4	Hydrocodone	Dihydrocodeinone, Dicodid®, Hycodan	1.6	15	Intermediate
5	Hydromorphone	Dihydromorphinone, Dilaudid®, Hymorphan, Dimorphid, and Dimorphone	0.15	2-4	High
6	Heroin		0.45	2-10	High
7	Nalorphine	Nalline®	4.8[f]	10	Low[g]
14	Etorphine	M-99®	0.001	0.05[h]	High[i]
16	Pethidine	Meperidine, Demerol®, Isonipecaine, Dolantin	4.7	80	High
17	Anileridine	Leritine	1.6	30	High
18	Piminodine		0.5	10	High
19	Phenoperidine		0.032	0.3-2	High
20	Alphaprodine	Nisentil, Prisilidine	0.9	40-60	High
21	Fentanyl	Sublimaze®	0.008	0.05	High
23	Methadone	Amidone, Dolophine®, Panalgen	0.8	5-10	High
25	Dipipanone	Diconal	1.4	20-25	High
27	Levorphanol	Dromoran®	0.25	2-3	High
29	Levallorphan		-	10	-[g]
30	Phenazocine	Narphen, Prinadol®, NIH 7519	0.1	2-3	Intermediate[j]
31	Pentazocine	Talwin®	4.7[f]	20-40	Low[g]
32	Cyclazocine		0.08[f]	0.025	Intermediate[g]
33	1-Etazocine	NIH 8178	1.17	8	Intermediate
34	1-Metazocine	NIH 7569	0.85	10	Intermediate

a) See reference 29.
b) Subcutaneous administration; Eddy-Leimbach method [Jacobson, A. E. and May, E. L., *J. Med. Chem.*, 8, 563, 1965, see references 8 and 9 therein].
c) Analgesic activity on parenteral administration (equivalence to 10 mg of morphine).
d) Drug dependence of opiate-type.
e) Abstinence-syndrome suppressant dose in monkeys, 3 mg/kg.
f) Subcutaneous administration; Nielsen method [Perrine, T. D., Atwell, L., Tice, I. B., Jacobson, A. E., and May, E. L., *J. Pharm. Sci.*, in press, 1971, see reference 8 and 9 therein].
g) Drug dependence of specific opiate antagonist type.
h) This dose level was used in cancer patients with severe pain.
i) Presumed "High" based on monkey studies.
j) Abstinence-syndrome suppressant dose in monkeys, 18 mg/kg.

derivative of morphine, is highly addictive and banned in this country for clinical use because of its abuse potential, but it is still being used in Britain.[4] Presumably, a more rapid onset of action can be obtained with heroin.

Replacement of the *N*-methyl group in morphine by an *N*-allyl group has produced an agonist-antagonist, nalorphine (*N*-allylnormorphine, Formula 7). Nalorphine was presumed to have been synthesized originally by McCawley, Hart and March,[11] clarification and definitive synthesis was achieved by Weijlard and Erickson.[12] Hart noted as early as 1941[13] that nalorphine antagonized the respiratory depression of morphine. This was not totally unexpected since much earlier work by Pohl[14] indicated that *N*-allylnorcodeine (Formula 8), the 3-methoxy relative of nalorphine, was an antagonist, albeit rather weak, to the respiratory depression of morphine, a report long buried in the literature and unearthed

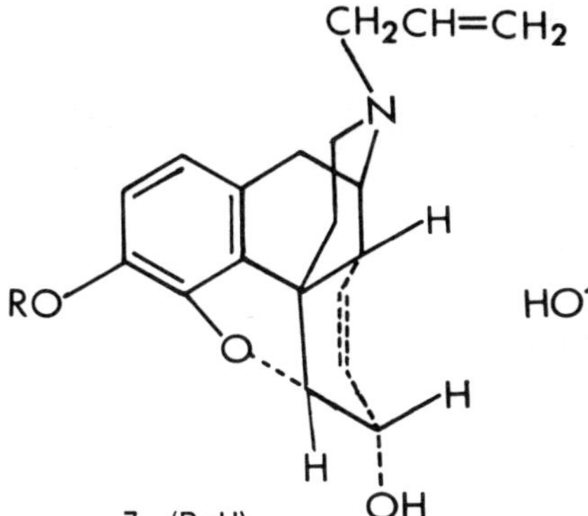

7 (R=H)
8 (R=CH3)

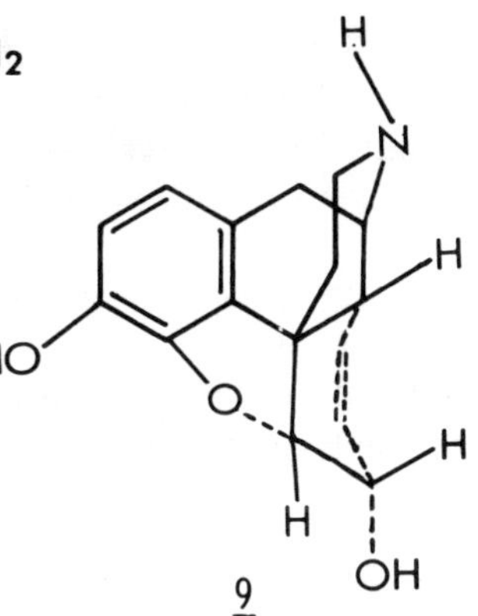

9

by Hart and McCawley. In a later paper, Hart and McCawley[15] stated that nalorphine was an analgesic as effective as morphine itself. It is possible, however, that they were testing a mixture of nalorphine and morphine; their intermediate in the synthesis, normorphine (Formula 9), was undoubtedly impure. The nalorphine obtained from their synthesis had a melting point of 92 to 93°, that from Weijlard and Erickson's synthesis melted at 208 to 209°. Although the idea of Hart and McCawley that nalorphine would be a compound which had both analgesic and antagonist properties was brilliant, it was discounted by the definitive synthesis of the pure nalorphine and the subsequent report by Unna[16] that nalorphine was inactive as an analgesic in the animal tests used at that time. Thus, most investigators logically assigned the reported analgesic property of nalorphine to the presumed impurity, morphine. For the next ten years pharmacological exploration of nalorphine was basically concentrated on its ability to antagonize the respiratory depression of narcotic analgesics. Eddy suggested[17] that nalorphine might prove advantageous in combination with morphine in man. He thought that the combination might retain the analgesic effectiveness of morphine, the side effects being antagonized by small quantities of nalorphine. This study was undertaken by Lasagna and Beecher.[18] Since the effect of the combination of two drugs was being observed, they carefully proceeded to study the individual drug nalorphine as a control on their results. The result, confirmed subsequently by Keats and Telford,[19] that nalorphine was as effective an analgesic as morphine in man, initiated the era of the remarkable agonist-antagonist.

Modification of another compound in this group of opium alkaloids, oxymorphone, has produced the very valuable naloxone (*N*-allyl-7,8-dihydro-14-hydroxynormorphinone, Formula 10).[20] The *N*-methyl group of oxymorphone is cleaved and is replaced by an *N*-allyl group. As alluded to in the Introduction, this type of replacement usually produces an agonist-antagonist. Naloxone, however, is not an analgesic at all. It is the only "pure" antagonist known. Since it is not a respiratory depressant, and has little toxic effect in man, it may, in the future, be widely used as the drug of choice in counteracting the respiratory depression of toxic doses of analgesics,[21] displacing the current drug of choice, nalorphine. Combinations of naloxone with narcotic analgesics are presently being studied for clinical efficacy.

Complex Derivatives of the Opium Alkaloids

Work with derivatives of the opium alkaloids was sporadic after 1939, due to the discovery of pethidine. Later, after the morphinans achieved considerable success, most medicinal chemists

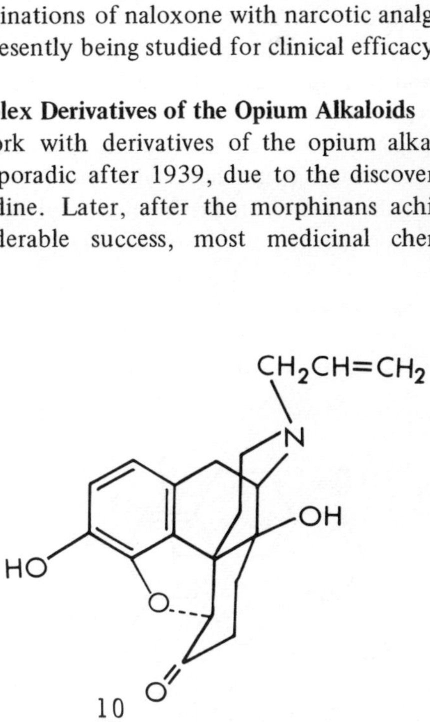

10

were occupied with removing as much of the morphine skeleton as possible in the hope of simultaneously removing the side effects of morphine. This work also met with success, and so the opium alkaloids were fairly neglected until Bentley and co-workers[22,23] decided to go in a direction opposite to that of most medicinal chemists. They reasoned that the separation of the desired from the undesirable properties of morphine might more easily be achieved by the preparation of more rigid and complex structures, claiming these structures would be more selectively adsorbed at the receptor sites. They began by using the opium alkaloid thebaine (Formula 11). A Diels-Alder reaction with dienophiles across the double bond system in thebaine produced compounds with activity comparable to pethidine, at first. Later, using different dienophiles with thebaine and then with the derived oripavine (Formula 12), they obtained compounds with about ten thousand times the activity of morphine in some animal tests.[24] These are, by far, the most active analgesics known. The parent compound of the series, 6,14-endoethenotetrahydrothebaine (Formula 13), a 6,14-ethano bridged derivative of codeine, is 40 times as potent as morphine.

Unfortunately, as the analgesic activity increased, the physical dependence liability and other side effects of the compounds increased commensurately. These drugs have found utility in the capture of wild game; charging rhinoceroses are said to stop "practically" in their tracks when injected *via* a specialized rifle. However, the compounds have not found clinical application for man, although Blane has stated that etorphine (tetrahydro-7*α*-(1-hydroxy-1-methylbutyl)-6,14-endoethenooripavine, see Formula 14) with paren-

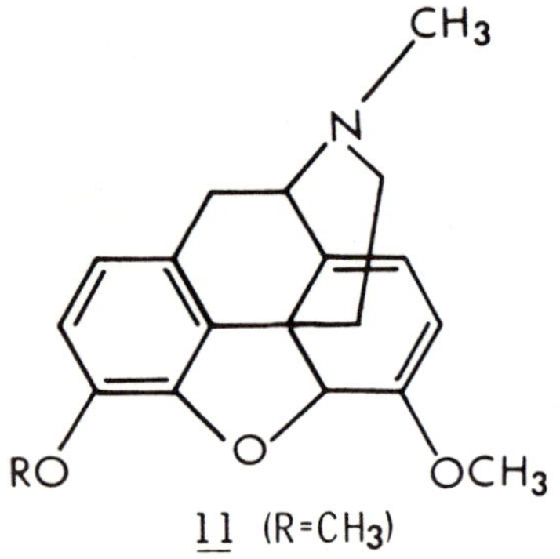

11 (R=CH3)
12 (R=H)

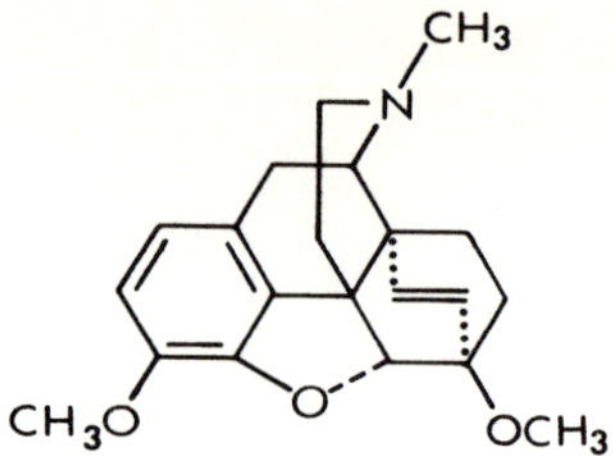

13

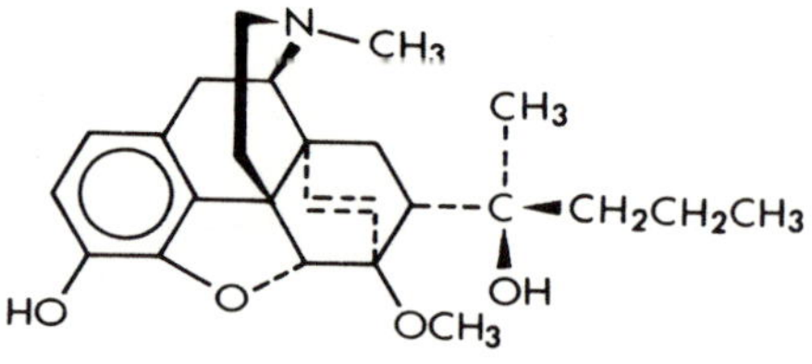

14

teral potency many times that of morphine in man should be used clinically.[25,26] The World Health Organization Expert Committee on Dependence-Producing Drugs disagrees with Blane's estimate, claiming etorphine to be a potentially dangerous drug, principally due to the low dosage necessary. This may be an unfair criterion, but a technician's displaced decimal point (from the usual 0.001mg/kg in man[25]) could cause havoc.

Lately, Bentley and co-workers[24,27] have prepared agonist-antagonists by *N*-substitution in an analogous endoethano series (Formula 15). The morphine antagonist (Formula 15) is said to be among the most potent known.[24] Again, as with the narcotic analgesics in the endoetheno or endothano series, the antagonists have not, as yet, achieved clinical utility.

PETHIDINE AND ITS CONGENERS

Eisleb and Schaumann[28] discovered, in 1939, that one of the piperidine derivatives synthesized

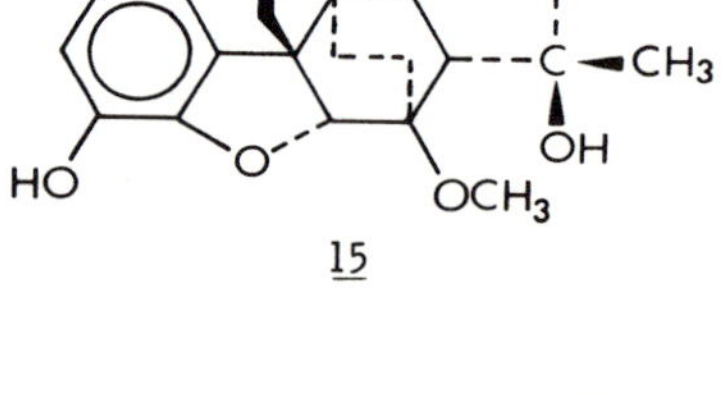

15

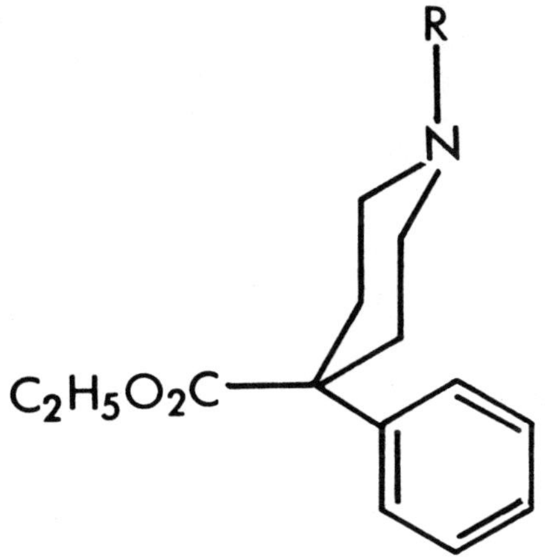

16 (R=CH_3)
17 (R=p-NH_2-$C_6H_5CH_2CH_2$-)
18 (R=$C_6H_5NHCH_2CH_2CH_2$-)
19 (R=$C_6H_5CH(OH)CH_2CH_2$-)

by them and tested primarily for spasmolytic activity was, in fact, a good analgesic. This sparked an intense effort among medicinal chemists who attempted to remove its undesirable characteristics of respiratory depression and drug dependence of the opiate type. The compound, now called pethidine[29] (meperidine, 1-methyl-4-carbethoxy-4-phenylpiperidine, Formula 16) is almost as popular among clinicians for the treatment of moderate to severe pain as morphine. The popularity of the drug is difficult to understand; in man, pethidine has one eighth the potency of morphine and retains most of morphine's undesirable features. Furthermore, pethidine has been known to cause psychic dependence in clinical use, such that the inefficiency of the drug in controlling pain is masked and a change to a more effective analgesic may be resisted by patients.

Pethidine meets most of the structure-activity relationships for narcotic analgesic activity, having a quaternary carbon atom, aromatic ring, and a tertiary amine in the correct juxtaposition. The fact that pethidine and its congeners are less conformationally rigid than the opium alkaloids has disturbed theoreticians who desire, for neatness perhaps, to place all strong analgesics in the same holes and hills of the "swiss cheese" type of receptor site. Thus, it has been of great interest to find the "actual" conformation of pethidine. This, after much speculation in the literature, was determined most precisely by x-ray crystallography[30] of a related compound. Previous to that determination it was assumed that pethidine could approximate the conformation of morphine, and a structure was drawn[31] (Figure 2) which might explain the biological activity of pethidine; it should fit the same "site" as morphine (i.e. compare Figure 2 and Formula 1).

Unfortunately, this conformational resemblance is based on an axially oriented phenyl group. The x-ray structure determination of *dl*-alphaprodine hydrochloride, a related compound, proved that the phenyl group existed in an equatorial conformation in the solid state (see Formula 20) in alphaprodine and, by analogy, in pethidine itself. However, it is now fairly well accepted that both a macromolecule which contains the receptor site, and a small drug molecule can interact and influence the conformation of the other. Whether such interaction can induce inversion through the boat form of pethidine's piperidine ring to a conformation of the pethidine molecule which might satisfy the unknown morphine receptor is, again, speculation. It would be helpful if information could be obtained about the macromolecule, or macromolecular system, with

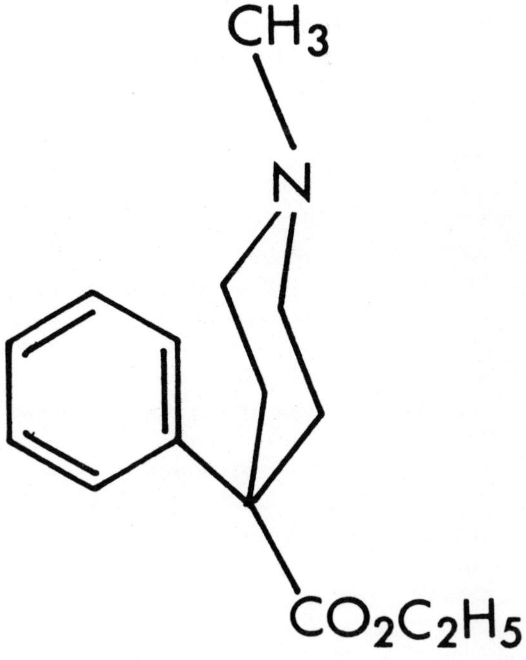

FIGURE 2. The presumed conformation of pethidine necessary for biological activity.

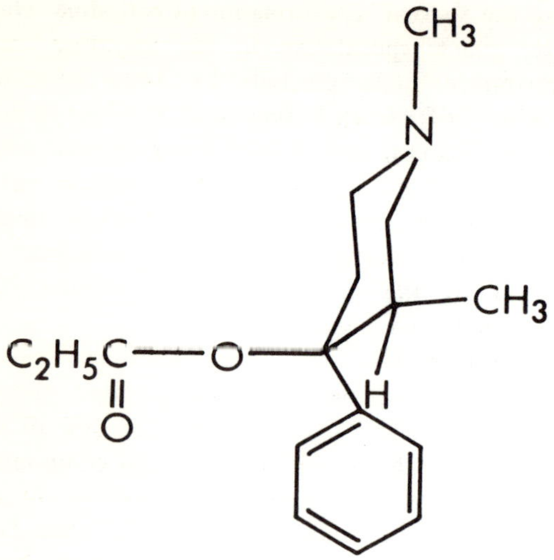

20

which analgesics interact to produce their biological effect. At least a rational start could then be made towards the determination of actual binding sites using, perhaps, the contemporary methods of electron paramagnetic resonance spectroscopy,[32] nuclear magnetic resonance spectroscopy,[33,34] and fluorescent antibody techniques.[35,36]

Over the last three decades several thousand derivatives of pethidine have been synthesized. Of these, only four or five have achieved clinical utility; pethidine remains the most popular and widely used drug[4] of its type and, indeed, of any other class of analgesic with the possible exception of morphine.

Three clinically useful compounds have been obtained by variation of the substituent of the nitrogen atom. The most popular of these is anileridine (1(*p*-aminophenethyl)-4-carbethoxy-4-phenylpiperidine, Formula 17). An *N*-*p*-aminophenethyl group was added to norpethidine as a substitute for the *N*-methyl group. The compound showed good activity, a surprise to medicinal chemists, anileridine being the first non-*N*-methyl pethidine to show such activity.[37] Anileridine is two to three times as active as pethidine orally or parenterally, and produces less circulatory depression. Although it is satisfactory for the mother in obstetric analgesia (in conjunction with scopolamine) it caused depression in 25% of the infants.[38] Piminodine (1-(3-phenylaminopropyl)-4-carbethoxy-4-phenylpiperidine, Formula 18), the *N*-3-phenylaminopropyl derivative of norpethidine, and phenoperidine (1-(3-phenylpropan-3-ol)-4-carbethoxy-4-phenylpiperidine, Formula 19), containing a 3-phenylpropan-3-ol moiety on the nitrogen atom, the latter available in Britain, are much less frequently prescribed. In terms of their overall spectrum of activity as opposed to their side effects, none show any great advantage over pethidine.[38] Piminodine is morphine-like in activity and perhaps causes less drowsiness; phenoperidine is very potent and short acting.

If the carbethoxy in the 4-position of pethidine is replaced by an acyloxy group a new series of analogs is produced. These "reversed esters" are called prodines,[1] and one of them has achieved some clinical utility, alphaprodine. Alphaprodine (α−1,3-dimethyl-4-phenyl-4-propionoxypiperidine, see Formula 20) has a rapid onset and a short duration of action and is three to five times as effective as pethidine in animals; it is used, infrequently due to its side effects, for the acute pain encountered in childbirth.[38]

The last of this group of analgesics based on piperidine is fentanyl[1] (1-phenethyl-4-*N*-propionylanilinopiperidine, see Formula 21), the only clinically used strong analgesic which does not follow the structure-activity rules enunciated in the Introduction. Fentanyl does not have a quaternary carbon atom; it is, however, one of the most potent analgesics known, having at least 100 times the activity of morphine in animals. Its effect is of short duration, and, once again, its advantages are far outweighed by its side effects.

The pethidine/prodine family of compounds, perhaps because they are not conformationally ridid, have not been convertible to clinically useful agonist-antagonists with *N*-substituents known to produce such antagonists in other classes of narcotic analgesics. In fact, 1,3-diallylnorprodine[3]

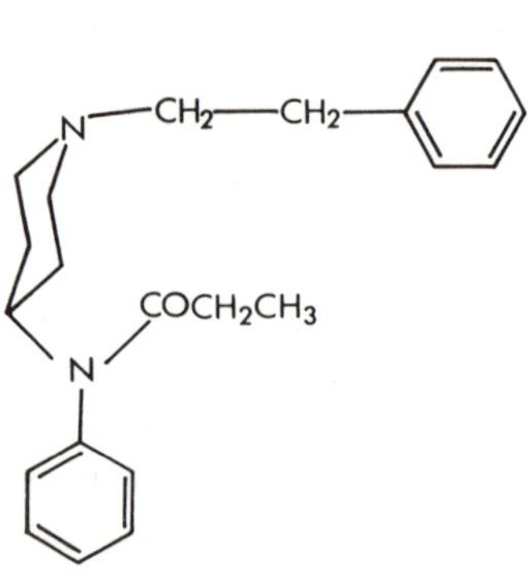

21

(Formula 22) shows high physical dependence capacity in monkeys.

METHADONE AND ITS COGNATES

A U.S. Commerce Department report[39] which related the synthesis of a new strong analgesic in Germany, during the second World War, started another stampede of synthesis which provided hundreds of derivatives. Bockmühl and Ehrhart[40] had synthesized methadone (6-dimethylamino-4,4-diphenyl-3-heptanone, see Formula 23), a drug which has become very useful indeed. Methadone

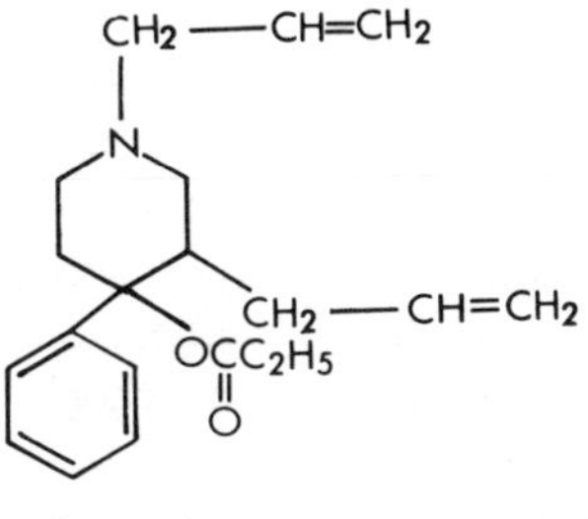

22

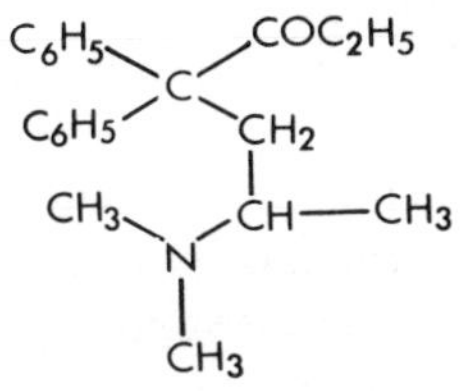

23

mimics the total pharmacological profile of morphine; it, like morphine and pethidine, has dependence liability of the opiate type, tolerance develops to its therapeutic action and side effects, cross-tolerance develops to other narcotic analgesics, and it elicits respiratory depression. However, psychic dependence does not seem to develop with methadone in clinical situations and the abstinence syndrome which is produced on withdrawal of the drug, or by the use of antagonists such as nalorphine and naloxone, is milder than that from morphine or pethidine.

The development of tolerance to a drug's therapeutic action and cross-tolerance to other analgesics, is usually considered a liability for an analgesic. However, it has been utilized in the case of methadone. Methadone has been used for the maintenance of addicts who are dependent on heroin, morphine, etc.; this is directly due to the cross-tolerance effect of methadone. A possible disadvantage of methadone for this use is that it must be given daily to maintain tolerance, although some experts believe that a more frequent appearance of an addict at a medical treatment center is, in fact, advantageous. Alpha-*levo*- acetylmethadol (*a-l*-4,4-diphenyl-6-dimethylamino-3-acetoxyheptane, see Formula 24)[1] might be used if a longer acting methadone-like drug is found to be desirable in the future.

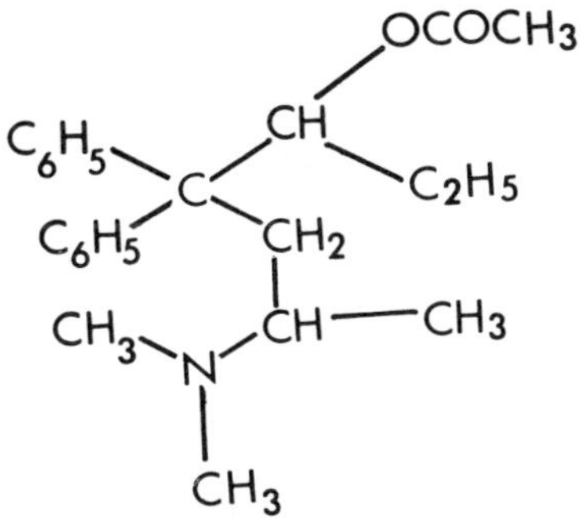

24

The acetylmethadols, exemplified by Formula 24, are obtained by acetylation of the reduction products of methadone. The formation of a new asymmetric carbon atom leads to additional isomers. Alpha-*l*-acetylmethadol can be obtained by a lithium aluminum hydride reduction of *d*-methadone, and subsequent acetylation of the newly formed secondary alcohol; the prefix alpha referring to the predominant product obtained. Chemical reduction of methadones (*via* sodium in propanol) gives, predominantly, *d*-betamethadol.[41]

Clinically, methadone is a very effective analgesic for moderate to severe pain both parenterally and orally;[38] it is more effective orally than pethidine, and is longer acting both orally and parenterally. The overall spectrum of activity *vs.* side effects is much more favorable for methadone than pethidine; its advantage over morphine lies in its totally synthetic character. If opium production could be totally halted worldwide any time in the future, a situation fervently desired by many, methadone would be one of the synthetic compounds which could serve as an effective replacement for the opium alkaloids until a new generation of agonist-antagonists replaces it. Naloxone production which is presently dependent on opium for its chemical source could be derived from plants in which alkaloidal biosynthesis stops at the thebaine stage; such plants are known.[42,43]

Only one narcotic analgesic methadone derivative, out of the several hundred known, has

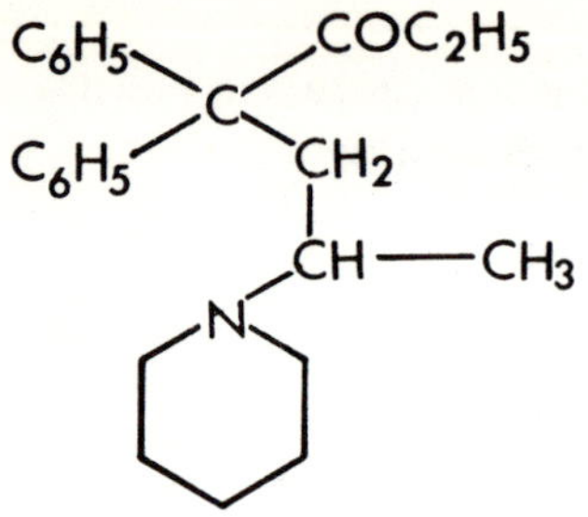

25

achieved some slight clinical utility, dipipanone (4,4-diphenyl-6-piperidino-3-heptanone, see Formula 25). In dipipanone the nitrogen atom has been tied into a piperidine ring. The drug is not available in the United States, but is utilized in Britain.[4] It displays a more rapid onset and shorter duration of action than methadone, and is useful for treating moderate pain at a 25mg dose level with minimal side effects; higher doses increase the side effects disproportionately.[38] Dipipanone, of course, has dependence liability.

Methadone meets the structure-activity requirements for narcotic analgesics, having a tertiary amine two carbon atoms away from a quaternary carbon which bears the aromatic ring. It, like pethidine, has a nonrigid structure and has received similar attention in attempts that have been made to relate its possible conformation with morphine. One such attempt, by Beckett, noted that interaction between the somewhat positive carbonyl carbon atom and the nitrogen's free electrons could aid in the retention of this conformation[44] (Figure 3).

However, a point still in some contention is whether the electrons on nitrogen are free. Methadone may exist at the active site, perhaps on a cell membrane, in cationic form. Initial transport at physiological pH to the active site should occur as the salt. Beckett considered this, and rearranged the proposed conformation of methadone to show interaction between the carbonyl oxygen's electrons and the positively charged nitrogen in what would now be a more favorable quasi-six-membered ring conformation[1] (Figure 4). All of this theory is subject to the same qualifications pointed out for the pethidine case. At the moment, such speculation serves pedagogical interest alone.

There are no reports in the literature on

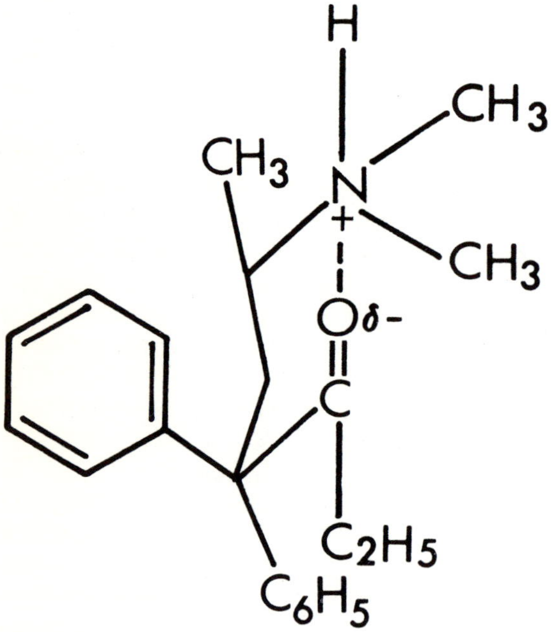

FIGURE 3. The presumed conformation of methadone (base) necessary for biological activity.

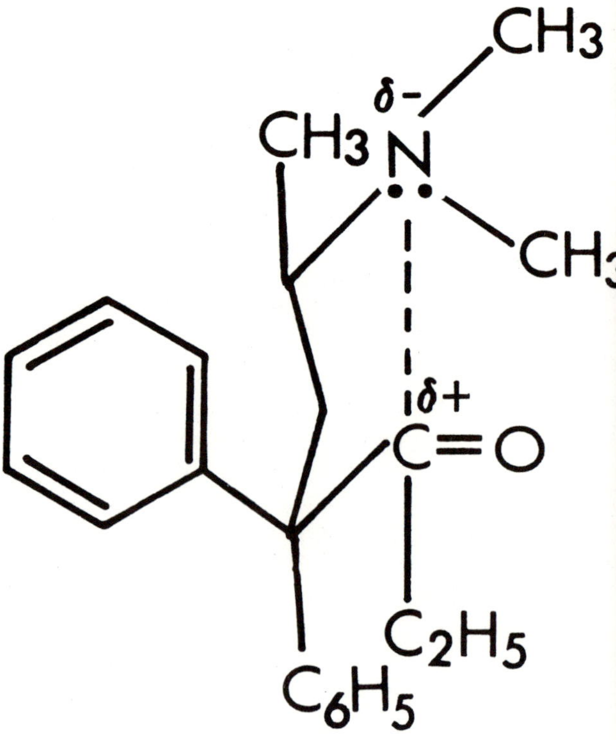

FIGURE 4. A presumed conformation of methadone (protonated) necessary for biological activity.

possible agonist-antagonist formation from the nonrigid methadone. It is likely that the *N*-allyl derivative of normethadone would be an analgesic similar to 1,3-diallylnorpethidine, rather than an antagonist. No doubt, such a synthesis will be reported in the near future.

THE MORPHINANS AND RELATIVES

Grewe's synthesis of *N*-methylmorphinan[45,46] (Formula 26) began the era of "simplified" morphines. Only a few clinically useful drugs have been obtained from research on morphinans. The hope of medicinal chemists that chemical dissection of the morphine molecule, rather than simple modification of the peripheral groups in morphine,[47,48] might result in the dissociation of analgesic activity from dependence liability began with the morphinans and finally culminated in E. L. May's 6,7-benzomorphans, which will be discussed in the next section.

N-Methylmorphinan can be looked at as a molecule of morphine from which the allylic alcohol moiety, the oxygen bridge and the phenolic hydroxyl group have been removed. Nevertheless, it retained one-fifth of the analgesic activity of morphine. This is a B/C *cis*-fused compound, as is morphine. The *trans*-fused diastereomeric *N*-methylisomorphinan is practically devoid of analgesic activity. When the phenolic hydroxyl group is incorporated in the molecule, to form racemorphan (*dl*-3-hydroxy-*N*-methylmorphinan, see Formula 27)[49-51] the analgesic potency becomes twice that of morphine in man. Thus, neither the presence of an oxygen bridge nor the allylic alcohol portion of morphine is necessary for its analgesic activity. The optical resolution of racemorphan, followed by etherification in the case of the *dextro* isomer, resulted in two clinically useful drugs; the analgesically active levorphanol (*levo*-3-hydroxy- *N*-methylmorphinan, *levo*, Formula 27) and the nonanalgesic, antitussive dextromethorphan[1] (*dextro*-3-methoxy-*N*-methylmorphinan, Formula 28).

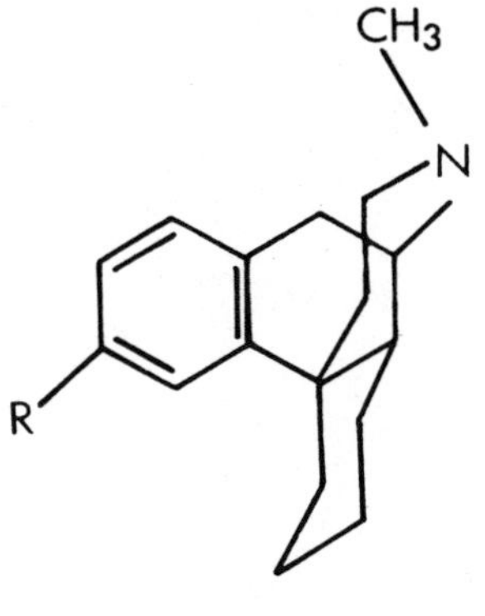

26 (R=H)
27 (R=OH)
28 (R=OCH3)

Levorphanol retains all of the analgesic activity of racemorphan and has, thus, four times the activity of morphine. It is highly effective orally. Levorphanol's side effects are very similar to those of morphine except for a decrease in the frequency of various types of spasms. The dependence liability of levorphanol is said to be as great as, and probably greater than that of morphine.[38]

It is of interest to note that a mixture of the *levo* (0.5mg) and *dextro* (0.5mg) isomers of 3-hydroxy-*N*-methylmorphinan does not raise the pain threshold to the point of the *levo* (0.5mg) compound alone. The activity of the admixture was expected, a priori, to be additive. The dimunition of analgesic activity of a *levo* compound by its *dextro* diastereomer pointed to a probable antagonistic behavior for the *dextro* compound.[38] This type of antagonism was noted by Slomka and associates.[52,53]

Analogs of levorphanol have been synthesized[1,3,54] but these compounds offer no advantage over the parent; its side effects do not appear to be eliminatable. However, the relatively rigid morphinan molecule does produce an agonist-antagonist. The *N*-desmethyl levorphanol has been converted to the *N*-allyl derivative [51] to form levallorphan (*l*-3-hydroxy-*N*-allylmorphinan, see Formula 29). Levallorphan displays analgesic activity in man equivalent to that of morphine, and is four times as potent as nalorphine in precipitating an abstinence syndrome in nonwithdrawn morphine-dependent monkeys.[55] Both levallorphan and nalorphine suffer from a psychotomimetic side effect which precludes general clinical use as analgesics. They are useful in counteracting respiratory depression caused by narcotic analgesics and precipitating a withdrawal syndrome in animals with narcotic analgesic dependence. It should be noted that levallorphan, nalorphine, and other agonist-antagonists themselves cause respiratory depression when administered to nondependent animals. This

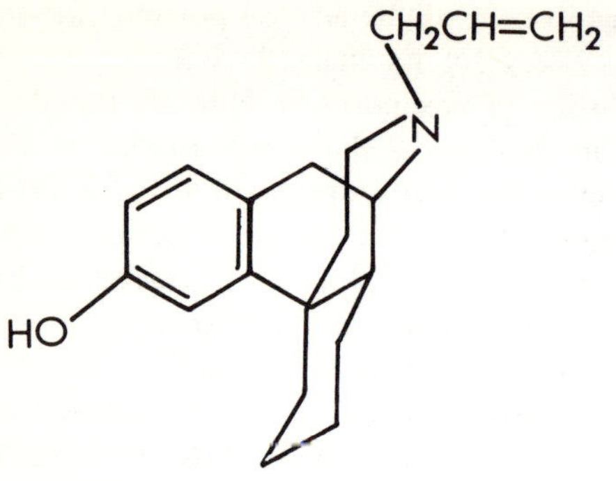

29

respiratory depression is moderate, and has never resulted in apnoea.[56]

THE 6,7-BENZOMORPHANS

6,7-Benzomorphans were initially synthesized at the National Institutes of Health by May and associates in 1954.[57] This work has been continued there and in various pharmaceutical companies and universities throughout the world. Widespread interest in this class of analgesic was engendered by the report that this was the first group of compounds in which there was evidence of complete dissociation of the hitherto undissociable twin parameters of analgesia and dependence liability.[58]

Evidence had been obtained from monkey species, an excellent prognosticator of dependence liability in man, for all of the previously discussed groups of analgesics. Unfortunately, with the benzomorphans, carryover to man was disappointing; evidently, monkeys are less sensitive to the benzomorphans, or they have somewhat different receptor sites for these analgesics than man. However, this series has produced drugs with lesser side effects than morphine, and agonist-antagonists have been prepared from them. One of these agonist-antagonists has attained considerable clinical utility as an analgesic. The search for others is the subject of much contemporary research.

The 6,7-benzomorphans are structurally related to the morphinans and, thus, morphine; they contain three out of the four rings of the morphinans. The C ring of the morphinan molecule is split to form alkyl substituents at what are now referred to as the C-5 and C-9 positions on the benzomorphan molecule. Actually, a large variety of substituents have been placed in these positions, including some aromatic moieties. Substituents at the 9-position can be oriented either towards the aromatic ring, denoted as alpha, or towards the nitrogen atom, the latter denoting the beta conformation. These are shown as R4 and R3 for the alpha and beta isomers, respectively, in Formulas 30 to 35. Almost invariably the beta compounds have greater analgesic activity than the corresponding alpha compounds. However, their toxicity is usually correspondingly greater.

The only benzomorphan to have achieved

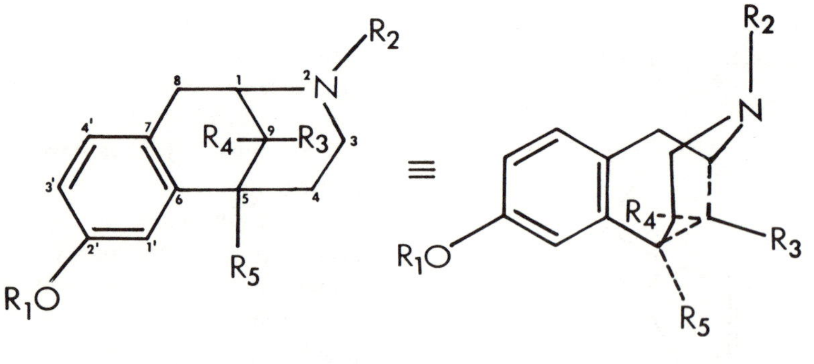

30 ($R_1=R_3=H$; $R_2=CH_2CH_2C_6H_5$; $R_4=R_5=CH_3$)
31 ($R_1=R_3=H$; $R_2=CH_2CH=C(CH_3)_2$; $R_4=R_5=CH_3$)
32 ($R_1=R_3=H$; $R_2=CH_2$–◁ ; $R_4=R_5=CH_3$)
33 ($R_1=R_3=H$; $R_2=CH_3$; $R_4=R_5=C_2H_5$)
34 ($R_1=R_3=H$; $R_2=R_4=R_5=CH_3$)
35 ($R_1=R_3=R_4=R_5=H$; $R_2=CH_3$)

clinical utility, except for the agonist-antagonists, is phenazocine[59] (α-2′-hydroxy-5,9-dimethyl-2-phenethyl-6,7,-benzomorphan, see Formula 30). This drug is available in Britain, no longer in the United States since its abuse potential in man precluded general availability.

Phenazocine is an effective analgesic both orally and parenterally for almost all types of severe pain, at about one third of the comparable dose of morphine. The side effects are fewer than with morphine and there is less circulatory depression. The development of tolerance is slower,[60] and the dependence liability of phenazocine is less than with morphine.[1] Nevertheless, although few untoward effects were observed in the treatment of chronic or postoperative pain in man in clinical practice,[61] the potential for abuse exists and the drug has been placed on the controlled narcotics list. It has been said that the synthetic phenazocine, together with methadone and, perhaps, levorphanol could be used to replace morphine, codeine, et al., if opium production ceased.

The fact that the benzomorphans as a class did not induce dependence liability in animal species, and the improvement of the activity vs. side effects spectrum with phenazocine over that seen with morphine, pethidine, et al., prompted an extensive effort to develop agonist-antagonists in this series. All of the moieties listed in the Introduction which have been found to confer antagonistic properties to analgetics have been used in various benzomorphans and a few of them have produced interesting drugs.[61]

Pentazocine (*dl*-α-5,9-dimethyl-2-(3,3-dimethylallyl)-2′-hydroxy-6,7-benzomorphan, Formula 31)[62] is the only clinically available agonist-antagonist in general use as an analgesic. In general, the dimethylallyl group (3-methyl-2-butenyl) produces weak antagonists when present on the nitrogen atom. Pentazocine is no exception to that rule, having only one fortieth the activity of nalorphine in precipitating an abstinence syndrome in nonwithdrawn morphine-dependent monkeys. It is not a particularly powerful analgesic, having perhaps one third the analgesic potency of morphine. In terms of its overall spectrum of activity vs. side effects it appears to be a good, clinically useful analgesic. Pentazocine has a low frequency of side effects, little respiratory depression, and very low abuse potential.[63] Although some drug-seeking behavior has been observed and a few cases of abuse have been recorded,[64] these have been insufficient, so far, to necessitate its restriction as a controlled narcotic.

A second, rather interesting agonist-antagonist, with little clinical utility due to its psychotomimetic side effect, is cyclazocine (dl-α-2-cyclopropylmethyl-5,9-dimethyl-2′-hydroxy-6,7-benzomorphan, see Formula 32). Cyclazocine has 140 times the antagonistic activity of pentazocine and 40 times the analgesic potency of morphine in man. Tolerance does develop to its subjective effects and cross-tolerance to the effect of nalorphine, but tolerance does not develop to its antagonism.[64] Interestingly, drug-seeking behavior was not observed upon abrupt withdrawal of cyclazocine after chronic administration to individuals prone to drug abuse, and the abstinence syndrome of the specific agonist-antagonist type was borne with equanimity.[64] Cyclazocine is under study as a rehabilitation agent and deterrent to illicit use of narcotics, in conjunction with naloxone.

Antagonistic behavior of a *dextro* isomer towards an analgesic *levo* diastereomer was mentioned in the morphinan series of compounds. May and Eddy[65] optically resolved α-*dl*-5,9-diethyl-2′-hydroxy-2-methyl-6,7-benzomorphan (etazocine, Formula 33) to see whether a similar effect could be observed. The benzomorphan was remarkable in that not only was the *levo* isomer nearly twice as analgesically effective (equivalent to morphine) as the racemate, but it precipitated abstinence of intermediate intensity in nonwithdrawn morphine-dependent monkeys. This was the first *N*-methyl analgesic to show nalorphine-like activity in animal species. The analogous *dextro* isomer had codeine-like analgesic activity and an intermediate capacity to support morphine dependence in monkeys; the latter indicated that the type of antipodal antagonsim which was observed with the morphinans (levorphanol and its *dextro* stereomer) was also occurring with the benzomorphan. The racemic benzomorphan (*dl*-Formula 33) displayed low dependence liability in monkeys.

The nalorphine-like antagonist property of Formula 33, observed in monkeys, does not appear to carry over completely to man. Trials with individuals physically dependent on narcotic analgesics appear to indicate that the compound does not precipitate an abstinence syndrome and these individuals do not seem to dislike it.[66] However, α-*l*-2′-hydroxy-2,5,9-trimethyl-6,7 benzomorphan (*l*-metazocine, Formula 34), equivalent to morphine in treating postoperative pain, is said to be little better than a placebo in supporting morphine dependence in man, but can produce morphine-like effects in postaddicts.[65]

Other benzomorphans have been optically resolved and display a similar pattern of effect,[3,67] although not all *levo* benzomorphans are agonist-antagonists.[68] The first, and only, *N*-methyl racemate to show nalorphine-like antagonist behavior was *dl*-2′-hydroxy-2-methyl-6,7-benzomorphan (Formula 35); both optical isomers (antipodes) of Formula 35 are good antagonists of morphine in monkeys. This is a nonquaternary carbon compound;[69,70] both the racemate and the *levo* isomer have pethidine-like analgesic activity in mice, the *dextro* isomer has half of the activity of codeine. These compounds may be examined for clinical utility in the near future.

CONCLUSION

The separation of dependence liability of the opiate type from analgesic activity has been achieved with angonist-antagonists in several series of compounds. These agonist-antagonists have great potential as a future generation of clinically useful analgesics. Some of these show a low frequency of side effects, a little respiratory depression (which has not been life-threatening, as it may be with the narcotic analgesics), and low abuse potential. Their dependence liability has been described[55,64] as a specific opiate antagonist type, the abstinence syndrome being qualitatively and quantitatively different than that from the narcotic analgesics although some symptoms are common to both. However, agonist-antagonists which show strong clinical analgesia always appear to have a concomitant psychotomimetic potential. If the analgesic effect of the agonist-antagonist is weak, this psychotomimetic effect is minimal; it may become pronounced if higher doses are given. Although it is believed that the psychotomimetic side effect will be separable from the analgesia provided by these compounds,[71] this has yet to be proven in any but the weakest antagonists. Future research will likely be very much concerned with the dissociation of this new side effect. Medicinal chemists have not quite jumped from the frying pan into the fire; quite satisfactory, albeit somewhat weaker, analgesics may be forthcoming from this group which have low psychotomimetic potential. These may not be the "perfect" analgesics we all seek; we may have to be satisfied with a happy medium.

The structure-activity correlations which have been presented have ex post facto use for purposes of classification and, indeed, satisfactorily correlate most clinically acceptable analgesics presently available. However, this is most likely a fortuitous happening. Too many effective analgesics do not fit this classification scheme although, admittedly, these have not met with commercial success, as yet. A better structure-activity analysis would be most desirable so that the activity of analgesics might be predicted; a start in this direction[72,73] has been made using partition coefficients, steric, and electronic factors in the Hansch program.[74] The partition coefficients simulate transport phenomena. These data are submitted to regression analysis. Thus far, only the benzomorphans have been treated in this way.[72] The equations which can be obtained from this approach equate biological activity with physicochemical parameters and are being used to predict the biological activity of new benzomorphans.

What is most lacking, and badly needed, is definitive knowledge of the biomacromolecular systems with which analgesics of various types interact. The suggestion that there is one common receptor site for analgesics,[75] or at least two active sites,[64,76,77] is of great interest but it is insufficient for theoretical evaluation of potential analgesics or evaluation of the macromolecular systems involved.

Acknowledgment

I would like to thank Drs. K. W. Bentley and G. F. Blane, Reckitt & Colman Limited, Hull, England, and Dr. E. L. May, N. I. H., for allowing me to preview a copy of their papers given at the Symposium on Agonist and Antagonist Actions of Narcotic Analgesic Drugs in Aberdeen, Scotland, 1971.

I would especially like to thank Drs. E. L. May and N. B. Eddy, Consultant, N. I. H., Bethesda, Md., for their invaluable recollections about the history of various analgesics, and their opinions on the current research in the field.

REFERENCES

1. de Stevens, G., Ed., *Analgetics*, Vol. 5, Academic Press, New York, 1965.

2. Janssen, P. A. J., Diphenylpropylamines, Hellerbach, J., Schnider, O., Besendorf, H., and Pellmont, B., Morphinans, in *Synthetic Analgesics*, Part I and II, Pergamon Press, New York, 1960, 1966.

3. Jacobson, A. E., May, E. L., and Sargent, L. J., Analgetics, in *Medicinal Chemistry*, Part II, 3rd ed., Burger, A., Ed., Wiley-Interscience, New York, 1970.

4. *Estimated World Requirements of Narcotic Drugs in 1971*, International Narcotics Control Board, United Nations, New York, 1970.

5. Weiss, U., Derivatives of morphine. I. 14-Hydroxydihydromorphinone, *J. Amer. Chem. Soc.*, 77, 5891, 1955.

6. Lister, R. E., The toxicity of some of the newer narcotic analgesics, *J. Pharm. Pharmacol.*, 18, 364, 1966.

7. Freund, M. and Speyer, E., Darstellung von 3 isomeren Reduktionsprodukten des Oxykodeinons, *Chem. Zentr.*, 88, Bd. 1, 716, 1917.

8. Small, L. F. and Lutz, R. E., *Chemistry of the Opium Alkaloids*, Supplement 103 to the Public Health Reports, U. S. Government Printing Office, Washington, D. C., 1932.

9. Mannich, C. and Löwenheim, H., Two new reduction products of codeine, *Arch. Pharm.*, 258, 295, 1920.

10. Knoll & Co. Chemische Fabrik, Darstellung von Ketoderivaten der Morphinreihe, *Chem. Zentr.*, 94, Bd. 2, 916, 1923.

11. McCawley, E. L., Hart, E. R., and March, D. F., The preparation of N-allylnormorphine, *J. Amer. Chem. Soc.*, 63, 314, 1941.

12. Weijlard, J. and Erickson, A. E., *N*-Allylnormorphine, *J. Amer. Chem. Soc.*, 64, 869, 1943.

13. Hart, E. R., *N*-Allyl-norcodeine and *N*-allyl-normorphine, *J. Pharmacol. Exp. Ther.*, 72, 19, 1941.

14. Pohl, J., Uber das *N*-allylnorcodein, einen antagonisten des morphin, *Z. Exp. Pathol. Ther.*, 17, 370, 1914.

15. Hart, E. R. and McCawley, E. L., The pharmacology of *N*-allylnormorphine as compared with morphine, *J. Pharmacol. Exp. Ther.*, 82, 339, 1944.

16. Unna, K., Antagonistic effect of *N*-allylnormorphine upon morphine, *J. Pharmacol. Exp. Ther.*, 79, 27, 1943.

17. Eddy, N. B., The chemopharmacological approach to the addiction problem, *Public Health Rept.* (U.S.), 78, 673, 1963.

18. Lasagna, L. and Beecher, H. K., The analgesic effectiveness of nalorphine and nalorphine-morphine combinations in man, *J. Pharmacol. Exp. Ther.*, 112, 356, 1954.

19. Keats, A. S. and Telford, J., Nalorphine, a potent analgesic in man, *J. Pharmacol. Exp. Ther.*, 117, 190, 1956.

20. Lewenstein, M. J. and Fishman, J., Morphine derivative, U.S. Patent 3,254,088, 1966.

21. Kallos, T. and Smith, T. C., Naloxone reversal of pentazocine-induced respiratory depression, *J.A.M.A.*, 204, 932, 1968.

22. Bentley, K. W. and Thomas, A. F., The morphine-thebaine group of alkaloids. Part VI. The condensation of thebaine with dienophiles, *J. Chem. Soc.*, 1863, 1956.

23. Bentley, K. W. and Hardy, D. G., New potent analgesics in the morphine series, *Proc. Chem. Soc.*, 220, 1963.

24. Bentley, K. W. and associates, Novel analgesics and molecular rearrangements in the morphine-thebaine group. I. to VI., *J. Amer. Chem. Soc.*, 89, 3267, 1967.

25. Blane, G. F. and Robbie, D. S., Trial of etorphine hydrochloride (M 99 Reckitt) in carcinoma pain: preliminary report, *Brit. J. Pharmacol.*, 39, 252P, 1970.

26. Blane, G. F., Compounds of the oripavine series, in *Agonists and Antagonists,* Kosterlitz, H., Villarreal, J., and Collyer, H.O.J., Eds., Macmillan Press, New York, in press.

27. Bentley, K. W. and Lewis, J. W., The relationship between structure and activity in the 6,14-endoethenotetrahydrothebaine series of analgesics, in *Agonists and Antagonists,* Kosterlitz, H., Villarreal, J., and Collyer, H.O.J., Eds., Macmillan Press, New York, in press.

28. Eisleb, O. and Schaumann, O., Dolantin, ein neuartiges Spasmolyticum und Analgetickum, *Deutsch. Med. Wschr.*, 65, 967, 1939.

29. All of the drug names used are, wherever possible, World Health Organization International non-proprietary names. Generic names are the same as these international names with the exception of pethidine, whose generic name is meperidine. A few common drug names are listed in Table 1. A more complete list of common names is given in reference 4, pg. XIII.

30. Kartha, G., Ahmed, F. R., and Barnes, W. H., The crystal and molecular structure of *dl*-alphaprodine hydrochloride. Addendum, *Acta Crystallogr.*, 14, 93, 1961, and 13, 525, 1960.

31. Beckett, A. H. and Casy, A. F., Synthetic analgesics: stereochemical considerations, *J. Pharm. Pharmacol.*, 6, 986, 1954.

32. Jost, P. and Griffith, O. H., Electron spin resonance and the spin labelling method, in *Methods in Pharmacology,* Vol. 2, Chignell, C., Ed., Appleton-Century-Crofts, New York, in press.

33. Fischer, J. J. and Jost, M. C., Nuclear magnetic resonance studies of drug-receptor interactions, *Molec. Pharmacol.*, 5, 420, 1969.

34. Bradbury, E. M. and Crane-Robinson, C., High resolution nuclear magnetic resonance studies of biopolymers, *Nature,* 220, 1079, 1968.

35. *Fluorescence Antibody Techniques and their Applications,* Kawamura, A., Ed., University Book Press, Baltimore, 1969.

36. Goldman, M., *Fluorescence Antibody Methods,* Academic Press, New York, 1969.

37. Weijlard, J., Orahovats, P. D., Sullivan, A. P., Jr., Purdue, G., Heath, F. K., and Pfister, K., III, A new synthetic analgesic, *J. Amer. Chem. Soc.,* 78, 2342, 1956.

38. Eddy, N. B., Halbach, H., and Braenden, O. J., Synthetic substances with morphine-like effect, *Bull. WHO,* 17, 569, 1957.

39. Kleiderer, E. C., Rice, J. B., Conquest, V., and Williams, J. H., Report No. PP—981, Office of the Publication Board, U. S. Department of Commerce, Washington, D. C., 1945.

40. Bockmühl, M. and Ehrhart, G., Über eine neue Klasse von spasmolytisch und analgetisch wirkenden Verbindungen, *Justus Liebigs Ann. Chem.,* 561, 52, 1948.

41. Eddy, N. B., May, E. L., and Mosettig, E., Chemistry and pharmacology of the methadols and acetylmethadols, *J. Org. Chem.,* 17, 321, 1952.

42. Sharghi, N. and Lalezari, I., *Papaver bracteatum* Lindl., a highly rich source of thebaine, *Nature,* 213, 1244, 1967.

43. Neubauer, Von D. and Mothes, K., Über *Papaver bracteatum, Planta Med.,* 11, 387, 1963.

44. Beckett, A. H., Analgesics and their antagonists: Some steric and chemical considerations, *J. Pharm. Pharmacol.,* 8, 848, 1956.

45. Grewe, R., Das Problem der Morphin-synthese, *Naturwissenschaften,* 33, 333, 1946.

46. Grewe, R. and Mondon, A., Synthesen in der Phenanthren-Reihe, VI. Mitteil.: Synthese des Morphinans, *Chem. Ber.*, 81, 279, 1948.

47. Small, L. F., Eddy, N. B., Mosettig, E., and Himmelsbach, C. K., Studies on drug addiction with special reference to chemical structure of opium derivatives and allied synthetic substances and their physiological action, Supplement No. 138 to Public Health Reports, U. S. Government Printing Office, Washington, D. C., 1938.

48. Villarreal, J. E., Recent advances in the pharmacology of morphine-like drugs, in *Advances in Mental Science*, Vol. 2 of *Drug Dependence*, Harris, R. T., Schuster, C. R., and McIsaac, W., Eds., University of Texas Press, Houston, 1970.

49. Schnider, O. and Grüssner, A., Synthese von Oxy-morphinanen, *Helv. Chim. Acta*, 32, 821, 1949.

50. Grewe, R., Pohlmann, H., and Schnoor, M., A new synthesis of morphinan, *Chem. Ber.*, 84, 527, 1951.

51. Schnider, O. and Hellerbach, J., Synthese von Morphinanen, *Helv. Chim. Acta*, 33, 1437, 1950.

52. Slomka, M. B. and Gross, E. G., An evaluation of the analgetic activity of the Dromoran isomers, *Proc. Soc. Exp. Biol. Med.*, 81, 548, 1952.

53. Slomka, M. B. and Sleeth, C. K., Analgetic activity of optical isomers of 3-hydroxy-*N*-methylmorphinan and 6-dimethylamino-4,4-diphenyl-3-heptanone, *Proc. Soc. Exp. Biol. Med.*, 84, 532, 1953.

54. Fraser, H. F. and Harris, L. S., Narcotic and narcotic antagonist analgesics, *Ann. Rev. Pharmacol.*, 7, 277, 1967.

55. Eddy, N. B. and Jacobson, A. E., Agonists-antagonists, *Curr. Med. Dialog*, 38, 330, 1971.

56. Keats, A. S. and Telford, J., Studies of analgesic drugs. X. Respiratory effects of narcotic antagonists, *J. Pharmacol. Exp. Ther.*, 151, 126, 1966.

57. May, E. L. and Murphy, J. G., Structures related to morphine. III. Synthesis of an analog of *N*-methylmorphinan, *J. Org. Chem.*, 20, 257, 1955.

58. Ager, J. H., Fullerton, S. E., and May, E. L., Structures related to morphine. XXV. 5-Propyl- and 5,9-dipropyl-6,7-benzomorphans and a pharmacologic summary, *J. Med. Chem.*, 6, 322, 1963.

59. May, E. L. and Eddy, N. B., Structures related to morphine. XII. (±)-2′-Hydroxy-5,9-dimethyl-2-phenethyl-6,7-benzomorphan (NIH 7519) and its optical forms, *J. Org. Chem.*, 24, 1435, 1959.

60. Fraser, H. F. and Isbell, H., Human pharmacology and addiction liabilities of phenazocine and levophenacylmorphan, *Bull. Narc.*, 12 (2), 15, 1960.

61. Eddy, N. B. and May, E. L., 6,7-Benzomorphans, in *Synthetic Analgesics*, Part IIB, Pergamon Press, New York, 1966.

62. Archer, S., Albertson, N. F., Harris, L. S., Pierson, A. K., and Bird, J. G., Pentazocine. Strong analgesics and analgesic antagonists in the benzomorphan series, *J. Med. Chem.*, 7, 123, 1964.

63. Jasinski, D. R., Martin, W. R., and Hoeldtke, R. D., Effects of short-and long-term administration of pentazocine in man, *Clin. Pharmacol. Ther.*, 11, 385, 1970.

64. Eddy, N. B. and Martin, W. R., Drug dependence of specific opiate antagonist type, *Pharmakopsychiatrie Neuro-Psychopharmakologie*, 3, 73, 1970.

65. May, E. L. and Eddy, N. B., Interesting pharmacological properties of the optical isomers of α-5,9-diethyl-2′-hydroxy-2-methyl-6,7-benzomorphan, *J. Med. Chem.*, 9, 851, 1966.

66. Jasinski, D. R. and Mansky, P., private communication, 1970.

67. Ager, J. H., Jacobson, A. E., and May, E. L., Separation of morphine-like effects by optical resolution. Levo isomers as strong analgetics and narcotic antagonists, *J. Med. Chem.*, 12, 288, 1969.

68. May, E. L. and Takeda, M., Optical isomers of miscellaneous strong analgetics, *J. Med. Chem.*, 13, 805, 1970.

69. Kanematsu, K., Parfitt, R. T., Jacobson, A. E., Ager, J. H., and May, E. L., Synthesis of 6,7-benzomorphan from 4-phenylpyridine, *J. Amer. Chem. Soc.*, 90, 1064, 1968.

70. Kanematsu, K., Takeda, M., Jacobson, A. E., and May, E. L., Synthesis of 6,7-benzomorphan and related nonquaternary carbon structures with marked analgetic activity, *J. Med. Chem.*, 12, 405, 1969.

71. Archer, S. and Harris, L. S., Narcotic antagonists, in *Progr. Drug Res.*, Jucker, E., Ed., Berkhaüsen Verlag, Basel, 1965.

72. Jacobson, A. E., unpublished data

73. Kaufmann, S. J., Jacobson, A. E., and Raub, W. F., Computer-assisted data management in Medicinal Chemistry - The use of a general purpose text editor, *J. Chem. Doc.*, 10, 248, 1970.

74. Hansch, C., A quantitative approach to biochemical structure-activity relationships, *Acc. Chem. Res.*, 2, 232, 1969.

75. Grumbach, L. and Chernov, H. I., The analgesic effect of opiate-opiate antagonist combinations in the rat, *J. Pharmacol. Exp. Ther.*, 149, 385, 1965.

76. Martin, W. R., Opioid antagonists, *Pharmacol. Rev.*, 19, 463, 1967.

77. Lewis, J. W., Bentley, K. W., and Cowan, A., Narcotic Analgesics and Antagonists, *Ann. Rev. Pharmacol.*, 11, 241, 1971.

BARBITURATES AND MINOR TRANQUILIZERS

S. Stolman

TABLE OF CONTENTS

INTRODUCTION

In view of the limited information available on the chemistry of the nonbarbiturate hypnosedatives such as paraldehyde, chloral hydrate, methyprylon, ethinamate, and glutethimide which are capable of causing tolerance, physical and psychological dependence, these agents will not be discussed. For a comprehensive review of the pharmacology and pharmacokinetics of the nonbarbiturate hypnosedatives, the reader is referred to the paper presented by Bush.[1]

In addition, no attempt was made to relate the addiction liability of a homologous series of compounds to a structural modification of a parent nucleus because of 1) the lack of experimental data and 2) the inability to demonstrate a relationship between the intensity of withdrawal reactions and dosage.

This chapter will be devoted primarily to a discussion of the physicochemical properties, synthesis, and structure-activity-relationships of the barbiturates, 1,3-propanodiols, and benzodiazepines.

CHEMISTRY OF CNS DEPRESSANTS

Barbiturates

Synthesis

The first barbituric acid derivative that was demonstrated to possess central nervous system depressant activity, was barbital, synthesized by Fischer and von Mering in 1903.[2]

Barbituric acid, like the monoureides, may be synthesized by a condensation of urea with malonic acid (see Figure 1).[3] The hexahydropyrimidine nucleus of barbituric acid contains three carbonyl groups which are capable of undergoing tautomeric transformations and four labile hydrogen atoms which may be substituted with different groups. To obtain barbituric acids with central nervous system depressant effects, the two labile hydrogens at the number 5 carbon may be replaced with either a straight or branched alkyl chain, an allyl, phenyl, or heterocyclic group.[1] Unlike the hydrogens at carbon number 5, the hydrogen atom at the number 1 nitrogen is substituted less readily.[4-6] Therefore, if a 5-monosubstituted barbituric acid is exposed to an alkyl substitution reaction as illustrated in Figure 2, the labile hydrogen at carbon 5 would be replaced first.

These reactions are widely used for the synthesis of N- or C-substituted barbituric acids because 1) the process occurs under gentle conditions, 2) provides good yields of the desired product, and 3) serves as a convenient procedure for introducing an unsaturated free radical to the barbiturate nucleus.[4-6]

Physicochemical Properties

As previously mentioned, the hexahydropyrimidine nucleus of barbituric acids contains three carbonyl groups which are capable of undergoing tautomeric transformations with an equilibrium existing between the lactam (keto) and lactim (enol) moieties (Figure 3).[2] In solution monosubstitued and disubstituted barbituric acid derivatives are considered to undergo only single enolization. For example, 1,3 disubstituted barbituric acid may exist in the following moieties (Figure 4).[7-9] The lactam moiety, stable in acidic solutions, is in equilibrium with lactim A and B, which are stable in an alkaline medium.[8] In the crystalline state, barbituric acid is in the lactam form. This was based on infrared spectral data which showed no absorption bands indicative of a -C=C-or-C=N- linkage, whereas an intense absorption band occurred for carbonyl groups.[1]

In general, the barbituric acid derivatives are sparingly soluble in water and readily soluble in nonpolar organic solvents like chloroform.[9-13] The sodium salts of these barbiturates which are

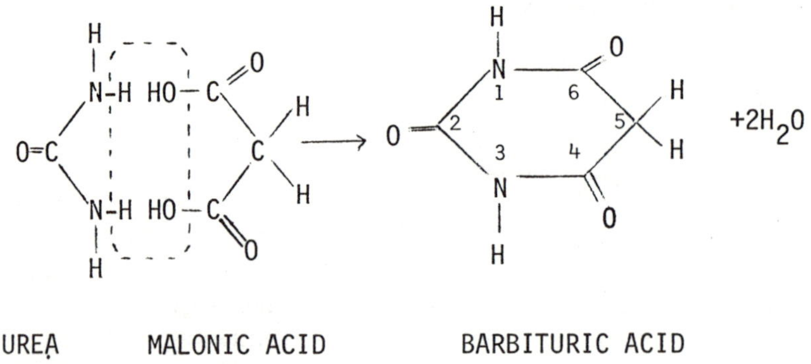

FIGURE 1. The synthesis of barbituric acid by a condensation reaction. (From Goodman, L.S. and Gilman, A., Eds., *The Pharmacological Basis of Therapeutics*, 4th ed., McMillan Co., New York, 1970, 99. With permission.)

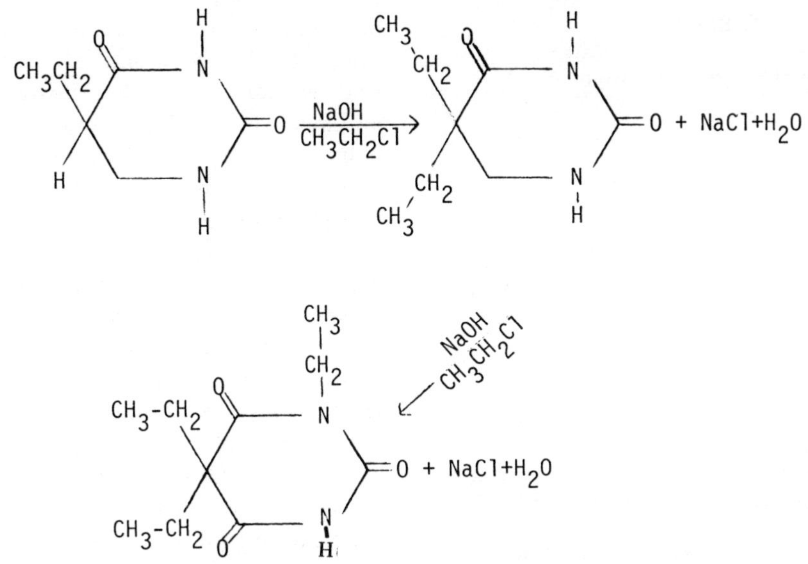

FIGURE 2. The synthesis of a 5-disubstituted barbituric acid derivative by an alkyl substitution reaction.

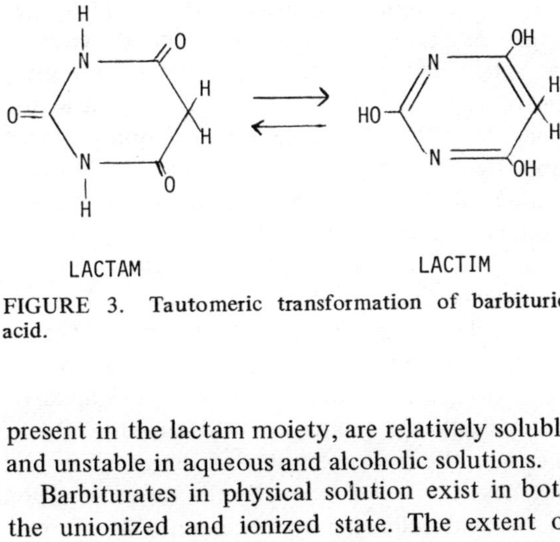

FIGURE 3. Tautomeric transformation of barbituric acid.

present in the lactam moiety, are relatively soluble and unstable in aqueous and alcoholic solutions.

Barbiturates in physical solution exist in both the unionized and ionized state. The extent of ionization of these weak acids is not only dependent on their pK_a, but the pH of their solution. Most barbiturates have a pK_a ranging from 7.4 to 8.0.[3] At a physiologic pH these compounds are primarily in the nonionized moiety which, unlike the ionized form, is highly lipid soluble. The high degree of lipid solubility in non-polar solvents is a characteristic feature of agents that have a pharmacologic effect on the central nervous system. As seen from the data presented in Table 1, the hypnotic activity of these agents is related to the degree of lipid solubility. Thiopental, an ultra short-acting agent used clinically as an intravenous anesthetic agent, is more lipid soluble than the agents listed in Table 1. This factor seemingly is attributed to the replacement of the number 2 carbon in the barbiturate nucleus with a sulfur atom.[13,15] The high degree of lipid solubility of this compound might be

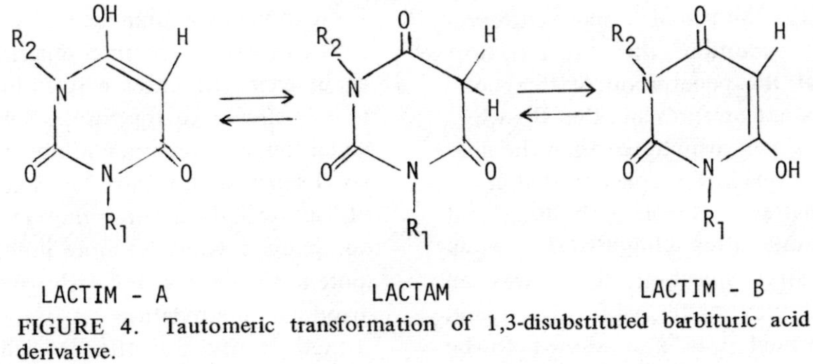

FIGURE 4. Tautomeric transformation of 1,3-disubstituted barbituric acid derivative.

TABLE 1

Physicochemical Properties of Barbiturates[14]

Compound	Log P[a]	pK_a	Log 1/C[b]
Barbital	0.65	7.75	3.09
Phenobarbital	1.42	7.26	3.46
Probarbital	0.95	7.90	3.30
Butabarbital	1.45	––	3.63
Butethal	1.65	7.76	3.72
Amobarbital	1.95	7.78	3.75

[a]Log P refers to the log of the lipid solubility ratio of these compounds in octanol : water.

[b]Log 1/C refers to the log of 1 divided by the drug concentration that produces a hypnotic effect at the 50% level.

(From Hansch, C., *J. Med. Chem.*, 10, 745, 1967. With permission.)

responsible for its rapid onset and short duration of action.[16] Goldstein and Aronow [17] have shown that the lightening of thiopental-induced anesthesia may be attributed to a redistribution of the compound from brain to other fluids and tissues and not due to the rate of biotransformation. In 1950 Butler[16] suggested that the lipid-to-water partition coefficient might be the physical factor for determining the rate of entrance of barbituric acids into brain. However, this physicochemical factor cannot always be utilized as an explanation of redistribution for all drugs, since ethanol can equilibrate with brain more rapidly than barbital, but has a lower partition coefficient than the latter compound.[16]

Roth and Barlow[18] reported that circulation, expressed as regional blood flow, is not decisive in influencing the entry or accumulation of exogenous substances in brain. The only compounds that have been demonstrated to be circulation-dependent are the extremely lipid soluble agents, thiopental and trifluoroiodomethane. In addition, these investigators demonstrated that the penetration of thiopental into cat brain was not uniform and that the white matter was more slowly penetrated than the gray matter. Thiopental was highly concentrated in the cortical gray matter, geniculate bodies, and colliculi, one minute after administration while thirty minutes after injection there was an equilibrium among gray matter, white matter, and plasma. Phenobarbital was also shown to be distributed nonuniformly in a fashion similar to thiopental in the brains of mature cats. These findings indicate that the penetration of this drug is hindered by white matter. However, in the brains of kittens, the primordial white areas were permeated more readily by phenobarbital. This was probobly due to an incomplete formation of laminated myelin sheaths. Goldberg and colleagues[19] also conducted experiments on the regional penetration characteristics of phenobarbital under conditions of respiratory acidosis (plasma pH 6.81) and alkalosis (plasma pH 7.68). Under the condition of hypercapnia, the penetration of this compound in brain was increased, while it was reduced under conditions of hypocapnia. Hypercapnia causes a higher concentration of the drug in white matter than gray matter, whereas the reverse situation occurs in a respiratory alkalotic state.

Structure-Activity-Relationships

Those barbituric acid derivatives which are active as central nervous system depressants are subdivided into four major categories: ultra short-, short-, intermediate-, and long-acting agents.[1,3,20,21] The duration of action of these subclasses is dependent on the substituent present at C-5 and N-1 of the hexahydropyrimidine nucleus.[1,3,22] If the two hydrogens at C-5 are replaced with two ethyl groups, the long-acting barbiturate barbital is formed. The replacement of one of the ethyl groups on this compound with an increasing lengthened straight or branched alkyl chain, aryl, or cycloalkenyl group up to 10 carbon atoms, increases the lipid solubility of the molecule and potency.[1,3,20] For example, the onset of action of barbital following an intravenous injection in mice is 22 minutes in contrast to a 2 minute induction elicited by butethal, which has an *n*-butyl group in place of an ethyl group at C-5.[1] Even though the branched alkyl substituents may have variable effects in comparison to the straight chain ones, the latter may induce pharmacologic effects similar to the former substituents with an equal number of carbon atoms. Furthermore, if an alkyl substituent is introduced at carbon 5 in place of an ethyl group, the resulting series of compounds would be more lipid soluble and more potent than the ethyl derivatives.[1] On the other hand, a methylation at the 3 position of a 1-methylbutlyl substituent will convert a CNS depressant derivative into a convulsant agent.[23-25] In addition, lengthening of the alkyl group at one or both nitrogens of the barbiturate nucleus will provide compounds that stimulate the CNS, as well as increasing the length of the alkyl chain at carbon 5 beyond 6 carbon atoms.[25]

Minor Tranquilizers

Pharmacology

The newer minor tranquilizers, such as the propanediol and benzodiazepine derivatives, were primarily introduced into clinical medicine in the 1950's to replace the barbiturates for their anxiolytic and sedative effects.[26] Like the barbiturates and alcohol, the minor tranquilizers are frequently abused and have been shown to cause tolerance to most of their effects upon repeated administration, physical dependence, and psychological dependence.[27]

Anticonvulsant Effects

Meprobamate, a 1,3-propanediol derivative, like many of the nonselective central nervous system depressants, has the ability to abolish convulsions by virtue of depressing the motor cortex.[26] The dose of this agent that is anticonvulsant produces a drug-induced sleep, while an agent like phenobarbital terminates convulsions at a dose that is approximately 1/3 the hypnotic dose.

The 1,4-benzodiazepines are capable of affording protection against pentylenetetrazol and strychnine-induced and electroshock-induced seizures in mice, rats, rabbits, cats, and monkeys.[28] These agents appear to have a broad spectrum of anitconvulsive properties in man, particularly petit mal and psychomotor seizures.[28,29] In the cat, nitrazepam was shown to be nine times more potent than diazepam, which was approximately four times as potent as chlordiazepoxide against pentylenetetrazol-induced seizures when given orally.[30] Unlike meprobamate, these agents do not produce hypnotic effects at the anticonvulsant dosage.

Muscle Relaxant Effects

In addition to anticonvulsant properties, the propanediol and benzodiazepine derivatives are capable of producing muscle relaxation which seemingly emanates from an inhibition of the internuncial neurons within the spinal cord.[26,31] Mephenesin, unlike meprobamate, has a shorter onset and duration of action, and is less effective when given by the enteral route of administration.[26] Chlordiazepoxide and diazepam, on the other hand, are more potent than meprobamate.[26,29,31-35] Even though these produce hypotonia in mice, rats, cats, and monkeys,[35] the muscle relaxation that occurs with the latter compound was qualitatively different from the former agent. Chlordiazepoxidized cats appeared relaxed when suspended by the scruff of the neck, in contrast to the protracted hindlimbs and stiff muscles noted in the meprobamatized animals.[31]

Taming Effects

The widespread use of the newer minor tranquilizing agents for the treatment of anxiety in man primarily arose from experimentation with monkeys.[36,37] These compounds have been used by veterinarians for quieting hard to handle animals and the taming effect of chlordiazepoxide has been demonstrated in lions, tigers, squirrels, as well as other species.[38] Schallek and colleagues demonstrated that chlordiazepoxide caused a taming of rats which were made vicious by a lesion in the septal region of the brain.[31,39] The dosage that evoked this pharmacological effect was less than the dose that causes sedation. Meprobamate, diazepam, and chlordiazepoxide also produced a taming of mice which were provoked to fight by electroshocks through a grid floor to the feet.[32] The latter two agents abolished the fighting behavior at a dose that was less than the muscle relaxant dose, whereas meprobamate abolished these fighting episodes at the muscle relaxant dose.[32] The barbiturates, unlike meprobamate, produce a taming effect below the muscle relaxant dose.[32]

The ability of the newer minor tranquilizers to produce their anxiolytic effects seems to be attributed to their depressant action on the limbic system, as well as other brain regions involved in the control of behavior.[31,39,40] In general, the benzodiazepines reduce aggression more than activity in animals, whereas the propanediols, barbiturates, and phenothiazines seemingly affect both actions to a similar degree[31,41]

Miscellaneous Effects

An unusual property of chlordiazepoxide is its ability to stimulate the appetite of animals and man in subataxic doses.[32] In a 90 day chronic study this compound was shown to cause an increase in the body weight of dogs and rats.[32]

The major advantage of the benzodiazepines over the major tranquilizers is their lack of an effect on the autonomic nervous system.[31] Moderate doses of the former derivatives do not cause a lowering of blood pressure or heart rate. Only large doses administered intravenously cause hypotension or bradycardia.[26]

1,3-Propanediols

Physicochemical Properties

Meprobamate, 2-methyl-2-*n*-propyl-1,3-propanediol dicarbamate, occurs as a white crystalline powder, which has a bitter taste, and is sparingly soluble in water and highly soluble in most organic solvents. This agent is stable in alkali and dilute acid and is not degraded by the gastrointestinal juices.[26]

Synthesis

The 2-disubstituted propanediol precursor which is needed for the formation of meprobamate was synthesized by Ludwig and Piech.[42] As shown in Figure 5, the precursor was made by a condensation of 2-methyl-valeraldehyde with formaldehyde. The former reactant is synthesized by a two-step reaction from propanal (Figure 5).[26] The dicarbamate derivative (meprobamate) was made by reacting the 2-substituted 1,3-propanediol derivative with phosgene in an inert medium consisting of a tertiary amine acceptor (see Figure 6). This phosgenation process, which was carried out at low temperatures, yields a chlorocarbonate derivative that is ultimately converted to the dicarbamate form. In order to avoid the formation of cyclic carbonates in the reaction vessel, an excess of phosgene must be present.

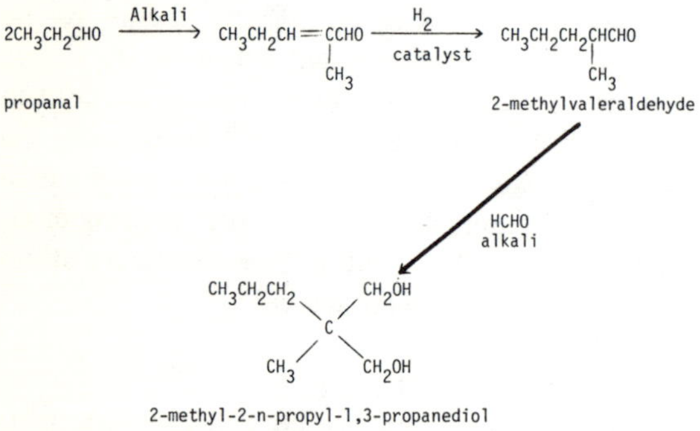

FIGURE 5. The synthesis of a 1,3-propanediol derivative from propanal. (From Berger, F. M. and Ludwig, B. J., *Psychopharmacological Agents,* Vol. 1, Gordon, M., Ed., Academic Press, New York, 1964, 103. With permission.)

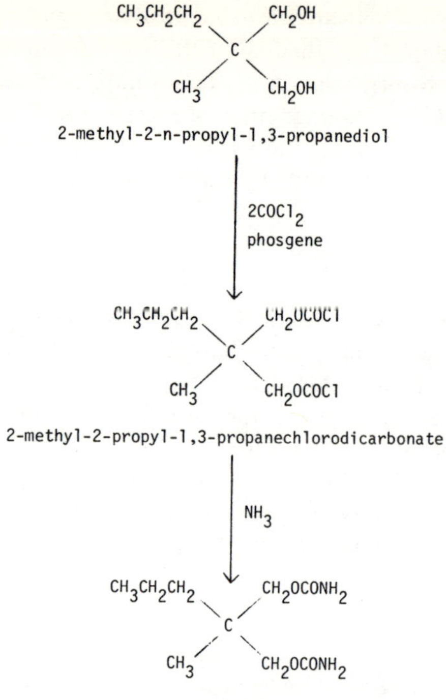

FIGURE 6. The synthesis of meprobamate from a 2-disubstituted 1,3-propanediol. (From Berger, F.M. and Ludwig, B.J., *Psychopharmacological Agents,* Vol. 1, Gordon, M., Ed., Academic Press, New York, 1964, 103. With permission.)

Structure-Activity-Relationships (SAR)

The most potent compound of the 2-disubstituted 1,3-propanediol series is meprobamate.[26] This agent not only has greater antianxiety properties, but is more effective than the other derivatives in abolishing seizures elicited by pentylenetetrazole, strychnine, and electroshock, as well as causing muscular paralysis.[25] Meprobamate, like the benzodiazepines, has minimal effects on the autonomic nervous system.[31] However, when the 2-*n*-propyl group is replaced with a butyl or isobutyl substituent, the resulting compound seems to act like a hypotensive agent.[26]

Other substitutions at the number 2 position yield compounds that are qualitatively similar to meprobamate in regards to biologic activity, but quantitatively dissimilar. Replacing the *n*-propyl group of meprobamate with a 2-chloroethyl, 2-bromopropyl, or a 2-chloropropyl group reduces the effectiveness of the parent molecule.[26] In addition, dicarbamate esters of 2-ethyl-2-*n*-butyl-1,3-propandiol, 2-isopropyl-2-*n*-butyl-1,3-propanediol, and 2-isobutyl-2-*n*-butyl-1,3-propanediol, are less potent.[43] This difference in potency was not attributed to a more rapid elimination of the drugs from the intact organism.[43] On the other hand, the addition of an alkyl substituent to the amide nitrogen of one of the carbamate groups may augment the pharmacologic activity of the parent molecule. The introduction of an isopropyl group at the amide nitrogen would yield the compound carisoprodol, which is more effective than meprobamate in blocking the activity of spinal reflexes.[44] The former compound is several times more effective than the latter agent on decerebrate rigidity.[45] However, carisoprodol, unlike meprobamate, is less potent in eradicating seizures induced by central nervous system stimulants or electroshock.[44] In contrast to the dicarbamate derivative, monocarbamate esters of 1,3-propanediol have a shorter duration of action.[46] Furthermore, an alkyl substitution on the amide nitrogen resembles the unesterified diol derivative, mephenesin, which has a short duration of action and weak anticonvulsant properties.[46]

The diacetate esters of 2,2-diethyl-1,3-propanediol are equally effective as the dicarbamate derivatives in terms of duration of action and anticonvulsant potency, whereas the dibenzoate and disuccinate esters are less effective.[47]

The *N*-dimethyl or *N*-diacetyl dicarbamate esters have an anticonvulsant action and duration of action that is very much like the *N*-unsubstituted derivatives.[46]

The difference in the duration of action of the mono- and dicarbamate esters seems to be attributed to the oxidation of the free alcoholic hydroxyl group.[48]

Benzodiazepines

In view of the comprehensive review presented by Archer and Sternbach[49] and Childress and Gluckman[50] on the chemistry of benzodiazepines, this section will be limited exclusively to a discussion of the 2-amino-1, 4-benzodiazepine-4-oxides and the 1,3-dihydro-1,4-benzodiazepin-2-ones. The major reason for this is that compounds belonging to these homologue series have been employed clinically for the treatment of anxiety, convulsions, and muscle spasms and have also been shown to cause tolerance, physical dependence, and psychological dependence.[27,29,51-53]

2-Amino-1,4-benzodiazepine-4-oxides

Physicochemical Properties

Chlordiazepoxide, which has the following chemical structure (see Figure 7):[30,51,52] is a colorless crystalline substance that is highly soluble in water, but unstable in solution.[29]

Synthesis

The major route of synthesis of chlordiazepoxide and other derivatives, as shown in Figure 8, is via a ring enlargement of quinazoline 3-oxides with either a primary aliphatic amine or hydrazine.[49,54-56] Several 2-amino-1,4-

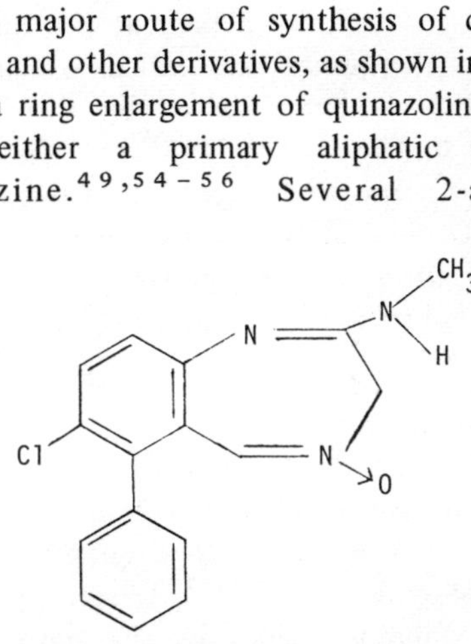

FIGURE 7. The chemical structure of chlordiazopoxide.

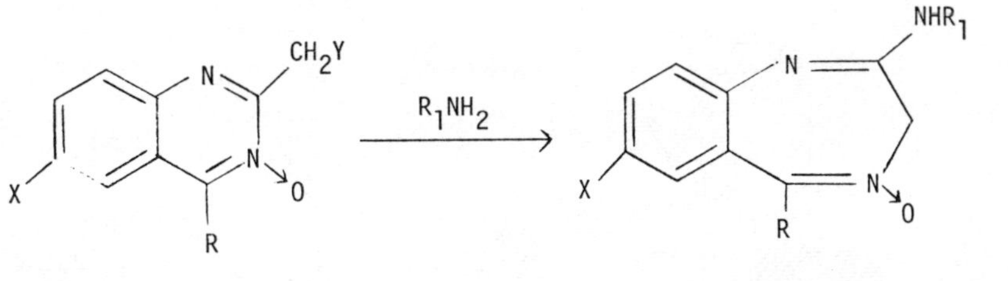

FIGURE 8. The synthesis of 2-amino-benzodiazepine-4-oxide. (From Archer, G. and Sternbach, L.H., *Chem. Rev.*, 68, 747, 1968. With permission.)

benzodiazepine derivatives may also be fabricated from this type of chemical reation by utilizing substituted quinazoline 3-oxides, in which R may be a phenyl or a substituted phenyl,[54-56] 2- or 4-pyridyl,[57] 2-thienyl,[56] hydrogen,[49] alkyl,[49] or cyclohexyl[56] group. In addition, X at the number 6 carbon may be a alkylthio,[58] chlorine,[54-56] bromine,[55] hydrogen,[55,56] methyl,[55,56] methoxycarbonyl,[49] nitro,[59] or a trifluoromethyl substituted group.[49] Although quinazoline 3-oxide derivatives are primarily reacted with primary amines to cause the enlargement of a ring from a 6 to a 7 membered structure, a similar reaction may occur with some secondary amines.[51] The two weak basic amines that have been utilized are dimethylamine[60] and pyrrolidine,[49] thereby resulting in a compound with a tertiary amine in the number 2 position. The leaving group at the number 2 position of quinazoline is usually chlorine.[54-56]

The mechanism involved in the ring enlargement, as shown in Figure 9, is attributed to a nucleophilic attack by a base at the number 2 position of the quinazoline nucleus which bears a partial positive charge caused by the inductive effects of the *N*-oxide.[49,50,61] The 3-*N*-oxide of quinazoline seems to be essential for this reaction, since quinazoline derivatives lacking this group are converted to a 2-amino-quinazoline compound when reacted with primary amines.[49]

Structure-Activity-Relationships

Chlordiazepoxide, in contrast to diazepam, a 1,3-dihydro-1,4-benzodiazepine-2-one, is the most potent derivative of the 2-amino-1,4-benzodiazepam-4-oxide series.[61,62] As seen in Table 2, this compound is formed by the addition of a methyl group at the R_2 position of the "B" ring, and a chloro group at position X. On the other hand, if the R_1 methyl is replaced with a longer, straight, or branched alkyl chain or an acyl substituent, the anxiolytic, anticonvulsant, and muscle relaxant effects are reduced. Furthermore, if the chloro group at position X of the "A" ring is substituted with either a bromo, methyl, or nitro group the potency of the resulting compounds is generally reduced, whereas a compound with a trifluoro methyl substituent has muscle relaxing properties quantitatively similar to chlordiazepoxide. However, a trifluoro methyl substituent is less effective than this compound regarding taming of fighting mice and eradicating seizures elicited by pentylenetetrazol. In addition, a replacement of the phenyl group at the 5 position of the "B" ring with a hydrogen, cyclohexyl, pyridyl, or a thiophenyl group reduces the effectiveness of the parent compound (not shown in Table 2).[62]

1,3-Dihydro-1,4-benzodiazepin-2-ones

Physicochemical Properties

Diazepam, unlike chlordiazepoxide, is a crystalline compound which is highly insoluble in water. This agent is available in the form of tablets and a syrup for oral usage.[29] For parenteral administration, the drug is dissolved in organic solvents consisting of propylene glycol, ethyl alcohol, and sodium benzoate in benzoic acid. This solution is slightly viscous and upon dilution with either saline or water, a transient cloudy solution may occur, however, without a loss of potency.[29] Oxazepam, on the other hand, is a white crystalline powder which is slightly soluble in water, ethanol, and chloroform,[29] whereas nitrazepam, a yellow crystalline agent, is insoluble in water and soluble in ethanol.[29]

Synthesis

There are approximately four methods that

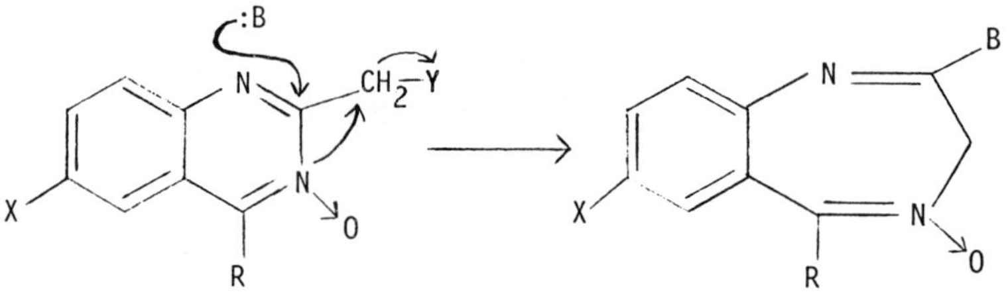

FIGURE 9. Organic mechanism for the conversion of a quinazoline nucleus into a benzodiazepine. (From Archer, G. and Sternbach, L.H., *Chem. Rev.*, 68, 747, 1968. With permission.)

TABLE 2

Structure Activity Relationship of 2-amino-1,4-benzodiazepine-4- Oxides Administered Orally to Mice

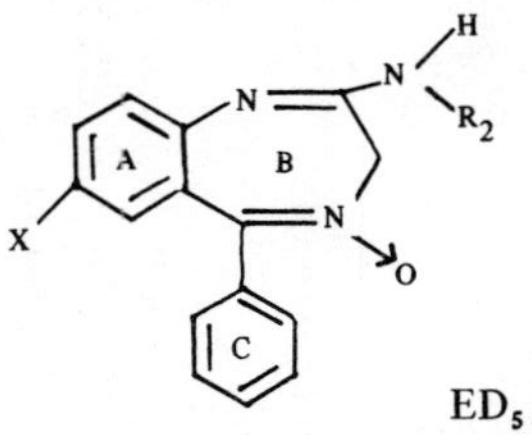

R_2	X	ED$_{50}$ mg/kg Muscle relaxant	Taming	Anticonvulsant[a]
H	Cl	158	80	83
CH_3	Cl	100	40	8
CH_2CH_3	Cl	228	80	37
$(CH_2)_2CH_3$	Cl	338	100	50
$CH(CH_3)_2$	Cl	500	100	700
CH_2-cyclopropyl	Cl	200	60	31
$CH_2C_6H_5$	Cl	500	100	65
$CH_2CH_2OCH_3$	Cl	250	100	100
$CH_2CH_2NH_2$	Cl	500	100	63
CH_3	H	150	100	800
CH_3	Cl	100	40	8
CH_3	Br	200	40	25
CH_3	NO_2	200	100	5
CH_3	CF_3	100	80	30
CH_3	CH_3	360	100	150

[a]Anticonvulsant action against pentylentetrazol-induced seizures.
(From Burger, A. Ed., *Drugs Affecting the Central Nervous System*, Vol. 2, Marcel Dekker, Inc., New York, 1968, Chap. 6. With permission.)

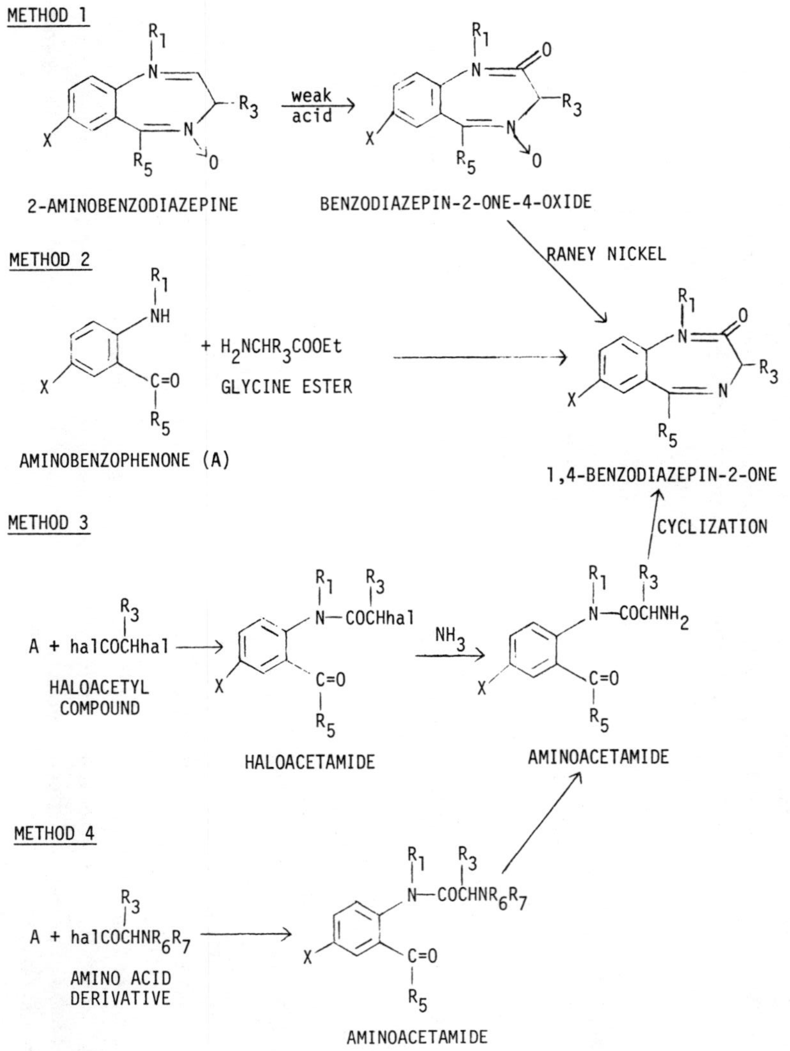

FIGURE 10. Four schematic methods for the synthesis of 1,4-benzodiazepin-2-ones. (From Archer, G. and Sternbach, L.H., *Chem. Rev.*, 68, 747, 1968. With permission.)

have been employed for the synthesis of benzodiazepin-2-ones, which are schematically presented in Figure 10. According to the first procedure, 2-amino-1,4-benzodiazepine-4-oxide derivatives may be reacted with a weak acid to yield benzodiazepin-2-one-4-oxides.[63] Deoxygenation of this product by catalytic hydrogenation over Raney nickel gives the corresponding benzodiazepin-2-one.[63] In the second method, aminobenzophenone is treated with a glycine ester to benzodiazepin-2-one directly.[64] The most versatile procedure is method 3, because it affords higher yields of product.[64,65] Here, aminobenzophenone is reacted with a haloacetyl compound to give haloacetamide, which on treatment with ammonia results in the formation of aminoacetamide. This product readily cyclizes to form benzodiazepin-2-one. In the last schematic reaction, aminobezophenone is acylated with a protected amino acid derivative such as carbobenzoxyglycine, carbobenzoxyglycylchloride, carbobenzoxyglycine anhydride, or phthalimidoacetyl chloride.[66] The protecting group is then removed to give the aminoacetamide compound which cyclizes to benzodiazepin-2-one.[66]

Although several benzodiazepin-2-one derivatives have been prepared by reacting an unsubstituted aminobenzophenone with sodium methoxide followed by an appropriate alkyl halide or sulfate,[49] many of these compounds may also be prepared via methods 2 through 4 (Figure 10) by treating a substituted aminobenzophenone in which R_5 may be an alkyl,[65] cyclohexyl, phenyl or substituted phenyl,[63-65] 2- or 4-pyridyl,[57] or a 2-thienyl group,[65] whereas X may be a hydrogen,[64,65] alkyl,[64,65] aryl,[63,64] alkoxyalkyl,[63] alkylthioalkyl,[63] or a dialkyl group.[64]

Structure-Activity-Relationships

As discussed in the preceding section, a modification of parent structure with different substitutents on the 1, 3, 5, and 7 position results in the formation of a variety of compounds with quantitative differences in pharmacologic activity.[34,49,50,61,62,67] If the hydrogen at the number 1 position of the "B" ring is replaced with an electron-withdrawing group (Table 3) such as a chloro, bromo, fluoro, cyano, nitro, or a trifluoromethyl group, the potency of the parent molecule is increased. A nitro group has stronger electron-withdrawing properties than a chloro group, and a molecule bearing the former substituent is more potent than the chloro derivative. The electron-releasing groups, like methyl and dimethylamino, tend to decrease the effectiveness of the molecule, whereas a mercapto group increases the po-

TABLE 3

Structure Activity Relationship of 1,4-benzodiazepin-2-ones Administered Orally to Mice

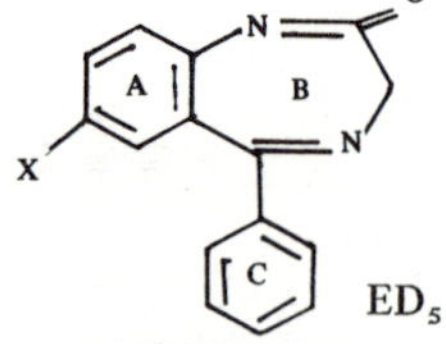

	ED$_{50}$ mg/kg		
X	Muscle relaxant	Taming	Anticonvulsant[a]
H	150	100	800.0
F	150	100	800.0
Cl	75	20	6.0
Br	25	20	2.0
CN	75	40	1.3
NO_2	15	5	0.7
CF_3	10	10	1.0
CH_3	500	100	175.0
$N(CH_3)_2$	500	100	40.0

[a]Anticonvulsant action against pentylenetetrazol-induced seizures.
(From Burger, A. Ed., *Drugs Affecting the Central Nervous System,* Vol. 2, Marcel Dekker, Inc, New York, 1968, Chap. 6. With permission.)

TABLE 4

Structure Activity Relationship of 1,4-benzodiazepin-2-ones Administered Orally to Mice

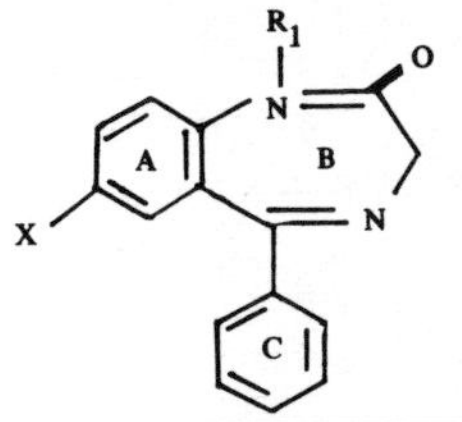

R_1	X	Muscle relaxant (ED_{50} mg/kg)	Taming (ED_{50} mg/kg)	Anticonvulsant[a] (ED_{50} mg/kg)
CH_3	Cl	30	10	1.4
CH_3	NO_2	10	2.5	0.7
CH_3	CN	20	5	1.0
CH_3	$N(CH_3)_2$	150	40	6.0
C_2H_5	Cl	75	20	3.8
CH_3CHCH_2	Cl	40	10	1.4
CH_2COCH_3	Cl	50	20	1.7
CH_2-◁	Cl	100	10	4.1
$(CH_2)_2C(CH_3)_2$	Cl	500	100	3.5
$(CH_2)_2N(CH_3)_2$	CF_3	250	80	3.4
$(CH_2)_2N(CH_3)_2$	Cl	250	100	6.3
$(CH_2)_2N(CH_3)_2$	NO_2	150	20	7.0
CH_2CONH_2	Cl	200	20	2.8
$CH_2CONHCH_3$	Cl	450	80	0.5
$CH_2CON(CH_3)_2$	Cl	275	20	1.6
$CH_2CONHCH_3$	NO_2	300	10	1.8
$CH_2CONHCH_3$	CF_3	250	80	3.4

[a]Anticonvulsant action against pentylenetetrazol-induced seizures.
(From Burger, A., Ed., *Drugs Affecting the Central Nervous System*, Vol. 2, Marcel Dekker, Inc., New York, 1968, Chap. 6. With permission.)

tency.[62] In addition, a saturation of the 4 to 5 double bond of the "B" ring by catalytic hydrogenation reduces the effectiveness of the compound when compared to compounds bearing the unsaturated double bond, regardless whether the derivative possesses an electron-withdrawing or releasing substituent.[62]

On the other hand, if the hydrogen on the number 1 nitrogen of the "B" ring is replaced with a methyl group (Table 4), the muscle relaxant effects, the taming of fighting mice, and the abolishment of convulsions evoked by prior treatment with pentylenetetrazol are enhanced. If, however, this methyl group is replaced by a straight or branched alkyl chain, as shown in Table 4, the potency of the molecule is diminished. The introduction of a cyclopropylmethyl, allyl, ethyl, or acetonyl group at the R_1 position does not seem to modify the activity of the unsubstituted compound, while larger groups such as alkylamino and 3-methylbutyl attenuate the pharmacologic activity. Although these derivatives are less effective than the R_1 methyl compounds, a strong electron-withdrawing group like nitro at the X position of the "A" ring will increase their potency. Furthermore, if an acetamide group is introduced at R_1, the anticonvulsant effects are either augmented or remain unchanged, while the taming and muscle relaxant properties are diminished. As seen from the results in Table 5, the addition of a methyl group at the R_3 position of the "B" ring of diazepam (R_1=methyl; R_3=hydrogen; R_5=phenyl; and X=chloro) increases its potency in terms of taming, muscle relaxant, and anticonvulsant effects. If the R_1 methyl of diazepam is replaced with a hydrogen atom, the taming and anticonvulsant potency is reduced, while the muscle relaxant effects remain unchanged. In addition, if the R_1 methyl and R_3 hydrogen of diazepam are removed and substituted with a hydrogen and hydroxyl group, respectively, the derivative oxazepam is formed. The latter com-

TABLE 5

Structure Activity Relationship of 1,4-benzodiazepin-2-ones Administered Orally to Mice

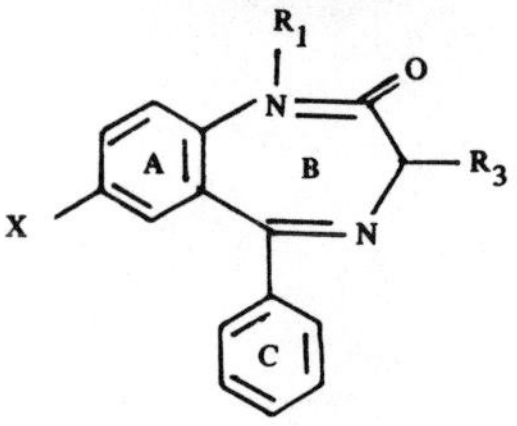

R_1	R_3	X	ED$_{50}$ mg/kg Muscle relaxant	Taming	Anticonvulsant[d]
H	CH_2CH_3	Cl	500	100	800.0
H	CH_3	Cl	80	60	20.0
CH_3	CH_3	Cl	30	10	3.4
H[a]	CH	Cl	225	40	0.9
CH_3[b]	H	Cl	30	10	1.4
H[c]	H	NO_2	15	5	0.5
H	H	Cl	75	20	6.0
H	NH_2	Cl	225	80	20.0
H	$OCOCH_3$	Cl	450	100	53.0
CH_3	$OCOCH_3$	Cl	500	100	22.5
CH_3	$OCOCH_3$	NO_2	100	40	0.98
H	phenyl	Cl	500	100	800.0
CH_3	OCH_3	Cl	20	10	1.6

[a]oxazepam;[b]diazepam;[c]nitrazepam
[d]Anticonvulsant action against pentylenetetrazol-induced seizures.
(From Burger, A., Ed., *Drugs Affecting the Central Nervous System,* Vol. 2, Marcel Dekker, Inc., New York, 1968, Chap. 6. With permission).

TABLE 6

Structure Activity Relationship of 1,4-benzodiazepin-2-ones Administered Orally to Mice

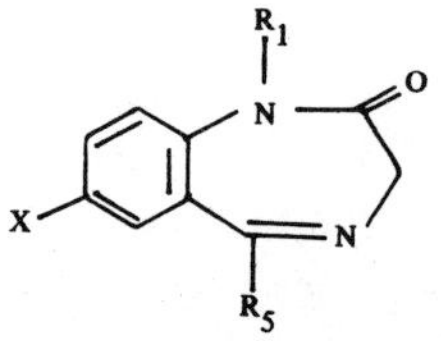

R_1	R_5	X	ED$_{50}$ mg/kg Muscle Relaxant	Taming	Anticonvulsant[a]
H	phenyl	Cl	75	20	3.0
H	methyl	Br	500	500	533.0
H	cyclohexyl	Cl	400	100	667.0
H	2-thienyl	Cl	500	100	100.0
H	pyridyl	H	200	100	400.0
H	pyridyl	Cl	75	10	0.53
H	pyridyl	Br	30	10	0.7
CH_3	pyridyl	Br	25	10	2.29
NH_2	pyridyl	Br	15	10	1.1
CH_2COCH_3	pyridyl	Br	20	10	1.2
$C_3H_7N(CH_3)_2$	pyridyl	Br	300	100	84.0
CF_3	pyridyl	H	10	10	1.0
H	phenyl	H	150	100	800.0

[a]Anticonvulsant action against pentylenetetrazol-induced seizures.
(From Burger, A., Ed., *Drugs Affecting the Central Nervous System,* Vol. 2, Marcel Dekker, Inc., New York, 1968, Chap. 6. With permission.)

pound, an endogenous metabolite of the former derivative, formed by hepatic metabolism in animals and man, is more potent in abolishing convulsions induced by pentylenetetrazol, but less potent as a muscle relaxant and antianxiety agent.[68,69] On the other hand, an introduction of a phenyl, acetyl, or amino group at R_3 decreases the effectiveness of diazepam, whereas a methoxy substituent has pharmacologic properties similar to the R_3 methyl derivative.

Like the 2-amino-1,4-benzodiazepine-4-oxides, the removal of the phenyl or substituted phenyl group at the R_5 position (Table 6) followed by the addition of a methyl, cyclohexyl, or 2-thienyl group, results in the formation of compounds which are exceedingly less effective than the parent molecule. However, after the introduction of a pyridyl group, these compounds seem to have more effective antianxiety and anticonvulsant properties, and variable muscle relaxant activities.

CONCLUSION (SAR)

Barbiturates

The potency and lipid solubility of barbituric acid may be increased by introducing an alkyl, aryl, allyl, or cycloalkenyl group at the number 5 carbon, or an alkyl group at the number 1 and/or 3 nitrogen.

1,3-Propandiols

An increase in size or length of an alkyl group or a substitution with a haloalkyl group at the number 2 position decreases the effectiveness of the parent 1,3-propandiol derivatives, whereas an *N*-monoalkyl substitution increases the potency of the parent molecule in regard to muscular relaxant activity. The *N*-monoalkyl derivatives have a shorter duration of action than meprobamate and are less effective for the treatment of anxiety and convulsions.

2-Amino-1,4-benzodiazepine-4-oxides

A compound which has a 2-aminomethyl, 5-phenyl, and a 7-chloro group is relatively the most potent antianxiety, anticonvulsant, and a muscle relaxant agent of the 2-amino-1,4-benzodiazepine-4-oxides series. Replacement of these groups at the 2, 5, and 7 position with a hydrogen, heterocyclic group, or other substituents, results in the formation of compounds that are generally less potent then chlordiazepoxide.

1,3-Dihydro-1,4-benzodiazepin-2-ones

The introduction of a strong electron-withdrawing group at position X of the "A" ring, a methyl group at R_1, a methyl or hydroxyl group at R_3, and a phenyl or substituted phenyl or pyridyl group at R_5, increases the potency of the unsubstituted derivative. On the other hand, some electron-releasing groups, substitutents other than methyl (excluding acetamido) at R_1 and hydroxyl at R_3, and a hydrogen, methyl, or heterocyclic group at R_5, generally reduce the antianxiety, anticonvulsant, and muscle relaxant activity of the parent molecule.

Acknowledgments

The author is extremely grateful to Drs. Roy Aston and Jay Goodman for their critical evaluation of this chapter. I am also deeply indebted to Mrs. Terry Blasen for typing the manuscript.

REFERENCES

1. Bush, M. T.,Sedatives and hypnotics, in *Physiological Pharmacology*, Vol. 1, Root, W. S. and Hofmann, F. G., Eds., Academic Press, New York, 1963, 185.

2. Levina, R. Y. and Velickko, F. K., Advances in the chemistry of barbituric acids, *Russ. Chem. Rev.*, 29, 437, 1960.

3. Sharpless, S. K., Hypnotics and sedatives. I. The barbiturates, in *The Pharmacological Basis of Therapeutics*, 4th ed., Goodman, L. S. and Gilman, A., Eds., The MacMillan Co., New York, 1970, 98.

4. Dox, A. W. and Jones, E. G., Direct substitution on the nitrogen of 5-5-dialkylbarbituric acids, *J. Amer. Chem. Soc.*, 51, 316, 1929.

5. Lyons, E. and Dox, A. W., The identification of alkylbarbituric acids, *J. Amer. Chem. Soc.*, 51, 288, 1929.

6. Doran, W. J. and Shonle, H. A., Some barbituric acids containing the 2-methylallyl group, *J. Amer. Chem. Soc.*, 59, 1625, 1937.

7. Stuckey, R. E., Ultraviolet absorption spectra of barbituric acid derivatives. III. Ionization and 5-monosubstituted barbituric acid derivatives, *Chem. Abs.*, 37, 2992, 1943.

8. Skinner, G. S., Krysiak, H. R., and Perregrino, J. A., Spiro-1′-benzene-sulfonylpiperidine-4′,5-barbituric acid and related derivatives of isonipecotic acid, *J. Amer. Chem. Soc.*, 77, 2248, 1955.

9. Dox, A. W., Ethylene-*N,N*-bisbarbital, a dimolecular barbital with hypnotic properties, *J. Amer. Chem. Soc.*, 55, 1230, 1933.

10. McElvain, S. M., 5,5-Diphenylbarbituric acid, *J. Amer. Chem. Soc.*, 57, 1303, 1935.

11. Schonle, H. A., Keltch, A. K., and Swanson, E. E., Dialkyl barbituric acids, *J. Amer. Chem. Soc.*, 52, 2240, 1930.

12. Tabern, D. L. and Volwiles, E. H., Sulfur-containing barbiturate hypnotics, *J. Amer. Chem. Soc.*, 57, 1961, 1935.

13. Tisher, M., Wellmann, J. W., and Ladenburg, K., The preparation of riboflavin. III. The synthesis of alloxazines and isoalloxazines, *J. Amer. Chem. Soc.*, 67, 2165, 1945.

14. Hansch, C. and Anderson, S. M., The structure-activity relationship in barbiturates and its similarity to that in other narcotics, *J. Med. Chem.*, 10, 745, 1967.

15. Dundee, J. W., Current views on the clinical pharmacology of barbiturates, *Int. Anesth. Clin.*, 7, 3, 1969.

16. Butler, T. C., The rate of penetration of barbituric acid derivatives into the brain, *J. Pharmacol. Exp. Ther.*, 100, 219, 1950.

17. Goldstein, A. and Aronow, L., The duration of action of thiopental, *J. Pharmacol. Exp. Ther.*, 128, 1, 1960.

18. Roth, L. J. and Barlow, C. F., Drugs in the brain, *Science*, 134, 22, 1961.

19. Goldberg, M. A., Barlow, C. F., and Roth, L. J., The effects of carbon dioxide on the entry and accumulation of drugs in the central nervous system, *J. Pharmacol. Exp. Ther.*, 131, 308, 1961.

20. Fitch, R. H. and Tatum, A. L., The duration of action of the barbituric acid hypnotics as a basis of classification, *J. Pharmacol. Exp. Ther.*, 44, 325, 1932.

21. Mark, L. C., Archaic classification of barbiturates, *Clin. Pharmacol. Ther.*, 10, 287, 1969.

22. Fuhrman, F. A. and Field, J., The relationship between chemical structure and inhibitory action of barbituric acid derivatives on rat brain respiration in vitro, *J. Pharmacol. Exp. Ther.*, 77, 384, 1943.

23. Koppanyi, T., Maling, H. M., Saul, W., and Brodie, B. B., Jumping activity by sodium 5-(1,3-dimethylbutyl)-5-ethyl barbiturate. II. The effects of age difference, *Proc. Soc. Exp. Biol. Med.*, 133, 813, 1970.

24. Koppanyi, T., Maling, H. M., Saul, W., and Brodie, B. B., Jumping activity induced by sodium 5-(1,3-dimethylbutyl)-5-ethyl barbiturate. I. The role of the sympathetic nervous system, *J. Pharmacol. Exp. Ther.*, 172, 170, 1970.

25. Downes, H., Perry, R. S., Ostlund, R. E., and Karler, R., A study of the excitatory effects of barbiturates, *J. Pharmacol. Exp. Ther.*, 175, 692, 1970.

26. Berger, F. M. and Ludwig, B. J., Meprobamate and related compounds, in *Psychopharmacological Agents*, Vol. 1, Gordon, M., Ed., Academic Press, New York, 1964, 103.

27. Jaffe, J. H., Drug addiction and drug abuse, in *The Pharmacological Basis of Therapeutics*, 4th ed., Goodman, L. S. and Gilman, A., Eds., The MacMillan Co., New York, 1970, 276.

28. Zbinden, G. and Randall, L. O., Pharmacology of benzodiazepines: laboratory and clinical correlations, *Advances Pharmacol.*, 5, 213, 1967.

29. Dundee, J. W. and Haslett, W. H. K., The benzodiazepines, a review of their actions and uses relative to anesthetic practice, *Brit. J. Anesth.*, 42, 217, 1970.

30. Straw, R. N., The effect of certain benzodiazepines on the threshold for pentylenetetrazol-induced seizures in the cat, *Arch. Int. Pharmacodyn.*, 175, 464, 1968.

31. Randall, L. O., Schallek, W., Heise, G. A., Keith, E. F., and Bagdon, R. E., The psychosedative properties of methaminodiazepoxide, *J. Pharmacol. Exp. Ther.*, 129, 163, 1960.

32. Randall, L. O., Pharmacology of chlordiazepoxide (Librium®), *Dis. Nerv. Syst.*, suppl. 7, 22, 7, 1961.

33. Hollister, L. E., Clinical use of psychotherapeutic drugs: current status, *Clin. Pharmacol. Ther.*, 10, 170, 1969.

34. Banziger, R. F., Anticonvulsant properties of chlordiazepoxide, diazepam and certain other 1,4-benzodiazepines, *Arch. Int. Pharmacodyn.*, 154, 131, 1965.

35. Randall, L. O., Heise, G. A., Schallek, W., Bagden, R. E., Banziger, R., Boris, A., Moe, R. A., and Abrams, W. B., Pharmacological and clinical studies on Valium,® a new psychotherapeutic agent of the benzodiazepine class, *Curr. Ther. Res.*, 3, 405, 1961.

36. Harris, T., Methaminodiazepoxide, J. A. M. A.. 172, 1162, 1960.

37. Tobin, J. M. and Lewis, W. D. C., New psychotherapeutic agent, chlordiazepoxide, *J. A. M. A.*, 174, 1242, 1960.

38. Hines, L. R., Methaminodiazepoxide (Librium®): a psychotherapeutic drug, *Curr. Ther. Res.*, 2, 277, 1960.

39. Schallek, W. and Jew, W., Effects of methaminodiazepoxide HCl on "Septal Rats" (Motion Picture), *Fed. Proc.*, 19, 24, 1960.

40. Kletzkin, M. and Berger, F. M., Effect of meprobamate on limbic system of the brain, *Proc. Soc. Exp. Biol. Med.*, 100, 681, 1959.

41. Svenson, S. E. and Gordon, L. E., Diazepam: a progress report, *Curr. Ther. Res.*, 7, 367, 1965.

42. Ludwig, B. J. and Piech, E. C., Anticonvulsant agents derived from 1,3-propanediols, *J. Amer. Chem. Soc.*, 73, 5779, 1951.

43. Delga, J., Labourne, J., and Olive, G., Study of the elimination and pharmacological properties of meprobamate and 3 of its homologs, *Ann. Pharm. Franc.*, 20, 121, 1962.

44. Berger, F. M., Kletzkin, M., Ludwig, B. J., Margolin, S., and Powell, L. S., Unusual muscle relaxant and analgesic properties of *N*-isopropyl-2-methyl-2-propyl-1, 3-propanediol dicarbamate (carisoprodol), *J. Pharmacol. Exp. Ther.*, 127, 66, 1959.

45. Berger, F. M., *The Pharmacology and Clinical Usefulness of Carisoprodol*, Wayne State Univ. Press, Detroit, Mich., 1959, 1.

46. Berger, F. M., Hendley, C. D., Ludwig, B. J., and Lynes, T. E., Central depressant and anticonvulsant activity of compounds isomeric with 2-methyl-2-propyl-1,3-propanediol dicarbamate, (Miltown®), *J. Pharmacol. Exp. Ther.*, 116, 337, 1956.

47. Berger, F. M. and Ludwig, B. J., The anticonvulsant action of 2,2-diethyl- 1,3-propanediol and some of its homologs and esters, *J. Pharmacol. Exp. Ther.*, 100, 27, 1950.

48. Berger, F.M., Anticonvulsant activity of carbamate ester of certain 2,2-disubstituted 1,3-propanediols, *J. Pharmacol. Exp. Ther.*, 104, 229, 1952.

49. Archer, G.A. and Sternbach, L. H., The chemistry of benzodiazepines, *Chem. Rev.*, 68, 747, 1968.

50. Childress, S. J. and Gluckman, M. I., 1,4-Benzodiazepines, *J. Pharm. Sci.*, 53, 577, 1964.

51. Feldman, H. S., The pill head menace: barbiturates and tranquilizers non-hardcore addicting drugs, *Psychosomatics*, 11, 99, 1970.

52. Essig, C. F., Addiction to nonbarbiturate sedative and tranquilizing drugs, *Clin. Pharmacol.*, 5, 334, 1964.

53. Seevers, M. H. and Deneau, G. A., Physiological aspects of tolerance and physical dependence, in *Physiological Pharmacology*, Vol. 1, Koot, W. S. and Hofmann, F. G., Eds., Academic Press, New York, 1963, 565.

54. Sternbach, L. H. and Reeder, E., Quinazolines and 1,4-benzodiazepines. II. The rearrangement of 6-chloro-2-chloromethyl-4-phenylquinazoline 3-oxide into 2-amino derivatives of 7-chloro-5-phenyl-3H-1,4-benzodiazepine 4-oxide, *J. Org. Chem.*, 26, 1111, 1961.

55. Sternbach, L. H., Reeder, E., Keller, O., and Metlesics, W., Quinazolines and 1,4-benzodiazepines. III. Substituted 2-amino-5-phenyl-3H-1,4-benzodiazepine 4-oxides, *J. Org. Chem.*, 26, 4488, 1961.

56. Bell, S. C., Gochman, C., and Childress, S. J., Some analogs of chlordiazepoxide, *J. Med. Pharm. Chem.*, 5, 63, 1962.

57. Fryer, R. I., Schmidt, R. A., and Sternbach, L. H., Quinazolines and 1,4-benzodiazepines. XVII. Synthesis of 1,3-dihydro-5-pyridyl-2H-1,4-benzodiazepine derivatives, *J. Pharm. Sci.*, 53, 265, 1964.

58. Keller, O., Steiger, N., and Sternbach, L. H., Aminobenzodiazepines, *C. A.*, 61, 5672, 1964.

59. Sternbach, L. H., Fryer, R. I., Keller, O., Metlesics, W., Sach, G., and Steiger, N., Quinazolines and 1,4-benzodiazepines. X. Nitro-substituted 5-phenyl-1,4-benzodiazepine derivatives, *J. Med. Chem.*, 6, 261, 1963.

60. Farber, S., Wuest, H. M., and Meltzer, R. I., Reactions of 6-chloro-2-chloromethyl-4-phenylquinazoline 3-oxide with dimethylamine, *J. Med. Chem.*, 7, 235, 1964.

61. Sternbach, L. H., Randall, L. O., and Gustafson, S., 1,4-Benzodiazepines (chlordiazepoxide and related compounds), in *Psychopharmacological Agents*, Vol. 1, Gorden, M., Ed., Academic Press, New York, 1964, 137.

62. Sternbach, L. H., Randall, L. O., Banziger, R., and Lehr, H., Structure-activity relationships in the 1,4-benzodiazepine series, in *Drugs Affecting The Central Nervous System*, Vol. 2, Burger, A., Ed., Marcel Dekker, Inc., New York, 1968, 237.

63. Sternbach, L. H. and Reeder, E., Quinazolines and 1,4-benzodiazepines. IV. Transformations of 7-chloro-2-methylamino-5-phenyl-3H,1,4-benzodiazepine 4-oxide, *J. Org. Chem.*, 26, 4936, 1961.

64. Sternbach, L. H., Fryer, R. I., Metlesics, E., Reeder, E., Sach, G., Saucy, G., and Stempel, A., Quinazolines and 1,4-benzodiazepines. VI. Halo-methyl-, and methoxy-substituted 1,3-dihydro-5-phenyl-2H,1,4-benzodiazepin-2-ones, *J. Org. Chem.*, 27, 3788, 1962.

65. Bell, S. C., Sulkowski, T. S., Gochman, C., and Childress, S. J., 1,3-Dihydro-2H-1,4-benzodiazepin-2-ones and their 4-oxides, *J. Org. Chem.*, 27, 562, 1962.

66. Stempel, A. and Zandgraf, F. W., Quinazolines and 1,4-benzodiazepines. IX. 2-Carbobenzoxyglycylamidobenzophenones and their conversion to 1,4-benzodiazepinones, *J. Org. Chem.*, 27, 4675, 1962.

67. Sternbach, L. H., Archer, G. A., Earley, J. V., Fryer, R. I., Reeder, E., Wasylim, N., Randall, L. O., and Banziger, R., Quinazolines and 1,4-benzodiazepines. XXV. Structure-activity relationships of aminoalkyl-substituted 1,4-benzodiazepin-2-ones, *J. Med. Chem.*, 8, 815, 1965.

68. Randall, L. O., Scheckel, C. L., and Banziger, R. F., Pharmacology of metabolites of chlordiazepoxide and diazepam, *Curr. Ther. Res.*, 7, 590, 1965.

69. Schwartz, M. A, Koechlin, B. A., Postma, E., Palmer, S., and Krol, G., Metabolism of diazepam in rats, dogs, and man, *J. Pharmacol. Exp. Ther.*, 149, 423, 1965.

ALCOHOL

C. S. Lieber

TABLE OF CONTENTS

INTRODUCTION

This chapter deals with the metabolism of ethanol and the associated biochemical changes. The widespread interest in the biochemical changes associated with the metabolism of ethanol originated, in part, with the realization that a number of pathologic effects of alcohol can be directly linked to its metabolism. Originally, these aspects were somewhat neglected, because the most apparent effects of alcohol abuse are functional changes of the central nervous system which are not conspicuously related to ethanol oxidation. Furthermore, several neurologic complications of alcoholism, such as polyneuropathy and Wernicke's syndrome, once thought to be due to a direct toxic effect of alcohol, were clearly recognized as consequences of vitamin deficiencies associated with alcoholism. The same trend of thought then led to the belief that diseases of the liver (and of other organs) associated with alcoholism are not due to ethanol per se, but merely to nutritional deficiencies so commonly associated with alcoholism. This point of view was exemplified by the statement that "there is no more evidence of a specific toxic effect of pure ethyl alcohol upon liver cells than there is for one due to sugar".[1] The subsequent discovery of the direct effect of alcohol on lipid metabolism in liver slices[2,3] and isolated perfused livers,[4] as well as the observation that alcohol consumption can lead to the development of fatty liver despite an otherwise adequate diet (both in man and in rats),[5,6] established ethanol itself as a direct cause for pathologic changes. This was substantiated by the observation that the fat accumulation of the liver was accompanied by striking ultrastructural abnormalities[7,8] which could not be prevented even by large dietary supplementation in protein, minerals, and vitamins, including choline.[9,10] This demonstration of a direct role of ethanol then prompted a series of investigations by several groups trying to unravel the biochemical mechanism involved in the pathologic changes produced by alcohol. Indeed, over the last decade, a number of deleterious effects of alcohol have been successfully linked to the biochemical alterations of intermediary metabolism produced by the oxidation of ethanol. These will be reviewed here although as yet they have not been firmly related to the development of alcohol dependence. It is not unreasonable to anticipate, however, that further progress in our knowledge of the metabolism of ethanol may ultimately unravel a biochemical connection between ethanol ingestion and the development of physical dependence, especially since several theories have already been proposed (based on some experimental evidence) linking biochemical changes to the development of dependence. These theories will be discussed in conjunction with the description of the corresponding biochemical changes. The actual signs of dependence and withdrawal will not be described, however, since these are dealt with in another chapter of this book.[11] Good descriptions of the alcohol withdrawal syndrome can also be found in experimental human studies by Isbell et al.[12] and Mendelson.[13] Similarly, the signs and symptoms of the pathologic effects resulting from or associated with the biochemical changes reviewed here (such as fatty liver, alcoholic hepatitis, cirrhosis, hematologic changes) will not be described. This would go beyond the scope of the chapter; detailed reviews are available elsewhere.[14-17]

SITE OF ABSORPTION AND METABOLISM OF ETHANOL

Although trace amounts of ethanol can originate endogenously from intestinal fermentation, alcohol is primarily an exogenous compound that can be readily absorbed from the gastrointestinal tract. Absorption, however, is more rapid in the small intestine than in the stomach, so that delay in gastric emptying (for instance, after a fat-containing meal) results in retardation of absorption. Once absorbed, the ethanol diffuses readily into the water space of the body. It is a common observation that regular drinkers usually become able to tolerate larger amounts of ethanol with repeated exposure. Measurements of alcohol concentrations in the brain have shown no difference between normal and tolerant animals,[18] indicating that delayed absorption or reduced entry into the brain does not play a role in the phenomenon of tolerance. Only 2 to 10% of the absorbed dose is eliminated in the breath, urine, and sweat.[19] There is no increased rate of excretion in an inebriated individual. There is, however, an increased rate of metabolism (so-called metabolic tolerance), the mechanism of which will be discussed subsequently. In addition, central nervous system tolerance develops. That is, for a given blood level, neurological effects of ethanol are less striking in a tolerant individual than in a nontolerant one. This aspect may be the most important one for the overall development of tolerance but will not be discussed further, since, unlike metabolic tolerance, no biochemical explanation is as yet available.

Most of the ethanol absorbed is oxidized in the body, and the main site for this is the liver. The rate of disappearance of ethanol from the blood is indeed remarkably decreased or halted by hepatectomy or procedures damaging the liver.[19] Moreover, the predominant role of the liver for ethanol metabolism was shown directly in individuals with portacaval shunts undergoing hepatic vein catheterization.[20] Extrahepatic metabolism of ethanol, although it occurs, is small.[21,22] This "organ specificity" probably explains why, despite the existence of intracellular mechanisms responsible for homeostasis, ethanol oxidation produces striking metabolic imbalances in the liver.

HEPATIC PATHWAYS FOR ETHANOL OXIDATION AND ASSOCIATED BIOCHEMICAL CHANGES

As illustrated in Figure 1, ethanol oxidation in the hepatocyte can proceed in at least two ways: a major pathway involving alcohol dehydrogenase (ADH) and a secondary pathway involving the microsomal ethanol oxidizing system (MEOS). In addition, and not represented in Figure 1, catalase-dependent ethanol oxidation has also been implicated and will be discussed subsequently together with MEOS.

Alcohol Dehydrogenase (ADH) Pathway and Effect of Excessive NADH Generation

The oxidation of ethanol by the ADH pathway results in the transfer of hydrogen to NAD (nicotinamide adenine dinucleotide) which is reduced to NADH, whereas ethanol is oxidized to acetaldehyde. In turn, acetaldehyde can exert some biochemical effects, as discussed in a subsequent paragraph, or it can be converted to acetate, again with transfer of hydrogen to NAD.

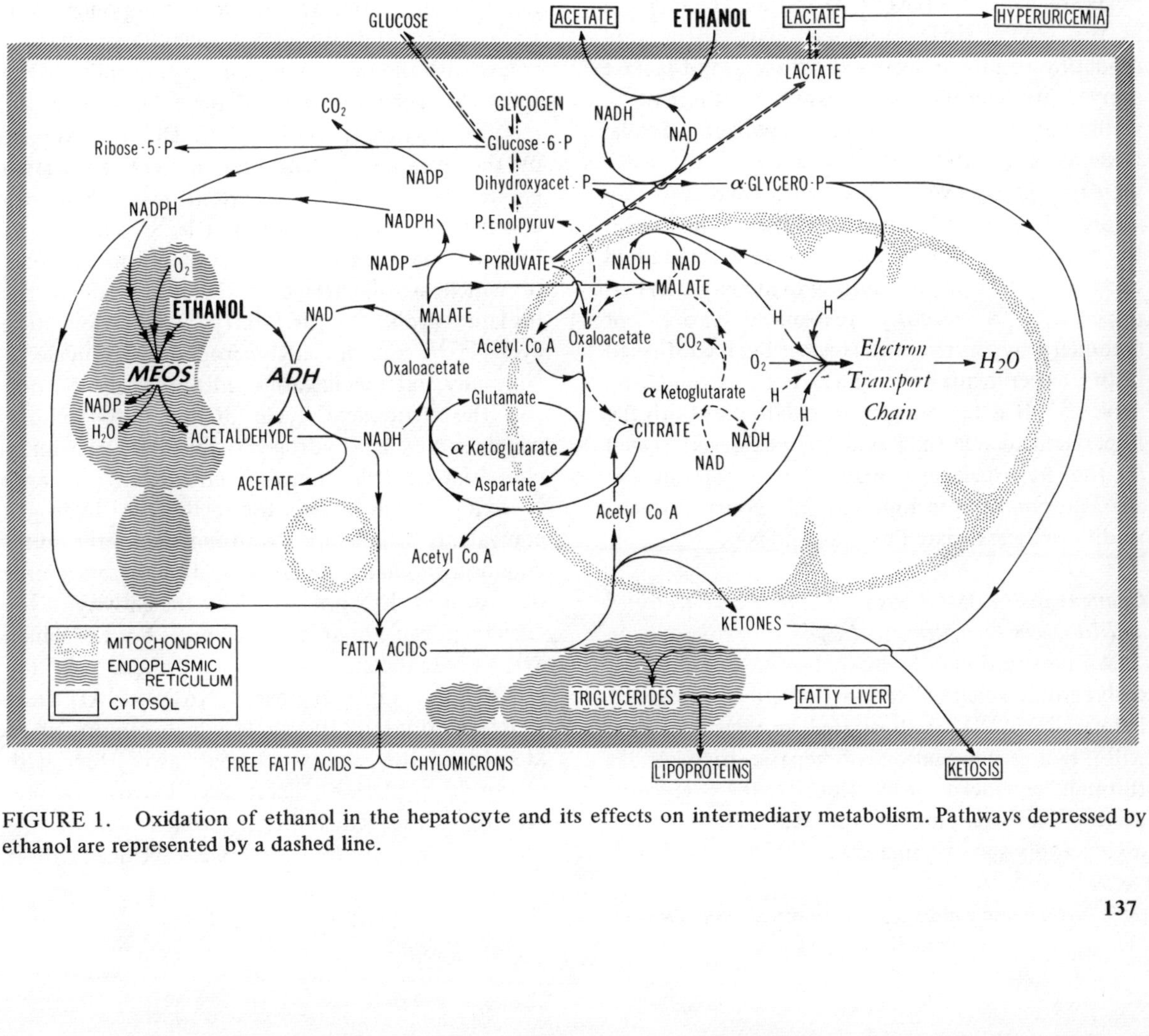

FIGURE 1. Oxidation of ethanol in the hepatocyte and its effects on intermediary metabolism. Pathways depressed by ethanol are represented by a dashed line.

The resulting acetate is primarily released in the bloodstream to be metabolized by other tissues. Thus, the most conspicuous result of ethanol oxidation in the liver is NADH generation. Because of the relative organ specificity for ethanol and the lack of an effective feedback mechanism to control rates of ethanol metabolism in the liver, ethanol oxidation results in a much greater NADH overload in the liver than is normally produced by the oxidation of other substrates (such as carbohydrates, amino acids, and fatty acids) which can be utilized not only in the liver, but in other tissues as well. Excess hepatic NADH generation reflects itself in an increased NADH/NAD ratio in the liver with a shift in the ratio of those metabolites whose reduction is determined by the NADH-NAD couple. This shift can explain a number of biochemical changes associated with ethanol oxidation and has been proposed as a major mechanism underlying pathological changes produced by ethanol.[23,24]

Hyperlactacidemia, Hyperuricemia, and Acidosis

The oxidation of lactate to pyruvate requires NAD and generates NADH. Therefore, the increase in the NADH/NAD ratio secondary to ethanol oxidation results in decreased utilization of lactate derived from extrahepatic tissues by the liver[25] with, as a consequence, hyperlactacidemia. Depending on the metabolic state of the liver, increased hepatic lactate production may also play a role. The resulting hyperlactacidemia contributes to acidosis[26] and reduced urinary uric acid excretion which in turn results in alcoholic hyperuricemia,[27] a recently recognized variety of secondary hyperuricemia. This has been confirmed both experimentally[28] and in a population survey.[29] It is tempting to speculate that both the hyperlactacidemia (and associated acidosis) as well as the hyperuricemia may play a role in the aggravation of precipitation of gouty attacks traditionally associated with alcoholism.

Changes in the Metabolism of Lipids and Ketones and Block in the Citric Acid Cycle

Administration of ethanol increases hepatic α-glycerophosphate,[30] again probably because of increased NADH, as illustrated in Figure 1. This will favor accumulation of hepatic triglycerides through enhanced production of their glycerol moiety and trapping of the fatty acid by the α-glycerophosphate. Increased NADH could also enhance fatty acid synthesis by the fatty acid elongation system of the outer mitochondria (Figure 1). Enhanced fatty acid synthesis was already suggested a decade ago with the observation that ethanol increases the incorporation of ^{14}C-acetate into hepatic fatty acids.[2,3] Moreover, if reduction of oxaloacetate to malate is coupled with the oxidation of ethanol, according to the scheme shown in Figure 1, enhanced NADH may result in increased NADPH, a building block needed for de novo fatty acid synthesis in the cytosol. As an overall result, increased lipogenesis can be theoretically considered as a means for disposing of the excess hydrogen produced upon ethanol oxidation in the liver.

Some of the excess hydrogen equivalents can also be transferred from the cytosol into the mitochondria. Since the mitochondrial membrane is normally impermeable to NADH, it is currently believed that the reducing equivalents of NADH are transferred to the mitochondrial respiratory chain via shuttle mechanisms. Thus, NADH reduces the oxidized partner of the shuttle pair in the presence of the cytoplasmic enzyme, thereby regenerating NAD. The reduced component now traverses the mitochondrial membrane where it reacts with the mitochondrial enzyme and NAD or FAD to generate NADH or FADH plus the reduced partner. FADH and NADH are oxidized by the respiratory chain and the reduced partner enters the cytoplasm where it is available for another round of the shuttle cycle. Several "shuttle" mechanisms have been proposed, three of which are illustrated in Figure 1, namely the malate cycle,[31] the fatty acid elongation cycle,[32,33] and the α-glycerophosphate cycle.[34] Normally, fatty acids are oxidized via β-oxidation and the citric acid cycle of the mitochondria, which serves as "hydrogen" donor for the mitochondrial electron transport chain. When ethanol is oxidized, however, the generated hydrogen equivalents which are "shuttled" into the mitochondria supplant the citric acid cycle as a source of hydrogen. Ethanol can block the activity of the citric acid cycle in at least two ways both of which are consequences of the changes in the NADH/NAD ratio. Increased NADH/ NAD slows those reactions of the cycle which require NAD. Moreover, the redox change associated with ethanol oxidation decreases hepatic oxaloacetate,[35] the availability of which controls the activity of citrate synthetase. Under these conditions, the mitochondria will utilize the hydrogen equivalents from the ethanol rather than oxidize the two carbon fragments derived from the fatty acids. The fatty acids, which normally represent the main mitochondrial fuel, are thus supplanted by ethanol. Inhibition of fatty acid oxidation was demonstrated both in liver slices[3] and in isolated perfused livers.[4] It explains the deposition in the liver of fatty acids derived from the diet, when ethanol is ingested with a fat-containing diet,[36,37] and may represent the main mechanism for the development of alcoholic fatty liver.[24] The importance of dietary fat was further illustrated by the fact that the capacity of a given amount of ethanol to produce fatty liver can be reduced by decreasing the fat content of the diet.[38] Even with a diet practically devoid of fat, however, isocaloric substitution of dietary carbohydrate by ethanol results in fat accumulation in the liver, consisting primarily of endogenously synthesized fatty acids.[36,37,39] The latter accumulate either because of a block in their oxidation, or through enhanced lipogenesis. In addition to the block in fatty acid oxidation due to the presence of ethanol itself which replaces the lipids as "preferred" fuel for the liver, decreased fatty acid oxidation can also result from the fact that prolonged ethanol consumption was found to be associated with a striking alteration in both mitochondrial structure[7-10] and function.[40,41] The mechanism for the striking alteration of mitochondrial morphology observed both in rats and in man after chronic ethanol ingestion is not known; it could be secondary to the decrease in mitochondrial protein synthesis recently described after ethanol.[42]

Increased availability of fatty acids in the liver may also contribute to the hyperketonemia and ketonuria observed during chronic alcohol consumption in association with fat-containing diets. Increased ketogenesis in the liver has been incriminated.[43] This may explain the recently described variety of "alcoholic ketoacidosis."[44]

Alcoholic Hypoglycemia and Hyperglycemia

Several amino acids enter gluconeogenetic pathways after deamination to either α-ketoglutarate or other compounds of the citric acid cycle such as oxaloacetate (figure 1). The decrease in citric acid cycle activity by ethanol could explain the reduction in gluconeogenesis from these precursors. Similarly, the diversion of pyruvate to lactate discussed before could explain the decreased utilization of amino acids (such as alanine) which must first be converted to pyruvate before serving for gluconeogenesis. By a combination of these and possibly other metabolic blocks, both in the extra- and intramitochondrial compartments (including decreased fatty acid oxidation) ethanol contributes to decreased gluconeogenesis which in turn is probably the cause of alcoholic hypoglycemia in individuals whose glycogen stores are already depleted, or who have preexistent abnormalities in carbohydrate metabolism.[45]

In addition to hypoglycemia, hyperglycemia has also been described in association with alcoholism. The mechanism of the hyperglycemia, however, is still obscure. Pancreatitis commonly occurs in alcoholics[16] and could be contributory. As discussed subsequently, an increase in circulating catecholamines is observed after ethanol abuse and could also result in some hyperglycemia. In some individuals, glucose intolerance develops after alcohol administration.[46] This may be due, at least in part, to decreased peripheral glucose utilization;[47,48] ethanol-induced ketosis[43] may also play a role.

Changes in the Metabolism of Galactose, Amines, Steroids, and Other Alterations Associated with the Enhanced NADH/NAD Ratio

As emphasized before,[23,24] a number of metabolic effects of alcohol can be attributed to the generation of NADH; these include interference with galactose, serotonin, and other amine metabolism. The increased availability of NADH also results in alteration of hepatic steroid metabolism in favor of the reduced compounds.[49,50]

Theoretically, to the extent that transhydrogenation from NADH to NADP occurs(either in the microsomes themselves or by the mechanism depicted in Figure 1), mixed function oxidase activity of the microsomes, which utilizes NADPH, will contribute to the disposal of excess hydrogen generated by ethanol oxidation in the cytosol. This may become of special importance after chronic ethanol consumption, which, as discussed subsequently, enhances mixed function oxidation in liver microsomes.

Catalase Pathway for Ethanol Oxidation

Catalase is an ubiquitous enzyme, found in

most animal tissues including the liver. In vitro, it can catalyze the peroxidative conversion of alcohols to the corresponding aldehydes.[51] Its role in vivo is still the subject of debate. It participates in the oxidation of methanol, at least in the rat, whereas in the monkey, alcohol dehydrogenase may play a greater role in that respect.[52] Which enzyme is involved in methanol oxidation in man has not been elucidated. Similarly, it is not known to what extent catalase participates in the in vivo oxidation of ethanol. Catalase was thought to have no role in ethanol metabolism in vivo,[53] an opinion supported by the observation that aminothiazole, a catalase inhibitor in vivo, does not affect rates of ethanol metabolism.[54]

The moderate oxidation of ethanol by mitochondria in vitro found by some[55] but not by others[56] may, when present, involve catalase.[57]

There is some debate whether in rats, ethanol feeding enhances catalase activity, with increases[58] or no change[59,60] reported. This question, however, may not be fully relevant to the problem of rates of ethanol metabolism since peroxidative metabolism of ethanol in the liver is probably limited by the rate of hydrogen peroxide formation rather than by the amount of available catalase.[61] As discussed subsequently, recent studies have shown that ethanol consumption enhances the activity of hepatic NADPH oxidase[62] which, as illustrated in Figure 2, is capable of H_2O_2 generation. It is not known, however, to what extent this mechanism contributes to ethanol metabolism in vivo and to its increase after chronic ethanol consumption.

Microsomal Ethanol Oxidizing System (MEOS)

The first indication of an interaction of ethanol with the microsomal fraction of the hepatocyte was provided by the morphologic observation that in rats, ethanol feeding results in a proliferation of the smooth endoplasmic reticulum (SER) which is part of the microsomal fraction.[63] This proliferation of SER was subsequently confirmed under a variety of conditions, both in rats[7,64] and in man[8-10] and has now been substantiated chemically.[65] This increase in SER resembles that seen after the administration of a wide variety of xenobiotic compounds including numerous therapeutic agents[66] and food additives.[67] Most of these substances, which induce a proliferation of the SER, are metabolized at least in part, in the microsomal fraction of the hepatocyte which comprises the SER. The observation that ethanol also produces proliferation of the SER suggested that, in addition to its oxidation by ADH in the cytosol, ethanol may also be metabolized by the

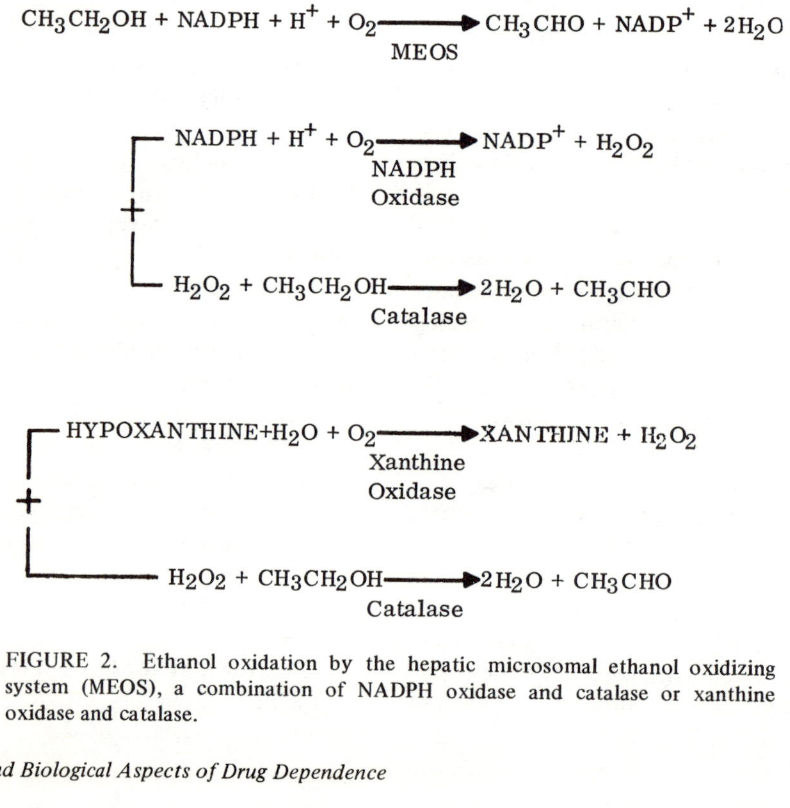

FIGURE 2. Ethanol oxidation by the hepatic microsomal ethanol oxidizing system (MEOS), a combination of NADPH oxidase and catalase or xanthine oxidase and catalase.

microsomes. This was corroborated by the observations that microsomes can oxidize methanol and, to a small extent, ethanol.[68] The difficulty of the very low rate of ethanol metabolism was subsequently overcome by the description of a new microsomal ethanol oxidizing system (MEOS) with a rate of ethanol oxidation ten times higher.[60,69] Furthermore, whereas the first system oxidizes methanol at a rate twice that of ethanol, this ratio is reversed for the latter.

Differentiation of MEOS from ADH

MEOS differs from ADH by a variety of characteristics:

Subcellular localization – ADH is part of the cytosol, not the microsomes.[60,70] No ADH activity is detectable in washed microsomes even when acetyl pyridine NAD (3-AP-NAD), which enhances the activity of ADH, is used as cofactor. Nevertheless, washed microsomes are still capable of ethanol oxidation.[60]

pH optimum in vitro – Contrasting with an optimum pH of 10 to 11 for ADH, the optimum pH for MEOS is in the physiological range.

Cofactor requirements and redox changes – ADH requires NAD, whereas in the microsomes only negligible ethanol oxidation occurs in the presence of NAD.[60] For MEOS activity, either NADPH or a NADPH generating system is needed. As a consequence, MEOS activity does not alter the redox potential, whereas ethanol oxidation via ADH increases the NADH/NAD ratio, as discussed before.

Effect of inhibitors – Pyrazole and pyrazole derivatives are potent ADH inhibitors. At high concentrations, pyrazole lacks specificity and affects a variety of other hepatic enzymes, both in the cytosol and the microsomes.[73] At low concentrations, it can serve to differentiate MEOS from ADH since it inhibits the former much less than the latter.[71,73]

Lack of energy conservation – Whereas ethanol oxidation by the ADH pathway generates NADH, the oxidation of which can be coupled with oxidative phosphorylation, MEOS activity results in NADPH oxidation by O_2, without apparent conservation of chemical energy.

Differentiation of MEOS from Catalase and NADPH Oxidase

Hepatic microsomes contain an enzyme, NADPH oxidase, which in the presence of NADPH and O_2, generates H_2O_2 (Figure 2). Addition of catalase to this system allows it to oxidize methanol.[74] Catalase resides primarily in the microbodies which are separated with the mitochondrial fraction. Other organelles, however, including the microsomes, contain traces of catalase. Therefore, it was postulated that the combination of H_2O_2 generation from NADPH oxidase and catalase could account for microsomal ethanol oxidation[75,76] (Figure 2), especially since a H_2O_2 generating system (glucose-glucose oxidase) can be substituted for NADPH. Actually, the latter is not unexpected, since not only do microsomes contain catalase, but commercial glucose oxidase is also contaminated with catalase and the combination of catalase, glucose oxidase, and glucose has been shown already by Keilin and Hartree[51] to be capable of ethanol oxidation. The question still remained whether normally, ethanol oxidation in the microsomes is due to a distinct microsomal ethanol oxidizing system (MEOS) or whether this activity can be accounted for by a combination of NADPH oxidase and catalase activity (Figure 2). Recently, it was reported that some inhibitors of NADPH oxidase (such as cholate) also reduce MEOS activity.[77,78] This does not mean that these two reactions are necessarily linked, since a nonspecific inhibitor such as cholate does indeed inhibit many unrelated reactions; including a variety of microsomal enzymes.[71] Nonspecific inhibitors, however, can be used for the dissociation of two reactions when these are differently affected by the inhibitor. Several experiments of this type have allowed differentiation of MEOS from catalase activity.[60] For instance, after administration of pyrazole in vivo, catalase activity of washed microsomes was reduced by 90%, whereas MEOS activity was unaffected. Under the same conditions, ethanol oxidation by a H_2O_2 generating system (hypoxanthine-xanthine oxidase) was reduced 80%. When azide (a catalase inhibitor) was added in vitro to microsomes of pyrazole-treated animals, activities of microsomal catalase and that of ethanol oxidation with the H_2O_2 generating system were virtually abolished, whereas 2/3 of the activity of MEOS remained. Thus, when microsomal ethanol oxidation is dependent upon H_2O_2 generation, it is also sensitive to catalase inhibition. Conversely, the relative insensitivity of MEOS activity to catalase inhibition suggests that catalase is not implicated in the activity of the system, at least for its major fraction.

Comparison of the Properties of MEOS with Those of Other Microsomal Drug Detoxifying Enzymes

MEOS shares many properties with other microsomal drug detoxifying enzymes, including the need for oxygen and requirement of NADPH. Feeding of substrates often results in increased activity of the corresponding detoxifying enzyme. This is also the case for MEOS, as discussed subsequently. Although MEOS activity is found in both rough (RER) and smooth (SER) endoplasmic reticulum, the increase after ethanol consumption occurs only in the SER.[65] The adaptive increase in the activity of MEOS results probably from a quantitative rather than a qualitative change in the enzyme system involved, because the apparent Km of the reaction remains unchanged at about 8mM.[60] Drugs which are oxidized by microsomes commonly "bind" to the microsomes and this is associated with spectral changes of two types (I or II). Addition of ethanol to microsomes produces a modified type II binding spectrum; the average magnitude of the spectral change tripled in animals pretreated chronically with ethanol.[79] The activities of many microsomal drug metabolizing enzymes are inhibited by SKF-525A. Some drugs, however, (especially those with type II binding characteristics) are metabolized by enzymes which are relatively insensitive to this inhibitor.[80] Similarly, MEOS activity is not affected by 1 mM SKF-525A in vitro. In view of the lack of effect of SKF-525A on MEOS activity in vitro, its ineffectiveness on ethanol metabolism in vivo[76] is not surprising.

Respective Roles of the Ethanol Oxidizing Systems in Vivo

"Normal" Ethanol Oxidation

Hitherto, the concept has prevailed that ADH is solely responsible for ethanol oxidation in vivo. This opinion is supported by recent observations that pyrazole, a potent ADH inhibitor, markedly reduces ethanol oxidation in vivo.[60,81] The inhibition, however, is not complete. Furthermore, when pyrazole is added in vitro either to liver slices[60] or to isolated perfused liver[82] at a concentration which virtually abolishes ADH activity, about 1/4 of the metabolism of ethanol persists. This probably reflects the activity of an alcohol oxidizing system other than ADH, most likely MEOS, especially since pyrazole in vivo is also a catalase inhibitor.[73] This concurs with the assessment of MEOS activity in vitro. When correction is made for microsomal losses, MEOS activity measured in vitro accounts for 20 to 25% of the rate of ethanol oxidation in vivo.[83] Moreover, the apparent "Km" of MEOS in vitro coincides with the apparent in vivo "Km" of blood ethanol disappearance after pyrazole.[83] Thus, although the respective roles of ADH and MEOS in vivo have not been settled, one can estimate that in individuals without a history of prior chronic exposure to alcohol, about 3/4 of the ethanol may be oxidized by the ADH pathway, whereas 1/4 may involve MEOS. The respective role of the two pathways will, of course, vary with the actual blood ethanol level achieved, and one must take into account that MEOS has a Km of 8 mM,[60] whereas that of ADH is about 2 mM[84] (which corresponds to alcohol concentrations of 37 and 9 mg%, respectively).

Recently,[85] a role for MEOS activity in vivo has been denied on the basis that CCl_4 reduced MEOS activity in vitro by 50 to 60%, without significantly affecting rates of ethanol metabolism in vivo. Actually, rates of blood ethanol disappearance appeared decreased 15 to 20%, but the results failed to reach a level of statistical significance and were offset by an unexplained increase in distribution space. Furthermore, no attempt was made to correct for microsomal losses during preparation, though these could be markedly affected by CCl_4. Moreover, another investigation did actually find a reduction in blood ethanol clearance after CCl_4.[86]

Tolerance to Ethanol and Increased Ethanol Metabolism after Chronic Ethanol Consumption

It is an old observation that regular drinkers acquire the capacity to tolerate large amounts of alcoholic beverages. Probably the most significant aspect of this phenomenon is increased central nervous system tolerance, that is, a progressive decrease in responsiveness in the central nervous system to a given level of alcohol.[18] The biochemical mechanism of this central nervous system adaptation, however, is unknown, and, therefore, we will not focus on this aspect of the adaptation phenomenon, though it is a very important one. Instead we will concentrate on that part of the adaptation which is due to increased rates of ethanol metabolism, so-called metabolic adaptation. Indeed, it has been found that alcoholics have higher rates of ethanol metabolism.[12,87] Moreover, experimental ethanol administration results in an increased rate of ethanol metabolism,[60,88-90] both in man and in rats, though some questioned this finding.[18] The mechanism of the acceleration has not been elucidated and could involve any of the pathways discussed before. There is a controversy on whether or not ethanol consumption affects activities of hepatic ADH with increases[88,91] or no change[59,60,89,92-95] (or even decreases) reported. Some who found a moderate initial increase subsequently observed a return to normal or a decrease after prolonged ethanol feeding.[96-98] Thus, an increase in ADH activity does not necessarily accompany the acceleration of ethanol metabolism. However, a marked decrease in ADH activity does slow ethanol oxidation. The effect of pyrazole has been discussed before. It is also possible that the reduced rate of ethanol metabolism produced by lack of dietary protein is due, at least in part, to the associated depression in ADH activity,[98] although lack of protein results in a general impairment of liver function. Actually, the question whether or not there is a moderate change in hepatic ADH activity may not have a direct bearing on the problem of rates of alcohol metabolism, since it is generally recognized that ADH is usually not the rate limiting step in that pathway. There are numerous examples of the lack of correlation between rates of ethanol oxidation and hepatic ADH activity. For instance, individuals with "atypical" ADH have enzyme activities seven times higher than normal, but this is not accompanied by an acceleration of the metabolism of ethanol in vivo.[99] This discrepancy supports the view that in the process of ADH mediated ethanol oxidation, ADH itself is not rate limiting but that velocities may depend on availability of the cofactor NAD and especially the speed of the reoxidation of the ADH-NADH complex. As an example of accelerated ethanol metabolism which may involve the ADH pathway, fructose can be cited; its moderate effect is probably due to a speeding up of the reoxidation of NADH.[100,101]

The reoxidation of NADH will also be increased if in some way the shuttling of the hydrogen equivalents from the cytosol into the mitochondria by any of the three mechanisms depicted in Figure 1 can be accelerated. It is not known whether this actually occurs, but that such a possibility is plausible was indicated by the recent experimental observation that CPIB, a hypocholesterolemic drug, was found to accelerate ethanol metabolism in rats; the associated five-fold increase in α-glycerophosphate dehydrogenase activity suggests that the corresponding shunt from the cytosol to the mitochondria may be stimulated.[102] Moreover, uncouplers, such as dinitrophenol, can stimulate the rate of ethanol metabolism in liver slices of normal rats,[94] suggesting that enhancement of electron transport chain activity may also accelerate ethanol metabolism.

In individuals with glycogen storage disease, ethanol metabolism is very rapid.[103,104] Since there is no increase of ADH[105] nor a striking shift in redox potential, as judged from the blood lactate, a non-ADH pathway may well be involved, possibly MEOS. Furthermore, since under our experimental conditions, the increase in blood ethanol clearance after chronic ethanol administration was associated with a rise in MEOS activity, the question also arises whether the latter can account for the increased rate of blood ethanol clearance. Calculations show indeed that when corrected for microsomal losses during the preparation procedure, the rise in MEOS activity can acount for 1/2 to 2/3 of the increase in blood ethanol clearance.[83] The unaccounted for difference may actually result from a secondary increase in oxidation via ADH, a pathway limited by the rate of NADH reoxidation. This indeed could be accelerated by an increase in MEOS activity, since the latter is associated with enhanced NADPH utilization and NADPH-NADP and NADH-NAD systems are linked.[105] Indirect evidence that MEOS activity may play a role in vivo can be derived from the fact that other drugs (such as barbiturates) which stimulate microsomes and increase total hepatic MEOS activity[106] were also found to enhance rates of blood ethanol clearance.[107] More recent studies failed to verify this effect.[76,108] In the latter investigations, however, longer-acting barbiturates were used and ethanol clearance was tested in close association with barbiturate administration, at a time when blood barbiturate levels were probably elevated. Under these conditions, it was found that barbiturates interfere with blood ethanol clearance.[83,109]

It must be pointed out that rates of ethanol metabolism never more than doubled after chronic ethanol consumption. Therefore, the metabolic adaptation may not much influence the early effects found after administration of large oral doses of ethanol or after ethanol injection. It will, however, significantly shorten the duration of the ethanol effect and may also influence the initial action of relatively small doses.

Interaction of Ethanol and Drug Metabolism

Interactions of the effects of ethanol and various drugs have been widely recognized.[110] In addition to developing tolerance to ethanol, alcoholics, when sober, appear to be more resistant to the action of a variety of drugs. Intoxicated individuals, however, are more susceptible to several medications.[111] These effects are usually attributed to central nervous system adaptation and to additive or synergistic effects of alcohol and various drugs on the central nervous system. However, the existence of an at least partially common microsomal system for ethanol and drug metabolism sheds new light on the interaction of ethanol and drug metabolism.

Stimulation of the Microsomal Drug Metabolizing Enzymes

Drug induced hypertrophy of SER is generally accompanied by an increase in microsomal protein and augmented activities of hepatic drug metabolizing enzymes located in the microsomal fraction.[66] Similarly, the proliferation of hepatic SER induced by ethanol has some functional counterpart: chronic administration of ethanol to man and rats results in an increased activity of a variety of microsomal drug detoxifying enzymes.[63,90,112,113] Ethanol also increases the activity of ALA synthetase[114-116] and the content of microsomal cytochrome P-450.[64,116] The increase in P-450 content occurs in the SER rather than in the RER.[65] The increase in hepatic microsomal drug detoxifying enzymes induced by ethanol ingestion offers a likely explanation for the recent observation that ethanol consumption enhances the rate of drug clearance in vivo.

Increased Drug Metabolism in Vivo: Drug Tolerance

The tolerance of the alcoholic to various drugs has been generally attributed to central nervous system adaptation.[117] The biochemical basis of this is unknown. In addition to central nervous systems adaptation, however, metabolic adaptation must be considered. Indeed, it has been shown recently that the rate of drug clearance from the blood is enhanced in alcoholics.[118] Of course this could be due to a variety of factors other than ethanol, such as effects of nutritional deficiency, congeners and use of other drugs, so commonly associated with alcoholism.[119] Recent studies showed, however, that administration of pure ethanol with nondeficient diets under metabolic ward conditions resulted in a striking increase in the rate of blood clearance of meprobamate and pentobarbital.[90] A similar effect was also observed in rats. Furthermore, the capacity of liver slices from animals fed ethanol to metabolize meprobamate was also increased, which clearly shows that ethanol consumption affects drug metabolism in the liver itself, independent of drug excretion or distribution.

Inhibition of Drug Metabolism by Ethanol

Contrasting with the increased tolerance of alcoholics in the sober state, intoxicated individuals are usually more susceptible to the action of a variety of drugs. This is caused by an additive or synergistic effect at the central nervous system level. Recent studies, however, have indicated that there may be a dissociation in the time course of the decreased drug sensitivity of the animal and the occurrence of central nervous system tolerance: the former was found to precede the latter.[120] The increased susceptibility of the inebriated individual could again be explained, at least in part, by the effect of ethanol on microsomal drug detoxifying enzymes. It has indeed been found that ethanol inhibits the metabolism of a variety of drugs in vitro.[112,113,116,121,122] These in vitro effects may explain the observation that in vivo, simultaneous administration of ethanol and drugs slows the rate of drug metabolism.[121,122]

Effect of Drug Administration on Ethanol Metabolism

As described before, administration of various drugs results in an increased activity of MEOS when expressed per gram of liver or per total body weight with an associated enhancement of blood ethanol clearance, when tested at a time when the drug has disappeared from the bloodstream.[107,109] In the presence of drugs, however, there is inhibition of ethanol metabolism,[83,109] the mechanism of which is not known. It could be due to an interference with microsomal ethanol metabolism in some cases, whereas in others, it has been traced to an inhibition of alcohol dehydrogenase.[123]

Effects of Ethanol on Lipid and Bilirubin Metabolism in the Endoplasmic Reticulum

Effect of Ethanol on Cholesterol Metabolism

In addition to its involvement in drug metabolism, the endoplasmic reticulum participates in many other functions, including cholesterol synthesis. The effects of ethanol on the microsomes may explain increased cholesterol synthesis after ethanol,[124] an effect probably akin to enhanced cholesterogenesis described after barbiturate administration.[125] This increased cholesterol synthesis may explain, in part, the accumulation of cholesterol ester observed in the liver after alcohol feeding,[5,126] especially when alcohol is given with a cholesterol-free diet. Administration of ethanol with cholesterol-containing diets, however, enhances the hepatic cholesterol accumulation.[124] This effect is probably due, in part, to decreased cholesterol catabolism, as evidenced by a reduction in bile acid production and turnover after alcohol feeding.[124] The mechanism by which ethanol inhibits bile acid formation has not yet been elucidated.

Effects of Ethanol on Fatty Acid, Glyceride, and Bilirubin Metabolism: Alcoholic Hyperlipemia

Both in man[5,127-132] and in rats[133] ethanol administration produces mild hyperlipemia and the most striking changes take place in the very low density lipoprotein fraction. The alcohol-induced hyperlipemia is exaggerated when alcohol is given with a fat-containing diet.[129] Incorporation into lipoprotein of intragastrically-administered ^{3}H-palmitate and intravenously-injected ^{14}C-lysine is increased to a great extent by alcohol administration.[133] This contrasts with choline deficiency, which produces the opposite effect.[134] These, as well as other studies, suggest that the ethanol-induced hyperlipemia results from enhanced lipoprotein production. Fatty acids are esterified and lipoproteins are formed in the endoplasmic reticulum. Moreover, ethanol consumption enhances the activity of hepatic microsomal L-α-glycerophosphate acyl transferase.[135] The mechanism of the alterations of these microsomal functions produced by ethanol has not been clarified. It could be linked directly to the fact that ethanol can be oxidized at this key metabolic site. Ethanol could also act indirectly by enhancing the availability of fatty acids by decreasing their oxidation or enhancing synthesis, as discussed before. This in turn can induce hepatic production of lipoproteins.[136] Contrasting with hepatic fatty acids, those derived from adipose tissue may be less available after alcohol. Short-term ethanol feeding produces a fall in the level of circulating free fatty acids (FFA) in man[127,137] with decreased FFA turnover and concomitant reduction in circulating glycerol.[139] This depression of FFA mobilization from adipose tissue was found to be mediated by acetate.[140] Acetate is the end product of ethanol metabolism in the liver and it is released into the bloodstream. With oral ethanol,[127,139] the fall of FFA was more sustained than after intravenous ethanol,[137] possibly because parenterally-administered ethanol may elicit hormonal responses (catecholamine release, vide infra) not produced by oral ethanol. The effects of one very large dose of ethanol on the circulating level of FFA is controversial, with reports of either an increase[141,142] or no change.[143] Since ethanol, when used at a stressful dose, probably both stimulates fatty acid mobilization (via catecholamine release, discussed subsequently) and depresses it (via acetate), the net effect may depend on particular experimental conditions. In man, even with amounts of ethanol as large as 300 g per day, concentration of circulating FFA do not increase; they rise only after ingestion of very large doses of ethanol (400 g per day).[5]

The hyperlipemia produced experimentally is much less pronounced than the marked lactescence observed in occasional alcoholics.[128] In these individuals the alcohol induced hyperlipemia is probably potentiated by an underlying defect in metabolism, such as diabetes, a low lipoprotein lipase activity[128] or coexisting pancreatitis;[144] the latter may on occasion be associated with a circulating lipoprotein lipase inhibitor.[145] In some of these cases hyperlipemia is inducible by ethanol but not by carbohydrates.[128,132] In addition to fatty liver, the hyperlipemia is sometimes accompanied by jaundice and hemolytic anemia[146] and the eponym "Zieve's Syndrome" has been used to characterize this clinical association.

Hepatic microsomes are responsible for a large

number of metabolic functions. On theoretical grounds one can postulate that several of these functions (which have not as yet been extensively studied) will be found to be affected by either acute or chronic ethanol consumption. One can now anticipate a number of reports, such as the prevention of hyperbilirubinemia of the newborn by ethanol,[147] attributed to induction of microsomal uridine-diphosphate-glucuronyl transferase.[148] The possible role of microsomal changes (induced by ethanol consumption) in the development of ethanol dependence is particularly intriguing, as discussed subsequently.

FACTORS OF ETHANOL DEPENDENCE

In addition to tolerance, the state of ethanol addiction is characterized by dependence. It has been traditional to distinguish between "physical" dependence and "psychic" or "psychological" dependence. Both reflect a state of discomfort produced by withdrawal of a drug from a subject who has been chronically or repeatedly exposed to it. The symptoms can be alleviated by renewed administration of that drug or another drug with similar pharmacological actions. Psychological dependence connotes a state of discomfort which consists of nonspecific dissatisfaction giving rise to a desire for the drug. When the discomfort includes more specific physiological disturbances, it is called physical dependence. Clinically, tolerance and physical dependence develop in a parallel way. The signs and symptoms of withdrawal of alcohol in man have been described elsewhere in this book and will not be reviewed here. It is noteworthy that virtually identical reactions have been reported in relation to withdrawal of barbiturates and of a variety of tranquilizers. As is the case for the problem of tolerance, our knowledge of the fundamental biological mechanisms of dependence is rudimentary. A number of changes have been described in association with dependence. However, their exact relationships are not known and it is often not possible to distinguish which effects are causes and which are consequences or merely concomitants. For instance, in animals made tolerant to ethanol, the activity of sodium- and potassium-dependent adenosine triphosphatase in brain was significantly increased and the rate of active transport of cations in brain tissue was enhanced when measured in the abscence of ethanol,[149] whereas in the presence of ethanol, they were depressed.[150,151] It is unknown, however, whether these findings have any bearing on the problem of central nervous system tolerance to ethanol. Similarly, the conflicting reports of the effects of ethanol on gamma amino butyric acid (GABA), reviewed elsewhere,[151] may reflect general metabolic changes produced on the central nervous system, rather than primary effects.

A variety of factors probably play important roles in the course of the development of both psychic and physical dependence. Only those theories will be reviewed here which are amenable to some experimental verification.

Role of Racial Factors in the Metabolism of Ethanol and the Development of Alcoholism

The incidence of alcoholism is steadily increasing. Although no group is immune, various segments of our society are differently affected. For instance, it is generally recognized that American Jews are relatively spared, whereas the American Indians seem to be more prone to alcoholism. These differences are attributed commonly to cultural factors, although genetic influences have not been ruled out. A hereditary link between alcoholism, cirrhosis, and color blindness has been implicated by some,[152] but denied by others.[153,154] Differences in rates of ethanol metabolism according to racial background, however, were recently reported by Fenna et al.[155] Prompted by the clinical observation that Eskimos and Indians take longer to sober up after an alcoholic debauch than do whites, Fenna et al. administered ethanol to volunteers with normal liver function tests and found that blood ethanol concentration fell significantly faster in whites than in Eskimos and Indians. The 50% difference could not be correlated with previous ethanol intake or dietary habits, leading the authors to conclude that genetic factors probably are implicated. Though absolute rates of ethanol metabolism were lower in Indians and Eskimos, their capacity to develop an accelerated blood ethanol clearance after chronic alcohol ingestion was much greater than in whites. One must wonder whether on the one hand, this apparent greater capacity for metabolic adaptation could in some way be linked to a higher incidence of alcoholism or whether on the other hand, it could also depend on genetic factors. A recent study conducted in identical twins has indeed revealed that individual differences in rates of ethanol elimination appear to be genetically controlled.[156] Ethanol administration increased the rate of metabolism of antipyrine,[156] as had been reported in another study with meprobamate and pentobarbital,[90] but considerable individual variations were noted despite control of environmental factors. The increase in rates of ethanol metabolism was even more variable, but the dose given in this study[156] was lower than in a preceding one.[90] Since genetic factors appear to play an important role in determining rates of ethanol and drug metabolism as well as the degree of the "inductive" response, one must wonder to what extent appetite for ethanol, as well as the propensity to develop dependence, is also determined by genetic factors. Genetic factors have been shown to play a role in affecting the appetite for alcohol in some strains of mice.[157] Apparently, however, ethanol intake was not sufficient in these strains to lead to the development of true dependence. Indeed, by conventional feeding techniques (incorporation of ethanol in drinking water), experimental animals refuse to spontaneously drink sufficient amounts of ethanol to consistently develop signs of dependence. Recently, this difficulty was overcome either by force feeding ethanol to dogs[158] and monkeys[159] or by the use of liquid diets in mice.[160] The technique of feeding ethanol as part of a totally liquid diet was first introduced to overcome the natural aversion of the rat for ethanol.[5] With usual feeding techniques, ethanol intake was indeed insufficient to produce consistent liver damage when the diet was adequate. By contrast, when ethanol was given as part of a totally liquid diet, ethanol intake was doubled, resulting in the development of fatty liver, despite an otherwise adequate diet.[5,6,126] During these studies, it was commonly observed that when ethanol intake was decreased (for instance because of intercurrent illness or of some interference with the delivery of the diet), some animals developed withdrawal symptoms such as seizures. Freund[160] has used similar liquid diets (preceded by starvation) to produce a model for ethanol withdrawal in mice. The animal models can be used to test various hypotheses concerning the mechanism of ethanol dependence.

Possible Microsomal Mechanism Contributing to Ethanol Dependence

Chronic ethanol consumption results not only in enhanced rates of ethanol clearance, but the alcoholic, when sober, also displays an accelerated metabolism of other compounds detoxified in the microsomes such as sedatives and tranquilizers.[90,95,118,156] It is plausible that the microsomal metabolism of some endogenous compounds, as yet unidentified, is also enhanced. The lack of these substances (or the excess of their metabolites) could produce adverse or unpleasant effects. However, in the presence of ethanol, the metabolism of other microsomal substrates is inhibited, presumably through competition for a partially shared microsomal detoxifying pathway. This is illustrated by the striking inhibition of drug metabolism in the presence of ethanol[95,112,113,116,121,122] observed both in vivo (in men and animals given drugs and ethanol) or in vitro in liver slices or isolated microsomes. If this inhibition by ethanol of microsomal metabolism applies to the postulated endogenous substrates, physical dependence on ethanol could perhaps be linked, at least in part, to the following theoretical sequence of events, illustrated in Figure 3: 1) chronic

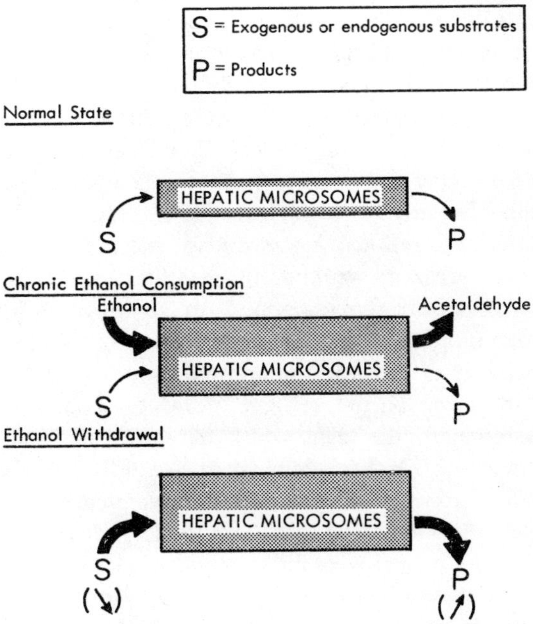

FIGURE 3. Theory of a microsomal contribution to the development of ethanol dependence.

ethanol consumption "induces" the activity of microsomal enzymes which metabolize exogenous as well as endogenous compounds; 2) as a result the alcoholic, upon sobering, experiences accelerated metabolism of these endogenous compounds with untoward effects; 3) these can be alleviated by further ethanol ingestion (the metabolism of which spares that of the postulated endogenous substrates), thereby promoting the craving for ethanol. Thus, one may wonder whether in addition to psychological and socioeconomic factors, an increased capacity of having one's metabolism "induced" by ethanol favors the development of alcoholism. This propensity of "induction" by ethanol could be influenced by both hereditary and acquired factors. In any event, physical dependence on ethanol probably has multiple determinants[161] and it is questionable whether a unitary mechanism explains all events associated with dependence. While it is proposed that hepatic microsomal changes may contribute to the development of dependence, it is not implied that these changes necessarily represent "the" sole or main mechanism responsible for the addictive process. Principal determinants of dependence may reside in the central nervous system. The proposed hypothesis, however, has the advantage of being consistent with a number of observed changes associated with dependence. If validated, it would indicate that drugs now commonly used for the treatment of withdrawal symptoms may affect not only the central nervous system but possibly could act by virtue of their being substrates, on the hepatic microsomal drug detoxifying systems. Furthermore, the microsomal theory of ethanol dependence has the advantage of offering a rational framework for the observation that ethanol withdrawal reactions (such as seizures) not only respond to treatment with barbiturates[162] but conversely, that ethanol is partially effective in the prevention of barbiturate withdrawal phenomena.[163] Moreover, as already mentioned, the signs which develop after withdrawal of either depressants or ethanol are remarkably similar. The clinical experience after alcohol withdrawal has been widely described. Similar findings were made in human experimental studies by Isbell et al.[12] and Mendelson.[13] The numerous studies describing similar symptoms after the withdrawal of barbiturates, tranquilizers, and a variety of hypnotics have been extensively reviewed by Kalant et al.[164]

Theories of Ethanol Dependence Linked to Acetaldehyde

Acetaldehyde is the first and major "specific" oxidation product of ethanol and its presence after the ingestion of alcohol has been demonstrated in the blood.[165] Acetaldehyde concentrations after alcohol ingestion, however, are small, except after Antabuse® administration. Nevertheless, it has long been speculated that acetaldehyde may contribute to the complications of alcoholism.[166] Although the exact pathways of its metabolism are still unknown, it is generally accepted that the oxidation of acetaldehyde results in the generation of NADH. Therefore, the hepatic metabolism of acetaldehyde could contribute to a number of pathologic effects through the mechanism of NADH generation, as discussed before for ethanol in this chapter. In addition, acetaldehyde could produce its effects through increased catecholamine release, the excretion[167-172] and production[173] of which was found to be enhanced by ethanol in various species. Excretion of other amines such as tryptamine[172] was also found increased after ethanol. An exception among the amines is histamine whose excretion in the urine remained unchanged, indicating that flushing associated with alcohol consumption is probably unrelated to this substance.[174] Acetaldehyde could be responsible for reduction in hepatic coenzyme A after ethanol, an effect attributed to an inactivation of the coenzyme by acetaldehyde.[175] However, the reduction in hepatic CoA has been questioned recently.[176] Some ethanol effects upon the brain have been attributed directly to acetaldehyde[166,177,178] and recently intriguing theories of ethanol dependence have been proposed with a key role for acetaldehyde. One of these theories exploits the fact that acetaldehyde can competitively inhibit the oxidation of other aldehydes. This was shown to be the case for the oxidation of 5 hydroxyindoleacetaldehyde to the corresponding acid,[179] which may explain (in addition to the excess NADH generation) the increased formation of the alcohol (5 hydroxytryptophol) in man[180,181] during alcohol ingestion. A similar mechanism probably explains the increased excretion of ^{14}C-3-methoxy-4-hydroxyphenylglycol with a reciprocal reduction in the acid (VMA) from ^{14}C-norepinephrine after ethanol administration.[182] Another possible consequence is the accumulation of intermediary aldehydes as discussed below.

Augmentation of Alkaloid Formation from Dopamine by Acetaldehyde

According to this theory, acetaldhyde, which results from the metabolism of ethanol, primarily in the liver, but possibly also in the brain[183] interferes with the biological disposition of a biogenic amine, namely dopamine. Normally, as shown in Figure 4, dopamine is converted to 3,4-dihydroxyphenyl acetaldehyde which is oxidized to its corresponding acid. Acetaldehyde, however, is a known inhibitor of the oxidation of aromatic aldehydes. Excess acetaldehyde originating from the ethanol may decrease the normal pathway of dopamine metabolism, thereby enhancing the condensation of 3,4-diphydroxyphenyl acetaldehyde with dopamine to form tetrahydropapaveroline. Indeed both ethanol and acetaldehyde significantly enhance tetrahydropapaveroline synthesis in brain stem homogenates.[184] In plants, tetrahydropapaveroline is a natural biosynthetic precursor of a vast complex of alkaloids which include morphine type compounds. It is conceivable that tetrahydropapaveroline could be formed as a consequence of alcohol abuse and then undergo similar biotransformation in mammalian systems, as illustrated in

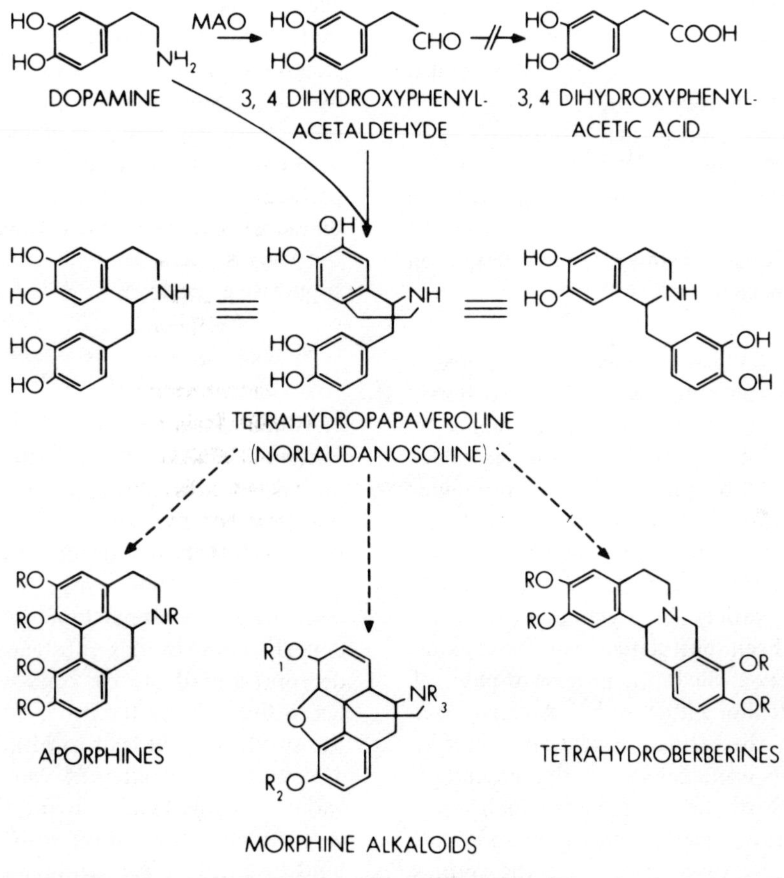

	R_1	R_2	R_3
NORMORPHINE	H	H	H
MORPHINE	H	H	CH_3
NORCODEINE	H	CH_3	H
CODEINE	H	CH_3	CH_3

FIGURE 4. Hypothesis for the relationship of ethanol mediated modification of dopamine metabolism to alcohol addiction. See explanations in the text. From Davis et al.[184] with permission.

Figure 4. In summary, it has been postulated by Davis et al.[184] that diversion of neuroamine metabolism with formation of biologically active alkaloid derivatives may then be involved in alcoholism. This theory has been the subject of vigorous criticism but thus far it has been neither conclusively proven nor disproven. An important objection raised was the striking clinical difference in the features of ethanol and morphine physical dependence,[185] but the hypothesis does not need to be relevant to all aspects of tolerance and physical dependence in alcoholism. Some of these could well be more directly related to other pharmacological actions of ethanol rather than to the proposed hypothesis. Other objections focused on the lack of direct evidence that tetrahydropapaveroline is formed in vivo.[186] It was also found that ethanol-dependent mice, when challenged with an opiate antagonist, do not develop opiate-dependent behavior.[187] Again, this latter criticism does not fully disprove the proposed theory, but indicates that the aspects of physical dependence in question are based on some different mechanism.

Condensation of Acetaldehyde with Neuroamines

Acetaldehyde can condense with neuroamines to form simple alkaloid derivatives. For instance, it has been shown that in adrenal tissue, acetaldehyde condenses with epinephrine and norepinephrine to form tetrahydroisoquinoline alkaloids. Since these alkaloids are similar in structure to a number of naturally occurring simple alkaloids which exhibit a variety of psychopharmacologic actions, it has been postulated that these compounds could play a role in the process of physical dependence in alcohol addiction.[188] An analogous reaction includes the formation of β-carbolines by condensation of acetaldehyde with indolethylamines.[189] Some of the compounds which result from a condensation reaction are known to inhibit monoamine oxidase or to antagonize the actions of serotonin. It is conceivable that, either by their direct effect on the central nervous system or by altering biogenic amine activity or function, these compounds may contribute to the central nervous system effects of ethanol.[188,190]

General Theories of Tolerance and Physical Dependence

A number of general theories which have been advanced to explain the development of tolerance to and physical dependence on drugs acting upon the central nervous system may have some application to the special case of ethanol as well. Most proposed hypotheses postulate some kind of homeostatic response to the effect of administered drugs. A self regulatory process is assumed to adapt to the drug effect in such a manner as to restore normal function if the drug is being administered. However, on drug withdrawal, the adaptive process then constitutes an uncompensated disturbance in its own right leading to withdrawal reaction. Various formulations of this hypothesis have been proposed. One of these is the denervation supersensitivity hypothesis of Jaffe and Sharpless.[191] This is based on the observation that many withdrawal phenomena represent an exaggeration of behavior which may be suppressed by the agent that induces dependence. It is postulated that during its administration, the agent induces an increase in excitability of nervous pathways that is masked by the depressing action of the drug on the same pathway or, alternatively, the drug induces depression through activation of suppressive pathways. Withdrawal will reveal a rebound excitability. The relevance of this theory to alcohol remains to be assessed.

Goldstein and Goldstein[192] have developed an enzyme induction theory which differs from the microsomal theory described before by the fact that ethanol (or any other drug producing dependence) does not act directly as the inducer but rather inhibits the synthesis of some substance essential for neuronal function. The reduction in concentration of this substance in turn results in derepression of the enzymes which synthesize it. On withdrawal of the drug, excessive synthesis of the substance will lead to withdrawal overactivity. The theory of Collier[193] can be considered as a variance of the Goldstein and Goldstein model. It is postulated that drugs with addictive potential bind to and "induce" an increase in receptor sites for an endogenous neurotransmitter substance in the central nervous system and possibly other tissues. When the drug is administered in increasing doses, additional receptor sites develop because the original ones are bound. When the drug is removed, an enhanced number of receptor sites are available to the endogenous transmitter and become active, hence withdrawal symptoms occur. Neither the essential substance postulated by Goldstein and Goldstein nor the activator of receptor sites proposed by Collier have been identified.

Psychoendocrine Factors

A number of hormonal changes are found consistantly to be altered in parallel with the development of dependence and can be considered as "biochemical correlates" of dependence. It is not known, however, whether there is a causal relationship between these hormonal changes and the dependence or whether the relationship is merely that of a parallel modification. As discussed before, acute alcohol administration increases urinary excretion of catecholamines and this could be mediated by the acetaldehyde formed upon ethanol oxidation.[194] An increase of catecholamine was also found during experimental ethanol administration to man,[161] and the levels remained elevated during withdrawal, which was also the case in clinical situations.[195] Thus, the changes in catecholamines do not fit any particular feedback system theory.

In addition to the activation of the adrenal medulla, alcohol produces a stimulation of the cortex. In the rat, intraperitoneal injection of ethanol was shown to stimulate adrenocortical function.[196,197] Hypophysectomy prevented the response. Repeated injections of ethanol may[198] or may not[197] alter this effect. Elevations of serum corticoids were also found in man after acute alcohol ingestion[199-202] and no such response was elicited in two subjects with pituitary lesions.[200] Growth hormone levels also increased after ethanol.[202] In alcoholic volunteers given ethanol for a four day period, a significant rise of serum cortisol was found which persisted in those subjects who showed withdrawal symptoms. Nonalcoholic subjects showed rises only when gastrointestinal symptoms developed while they were drinking; none of these subjects, however, developed withdrawal symptoms and serum cortisol levels were normal during the postalcohol period.[203]

The mechanism of the stimulation of adrenocortical function by ethanol is not known. The hypophysis is apparently involved. Theoretically, alcohol could also decrease steroid metabolism by inhibiting hepatic microsomal breakdown, but this remains to be tested. Whatever its pathogenesis, the increased adrenocortical response could conceivably play a role in ethanol dependence. Kakihana and associates[204] have indeed found a correlation between the magnitude of the plasma corticosterone response after ethanol ingestion and the level of behavioral tolerance to ethanol in various strains of mice. The greatest tolerance for ethanol was found in the animals with the highest plasma corticosterone response after ethanol administration.

In addition to the adrenoglucocorticoid response after ethanol, there is now evidence that adrenal mineralocorticoid activity may also be increased,[205,206] but the mechanism of this and its relevance to the phenomenon of dependence are not known.

SUMMARY

The pathogenesis of many of the effects of ethanol on lipids, drug, and intermediary metabolism has now been elucidated: these changes are either mediated by metabolites of alcohol, such as acetaldehyde and acetate, or are the result of hepatic generation of NADH (when ethanol is metabolized by hepatic ADH), or are closely similar to processes of microsomal drug detoxification in the liver upon oxidation of ethanol via a new pathway, the microsomal ethanol oxidizing system (MEOS). These effects of ethanol enable us to understand the development of fatty liver, hyperlipemia, hyperlactacidemia, hyperuricemia, ketosis, acidosis, hypoglycemia, metabolic tolerance to ethanol, increased tolerance to drugs in the alcoholic (when sober), and enhanced susceptibility to sedatives and tranquilizers in inebriated individuals. The pathogenesis of ethanol dependence is still not understood but several theoretical mechanisms have been proposed.

REFERENCES

1. Best, C. H., Hartroft, W. S., Lucas, C. C., and Ridout, J. H., Liver damage produced by feeding alcohol or sugar and its prevention by choline, *Brit. Med. J.*, 2,1001, 1949.

2. Lieber, C. S., DeCarli, L., and Schmid, R., Effect of ethanol on fatty acid metabolism in liver slices, *Biochem. Biophys. Res. Commun.*, 1, 302, 1959.

3. Lieber, C. S. and Schmid, R., The effect of ethanol on fatty acid metabolism; stimulation of hepatic fatty acid synthesis in vitro, *J. Clin. Invest.*, 40, 394, 1961.

4. Lieber, C. S., Lefèvre, A., Spritz, N., Feinman, L., and DeCarli, L. M., Difference in hepatic metabolism of long - and medium-chain fatty acids: the role of fatty acid chain length in the production of the alcoholic fatty liver, *J. Clin. Invest.*, 46, 1451, 1967.

5. Lieber, C. S., Jones, D. P., Mendelson, J., and DeCarli, L. M., Fatty liver hyperlipemia and hyperuricemia produced by prolonged alcohol consumption despite adequate dietary intake, *Trans. Ass. Amer. Physicians*, 76, 289, 1963.

6. Lieber, C. S., Jones, D. P., and DeCarli, L. M., Effects of prolonged ethanol intake: production of fatty liver despite adequate diets, *J. Clin. Invest.*, 44, 1009, 1965.

7. Iseri, O. A., Lieber, C. S., and Gottlieb, L. S., The ultrastructure of fatty liver induced by prolonged ethanol ingestion, *Amer. J. Path.*, 48, 535, 1966.

8. Lane, B. P. and Lieber, C. S., Ultrastructural alterations in human hepatocytes following ingestion of ethanol with adequate diets, *Amer. J. Path.*, 49, 593, 1966.

9. Lieber, C. S. and Rubin, E., Alcoholic fatty liver in man on a high protein and low fat diet, *Amer. J. Med.*, 44, 200, 1968.

10. Rubin, E. and Lieber, C. S., Alcohol-induced hepatic injury in non-alcoholic volunteers, *New Eng. J. Med.*, 278, 869, 1968.

11. Aston, R., Characteristics of drug dependence to barbiturates, alcohol, and tranquilizers, in *Chemical and Biologic Aspects of Drug Dependence*, Mulé, S. J. and Brill, H., Eds., Chemical Rubber Co., Cleveland, 1972, Chap. 2.

12. Isbell, H., Fraser, H. F., Wikler, A., Belleville, R. E., and Eisenman, A. J., An experimental study of the etiology of "rum fits" and delirium tremens, *Quart. J. Stud. Alcohol*, 16, 1, 1955.

13. Mendelson, J. H., Experimentally induced chronic intoxication and withdrawal in alcoholics, *Quart. J. Stud. Alcohol*, Suppl. 2, 1964, 14.

14. Lieber, C. S., Rubin, E., and DeCarli, L. M., Effects of ethanol on lipid, uric acid intermediary and drug metabolism, including pathogenesis of the alcoholic fatty liver, in *The Biology of Alcoholism*, Vol. 1, Kissin, B. and Begleiter, H., Eds., Plenum Press, New York, 1971, 263.

15. Feinman, L. and Lieber, C. S., Liver disease in alcoholism, in *The Biology of Alcoholism*, Vol. 3, Kissin, B. and Begleiter, H., Eds., Plenum Press, New York, 1972, in press.

16. Pirola, R. and Lieber, C. S., Acute and chronic pancreatitis, in *The Biology of Alcoholism*, Vol. 3, Kissin, B. and Begleiter, H., Eds., Plenum Press, New York, 1972, in press.

17. Lindenbaum, J. and Lieber, C. S., Effects of ethanol on the blood, bone marrow, and small intestine in man, in *Biological Aspects of Alcohol*, Roach, M. K., McIsaac, W. M., and Creaven, P. J., Eds., University of Texas Press, Austin, 1971, 27.

18. Levy, J., Contribution à l'étude de l'accoutumance expérimentale aux poisons. II. Alcoolisme expérimental. Fixation de l'alcool sur les tissus de l'organisme accoutumé à cette substance, *Bull. Soc. Chim. Biol.*, 17, 27, 1935.

19. Thompson, G. N., *Alcoholism*, Charles C Thomas, Springfield, Illinois, 1956.

20. Winkler, K., Lundquist, F., and Tygstrup, N., The hepatic metabolism of ethanol in patients with cirrhosis of the liver, *Scand. J. Clin. Lab. Invest.*, 23, 59, 1969.

21. Forsander, O. A., Räihä, N., and Suomalainen, H., Oxydation des Athylalkohols in isolierter Leber und isoliertem Hinterkörper der Ratte, *Hoppe Seyler Z. Physiol. Chem.*, 318, 1, 1960.

22. Larsen, J. A., Extrahepatic metabolism of ethanol in man, *Nature*, 184, 1236, 1959.

23. Lieber, C. S. and Davidson, C. S., Some metabolic effects of ethyl alcohol, *Amer. J. Med.*, 33, 319, 1962.

24. Lieber, C. S., Metabolic effects produced by alcohol in the liver and other tissues, *Advances Intern. Med.*, 14, 151, 1968.

25. Krebs, H. A., Effects of ethanol on gluconeogenesis in the perfused rat liver, in *Konferenz der Gesellschaft fur Biologische Chemie,* Springer Verlag, Berlin, 1967, 216.

26. Daughaday, W. H., Lipicky, R. J., and Rasinski, D. C., Lactic acidosis as a cause of nonketotic acidosis in diabetic patients, *New Eng. J. Med.*, 267, 1010, 1962.

27. Lieber, C. S., Jones, D. P., Losowsky, M. S., and Davidson, C. S., Interrelation of uric acid and ethanol metabolism in man, *J. Clin. Invest.*, 41, 1863, 1962.

28. Maclachlan, M. J. and Rodnan, G. P., Effects of food, fast and alcohol on serum uric acid and acute attacks of gout, *Amer. J. Med.*, 42, 38, 1967.

29. Evans, J. G., Prior, I.A.M., and Harvey, H.P.B., Relation of serum uric acid to body bulk, haemoglobin, and alcohol intake in two South Pacific Polynesian populations, *Ann. Rheum. Dis.*, 27, 319, 1968.

30. Nikkila, E. A. and Ojala, K., Role of hepatic L-α-glycerophosphate and triglyceride synthesis in production of fatty liver by ethanol, *Proc. Soc. Exp. Biol. Med.*, 113, 814, 1963.

31. Chappell, J. B., Systems used for the transport of substrates into mitochondria, *Brit. Med. Bull.*, 24, 150, 1968.

32. Whereat, A. F., Orishimo, M. W., and Nelson, J., The location of different synthetic systems for fatty acids in inner and outer mitochondrial membranes from rabbit heart, *J. Biol. Chem.*, 244, 6498, 1969.

33. Grunnet, N., Oxidation of extramitochondrial NADH by rat liver mitochondria: possible role of acyl SCoA elongation enzymes, *Biochem. Biophys. Res. Commun.*, 41, 909, 1970.

34. Bücher, T. and Klingenberg, M., Wege des Wasserstoffs in der'lebendigen Organisation, *Angew. Chem.*, 70, 552, 1958.

35. Williamson, J. R., Scholz, R., Browning, E. T., Thurman, R. G., and Fukami, M. H., Metabolic effects of ethanol in perfused rat liver, *J. Biol Chem.*, 244, 5044, 1969.

36. Lieber, C. S., Spritz, N., and DeCarli, L. M., Role of dietary, adipose and endogenously synthesized fatty acids in the pathogenesis of the alcoholic fatty liver, *J. Clin. Invest.*, 45, 51, 1966.

37. Lieber, C. S. and Spritz, N., Effects of prolonged ethanol intake in man: role of dietary, adipose and endogenously synthesized fatty acids in the pathogenesis of the alcoholic fatty liver, *J. Clin. Invest.*, 45, 1400, 1966.

38. Lieber, C. S. and DeCarli, L. M., Quantitative relationship between the amount of dietary fat and the severity of the alcoholic fatty liver, *Amer. J. Clin. Nutr.*, 23, 474, 1970.

39. Lieber, C. S., Spritz, N., and DeCarli, L. M., Fatty liver produced by dietary deficiencies: its pathogenesis and potentiation by ethanol, *J. Lipid Res.*, 10, 283, 1969.

40. Kiessling, K. H. and Tilander, K., The effect of prolonged alcohol treatment on the respiration of liver and brain mitochondria from male and female rats, *Exp. Cell Res.*, 30, 476, 1963.

41. Rubin, E., Beattie, D. S., Toth, A., and Lieber, C. S., Structural and functional effects of ethanol on hepatic mitochondria, *Fed. Proc.*, 31, 131, 1972.

42. Rubin, E., Beattie, D. S., and Lieber, C. S., Effects of ethanol on the biogenesis of mitochondrial membranes and associated mitochondrial functions, *Lab. Invest.*, 23, 620, 1970.

43. Lefèvre, A., Adler, H., and Lieber, C. S., Effect of ethanol on ketone metabolism, *J. Clin. Invest.*, 49, 1775, 1970.

44. Jenkins, D. W., Eckel, R. E., and Craig, J. W., Alcoholic ketoacidosis, *J.A.M.A.*, 217, 177, 1971.

45. Freinkel, N. and Arky, R. A., Effects of alcohol on carbohydrate metabolism in man, *Psychosom. Med.*, 28, 551, 1966.

46. Phillips, G. B. and Safrit, H. F., Alcoholic diabetes. Induction of glucose intolerance with alcohol, *J.A.M.A.*, 217, 1513, 1971

47. Lochner, A., Wulff, J., and Madison, L. L., Ethanol-induced hypoglycemia. 1. The acute effects of ethanol on hepatic glucose output and peripheral glucose utilization in fasted dogs, *Metabolism*, 16, 1, 1967.

48. Kreisberg, R. A., Siegal, A. M., and Owen, W. C., Glucose-lactate interrelationships: effect of ethanol, *J. Clin. Invest.*, 50, 175, 1971.

49. Cronholm, T. and Sjövall, J., Effect of ethanol metabolism on redox state of steroid sulphates in man, *Europ. J. Biochem.*, 13, 124, 1970.

50. Admirand, W. H., Cronholm, T., and Sjövall, J., Reduction of dehydroepiandrosterone sulfate in the liver during ethanol metabolism, *Biochim. Biophys. Acta*, 202, 343, 1970.

51. Keilin, D. and Hartree, E. F., Properties of catalase. Catalysis of coupled oxidation of alcohols, *Biochem. J.*, 39, 293, 1945.

52. Makar, A. B., Tephly, T. R., and Mannering, G. J., Methanol metabolism in the monkey, *Molec. Pharmacol.*, 4, 471, 1968.

53. Barlett, G. R., Does catalase participate in the physiological oxidation of alcohols? *Quart. J. Stud. Alcohol*, 13, 583, 1952.

54. Tephly, T. R., Parks, R. E., Jr., and Mannering, G. J., Methanol metabolism in the rat, *J. Pharmacol. Exp. Ther.*, 143, 292, 1964.

55. Kiessling, K. H., Ethanol oxidation in rat liver mitochondria, *Chem. Biol. Interact.*, 1, 165, 1970.

56. Thore, A. and Baltscheffsky, H., Inhibitory effects of lower aliphatic alcohols on electron transport phosphorylation systems. I. Straight-chain, primary alcohols, *Acta Chem. Scand.*, 19, 1591, 1965.

57. McGuire, J. S., Coupled aldehyde dehydrogenase and catalase in mitochondrial extracts, *Arch. Biochem. Biophys.*, 110, 104, 1965.

58. Ugarte, G., Pereda, T., and Iturriaga, H., Influence of chronic alcohol administration on catalase activity of rat liver, *Arch. Biol. Med. Exp.*, 6, 56, 1969.

59. von Wartburg, J. P. and Rothlisberger, M., Enzymatische Veränderungen in der Leber nach langdauernder Belastung mit Aethanol und Methanol bei der Ratte, *Helv. Physiol. Acta*, 19, 30, 1961.

60. Lieber, C. S. and DeCarli, L. M., Hepatic microsomal ethanol oxidizing system: in vitro characteristics and adaptive properties in vivo, *J. Biol. Chem.*, 245, 2505, 1970.

61. Portwich, F. and Aebi, H., Erfassung der Peroxydbildung tierischer Gewebe mittels peroxydatischer Umsetzungen, *Helv. Physiol. Acta*, 18, 312, 1960.

62. Lieber, C. S. and DeCarli, L. M., Reduced nicotinamideadenine dinucleotide phosphate oxidase: activity enhanced by ethanol consumption, *Science*, 170, 78, 1970.

63. Iseri, O. A., Gottlieb, L. S., and Lieber, C. S., The ultrastructure of enthanol-induced fatty liver, *Fed. Proc.*, 23, 579, 1964.

64. Rubin, E., Hutterer, F., and Lieber, C. S., Ethanol increases hepatic smooth endoplasmic reticulum and drug-metabolizing enzymes, *Science*, 159, 1469, 1968.

65. Ishii, H., Joly, J. G., and Lieber, C. S., Effect of ethanol on hepatic rough (RER) and smooth (SER) endoplasmic reticulum, *Clin. Res.*, 19, 351, 1971.

66. Conney, A. H., Pharmacological implications of microsomal enzyme induction, *Pharmacol. Rev.*, 19, 317, 1967.

67. Lane, B. P. and Lieber, C. S., Effects of butylated hydroxytoluene on the ultrastructure of rat hepatocytes, *Lab. Invest.*, 16, 342, 1967.

68. Orme-Johnson, W. H. and Ziegler, D. M., Alcohol mixed function oxidase activity of mammalian liver microsomes, *Biochem. Biophys. Res. Commun.*, 21, 78, 1965.

69. Lieber, C. S. and DeCarli, L. M., Ethanol oxidation by hepatic microsomes: adaptive increase after ethanol feeding, *Science*, 162, 917, 1968.

70. Nyberg, A., Schuberth, J., and Anggard, L., On the intracellular distribution of catalase and alcohol dehydrogenase, *Acta Chem. Scand.*, 7, 1170, 1953.

71. Lieber, C. S., Rubin, E., and DeCarli, L. M., Hepatic microsomal ethanol oxidizing system (MEOS): differentiation from alcohol dehydrogenase and NADPH oxidase, *Biochem. Biophys. Res. Commun.*, 48, 858, 1970.

72. Theorell, H., Die Alkoholdehydrogenase: Ihre Wirkungsweisen und Komplexverbindungen, *Experientia*, 21, 553, 1965.

73. Lieber, C. S., Rubin, E., DeCarli, L. M., Misra, P., and Gang, H., Effects of pyrazole on hepatic function and structure, *Lab. Invest.*, 22, 615, 1970.

74. Gillette, J. R., Brodie, B. B., and La Du, B. N., The oxidation of drugs by liver microsomes: on the role of TPNH and oxygen, *J. Pharmacol. Exp. Ther.*, 119, 532, 1957.

75. Roach, M. K., Reese, W. N., Jr., and Creaven, P. J., Ethanol oxidation in the microsomal fraction of rat liver, *Biochem. Biophys. Res. Commun.*, 36, 596, 1969.

76. Tephly, T. R., Tinelli, F., and Watkins, W. D., Alcohol metabolism: role of microsomal oxidation in vivo, *Science*, 166, 627, 1969.

77. Isselbacher, K. J. and Carter, E. A., Ethanol oxidation by liver microsomes: evidence against a separate and distinct enzyme system, *Biochem. Biophys. Res. Commun.*, 39, 530, 1970.

78. Khanna, J. M., Kalant, H., and Lin, G., Metabolism of ethanol by rat liver microsomal enzymes, *Biochem. Pharmacol.*, 19, 2493, 1970.

79. Rubin, E., Lieber, C. S., Alvares, A. P., Levin, W., and Kuntzman, R., Ethanol binding to hepatic microsomes: its increase by ethanol consumption, *Biochem. Pharmacol.*, 20, 229, 1971.

80. Anders, M. W., Enhancement and inhibition of drug metabolism, *Ann. Rev. Pharmacol.*, 11, 37, 1971.

81. Lester, D., Keokosky, W. Z., and Felzenberg, F., Effect of pyrazoles and other compounds on alcohol metabolism, *Quart. J. Stud. Alcohol*, 29, 449, 1968.

82. Papenberg, J., von Wartburg, J. P., and Aebi, H., Metabolism of ethanol and fructose in the perfused rat liver, *Enzym. Biol. Clin.*, 11, 237, 1970.

83. Lieber, C. S. and DeCarli, L. M., The role of the hepatic microsomal ethanol oxidizing system (MEOS) for ethanol metabolism in vivo, *J. Pharmacol. Exp. Ther.*, 1972, in press.

84. Lundquist, F. and Wolthers, H., The influence of fructose on the kinetics of alcohol elimination in man, *Acta Pharmacol.*, 14, 290, 1958.

85. Khanna, J. M., Kalant, H., Lin, G., and Bustos, G. O., Effect of carbon tetrachloride treatment on ethanol metabolism, *Biochem. Pharmacol.*, 20, 3269, 1971.

86. Fischer, H. D., Zur Alkoholelimination bei Kaninchen nach CCl_4-Vergiftung, *Med. Pharmacol. Exp.*, 17, 60, 1967.

87. Kater, R. M. H., Carulli, N., and Iber, F. L., Differences in the rate of ethanol metabolism in recently drinking alcoholic and nondrinking subjects, *Amer. J. Clin. Nutr.*, 22, 1608, 1969.

88. Hawkins, R. D., Kalant, H., and Khanna, J. M., Effects of chronic intake of ethanol on rate of ethanol metabolism, *Canad. J. Physiol. Pharmacol.*, 44, 241, 1966.

89. Tobon, F. and Mezey, E., Effect of ethanol administration on hepatic ethanol and drug-metabolizing enzymes and on rates of ethanol degradation, *J. Lab. Clin. Med.*, 77, 110, 1971.

90. Misra, P. S., Lefèvre, A., Ishii, H., Rubin, E., and Lieber, C. S., Increase of ethanol, meprobamate and pentobarbital metabolism after chronic ethanol administration in man and in rats, *Amer. J. Med.*, 51, 346, 1971.

91. Mistilis, S. P. and Garske, A., Induction of alcohol dehydrogenase in liver and gastro-intestinal tract, *Aust. Ann. Med.*, 18, 227, 1969.

92. Greenberger, N. J., Cohen, R. B., and Isselbacher, K. J., The effect of chronic ethanol administration on liver alcohol dehydrogenase activity in the rat, *Lab. Invest.*, 14, 264, 1965.

93. Morrison, G. R. and Brock, F. E., Quantitative measurement of alcohol dehydrogenase activity within the liver lobule of rats after prolonged ethanol ingestion, *J. Nutr.*, 92, 286, 1967.

94. Videla, L. and Israel, Y., Factors that modify the metabolism of ethanol in rat liver and adaptive changes produced by its chronic administration, *Biochem. J.*, 118, 275, 1970.

95. Carulli, N., Manenti, F., Gallo, M., and Salvioli, G. F., Alcohol-drugs interaction in man: alcohol and tolbutamide, *Europ. J. Clin. Invest.*, 1, 421, 1971.

96. Dajani, R. M., Danielski, J., and Orten, J. M., The utilization of ethanol. II. The alcohol-acetaldehyde dehydrogenase system in the livers of alcohol-treated rats, *J. Nutr.*, 80, 196, 1963.

97. Figueroa, R. B. and Klotz, A. P., Alterations of alcohol dehydrogenase and other hepatic enzymes following oral alcohol intoxication, *Amer. J. Clin. Nutr.*, 11, 235, 1962.

98. Bode, C. H., Goebell, H., and Stahler, M., Anderungen der Alkoholdehydrogenase-Aktivitat in der Rattenleber durch Eiweissmangel und Athanol, *Z. Ges. Exp. Med.*, 152, 111, 1970.

99. Edwards, J. A. and Evans, D. A. P., Ethanol metabolism in subjects possessing typical and atypical liver alcohol dehydrogenase, *Clin. Pharmacol. Ther.*, 8, 824, 1967.

100. Holzer, H. and Schneider, S., Zum Mechanismus der Beeinflussung der Alkoholoxydation in der Leber Durch Fructose, *Klin. Wschr.*, 33, 1006, 1955.

101. Lowenstein, L. M., Simone, R., Boulter, P., and Nathan, P., Effect of fructose on alcohol concentrations in the blood in man, *J.A.M.A.*, 213, 1899, 1970.

102. Kahonen, M. T., Ylikahri, R. H., and Hassinen, I., Ethanol metabolism in rats treated with ethyl-α-p-chlorophenoxy-isobutyrate (clofibrate), *Life Sci.*, 10, 661, 1971.

103. Lowe, C. U. and Mosovich, L. L., The paradoxical effect of alcohol on carbohydrate metabolism in four patients with liver glycogen disease, *Pediatrics*, 35, 1005, 1965.

104. Papenberg, J., Ethanol metabolism, in *Alcohol and the Liver*, Gerok, W., Sickinger, K., and Hennekeuser, H. H., Eds., F. K. Schattauer Verlag, New York, 1971, 45.

105. Veech, R. L., Eggleston, L. V., and Krebs, H. A., The redox state of free nicotinamide-adenine dinucleotide phosphate in the cytoplasm of rat liver, *Biochem. J.*, 115, 609, 1969.

106. Lieber, C. S. and DeCarli, L. M., Effect of drug administration on the activity of the hepatic microsomal ethanol oxidizing system, *Life Sci.*, 9, 267, 1970.

107. Fischer, H. -D., The influence of barbiturates on the rate of detoxication of ethyl alcohol, *Biochem. Pharmacol.*, 11, 307, 1962.

108. Klassen, C. D., Ethanol metabolism in rats after microsomal metabolizing enzymes induction, *Proc. Soc. Exp. Biol. Med.*, 132, 1099, 1969.

109. Lieber, C. S. and DeCarli, L. M., Paradoxical effects of barbiturates on ethanol metabolism, *Gastroenterology*, 60, 177, 1971.

110. Forney, R. B. and Hughes, F. W., *Combined Effects of Alcohol and Other Drugs*, Charles C Thomas, Springfield, Ill. 1968.

111. Soehring, K. and Schüppel, R., Wechselwirkungen zwischen Alkohol und Arzneimitteln, *Deusch. Med. Wschr.*, 91, 1892, 1966.

112. Rubin, E. and Lieber, C. S., Hepatic microsomal enzymes in man and rat: induction and inhibition by ethanol, *Science*, 162, 690, 1968.

113. Ariyoshi, T., Takabatake, E., and Remmer, H., Drug metabolism in ethanol induced fatty liver, *Life Sci.*, 9, 361, 1970.

114. Shanley, B. C., Zail, S. S., and Joubert, S. M., Effect of ethanol on liver delta-aminolevulinate synthetase in rats, *Lancet*, 1, 70, 1968.

115. Shanley, B. C., Zail, S. S., and Joubert, S. M., Effect of ethanol on liver delta-aminolaevulinate synthetase activity and urinary porphyrin excretion in symptomatic porphyria, *Brit. J. Haemat.*, 17, 389, 1969.

116. Rubin, E., Bacchin, P., Gang, H., and Lieber, C. S., Induction and inhibition of hepatic microsomal and mitochondrial enzymes by ethanol, *Lab. Invest.*, 22, 569, 1970.

117. Kalant, H., Khanna, J. M., and Marshman, J., Effect of chronic intake of ethanol on pentobarbital metabolism, *J. Pharmacol. Exp. Ther.*, 175, 318, 1970.

118. Kater, R. M. H., Roggin, G., Tobon, F., Zieve, P., and Iber, F. L., Increased rate of clearance of drugs from the circulation of alcoholics, *Amer. J. Med. Sci.*, 258, 35, 1969.

119. Devenyi, P. and Wilson, M., Barbiturate abuse and addiction and their relationship to alcohol and alcoholism, *Canad. Med. Ass. J.*, 104, 215, 1971.

120. Ratcliffe, F., The effect of chronic ethanol administration on the responses to amylobarbitone sodium in the rat, *Life Sci.*, 8, 1051, 1969.

121. Rubin, E., Gang, H., Misra, P. S., and Lieber, C. S., Inhibition of drug metabolism by acute ethanol intoxication. A hepatic microsomal mechanism, *Amer. J. Med.*, 49, 801, 1970.

122. Schüppel, R., Wirkungen von Alkohol auf den Arzneistoffwechsel, in *Alcohol and the Liver*, Gerok, W., Sickinger, K., and Hennekeuser, H. H., Eds., Schattauer Verlag, New York, 1971, 227.

123. Sutherland, V. C., Burbridge, T. N., Adams, J. E., and Simon, A., Cerebral metabolism in problem drinkers under the influence of alcohol and chlorpromazine hydrochloride, *J. Appl. Physiol.*, 15, 189, 1960.

124. Lefèvre, A. F., DeCarli, L. M., and Lieber, C. S., Effect of ethanol on cholesterol and bile acid metabolism, *J. Lipid. Res.*, 13, 48, 1972.

125. Jones, A. L. and Armstrong, D. T., Increased cholesterol biosynthesis following phenobarbital induced hypertrophy of agranular endoplasmic reticulum in liver, *Proc. Soc. Exp. Biol. Med.*, 119, 1136, 1965.

126. DeCarli, L. M. and Lieber, C. S., Fatty liver in the rat after prolonged intake of ethanol with a nutritionally adequate new liquid diet, *J. Nutr.*, 91, 331, 1967.

127. Jones, D. P., Losowsky, M. S., Davidson, C. S., and Lieber, C. S., Effects of ethanol on plasma lipids in man, *J. Lab. Clin. Med.*, 62, 675, 1963.

128. Losowsky, M. S., Jones, D. P., Davidson, C. S., and Lieber, C. S., Studies of alcoholic hyperlipemia and its mechanism, *Amer. J. Med.*, 35, 794, 1963.

129. Brewster, A. C., Lankford, H. G., Schwartz, M. G., and Sullivan, J. F., Ethanol and alimentary lipemia, *Amer. J. Clin. Nutr.*, 19, 255, 1966.

130. Barboriak, J. J. and Meade, R. C., Enhancement of alimentary lipemia by preprandial alcohol, *Amer. J. Med. Sci.*, 255, 245, 1968.

131. Wilson, D. E., Schreibman, P. H., Brewster, A. C., and Arky, R. A., The enhancement of alimentary lipemia by ethanol in man, *J. Clin. Lab. Med.*, 75, 264, 1970.

132. Kudzma, D. J. and Schonfeld, G., Alcoholic hyperlipidemia: induction by alcohol but not by carbohydrate, *J. Lab. Clin. Med.*, 77, 384, 1971.

133. Baraona, E. and Lieber, C. S., Effects of chronic ethanol feeding of serum lipoprotein metabolism in the rat, *J. Clin. Invest.*, 49, 769, 1970.

134. Oler, A. and Lombardi, B., Further studies on a defect in the intracellular transport and secretion of proteins by the liver of choline deficient rats, *J. Biol. Chem.*, 245, 1282, 1970.

135. Joly, J. -G., Feinman, L., Ishii, H., and Lieber, C. S., Stimulation of hepatic L-α-glycerophosphate acyl transferase (GPAT) activity by ethanol; its submicrosomal site, *Clin. Res.*, 19, 395, 1971.

136. Alcindor, L. G., Infante, R., Soler-Argilaga, C., Raisonnier, A., Polonovski, J., and Caroli, J., Induction of the hepatic synthesis of β-lipoproteins by high concentrations of fatty acids. Effect of actinomycin D, *Biochim. Biophys. Acta*, 210, 483, 1970.

137. Lieber, C. S., Leevy, C. M., Stein, S. W., George, W. S., Cherrick, G. R., Abelmann, W. H., and Davidson, C. S., Effect of ethanol on plasma free fatty acids in man, *J. Lab. Clin. Med.*, 59, 826, 1962.

138. Jones, D. P., Perman, E. S., and Lieber, C. S., Free fatty acid turnover and triglyceride metabolism after ethanol ingestion in man, *J. Lab. Clin. Med.*, 66, 804, 1965.

139. Feinman, L. and Lieber, C. S., Effect of ethanol on plasma glycerol in man, *Amer. J. Clin. Nutr.*, 20, 400, 1967.

140. Crouse, J. R., Gerson, C. D., DeCarli, L. M., and Lieber, C. S., Role of acetate in the reduction of plasma free fatty acids produced by alcohol in man, *J. Lipid Res.*, 9, 509, 1968.

141. Brodie, B. B., Butler, W. M., Horning, M. G., Maickel, R. P., and Maling, H. M., Alcohol-induced triglyceride deposition in liver through derangement of fat transport, *Amer. J. Clin. Nutr.*, 9, 432, 1961.

142. Mallov, S., Effect of ethanol intoxication on plasma free fatty acids in the rat, *Quart. J. Stud. Alcohol*, 22, 250, 1961.

143. Elko, E. E., Wooles, W. R., and DiLuzio, N. R., Alterations and mobilization of lipids in acute ethanol-treated rats, *Amer. J. Physiol.*, 201, 923, 1961.

144. Albrink, M. J. and Klatskin, G., Lactescence of serum following episodes of acute alcoholism and its probable relationship to acute pancreatitis, *Amer. J. Med.*, 23, 26, 1957.

145. Kessler, J. I., Kniffen, J. C., and Janowitz, H. D., Lipoprotein lipase inhibition in the hyperlipemia of acute alcoholic pancreatitis, *New Eng. J. Med.*, 269, 943, 1963.

146. Zieve, L., Jaundice, hyperlipemia and hemolytic anemia: a heretofore unrecognized syndrome associated with alcoholic fatty liver and cirrhosis, *Ann. Intern. Med.*, 48, 471, 1958.

147. Waltman, R., Nigrin, G., Bonura, F., and Pipat, C., Ethanol in prevention of hyperbilirubinaemia in the new born, *Lancet*, 2, 1265, 1969.

148. Ideo, G., De Franchis, R., Del Ninno, E., and Dioguardi, N., Ethanol increase liver uridine-diphosphate-glucuronyltransferase, *Experientia*, 27, 24, 1971.

149. Israel, Y., Kalant, H., LeBlanc, E., Bernstein, J. C., and Salazar, I., Changes in cation transport and (Na +K)-activated adenosine triphosphatase produced by chronic administration of ethanol, *J. Pharmacol. Exp. Ther.*, 174, 330, 1970.

150. Jarnefelt, J., Inhibition of the brain microsomal adenosinetriphosphatase by depolarizing agents, *Biochim. Biophys. Acta*, 48, 111, 1961.

151. Israel, Y., Cellular effects of alcohol, *Quart J. Stud. Alcohol*, 31, 293, 1970.

152. Ugarte, G. R., Cruz-Coke, R. L., Rivera, L., Altschiller, H., and Mardones, J., Relationship of color blindness to alcoholic liver damage, *Pharmacology*, 4, 297, 1970.

153. Fialkow, P. J., Thuline, H. C., and Fenster, L. F., Lack of association between cirrhosis and the common types of color blindness, *New Eng. J. Med.*, 275, 584, 1966.

154. Riffenburg, R. S. and Shea, J. F., Lack of association between color blindness and alcoholism, *Eye Ear Nose Throat Monthly*, 49, 240, 1970.

155. Fenna, A., Mix, L., Schaefer, O., and Gilbert, J. A. L., Ethanol metabolism in various racial groups, *Canad. Med. Ass. J.*, 105, 472, 1971.

156. Vesell, E. S., Page, J. G., and Passananti, G. T., Genetic and environmental factors affecting ethanol metabolism in man, *Clin. Pharmacol. Ther.*, 12, 192, 1970.

157. Rodgers, D. A., Factors underlying differences in alcohol preference among inbred strains of mice, *Psychosom. Med.*, 28, 498, 1966.

158. Essig, C. F. and Lam, R. C., Convulsions and hallucinatory behavior following alcohol withdrawal in the dog, *Arch. Neurol.*, 18, 626, 1968.

159. Ellis, F. W. and Pick, J. R., Experimentally induced ethanol dependence rhesus monkeys, *J. Pharmacol. Exp. Ther.*, 175, 88, 1970.

160. Freund, G., Alcohol withdrawal syndrome in mice, *Arch. Neurol.*, 21, 315, 1969.

161. Mendelson, J. H., Biologic concomitants of alcoholism, *New Eng. J. Med.*, 283, 24, 1970.

162. Essig, C. F., Jones, B. E., and Lam, R. C., The effect of pentobarbital on alcohol withdrawl in dogs, *Arch Neurol.*, 20, 553, 1969.

163. Fraser, H. F., Wikler, A., Isbell, H., and Johnson, N. K., Partial equivalence of chronic alcohol and barbiturate intoxications, *Quart J. Stud. Alcohol.*, 18, 541, 1957.

164. Kalant, H., LeBlanc, A. E., and Gibbins, R. J., Tolerance to, and dependence on some non-opiate psychotropic drugs, *Pharmacol. Rev.*, 23, 135, 1971.

165. Forster, B., Die Veränderungen des Acetaldehydspiegels im Blute nach Alkoholaufnahme, *Deutsch. Z. Ges. Gerichtl. Med.*, 45, 221, 1956.

166. Truitt, E. B., Jr. and Duritz, G., The role of acetaldehyde in the actions of ethanol, in *Biochemical Factors in Alcoholism*, Maickel, R. P., Ed., Pergamon Press, New York, 1967.

167. Klingman, G. I. and Haag, H. B., Studies on severe alcohol intoxication in dogs, *Quart. J. Stud. Alcohol*, 19, 203, 1958.

168. Perman, E. S., The effect of ethyl alcohol on the secretion from the adrenal medulla in man, *Acta Physiol. Scand.*, 44, 241, 1958.

169. von Wartburg, J. P., Berli, W., and Aebi, H., Der Einfluss langdauernder Athylalkoholbelastung auf die Katecholaminausscheidung im Harn der Ratte, *Helv. Med. Acta,* 28, 89, 1961.

170. Abelin, I., Herren, C., and Berli, W., Uber die erregende Wirkung des Alkohols auf den Adrenalin und Noradrenalinhaushalt des menschlichen Organismus, *Helv. Med. Acta,* 25, 591, 1958.

171. Anton, A. H., Ethanol and urinary catecholamines in man, *Clin. Pharmacol Ther.,* 6, 462, 1965.

172. Schenker, V. J., Kissin, B., Maynard, L. S., and Schenker, A. C., Adrenal hormones and amine metabolism in alcoholism, *Psychosom. Med.,* 28, 564, 1966.

173. Perman, E. S., The effect of ethyl alcohol on the secretion from the adrenal medulla of the cat, *Acta Physiol. Scand.,* 48, 323, 1960.

174. Perman, E. S., Observations on the effect of ethanol on the urinary excretion of histamine, 5-hydroxyindole acetic acid, catecholamines and 17-hydroxycorticosteroids in man, *Acta Physiol. Scand.,* 51, 62, 1961.

175. Ammon, H. P. T., Estler, C. -J., and Heim, F., Der Einfluss von Acetaldehyd auf Coenzym A-Aktivitat und Atmung von Leber-und Hirnmitochondrien, *Biochem. Pharmacol.,* 16, 769, 1967.

176. Bode, CH. Stahler, E., Kono, H., and Goebell, H., Effects of ethanol on free coenzyme A, free carnitine and their fatty acid esters in rat liver, *Biochim Biophys. Acta,* 210, 448, 1970.

177. Duritz, G. and Truitt, E. B., Jr., Importance of acetaldehyde in the action of ethanol on brain norepinephrine and 5-hydroxytryptamine, *Biochem. Pharmacol.,* 15, 711, 1966.

178. Towne, J. C., Effect of ethanol and acetaldehyde on liver and brain monoamine oxidase, *Nature,* 201, 709, 1964.

179. Lahti, R. A. and Majchrovicz, E., The effects of acetaldehyde on serotonin metabolism, *Life Sci.,* 6, 1399, 1967.

180. Davis, V. E., Brown, H., Huff, J. A., and Cashaw, J. L., The alteration of serotonin metabolism to 5-hydroxytryptophol by ethanol ingestion in man, *J. Lab. Clin. Med.,* 69, 132, 1967.

181. Feldstein, A., Hoagland, H., Freeman, H., and Williamson, O., The effect of ethanol ingestion on serotonin-C^{14} metabolism in man, *Life Sci.,* 6, 53, 1967.

182. Davis, V. E., Brown, H., Huff, M.J.A., and Cashaw, J. L., Ethanol-induced alterations of norepinephrine metabolism in man, *J. Lab. Clin. Med.,* 69, 787, 1967.

183. Raskin, N. H. and Sokoloff, L., Alcohol dehydrogenase activity in rat brain and liver, *J. Neurochem.,* 17, 1677, 1970.

184. Davis, V. E., Walsh, M. J., and Yamanaka, Y., Augmentation of alkaloid formation from dopamine by alcohol and acetaldehyde in vitro, *J. Pharmacol, Exp. Ther.,* 174, 401, 1970.

185. Seevers, M. H., Morphine and ethanol physical dependence: a critique of a hypothesis, *Science,* 170, 1113, 1970.

186. Halushka, P. V. and Hoffmann, P. C., Alcohol addiction and tetrahydropapaveroline, *Science,* 169, 1104, 1970.

187. Goldstein, A. and Judson, B. A., Alcohol dependence and opiate dependence: lack of relationship in mice, *Science,* 172, 290, 1971.

188. Cohen, G. and Collins, M., Alkaloids from catecholamines in adrenal tissue: possible role in alcoholism, *Science,* 167, 1749, 1970.

189. Taborsky, R. S. and McIssac, W. M., The synthesis and preliminary pharmacology of some 9H-pyrido (3,4-b) idoles (β-carbolines) and tryptamines related to serotonin and melatonin, *J. Med. Chem.,* 7, 135, 1964.

190. Davis, V. E. and Walsh, M. J., Effect of ethanol on neuroamine metabolism, in *Biological Basis of Alcoholism,* Israel, Y. and Mardones, J., Eds., John Wiley & Sons, Inc., New York, 1971, 73.

191. Jaffe, H. H. and Sharpless, S. K., Pharmacological denervation supersensitivity in the central nervous system: a theory of physical dependence, in *Addictive States* Wikler, A., Ed., Res. Publ. Ass. Nerv. Ment. Dis., Williams & Wilkins, Baltimore, 1968, 226.

192. Goldstein, A. and Goldstein, D. B., Enzyme expansion theory of drug tolerance and physical dependence, in *Addictive States,* Wikler, A., Ed., Res. Publ. Ass. Nerv. Ment. Dis., Williams & Wilkins, Baltimore, 1968, 265.

193. Collier, H. O., A general theory of the genesis of drug dependence by induction of receptors, *Nature,* 108, 181, 1965.

194. Eade, N. R., Mechanism of sympathomimetic action of aldehydes, *J. Pharmacol. Exp. Ther.,* 127, 29, 1959.

195. Carlsson, C. and Haggendal, J., Arterial noradrenaline levels after ethanol withdrawal, *Lancet,* 2, 889, 1970.

196. Czaja, C. and Kalant, H., The effect of acute alcoholic intoxication on adrenal ascorbic acid and cholesterol in the rat, *Canad. J. Biochem. Physiol.,* 39, 327, 1961.

197. Ellis, F. W., Effect of ethanol on plasma corticosterone levels, *J. Pharmacol. Exp. Ther.,* 153, 121, 1966.

198. Kakihana, R., Butte, J. C., Hathaway, A., and Noble, E. P., Adrenocortical response to ethanol in mice: modification by chronic ethanol consumption, *Acta Endocr.,* 67, 653, 1971.

199. Kissin, B., Schenker, V., and Schenker, A. C., The acute effect of ethanol ingestion on plasma and urinary 17-hydroxycorticoids in alcoholic subjects, *Amer. J. Med. Sci.,* 239, 960, 1960.

200. Jenkins, J. S. and Connolly, J., Adrencortical response to ethanol in man, *Brit. Med. J.,* 2, 804, 1968.

201. Bellet, S., Roman, L., DeCastro, O., and Herrera, M., Effect of acute ethanol intake on plasma II hydroxycorticosteroid levels, *Metabolism,* 19, 664, 1970.

202. Bellet, S., Yoshimine, N., DeCastro, O.A.P., Roman, L., Parmar, S. S., and Sandberg, H., Effects of alcohol ingestion on growth hormone levels: their relation to II-hydroxycorticoid levels and serum FFA, *Metabolism,* 20, 762, 1971.

203. Mendelson, J. H. and Stein, S., Serum cortisol levels in alcoholic and nonalcoholic subjects during experimentally induced ethanol intoxication, *Psychosom. Med.,* 28, 616, 1966.

204. Kakihana, R., Noble, E. P., and Butte, J. C., Corticosterone response to ethanol in inbred strains of mice, *Nature,* 218, 360, 1968.

205. Ogata, M., Mendelson, J. H., and Mello, N. K., Electrolytes and osmolality in alcoholics during experimentally induced intoxication, *Psychosom. Med.,* 30, 463, 1968.

206. Sereny, G., Rapoport, S. A., and Husdan, H., The effect of alcohol withdrawal on electrolyte and acid-base balance, *Metabolism,* 15, 896, 1966.

HALLUCINOGENS, CNS STIMULANTS, AND CANNABIS

A. T. Shulgin

TABLE OF CONTENTS

COMMON CHARACTERISTICS OF SOME DRUGS

The drugs known variously as the hallucinogens, the Central Nervous System (CNS) stimulants, and cannabis are by name and reputation a varied collection of materials. A hallucinogen is, broadly, a substance that creates some unexplained and unconfirmable imagery, a CNS stimulant clearly invokes some anatomical or physiological site of action, and cannabis is the generic name of a plant. Also included in this apparently disparate group are substances which are best referred to as delusionary agents; drugs that induce sensory deprivation and distortion that effectively achieve a clinical state of anesthesia. However, there are unifying features of this heterogeneous collection that all share in common:

1. They are drugs that are being used by an increasingly large minority within the society as psychotropic agents;

2. They are drugs that are being used for their effective modification of sensory integrity, whether for believed virtues of self-understanding, self-instruction, religious insight, or simple escape;

3. They are drugs that are disapproved of by the majority within the society and which have, in several instances, been made illegal;

4. They are drugs that are certainly habituating, thus leading to a degree of psychological dependence, but drugs which appear to be, without exception, free of known capability of leading to a physiologically dependent state or addiction, seen frequently with the three classes discussed earlier; the narcotics, the barbiturates, and alcohol;

5. Except for the phenethylamine analogues, they are drugs that have not received official recognition of medical utility and are only rarely employed in medical practice;

6. They are drugs that have evolved from the plant kingdom, although many of the currently employed substances are synthetic modifications of the parent botanical prototypes.

Consideration of the dosage must be made concerning a number of these drugs. With some, primarily the stimulants, usage at low levels is medically acceptable and encouraged for both anorexogenic and mood modifying effects. It is only when the user has become tolerant of excitatory properties and increases the dosage to the level that produces a psychotomimetic intoxication, that the drug is generally condemned. With others, there may be such expressions of excitation or perhaps some sedative depression at large dosages, but the sought after intoxication and sensory distortion syndrome is expressed at smaller levels of use. External, obvious symptoms of physical change are evident only in instances of overdosage.

The discussion that follows is based on chemical, rather than pharmacological lines. Where appropriate, some comparative descriptions of the nature of action will be made, but to a large measure this presentation is intended to serve as a reference body of chemical structure, botanical source, and terminology.

THE INDOLE FAMILY

The most potent, the most famous, and the most notorious of all the drugs to be discussed in this chapter are chemically based on the indole nucleus. These are chemical substances that are, at least in origin, completely derived from the plant kingdom. There are the ergot-like alkaloids from the fungi and the *Convolvulaceae* families, the carboline group of bases stemming primarily from the South American vines of the genus *Banisteriopsis,* and the compounds that account for the activity of the New World snuffs; relatives of a compact family of compounds related to the parenterally active tryptamine bases.

The most widely known drug of this entire group is the semisynthetic compound, lysergic acid diethylamide, LSD-25. The stereochemical structure of the active (*d*-) isomer is shown in Figure 1. Although the chemical was first synthesized in 1937, its extraordinary activity was not recognized until 1943,[1] and not reported until 1947.[2,3] Within a few years, it had been introduced and received broad experimental evaluation within both medical and experimental social circles of the U. S.

Hundreds of minor chemical variations of LSD have been synthesized, and a number of these have been evaluated in human subjects. One of the first extensive reports of such a study[4] has shown the exquisite sensitiveness of the relationship of chemical structure to biological activity. Shortening one of the two amide ethyl groups to a methyl group (LME, Figure 2; R^1=methyl, ethyl; R^2, R^3 = H) or lengthening one to a propyl group (Figure 2 LEP, R^1 = ethyl, propyl; R^2, R^3 = H) greatly reduces its activity as a psychotomimetic. The LSD isomer, the *N*-methyl-*N*-propyl counterpart, or the mono-ethyl homolog (LAE) are virtually without activity. Bromination at the indolic 2-position (Figure 2, R^1 = ethyl; R^2 = Br; R^3 = H) reduced the high potency of LSD. Changes within the D-ring, either the hydrogenation of the double bond, conversion to the *l*-isomer, or structural rearrangement to the *cis*-configuration, all result in an inactivo molcculc.

It is only with substitution on the indolic nitrogen, that psychotomimetic potency is maintained or enhanced. The methyl and acetyl counterparts (Figure 2; R^1 = ethyl; R^2 = H; R^3 = CH_3, $COCH_3$) are comparable to LSD in human potency.[5]

Another group of highly potent alkaloids, closely related to LSD chemically, but total strangers in the botanical sense, are the ergot-like bases isolated from the various *Convolvulaceae* of the morning glory group.

The New World drug, Ololiuqui is known to

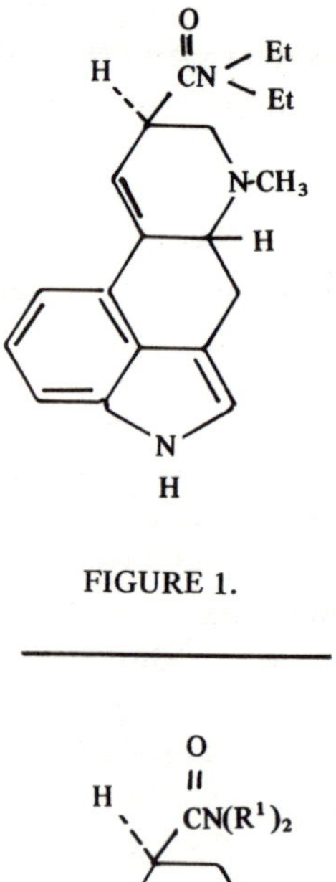

FIGURE 1.

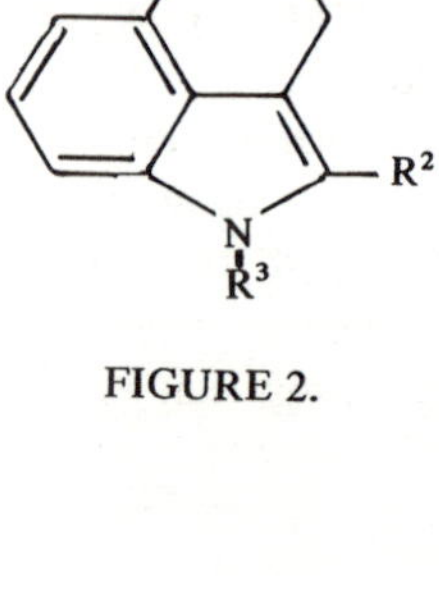

FIGURE 2.

come from the seeds of the plant *Rivea corymbosa.*[6] These are brown in color and are known locally as "badoh", but they are used interchangeably with the black seeds (badoh negro) of the larger and more dramatic morning glory, *Ipomoea violacea.* The composition of these two species has been found to be essentially identical.[7] The major alkaloids present were found to be ergine (*d*-Lysergic acid amide, Figure 2; R^1, R^2, R^3 = H) and the enantiomorph isoergine (*d*-Isolysergic acid amide, identical with ergine, but with the opposite epimeric configuration on the carbon atom that carries the amide carbonyl group). These two compounds have been shown to have some activity in man, but it is possible that their presence in the natural seed as the extremely labile acetaldehyde condensates (the hydroxyethylamides) may explain the activity of the seed compared to the lack of activity of the ergot isolates.[8]

A third major alkaloid present in both species is Chanoclavine (Figure 3), an open ring analog of the ergoline series of compounds, which is present to about 10% in the ergine-isoergine content, but completely unexplored in humans.

Yet, another morning glory relative, the Hawaiian Baby Woodrose, or *Argyreia nervosa,* has found extensive usage as a hallucinogenic plant source. Both ergine and isoergine have been shown to be present in exceptionally large amounts,[9,10] but penniclavine (Figure 4), a minor component of both the *Rivea* and *Ipomoea* species, is also present as a major component. Again, its pharmacology in man is unknown. A recent study of this potent plant material[11] revealed the presence of more than a dozen additional alkaloids, and it is certain that some of them must play some role in the explanation of the hallucinogenic

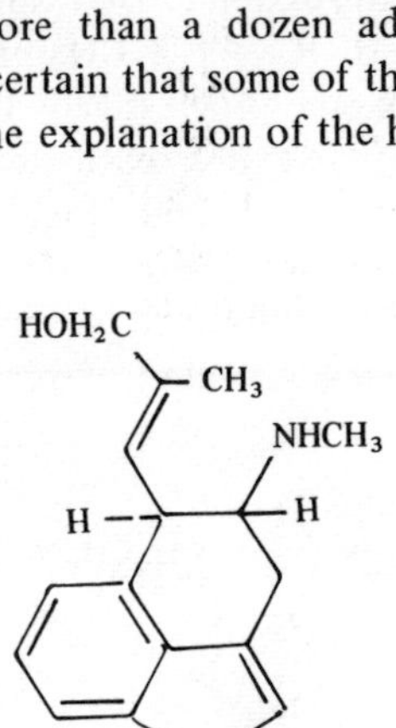

FIGURE 3.

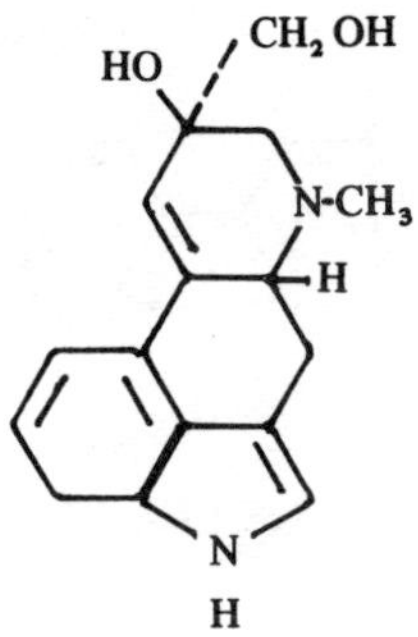

FIGURE 4.

effectiveness of this plant. The large Hawaiian Wood Rose (*Ipomoea tuberosa*) is interestingly without alkaloids and biological activity.

Ibogaine is yet another indole alkaloid that should be mentioned briefly under this heading. Basically, it is an indole in structure (Figure 5) and has a polycyclic structure superficially similar to that of LSD. Second, it shows psychotomimetic properties at large dosages[12] and due to a brief, but active flurry of illegal appearance as a street drug, has been included into the BNDD listings of dangerous drugs. It is synthetically unobtainable, being isolated only from the African plant, *Tabernanthe iboga.* Modifications of the structure are unknown, both chemically and pharmacologically.

The carbolines represent a chemical class of simpler chemical structure and some biochemical logic from the point of view of rationale of action. They are tricyclic indole substances represented by the general structural formula in Figure 6.

Of these substances the best studied are those of the harmine family, found in the plants of the genera *Peganum* (of the Old World) and *Banisteriopsis* (formerly *Banisteria,* of the New World). The extract of this latter vine is known as Ayahuasca (or Caapi or Yaje), and has been used for generations by Indians in the Amazon and Orinoco river basins, as an orally active hallucinogen.

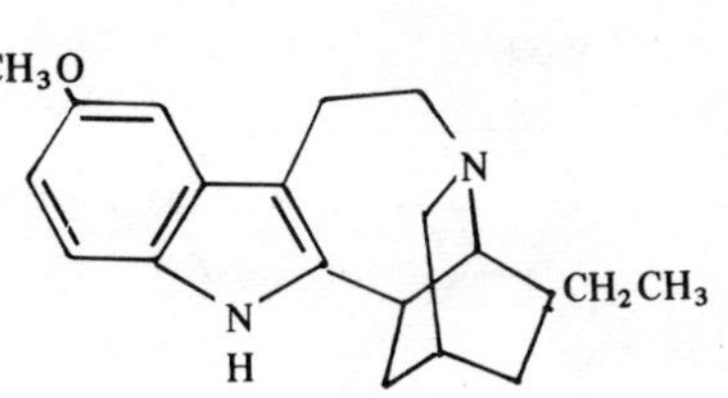

FIGURE 5.

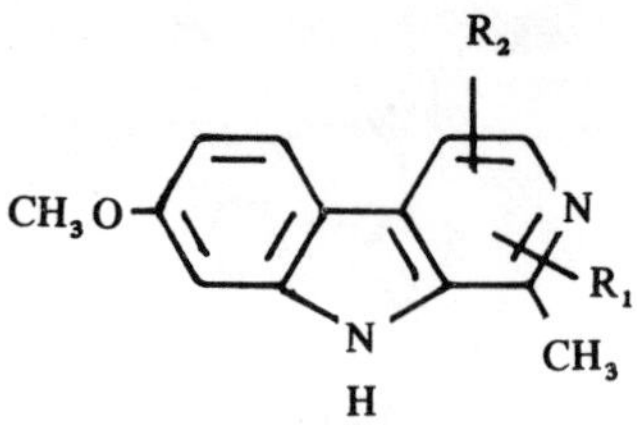

FIGURE 6.

The principal alkaloids of this plant group were recognized early as being related to harmine (Figure 6) through various degrees of hydrogenation in the pyridine ring. The major alkaloid in *Banisteriopsis caapi* has been reported to be the dihydro counterpart, harmaline (Figure 6, R^2 = H_2).[13] This isomer may be the major contributor to the action of the plant product Ayahuasca, as the tetrahydro analog (tetrahydroharmine, Leptoflorin, Figure 6, R_1, R_2 = H_2). Although clearly present as an alkaloidal component,[14] it appears be less active than harmaline in humans.[15]

A parallel family of compounds carries the methoxy group in the indolic 5-position (Figure 7). This group is implicated more logically in human metabolism (as analogs of serotonin) but has been identified as components of plant intoxicants only very recently.

The *Virola* snuffs of northern South America have long been associated with the *Piptadenia* group of intoxicants known as Yaje. Although originally thought to be related to nutmeg, these are now known to contain alkaloids.[16] These are positional isomers of the harmaline series and are more potent. Here, the major alkaloid is the tetrahydro isomer[17] (Figure 7, R^1 = CH_3, R^2 = H), but the two dehydrogenation products (6-methoxyharmalan and 6-methoxyharman, Figure 7, with one and two double bonds in the pyridine ring) are clearly present.[18] Theoretically, these plant products are derivable from the brain hormone melatonin. This potential route to an endogenously-produced psychotogen has been advanced as a clear and simple explanation of mental illness,[19] but it has not yet received experimental support.

A recent report describes two *N*-methylated carbolines present in Virola (Figure 7, R^1 = H, R^2 = CH_3 and R^1 = R^2 = CH_3).[20] Their contribution to the hallucinogenic effects of the plant are not known.

A major alkaloid of this snuff, and of many other South American plant medicines such as Parica (Epena)[21] and the Caribbean counterpart Cohoba is the simple indole, dimethyltryptamine (DMT). This base (Figure 8, R^1, R^2 = H, R^3 = CH_3) has been identified as a component of a large number of New World hallucinogens and has been extensively evaluated in clinical studies.[22] It has been detected in the urine of schizophrenic patients[23] and may be involved in the abnormal metabolism associated with mental illness.

There are a large number of hallucinogens closely related to dimethyltryptamine chemically. 5-Methoxydimethyltryptamine (Figure 8, R^1 = H, R^2 = OCH_3, R^3 = CH_3) which accompanies DMT in many of the South American snuffs, is an extremely rapidly acting chemical (effective within seconds), and like DMT, is only active parenterally. The phenolic analog, 5-hydroxy-*NN*-dimethyltryptamine is known as bufotenine. Although it is legally classified as an hallucinogenic substance, there is little medical justification for this assignment.[24]

The alkyl homologs of DMT (diethyltryptamine and dipropyltryptamine, DET and DPT, Figure 8, R^1 = R^2 = H, R^3 = CH_2CH_3 and $CH_2CH_2CH_3$, respectively), are progressively longer-acting and less potent.[25] It has been reported that the diisopropyl isomer and the *N*-monotertbutyl homolog are active orally, but this has not been confirmed in the published literature.

An unusual compound within the dialkyltryp-

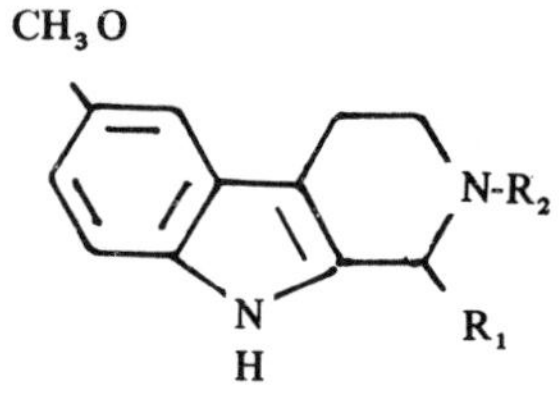

FIGURE 7.

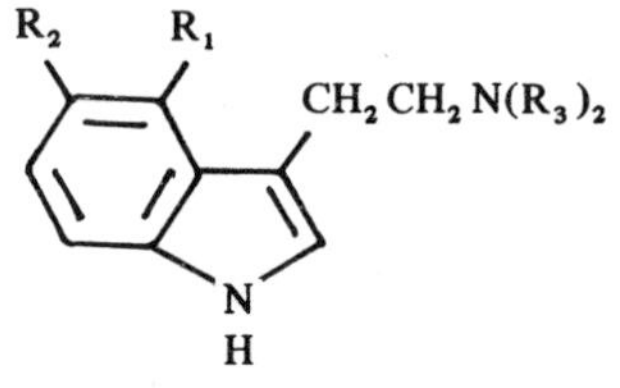

FIGURE 8.

tamine family is the 4-hydroxy analog, psilocin, and its pharmacologically equivalent phosphate ester, psilocybin (Figure 8, R^1 = OH or $OPO(OH)_2$, R^2 = H, R^3 = CH_3). These orally active hallucinogens have been isolated from, and completely account for, the central activity of the Mexican sacred mushroom, Teonanacatl.[26] These mushrooms were found to be of the Genus *Psilocybe*,[27] but recently a number of other fungi have been identified as sources of these alkaloids.[28] Synthetic modifications of these basic structures have indicated that the diethyl homolog of psilocin (SZ-74, Figure 8, R^1 = OH, R^2 = H, R^3 = CH_2CH_3) is somewhat less potent than psilocin, but acts more rapidly, quite the opposite action of DET compared to DMT.[29] There are no reports of studies in humans of the higher homologs.

THE PHENETHYLAMINE FAMILY

The simplest of the central stimulants and the parent structure to a large number of active compounds, both as sympathomimetic stimulants and as psychotomimetics, is the chemical phenethylamine (Figure 9, R^1 = R^2 = R^3 = R^4 = R^5 =H). Although this compound is not active in the human due to its extremely rapid metabolic removal, modifications of it have proven to be resistant to in vivo destruction. Alkalylation of the carbon next to the amine group (Figure 9, R^4) leads to central stimulants, whereas ether substitution upon the aromatic ring (R^1,R^2,R^3) leads to hallucinogenic compounds. The latter pharmacological property appears to be the more dominant, as changes simultaneously in both areas of the molecule yield hallucinogens that are of increased potency, but do not promote appreciable stimulation.

One of the best documented hallucinogenic plants known is the Peyote cactus (*Anhalonium lewinii, Lophorphora williamsii*) which contains mescaline as its principal alkaloid. (Figure 9, R^1 = R^2 = R^3 = OCH_3, R^4 = R^5 = H). A number of nitrogen substituted analogs are also present, the *N*-methyl and the *N*-acetyl analogs, but they are known to be biologically inert, and probably do not contribute to the reported pharmacology of the entire plant.

Several tetrahydroisoquinoline derivatives are biosynthetically derivable from mescaline and its precursors, and some of these have been observed as plant components. Of the four best-studied compounds, two are phenolic (anhalonidine, Figure 10, R^1 = R^2 = OCH_3, R^3 = OH, R^4 = CH_3, R^5 = H; and pellotine, R^1 = R^2 = OCH_3, R^3 = OH, R^4 = R^5 = CH_3) and 2 are methylenedioxy ethers (anhalonine, Figure 10, R^1 = OCH_3, R^2, R^3 = -OCH_2O-, R^4 = CH_3, R^5 = H; and lophophorine, R^1 = OCH_3, R^2, R^3 = -OCH_2O-, R^4 = R^5 = CH_3). The best accumulation of the sparse-known pharmacology of these peyote components can be found in the appendices of La Barre's study of the peyote cult.[30]

Structure modifications of the mescaline molecule can be arranged in two pharmacologically justified groups. One, accepting the α-methyl substitution pattern as a necessity to circumvent the metabolic clearing of the drug, has led to the discovery of a wealth of aromatic substitution derivatives that have uncovered many active hallucinogens. The other, exploiting the excitatory consequence of the α-methyl substitution pattern, has led to a family of sympathomimetic stimulants.

The first of these modifications, the presentation of the amphetamine carbon skeleton, coupled with a freedom of rearrangement of the groupings of mescaline, has led first to the discovery of TMA (Figure 11, R^1 = H, R^2 = R^3 = R^4 = OCH_3)[31] followed by positional isomers, the most potent of which has been the 2,4,5-counterpart (TMA-2, R^1 = R^3 = R^4 = OCH_3, R^2 = H).[32] The incorporation of the methylenedioxy ring into this general structure, a feature found regularly in the peyote tetrahydroisoquinoline alkaloids, leads to a further increase in potency.[33] The retention of the

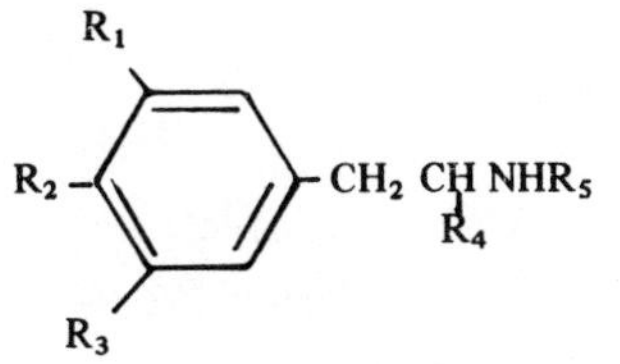

FIGURE 9.

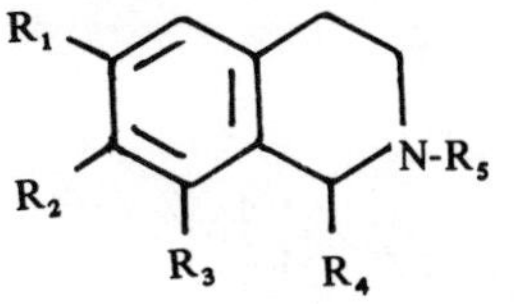

FIGURE 10.

2,4,5-substitution pattern, but with the incorporation of unusual groups into the 4-position, has led to several extremely potent compounds.

The 4-methyl and the 4-ethyl homologs of 2,5-dimethoxy-phenylisopropylamine (DOM, STP, Figure 11, $R^1 = R^4 = OCH_3$, $R^2 = H$, $R^3 = CH_3$; and DOET, $R^1 = R^4 = OCH_3$, $R^2 = H$, $R^3 = CH_2CH_3$) are both effective antidepressants at modest levels (15 μg/kg) and clearly psychotomimetic at higher dosages.[34] The 4-bromo analog (Figure 11, $R^1 = R^4 = OCH_3$, $R^2 = H$, $R^3 = Br$), effective at 4 μg/kg in man, is the most potent of the substituted phenethylamines described in the medical literature.[35]

The second of the structure-modification groups stemming from the skeleton of phenethylamine modified by an alpha-methyl substituent has emphasized changes on the aliphatic chain portion of the molecule, with no substitution whatsoever on the aromatic ring. The results of this have been the development of a number of sympathomimetic stimulants which do not present central distortions, at least within reasonable dosages.

A host of α- and N-alkyl substituted derivatives have been prepared by the pharmaceutical chemist, evaluated by the experimental pharmacologist, and promptly exploited and abused by the socially active drug subculture. The N-methyl homolog of amphetamine (Benzedrine and Dexadrine, Figure 12, $R^1 = R^2 = R^3 = H$) is methamphetamine (Figure 12, $R^1 = R^2 = H$, $R^3 = CH_3$). This chemical has no medical virtue over amphetamine itself, but has been abused greatly for its stimulant action. In an effort to circumvent abuse, the homolog mephentermine has been substituted as a decongestant inhalent, but this chemical (Wyamine®, Figure 12, $R^1 = H$, $R^2 = R^3 = CH_3$) promptly found an abuse market as an excitant.[36] The beta-hydroxy analogs of these chemicals, members of the *Ephedra* botanical group, have been long known as stimulants. A number of these have come into the pharmacological literature (ephedrine and phenylpropanolamine, Figure 12, $R^1 = OH$, $R^2 = H$, $R^3 = H$ or CH_3) and encountered the illicit drug trade.

Most frequently noted are those drugs that are distributed as prescribed chemicals and are employed as acceptable stimulants, but which are found in broad abuse through simple overavailability. Ritalin® (methylphenidate) (Figure 13) has become a major problem in Sweden, and is frequently a "street" problem in the U.S. Preludin® (phenmetrazine, Figure 14) is also occasionally encountered and deserves additional attention.

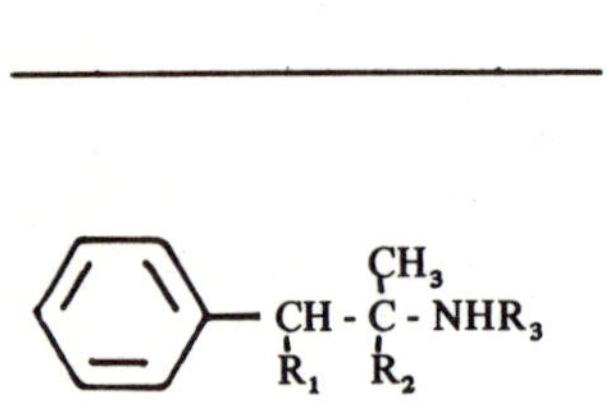

FIGURE 11.

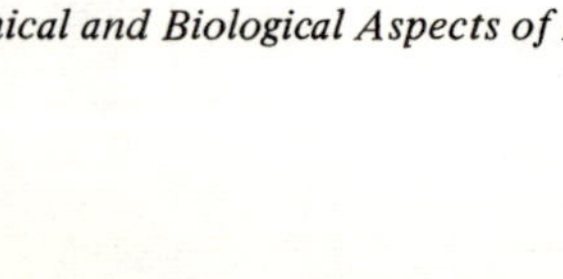

FIGURE 12.

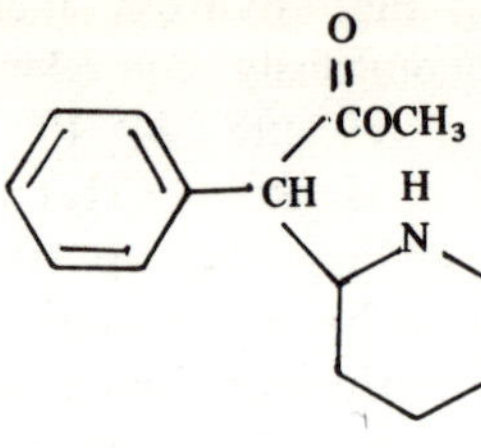

FIGURE 13.

HETEROCYCLIC SYSTEMS

The only heterocyclic system mentioned so far has been the indole system and it is indeed paramount in most alkaloidal chemical systems. However, many other heterocyclic systems are known in the plant kingdom and many have evolved intoxicants that are extremely effective in man.

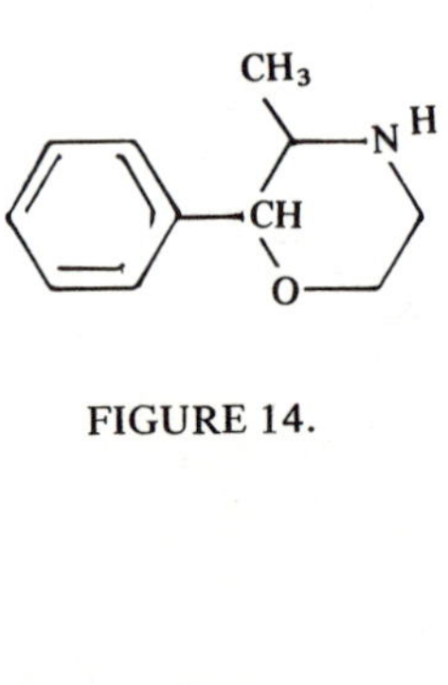

FIGURE 14.

The tropane family of alkaloids is represented in two classes of drugs, the local anesthetics and central stimulants associated with cocaine and the parasympatholytics related to scopolamine. Other natural alkaloid families are the purines (caffeine) and the isooxazoles (active components of the *Amanita muscaria* mushroom). Only a very few synthetic heterocyclics that are unrelated to some plant source, are known.

Cocaine (Figure 15, $R^1 = CH_3$, $R^2 = OCOC_6H_5$ [benzoyl]) is obtained from the leaves of the South American plant, *Erythroxylon coca*. For many centuries, it has been used as a stimulant by the Andean Indians, and the knowledge of its effectiveness as a local anesthetic is over 100-years old. From the medical viewpoint, cocaine has served valuably both per se as a topical anesthetic and as a chemical model that has led to the synthesis of a wealth of related anesthetics that are much safer for injection. Procaine (Figure 16) exemplifies this family of benzoate esters and has been known for 65 years. The social use (misuse?) of cocaine can be considered in two lights. The native use (mentioned above) is restricted to the mountainous areas of western South America and has recently been summarized in an extensive report.[37]

A clearer abuse of cocaine has stemmed from its popularization during the pre-World War II period as an intoxicant. It was popularly administered parenterally by direct inhalation of the crystalline alkaloid.

In the last year or two, cocaine has become a widely touted fad in the drug subculture, but its inherent expense, rather than its illegal classification (along with the parent compound ecgonine, Figure 15, $R^1 = R^2 = H$, as a schedule 2 controlled substance[38]) appears to be limiting its use. The more readily obtainable anesthetic phencyclidine (vide infra) is commonly offered and frequently accepted as "inexpensive cocaine".

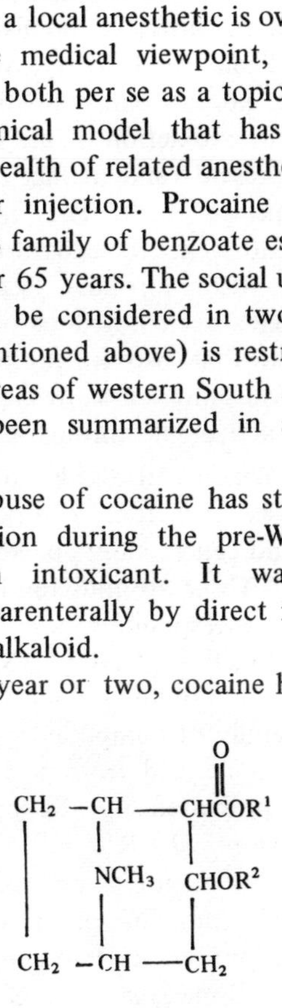

FIGURE 15.

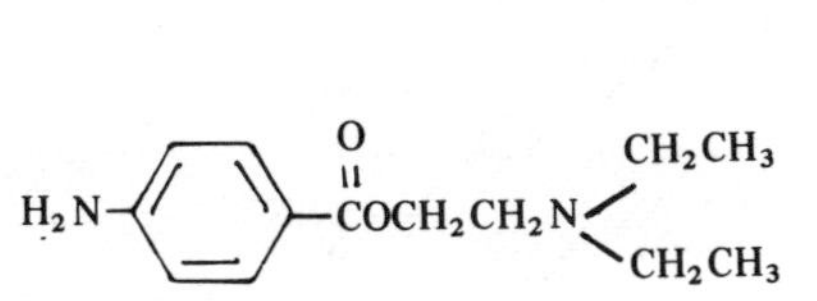

FIGURE 16.

A second family of drugs that stems from the tropane carbon skeleton is based on the structure of scopolamine (Figure 17, R^1, R^2 is an epoxide ring). It and the related base atropine (Figure 17, $R^1 = R^2 = H$) are the principal alkaloids in a variety of intoxicating plants. A number of species of the *Datura* genus have been employed as intoxicants and for religious purposes both in North[39] and South[40] America. Henbane (*Hyosyamus niger*) and Nightshade (*Atropa belladonna*) are native to the eastern Mediterranean regions and Mandrake (*Mandragora officinarum*) probably had its origins in western Asia; these have been known and used since prehistoric times. Even on the Australian continent, intoxicating members of the *Solanaceae* family are found. Pituri (*Duboisia hopwoodii*) also contains the belladonna alkaloids and its leaves are chewed or smoked for their hallucinogen potential.[41] A recent report describes the presence of a tropane alkaloid identical to atropine, but with a 3,4,5-trimethoxycinnamyl acid moiety, rather than tropic acid.[42] The plant, which is native to Australia, is interestingly of the genus that provides cocaine (*Erythroxylon*).

There has been only a small degree of recent social abuse of such plants, although the presence of "stramonium" in a number of over-the-counter medications has led to the expected amount of exploration. Of more concern, is the growing availability of a large number of synthetic substitutes for scopolamine, which although of similar pharmacology, are immensely more potent and easily manufactured.[43] A number of such

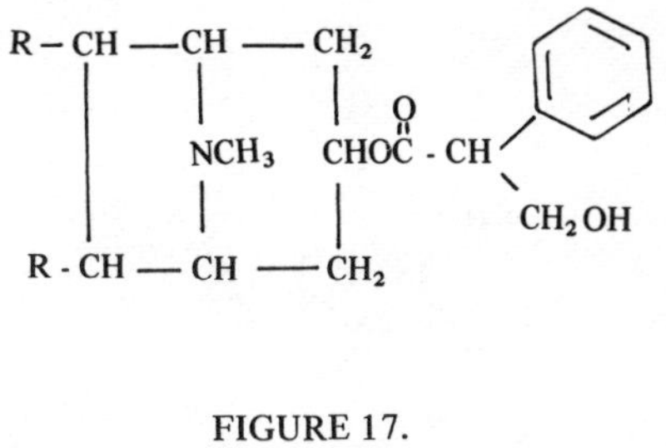

FIGURE 17.

compounds have been developed by the Lakeside Laboratories, and have been extensively explored in human subjects, both clinically and illegally. Examples of this family are JB-329 (Ditran®, Figure 18, $R^1 = C_2H_5$, R^2 = cyclopentyl), JB-318 (Figure 18, $R^1 = C_2H_5$, R^2 = phenyl) and JB-336 (Figure 18, $R^1 = CH_3$, R^2 = phenyl). The latter two homologs have received wide distribution in the eastern regions of the U.S. and have recently been included in the listing of drugs subject to control by the Bureau of Narcotics and Dangerous Drugs.

The best known of all the heterocyclic stimulants is the ubiquitous purine, caffeine. It is a mild euphoriant, yet by no means can be called a psychotomimetic and is a major component of a large number of socially acceptable drinks, yet it cannot gracefully be classified as a drug. Coffee and tea are major sources (containing perhaps 2% caffeine) found in our society; cacao, Maté, and kola are drinks of comparable strength used elsewhere.

Caffeine (Figure 19, $R = CH_3$) is the most effective stimulant of the methylated xanthines. However, a number of compounds are being explored which are 7-substituted theophylline derivatives and show potentially disruptive central effects at higher levels of use. Dimethazan (Figure 19, $R = CH_2CH_2N(CH_3)_2$) is being explored as an antidepressive in geriatric patients, and Fenethylline (Captagon, Figure 19, $R = CH_2CH_2NHCH(CH_3)CH_2C_6H_5$), an amalgamation of the structures of caffeine and of

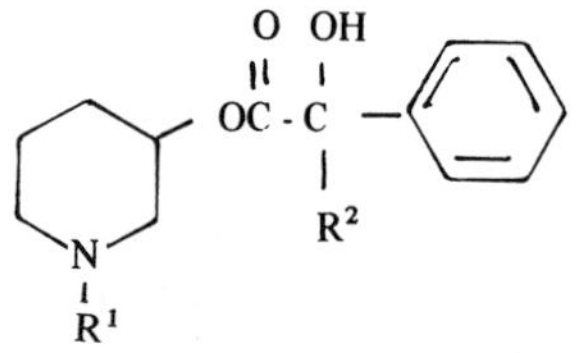

FIGURE 18.

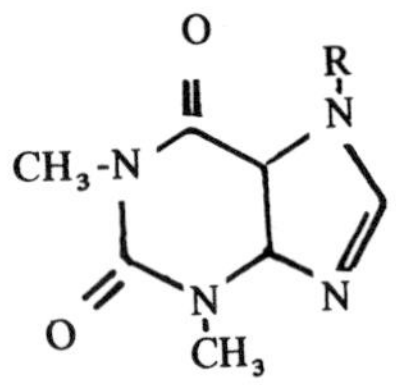

FIGURE 19.

methamphetamine which has been sold through the over-the-counter market in Germany as a psychostimulant and antidepressant. Recent abuse through overuse has caused it to be withdrawn.

An unusual family of heterocyclics, identified as components of the hallucinogenic mushroom *Amanita muscaria* (fly agaric), is the isooxazoles. The thesis of a masterful study[44] is that the legendary drink Soma can be identified with this mushroom but the discrepancies between the reported pharmacology of intoxication following use of the isooxazole alkaloids and the excesses associated through use of Soma (according to the *Rig Veda*) still leave the assignment open to question. The chemistry of the plant has, however, been worked out well. Early, it was felt that muscarine, a potent parasympathomimetic, was responsible for the action of the mushroom, as it was clearly present (and in fact derived its name from the species title). The amounts present, however, cannot begin to account for the action of the fungus. Also, atropine, scopolamine, and bufotenine have been noted to be present in the plant, but the first two are present in too small amounts to account for activity, and the last is known to be active only through parenteral routes.

Two isooxizole alkaloids have been well established as principal components of the mushroom and can account for a large measure of its activity.[45] These are muscimol (Figure 20, R = H) and the corresponding amino acid, ibotenic acid (Figure 20, R = COOH).[46] Variants of these two structures are unknown and thus unexplored.

A small family of compounds, unnatural in the sense that it is derived from no known botanical source, is represented by the compound phencyclidine (Figure 21, R^1, R^2 = $(CH_2)_5$). This compound is not psychotomimetic or "psychedelic" from any point of view, but has become broadly used for two simple reasons; it is potent (5 to 10 mg is a thorough dose producing anesthesia without loss of consciousness) and it is exceptionally inexpensive to synthesize in large quantities, with neither skill nor expert equip-

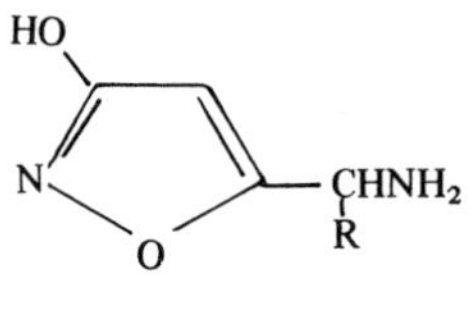

FIGURE 20.

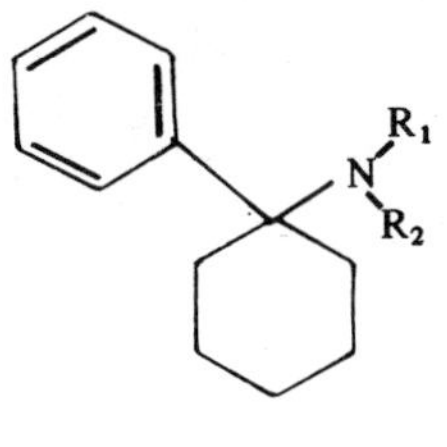

FIGURE 21.

ment. A large number of variations are potentially available through minor variations in the molecule. A recent report from the BNDD indicates the appearance of the mono-ethyl analog (Figure 21, $R^1 = H$, $R^2 = CH_2CH_3$), an analog of phencyclidine that is reported to be of equivalent potency in humans.[47] Another chemically related psychotomimetic and anesthetic (Ketamine, Figure 22) has been introduced into human clinical studies,[48] and has served to show the chemical versatility potentially available within this family. It is only 1/10 the potency of phencyclidine.

NONNITROGENOUS SYSTEMS

A number of intoxicants, psychotomimetics or hallucinogens, are known that do not fit any simple classification. These include the terpenacious or etherial fractions of many plants, the broad problem of *Cannabis* (marijuana) and its currently assumed active components, and last but not least, the unending list of fads, rumors, put-ons, and fables that are believed active by the young drug-oriented subject.

A great number of plants have the reputation of leading to some form of intoxicated state following the ingestion of some reasonable quantity of their oil-rich portions. These range from the Oil of Calamus, noted in biblical times,[49] to the oils of absinthe to zingiber, all of which have found their way into the pharmacopoeias and dispensatories of the last century. They all share in common a distillation fraction that is rich in nitrogen-free aromatic ethers, usually carrying an allyl or propenyl side chain.

Little is known specifically about these neutral compounds in human pharmacology, but studies have been made on the many amination products that are easily derived from them chemically, and to a large measure they have proven to be active as psychotomimetics.[50] The mechanism of action of intoxication of the essential oils is completely unclear, but it has been shown that at least one of the group of essential oils, safrole, is not converted to an amphetamine, but to one of several tertiary amino-methylenedioxypropiophenones.[51] If these are proven to be centrally active, they well may account for the chemistry of plant oil intoxication.

The question of pharmacological mechanism of marijuana intoxication and the medical significance of the many components that have been reported in the extracts of the parent plant (*Cannabis sativa*) has prompted a bewildering body of largely trivial information. A number of historical and scientific reviews have recently appeared and symposia representing the current state of the art occur about once a month. The following points seem to be well established, and are generally agreed upon. Delta-*l*-tetrahydrocannabinol (Figure 23, R = amyl) is clearly a major component of the resin fraction of the marijuana plant; it is biologically active in man, and certainly contributes to, if not accounts for, the primary action of the entire plant. A principal companion is the two-ring counterpart cannabidiol (Figure 24, R = amyl) which is capable of generating tetrahydrocannabinol under certain conditions and

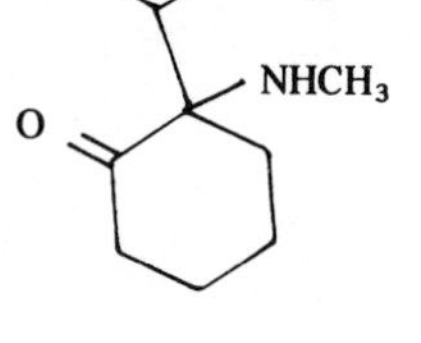

FIGURE 22.

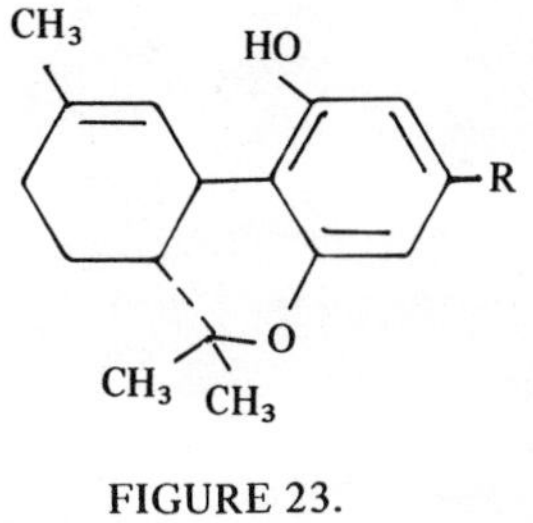

FIGURE 23.

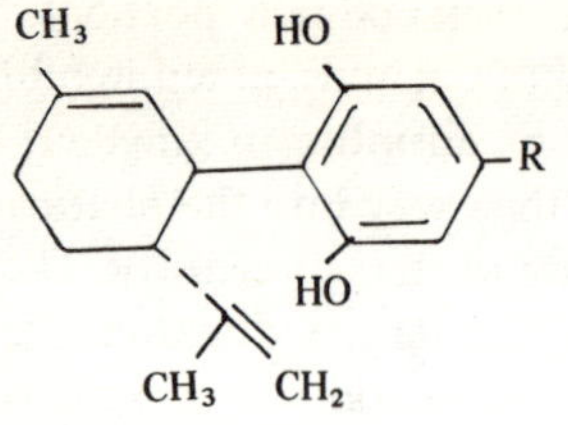

FIGURE 24.

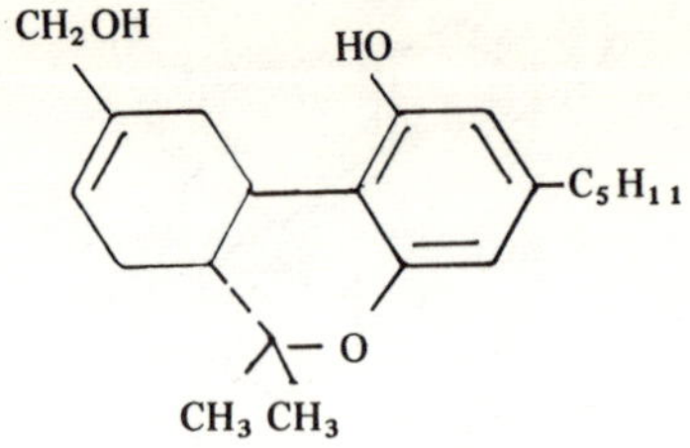

FIGURE 25.

might influence the latter's metabolic disposition. The propyl homologs of both of these compounds occur in the *Cannabis* resin (Figures 23, 24; R = propyl), but only to a small degree. They are of reduced activity and probably do not contribute to the activity of the resin to a significant extent. A principal metabolite of tetrahydrocannabinol (THC) is the isomeric hydroxylation product (Figure 25). This is produced rapidly, but is still controversial as to whether this represents an active form of the drug. A proven component of the original plant, and at least one of the metabolic end products, is cannabinol (Figure 26), but it is not felt to contribute to the overall pharmacological picture of marijuana intoxication.

A large number of extremely active cannabinoid analogs have been prepared with the double bond located in the 3,4-position (Figure 27) and their action in animal and in man appears to be extremely sensitive to the exact identity of the alkyl group R. The homolog with nine carbons (R = $-CH(CH_3)CH(CH_3)CH_2CH_2CH_2CH_2CH_3$) is probably the most potent, but does not imitate the human pharmacology of marijuana with any clinical satisfaction. None of these latter compounds occur in nature. Recent reviews have summarized the chemical[52] and the metabolic[53] research in the marijuana area.

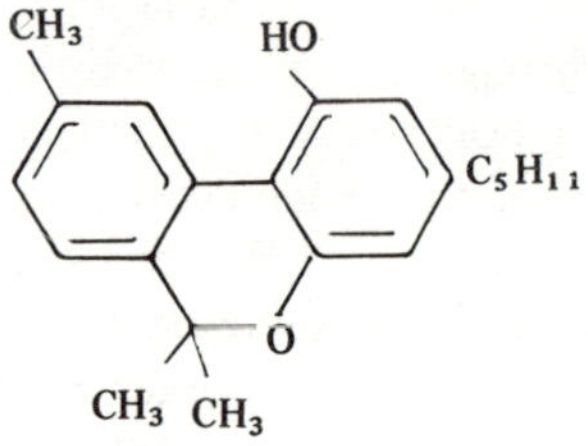

FIGURE 26.

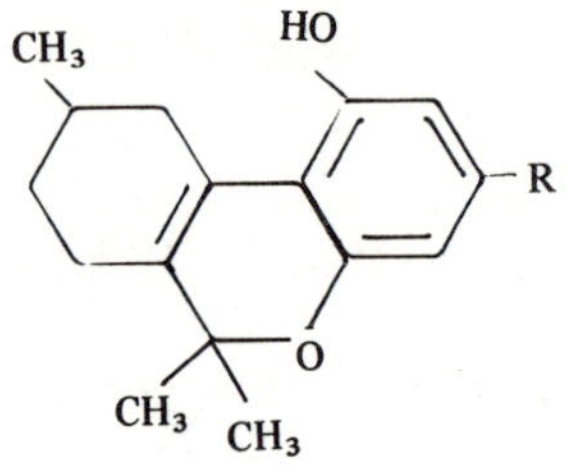

FIGURE 27.

REFERENCES

1. Hofmann, A., Notes and documents concerning the discovery of LSD, *Agents and Actions*, 1, 148, 1970.

2. Stoll, W. A., Ein neues in sehr kleinen mengen wirksames Phantastikum, *Arch. Neurol.*, 64, 483, 1949. (Presented at the 108th meeting of the Swiss Soc. Psychiat., Nov. 22, 1947, Zurich.)

3. Stoll, W. A., Lysergsäure-diäthylamid, ein Phantastikum aus der Mutterkorngruppe, *Schweiz. Arch. Neurol. Neurochir. Psychiat.*, 60, 279, 1947.

4. Abramson, H. A. and Rolo, A., Comparison of LSD with Methysergide and Psilocybin on test subjects, in *The Uses of LSD in Psychotherapy and Alcoholism*, Abramson, H. A., Ed., Bobbs-Merrill Co., New York, 1967.

5. Hofmann, A., Psychotomimetic Agents, in *Drugs Affecting the Central Nervous System*, Medicinal Research Series, Vol. 2, Burger, A., Ed., Marcel Dekker, New York, 1968.

6. Schultes, R. E., A contribution to the knowledge of *Rivea corymbosa:* the narcotic Ololiuqui of the Aztecs, Bot. Museum, Harvard, 1941.

7. Hofmann, A., The active principles of the seeds of *Rivea corymbosa* and *Ipomoea violacea, Psychedelic Rev.*, 1, 302, 1964.

8. Hofmann, A., Teonanácatl and Ololiuqui, two ancient magic drugs of Mexico, *Bull. Narc.*, 23, 3, 1971.

9. Hylin, J. W. and Watson, D. P., Ergoline alkaloids in tropical wood roses, *Science*, 148, 499, 1965.

10. Miller, M. D., Isolation and identification of lysergic acid amide and isolysergic acid amide as the principal ergoline alkaloids in *Argyreia nervosa*, a tropical wood rose, *J.A.O.A.C.*, 53, 123, 1970.

11. Der Marderosian, A. H. and Chao, J., The indole alkaloid constituents of *Argyreia nervosa* Burm. f. Bojer. (convolvulaceae), *Die Gesellschaft Arzneipflanzenforschung* (abs.), Vienna, 1970.

12. Naranjo, C., Ibogaine: A psychotherapeutic picture of its use in humans, *Clin. Toxicol.*, 2, 209, 1969.

13. Hochstein, F. A. and Paraoies, A. M., Alkaloids of *Banisteria caapi* and *Prestonia amazonicum*, *J. Amer. Chem. Soc.*, 79, 5735, 1957.

14. Bernauer, K., Notiz über die Isolierung von Harmin und (+)-1,2,3,4-Tetrahydro-harmin aus einer indianischen Schnupfdroge, *Helv. Chim. Acta*, 47, 1075, 1964.

15. Naranjo, C., Psychotropic Properties of the Harmala Alkaloids, in *Ethnopharmacologic Search for Psychoactive Drugs*, Efron, D. H., Ed., U.S. Government Printing, Washington, D.C., 1967, 385.

16. Schultes, R. E. and Homstedt, B., *De Plantis Toxicariis e Mundo Novo Tropicale Commentationes II* (The vegetal ingredients of the myristicaceous snuffs of the northwest Amazon), *Rhodora*, 70, 781, 1968.

17. Cassady, J. M., Tyler, V. E., Williams, M., and Blair, G. E., The isolation of 6-methoxytetrahydroharman from *Virola cuspidata* and *N*-monomethyltryptamine from *Virola theiodora, Proc. Sym. Biochem. Physiol. Alkaloids*, Halle (Saale), 1970.

18. Cassady, J. M., Blair, G. E., Raffauf, R. F., and Tyler, V. E., The isolation of 6-methoxyharmalan and 6-methoxyharman from *Virola cuspidata, Lloydia*, 34, 161, 1971.

19. McIsaac, W. M., A biochemical concept of mental disease, *Postgrad. Med.*, 30, 111, 1961.

20. Agurell, S., Holmstedt, B., Lindgren, J.-E., and Schultes, R. E., Identification of two new β-carboline alkaloids in South American hallucinogenic plants, *Biochem. Pharmacol.*, 17, 2487, 1968.

21. Wassén, S. H. and Holmstedt, B., The use of Paricá, an ethnological and pharmacological review, *Ethnos*, 5, 1, 1963.

22. Szara, S., Dimethyltryptamine: its metabolism in man; the relation of its psychotic effect to the serotonin metabolism, *Experientia,* 12, 441, 1956.
Arnold, O. H. and Hofmann, G., Zur Psychopathologie des Dimethyltryptamine: ein weiterer Beitrag zur Pharmakopsychiatrie: vorlaufige Mitteilung, *Wein Z. Nervenheilk*, 13, 438, 1957.

23. Tanimukai, H., Ginther, R., Spaide, J., Bueno, J. R., and Himwich, H. E., Detection of psychotomimetic N,N-dimethylated indoleamines in the urine of four schizophrenic patients, *Brit. J. Psychiat.*, 117, 421, 1970.

24. Fabing, H. D. and Hawkins, R. J., Intravenous bufotenine injection in the human being, *Science*, 123, 886, 1956.
Turner, W. J. and Merlis, S., Effect of some indolealkylamines on man, *Arch. Neurol. Psychiat.*, 81, 121, 1959.

25. Szara, S., DMT (N,N-dimethyltryptamine) and homologues: clinical and pharmacological considerations, in *Psychotomimetic Drugs*, Efron, D. H., Ed., Raven Press, New York, 1970, 275.

26. Hofmann, A., Heim, R., Brack, A., and Kobel, H., Psilocybin, ein psychotroper Wirkstoff aus dem mexikanischen Rauschpilz, *Psilocybe mexicana*, Heim, *Experientia*, 14, 107, 1958.

27. Heim, R. and Wasson, R. G., Les champignons hallucinogénes du Mexique, Ed. du Muséum National d'Histoire Naturelle, Paris, 1958.

28. Hofmann, A., Teonanácatl and Ololiuqui, two ancient magic drugs of Mexico, *Bull. Narc.*, 23, 3, 1971.

29. Leuner, H. and Baer, G., Two new short-acting hallucinogens of the psilocybin group, *Neuro-psychopharm.*, 4, 471, 1965.

30. La Barre, W., *The Peyote Cult*, Schocken Books, New York, 1969.

31. Peretz, D. I., Smythies, J. R., and Gibson, W. C., A new hallucinogen: 3,4,5-trimethoxyphenyl-β-aminopropane, with notes on the stroboscopic phenomenon, *J. Ment. Sci.*, 101, 317, 1955.
Shulgin, A. T., Bunnel, S., and Sargent, T., The psychotomimetic properties of 3,4,5-trimethoxyamphetamine, *Nature*, 189, 1011, 1961.

32. Shulgin, A. T., The six trimethoxyphenylisopropylamines (trimethoxyamphetamines), *J. Med. Chem.*, 9, 445, 1966.

33. Shulgin, A. T., Psychotomimetic Amphetamines: Methoxy 3,4-dialkoxyamphetamines, *Experientia*, 20, 366, 1964.

34. Snyder, S. H., Faillace, L. A., and Weingartner, H., DOM (STP), a new hallucinogenic drug, and DOET: effects in normal subjects, *Amer. J. Psychiat.*, 125, 113, 1968.
Hollister, L. E., Macnicol, M. F., and Gillespie, H. K., An hallucinogenic amphetamine analog (DOM) in man, *Psychopharmacologia*, 14, 62, 1969.

35. Shulgin, A. T., Sargent, T., and Naranjo, C., 4-Bromo-2,5-dimethoxyphenylisopropylamine, a new centrally active amphetamine analog, *Pharmacology*, 5, 103, 1971.
Barfknecht, C. F. and Nichols, D. E., Potential Psychotomimetics. Bromomethoxyamphetamines, *J. Med. Chem.*, 14, 370, 1971.

36. Angrist, B. M., Schweitzer, J. W., Gershon, S., and Friedhoff, A. J., Mephentermine psychosis: misuse of the Wyamine inhaler, *Amer. J. Psychiat.*, 126, 149, 1970.

37. United Nations, Report of the Commission of Enquiry on the Coca Leaf, Economic and Social Council, 1950, Special Supplement No. 1, Lake Success, New York.

38. Public Law 91-513, Schedules of Controlled Substances, U.S. Government Printing Office, Washington, D.C., 1971.

39. Gayton, A. H., Ph.D. Thesis, University of California, 1928.

40. Bristol, M. L., Tree datura drugs of the Colombian Sibundoy, *Botan. Mus. Leafl., Harvard Univ.*, 22, 165, 1969.

41. Lewin, L., *Phantastica, Narcotic and Stimulating Drugs*, Routledge and Kegan Paul, London, 1964, 138.

42. Johns, S. R., Lamberton, J. A., and Sioumis, Tropine 3,4,5-trimethoxycinnamate., a new alkaloid from *Erythroxylum ellipticum (Erythroxylaceae), Aust. J. Chem.*, 23, 421, 1970.

43. Abood, L. G., The psychotomimetic Glycolate esters, in, *Drugs Affecting the Central Nervous System*, Medicinal Research Series, Vol. 2, Burger, A., Ed., 1968, 127.

44. Wasson, G., *Soma: Divine Mushroom of Immortality*, Harcourt, Brace and World, New York, 1970.

45. Waser, P. G., The pharmacology of *Amanita muscaria*, in *Ethnopharmacologic Search for Psychoactive Drugs*, Efron, D. H., Ed., U.S. Government Printing Office, Washington, D.C., 1967, 419.

46. Catalfomo, P. and Eugster, C. H., *Amanita muscaria*: present understanding of its chemistry, *Bull. Narc.*, 22, 33, 1970.

47. Godefroi, E. F., Maddox, V. H., and Parcell, R. F., Process for producing a depressant-like effect on the central nervous system, U.S. Patent 3,097,136, 1963.

48. Domino, E. F., Chodoff, P., and Corssen, G., Human pharmacology of CI-581, a new intravenous agent chemically related to phencyclidine, *Fed. Proc.*, 24, 268, 1965.

49. Exodus 30:23.

50. Shulgin, A. T., Sargent, T., and Naranjo, C., The chemistry and psychopharmacology of nutmeg and of several related phenylisopropylamines, in, *Ethnopharmacologic Search for Psychoactive Drugs*, Efron, D. H., Ed., U.S. Government Printing Office, Washington, D.C., 1967, 202.

51. Oswald, E. O., Fishbein, L., Corbett, B. J., and Walker, M. P., Identification of tertiary aminomethylenedioxy-propiophenones as urinary metabolites of safrole in the rat and guinea pig, *Biochim. Biophys. Acta*, 230, 237, 1971.

52. Mechoulam, R. and Gaoni, Y., Recent advances in the chemistry of hashish, *Fortsch. Chem. Org. Naturst.*, 25, 175, 1967.

53. Mechoulam, R., Marijuana chemistry, *Science*, 168, 1159, 1970.

INTERACTION OF DRUGS OF DEPENDENCE WITH RECEPTORS

S. Ehrenpreis and D. N. Teller

TABLE OF CONTENTS

INTRODUCTION

The most important drugs of abuse consist of a heterogeneous group of compounds that have little in common pharmacologically except for their profound effects on CNS activity. In view of the specificity of these effects, it may be concluded that at least some result from interaction with cellular receptors. The extent to which these effects can be interpreted in terms of receptor concepts constitutes the subject of this discussion. Wherever possible, the ability of these drugs to cause tolerance, physical dependence, and withdrawal symptoms will also be discussed within the framework of the receptor concept.

The drugs considered will include the potent analgesics, hallucinogens (LSD, mescaline, tryptamines, amphetamines), barbiturates, and alcohol.

We begin by defining as precisely as possible what we consider to be a "receptor." In the case of these drugs, the definition necessarily differs somewhat from that of Ehrenpreis et al.[1] who recently defined a receptor as a genetically-determined tissue component which has been designed to interact with a naturally-occurring substance, this interaction initiating a series of events culminating in an effect. The naturally-occurring substance is generally a neurohormone or another exceedingly potent compound, e.g., acetylcholine (ACh), norepinephrine (NE), serotonin (5-HT), histamine, various polypeptides, etc. Innumerable synthetic compounds combine with such receptors causing both positive and negative effects, i.e., mimic or antagonize the naturally-occurring substance. However, there are other kinds of cellular macromolecules with which potent neurotropic drugs combine with great specificity. Interaction with these "receptors" also initiates a sequence of events that generally results in an alteration of synaptic function. We term the first group "physiological receptors" and the latter "drug receptors." While the physiological receptors are located within postsynaptic membranes of nerves and muscle, the drug receptors are mainly in *nerve terminals,* i.e., within presynaptic sites. For the most part, there is little, if any, direct interaction between drug and transmitter, despite the fact that the drugs under consideration influence virtually all types of transmission mechanisms, electrogenic and chemical. Therefore, one of the most important tests of a receptor mechanism, namely, the ability of a transmitter to compete with drugs blocking such receptors, cannot be utilized in evaluating the specificity of action of these drugs; other criteria must be used.

As a further distinction, we suggest that drugs which have as a *primary site* of action the *physiological receptor* apparently *do not give rise to dependence and addiction,* whereas those which act indirectly, i.e., with pharmacological or drug receptors, are potentially capable of producing such effects. Upon continuous administration of the drug, distinct changes in the properties of the physiological receptors may occur, changes which might be involved in supersensitivity and tolerance.

The nerve terminal contains a number of important sites of potential interaction for drugs; combination of drugs with components at these points could profoundly alter transmission at the particular junction. Whether these sites constitute receptors in the sense defined previously has been established with certainty for only a few of these drugs. In studying these drugs, specificity of effect is most readily determined by using specific antagonists or structure-activity relationship (SAR) studies, particularly if optical isomers can be employed.

The various neuronal sites which could function as drug receptors, as well as the consequences of drug interaction, will now be discussed in some detail (See Figure 1 for diagramatic representation).

The Transmitter Storage Vesicle

Neurotransmitters are present in nerve terminals in a bound form, mainly confined within ultramicroscopic particles termed synaptic vesicles. In the case of ACh, these are about 400 Å in diameter and contain from 10^4 to 10^5 ACh molecules. Little is known about the exact content of NE molecules. It is uncertain whether ACh exists in a free solution within its vesicles or bound to a macromolecule. Smythies et al.[2] considered that ACh is bound to "a stacked array of cytidine monophosphate molecules stabilized by divalent cations." NE is bound to an ATP-protein (chromogranin?) complex which is released in its entirety upon nerve stimulation. Smythies et al.[2] believed that 5-HT is stored in a similar manner.

Many drugs are known to interact with these storage sites, thereby displacing the transmitter and preventing subsequent binding of newly-synthesized transmitters. The physiological effect

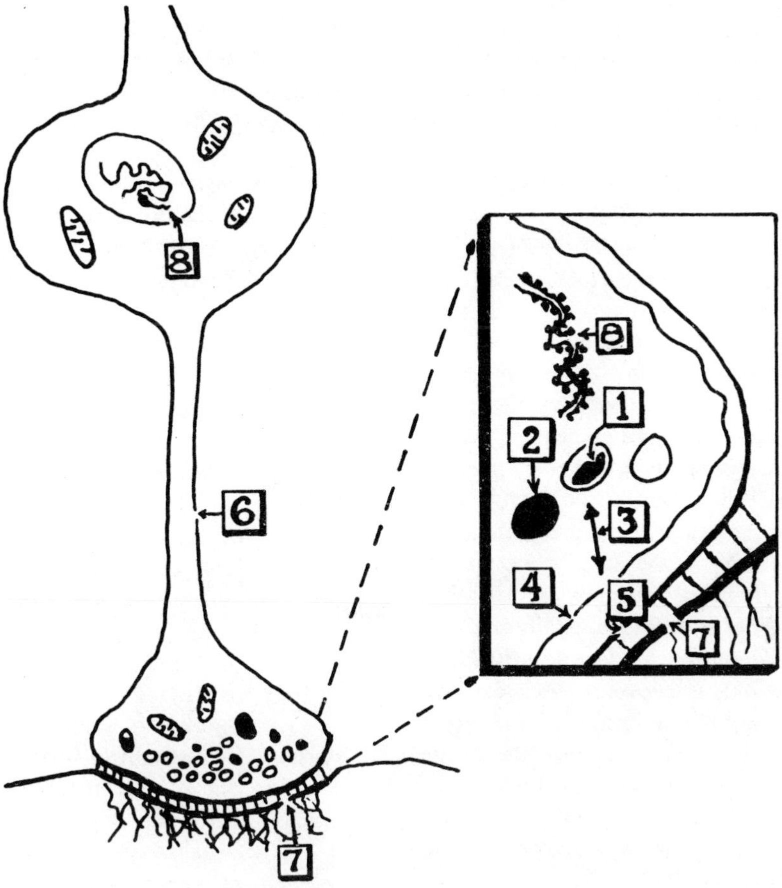

FIGURE 1. Possible neuronal sites for receptors for drugs of dependence. (1) Binding site for neurotransmitter within synaptic vesicle. (2) Vesicle membrane. (3) Extra-vesicular transport system, MAO, and neurotransmitter synthesizing enzymes. (4) Reuptake mechanism in nerve terminal membrane. (5) Presynaptic nerve surface membrane. (6) Nerve axon. (7) Physiological (neurotransmitter) postsynaptic receptor. (8) Ribosomal particles and nucleoprotein.
NOTE: Inset is schematic expansion of synaptic region.

of a released transmitter often is followed by its depletion from the particular nerve terminal and inhibition of further transmission. Drugs which act in this manner are called indirectly acting agents. A prime example of this type of drug is amphetamine, which produces at least some of its effects by releasing catecholamines in the CNS.

The vesicle membrane is another possible target for drugs. It has been established that NE, in particular, is taken up into its storage sites by an active process that probably occurs both in the vesicular wall as well as across the nerve terminal membrane.

Binding of a drug to the vesicular membrane might also inhibit release of the particular transmitter during nerve stimulation. This would occur if the drug is a membrane "stabilizer" as has been described by Shanes[3] for local anesthetics and by Seeman[4] for many types of drugs interacting with R.B.C. membranes. Binding could also produce disruption of the vesicular wall with discharge of its contents; such agents have been termed "labilizers" by Shanes; examples are aconitine and the veratrum alkaloids which destabilize membranes present in nerve axons, cardiac cells, etc. Whether drugs act in a similar manner on synaptic vesicles has not been determined. Moreover, Seeman has demonstrated that stabilizers become labilizers at high concentrations. A possible example of a labilizer of nerve terminal vesicles is mescaline which, as shown by Teller and Denber,[5] produces a type of disorganization or disruption of formed elements present in nerve terminals. It is conceivable that with other drugs such an effect would be extremely long lasting, requiring synthesis of the vesicular membrane components to repair the "lesion" caused by disruption of the membrane.

A third type of interaction which might occur at the vesicular membrane may not result in an overt effect. This would be an example of a "silent receptor." Binding of morphine in this manner has been postulated to occur to vesicles present in postganglionic elements of the guinea pig ileum.[6]

The vesicle membrane is a site of uptake of neurotransmitters, particularly NE and ACh. Choline may also be taken up actively into ACh vesicles, since much of the cholineacetylase is present in bound form, possibly within these vesicles.[7] Such carrier systems are readily inhibited in a specific manner by many drugs, and thus these might be considered as receptor sites for such drugs. Not only would inhibition of the carrier affect uptake and binding of the neurotransmitter, but also its synthesis. Some steps in the synthesis of transmitter take place within the vesicle itself. If some intermediate is prevented from entering the vesicle by drug inhibition of a carrier, ultimately the content of stored transmitter would be depleted. Moreover, some other metabolic pathway may supersede, bypassing the block caused by lack of intermediate; in such cases a "false transmitter" may result. This has been the explanation for many of the pharmacological effects of the potent MAO inhibitors, tryptamine derivatives, and amphetamines, particularly in the peripheral nervous system. The metabolic pathways in the central nervous system appear to be somewhat different from peripheral sites since few of the false transmitters produced or stored peripherally are produced in significant quantity in the CNS.

The Nerve Terminal Membrane

The nerve terminal membrane is the site of many biochemical and physiological events[8] and increasingly has been proposed as the primary, if not exclusive, site of action for many types of pharmacological agents. Indeed, in the view of one school,[9] virtually all drugs acting at cholinergic synapses do so via the nerve terminal to the exclusion of the postsynaptic elements (physiological receptors). We do not completely agree with this proposal as applied to striated muscle synapses; however, there is little doubt in the case of many of the drugs of abuse that the presynaptic nerve ending membrane is a primary site of action.

The following processes which occur within or across the nerve terminal membrane are possible points of attack of drugs of abuse:

1. Depolarization of the membrane upon nerve stimulation, i.e., increased permeability to Na and K. Depolarization may occur directly by the conducted impluse from the axon or by "reflux" of transmitter, in particular ACh.[10]
2. Link between depolarization and liberation of transmitter. This may involve Ca^{++} release within the nerve terminal.
3. Uptake of transmitter after its release (mainly for NE).
4. Uptake of metabolites required for resynthesis of transmitter (mainly for ACh).
5. Uptake of metabolites for generalized metabolic processes, e.g., into mitochondria.

Each of these involves a specific molecular membrane component, e.g., sites controlling ion flux or a carrier molecule. Interaction of a drug with any one of these sites would result in an immediate or delayed transmission block. When this occurs, any or all metabolic pathways in the affected synaptic region could be altered; these would clearly be secondary effects. Therefore, evaluation of changes in carbohydrate, protein, nucleic acid, etc., metabolism produced by a particular drug may not be relevant to understanding its basic mode of action.

There are several approaches for investigating the presynaptic sites of actions of drugs in the CNS. These include:

1. Morphological – use of electron microscope to examine changes in thickness of nerve terminal walls, disappearance of boutons, etc.
2. Biogenic amine levels and turnover.
3. Effects of drugs on uptake of biogenic amines into brain slices* or synaptosomes (NEPs).

*It is generally considered that NE in particular is largely taken up by nerve terminals. However, recent evidence has been obtained that post-synaptic sites can also accumulate NE and catecholamines by a mechanism involving physiological adrenergic receptors. Hendley and Snyder[11] have shown how it is possible to distinguish pre- and post-synaptic binding to elements of brain slices.

4. Binding of drugs to synaptosomes or to presynaptic membranes.

The Axonal Membrane

The axonal membrane contains receptors for many types of neurotropic drugs; for some, the axon proper as well as nerve terminal are regions of attachment, e.g., local anesthetics, the barbiturates, and the phenothiazines. For most, however, the axon is excluded as a site of interaction, while the terminal is highly susceptible. Examples include morphine, amphetamines, mescaline, and LSD. Since these drugs are all fairly hydrophobic, the lipids surrounding the axonal membrane (e.g., myelin) should not prevent their penetration to the active membrane where the receptors are located. The fact that most of these drugs have minimal axonal blocking action strongly suggests the presence of specific terminal receptor sites which are different from those in the axon.

A drug which clearly alters axonal conduction is alcohol. The effect is complex, initially enhanced stimulation followed by block;[12] however, it is doubtful whether this comes about by interaction with axonal receptors. Ehrenpreis[13,14] proposed that alcohol blocks conduction by promoting the binding of Ca^{++} and Mg^{++} to nerve phospholipids; this opposes depolarization which is initiated by the dissociation of these cations. Promotion by alcohol of divalent cation binding to macromolecules isolated from nerve tissue could be demonstrated.[13] Similarly alcohol produces complex effects postsynaptically, initially causing a depolarization. This too could be an indirect effect due to enhanced binding of transmitters to their receptors perhaps via stabilized cations.

Using the technique of subcellular fractionation, investigators recently have attempted to localize the receptors with which these various drugs interact in a direct way. Autoradiography and studies on interactions with well-known macromolecules have provided some information. The problems associated with determining the nature of receptors by these and other techniques have been discussed in detail elsewhere.[1] Despite the shortcomings of the above approaches, they have provided at least some insight into the nature and localization of important binding sites in tissue for these drugs and are thus helpful in explaining some of their pharmacological actions. Thus, an analysis of the data obtained in these investigations will constitute an important part of our discussion.

THE POTENT ANALGESICS

The actions of the potent analgesics have been the subject of many review articles,[15-21] most of which discuss mechanisms of analgesia, tolerance, and addiction in terms of changes in cell biochemistry (i.e., metabolism) caused either after the drug is administered to an animal or added to the medium bathing brain slices. It is our contention that many of the extensive metabolic effects observed are consequences of the action of the drugs in blocking synaptic transmission. Thus, an evaluation of these agents as inhibitors of important metabolic enzymes may not reveal their primary site or mechanism of action. On the other hand, certain biochemical changes which do occur when the drugs are given chronically, such as receptor induction or supersensitivity,[22] may play an important role in the development of tolerance and dependence.

In the following discussion, we will evaluate the effects of these drugs, and particularly morphine, on cholinergic, adrenergic, and serotonergic pathways from the receptor standpoint. A new mechanism of morphine tolerance based on the receptor concept will be presented.

Sites of Interaction in Tissues

Receptors for Neurohormones

Despite the fact that morphine and related compounds are extremely potent in influencing cholinergic and adrenergic transmission, there is little doubt that for the most part these effects do not occur through combination with the physiological receptors located in postsynaptic membranes. The best test for distinguishing presynaptic from postsynaptic sites of action is whether the particular transmitter is still effective when applied exogenously. Thus, when morphine blocks striated or smooth neuromuscular junctions, exogenous ACh still produces a contraction.[6,23,24] Some exceptions may exist; e.g., morphine inhibition of certain spinal neurons is said to occur both pre- and postsynaptically.[25a,25b] The antagonism of serotonin by morphine on various smooth muscles most likely takes place at postsynaptic (i.e., muscle) sites, but there may also be an important presynaptic component since serotonin contractions are

TABLE 1

Potency of a Series of Drugs as Analgesics in Mice and Man and as Inhibitors of Contractions of the Isolated Guinea Pig Ileum*

Drug	50% depression of contractions of the ileum: molar potency relative to morphine	Analgesia in mice (hot plate method): molar potency relative to morphine	Analgesia in man: molar potency relative to morphine
Fentanyl	10,000	250	100
Phenoperidine	2,000	42	10
Oxymorphone	500	13	7.1
Nalorphine	2	0.03	1.1
Diamorphine	1.7	2.8	2.4
Normorphine	1.4	0.05	0.25
Phenazocine	1.2	19	4.0
Morphine	1.0	1.0	1.0
Pentazocine	0.6	0.3	0.42
Codeine	0.15	0.16	0.09
Morphine-*N*-oxide	0.05	0.10	-
Dextrorphan	inactive		inactive

*Compiled by Fennessey et al.[28]

mediated in part by the release of neuronal ACh. The ability of morphine to block ACh release in smooth muscle has been long established.

Cholinergic Neurone Receptors

Following the early studies of Paton[23] and Schaumann,[26] much evidence has accumulated suggesting that the neuronal elements of various smooth muscles have specific morphine receptors. The most sensitive tissue is the guinea pig ileum in which contractions induced by electrical stimulation are abolished by 10^{-8} *M* morphine. In view of the highly significant correlation (r = 0.99)[27] between the potency of many drugs in inhibiting contractions and their action as potent analgesics (Table 1), this tissue has been proposed as a useful experimental model to substitute for the CNS when investigating the mode of action of these drugs.[6,23,27] The following discussion is concerned with the mechanism of action of these drugs on the ileum, their antagonism by naloxone, and the properties of intestines removed from animals which were given repeated injections of morphine.

The guinea pig ileum possesses a multiplicity of potential receptor sites for morphine; combination with any one of these would result in blockade of the cholinergic pathway. These include the preganglionic nerve axon, its terminals, postganglionic receptors, postganglionic neuron or axon, its nerve terminal, postsynaptic ACh receptors, the transport mechanism for choline, and cholinesterase (ChE). All but one may be ruled out as a possible receptor site. The entire pathway from preganglionic fibers to ganglion may be blocked by either hexamethonium, chlorisondamine, or nicotine without changing the action of morphine in any way. AChE affinity for morphine is too weak to account for its effect on transmission; indeed, ChE inhibitors would potentiate rather than inhibit transmission. Addition of choline does not influence inhibition by morphine.[29] Finally, at a time when transmission is completely blocked, response of the tissue to ACh is totally unaltered.[6,23] Therefore, the effect of morphine is relegated to the postganglionic neuron. In view of the weak local anesthetic activity of morphine, it is anticipated that at the concentrations used to block contractions, the drug would have little, if any, effect on conduction in postganglionic elements. The evidence strongly suggests that the site of morphine action is in the nerve terminal. At this site morphine inhibits the release of ACh either at rest or upon electrical stimulation.[23,26]

The specificity of the nerve terminal site for morphine and related compounds has been investigated in many laboratories. On this basis, there is little doubt that the presynaptic analgesic binding does indeed occur with a true receptor. One of the most convincing arguments is that dextrorphan and dextromethorphan are totally inert in producing a block of contraction, whereas the levo isomers are exceedingly potent.[27]

Another indication of specificity is the antagonism of blockade by various specific antagonists, in particular naloxone. As shown in Figure 2, this compound reverses the blockade of electrical stimulation produced by morphine at extremely low concentrations (1 to 2 ng/ml). Specificity of this antagonism is indicated by the fact that naloxone does not reverse the blockade of electrical stimulation produced by barbiturates, diphenylhydantoin, strychnine, and metrazole.[6]

Antagonism of morphine by naloxone has led to the conclusion that there are two major neuronal receptor sites for morphine.[6,30] These two sites have been termed the "T" site and the "I" site, the former being the presynaptic site involved in the release of ACh upon nerve stimulation, the other binding morphine specifically, but not concerned directly with release of ACh. This second site of binding was discovered through the use of naloxone. Figure 3 shows what happens when 16 ng of naloxone/ml is added to a tissue previously exposed to morphine. Along with recovery of electrically induced contractions, there is a very marked contracture (increase in tension) of the tissue.

These two actions of naloxone following morphine – reversal of blockade of electrically stimulated contractions and appearance of contracture – have been shown to be independent in several ways. After addition of an appropriate concentration of morphine, the tissue is washed and often recovers within a few minutes, i.e., the block of transmission is reversed. However, if naloxone is added, the contracture may still be observed (Figure 4) even if the tissue is exposed to morphine for only a short time. Naloxone, even in the presence of morphine, produces recovery without contracture (Figure 5). Finally, if a very low concentration of naloxone is added, recovery may be observed to be unaccompanied by contracture. If a high concentration of naloxone is added at this time, contracture is clearly observed without any further recovery of contraction amplitude.

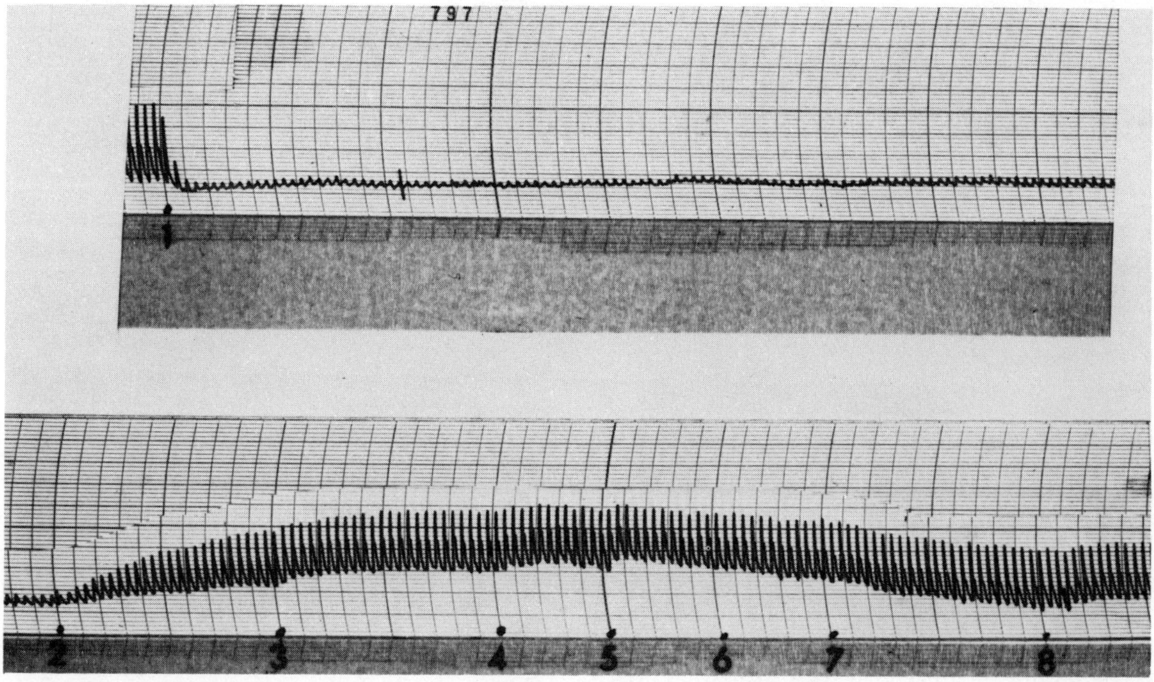

FIGURE 2. Morphine-naloxone antagonism: lower limit of sensitivity to naloxone. Electrically stimulated guinea pig ileum: 0.2 Hz, 40 V, 0.4 msec. current duration.

(1) Morphine, 25 ng/ml. (2) Naloxone (final concentration) 0.4 ng/ml; note distinct evidence of recovery of contractions. (3) 0.8 ng/ml. (4) 1.6 ng/ml. (5) 3.2 ng/ml. (6) 6.4 ng/ml. (7) 12.8 ng/ml. (8) 52.8 ng/ml.

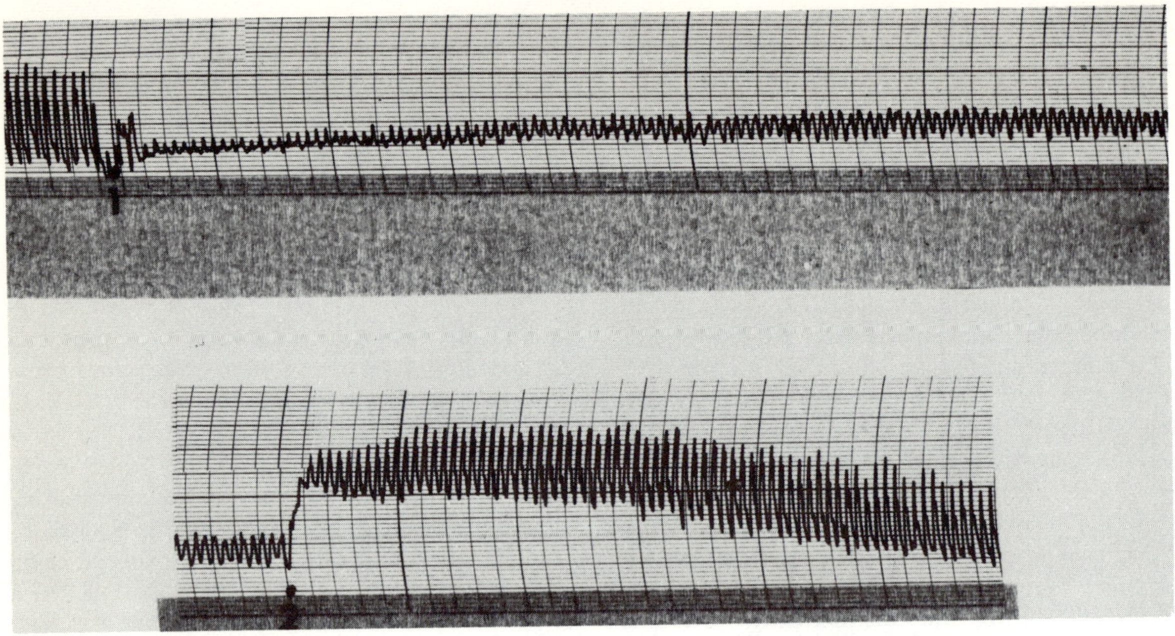

FIGURE 3. Naloxone-induced contracture of guinea pig ileum after morphine in vitro. (1) Morphine, 12 ng/ml applied for 10 min. (2) Naloxone, 16 ng/ml.

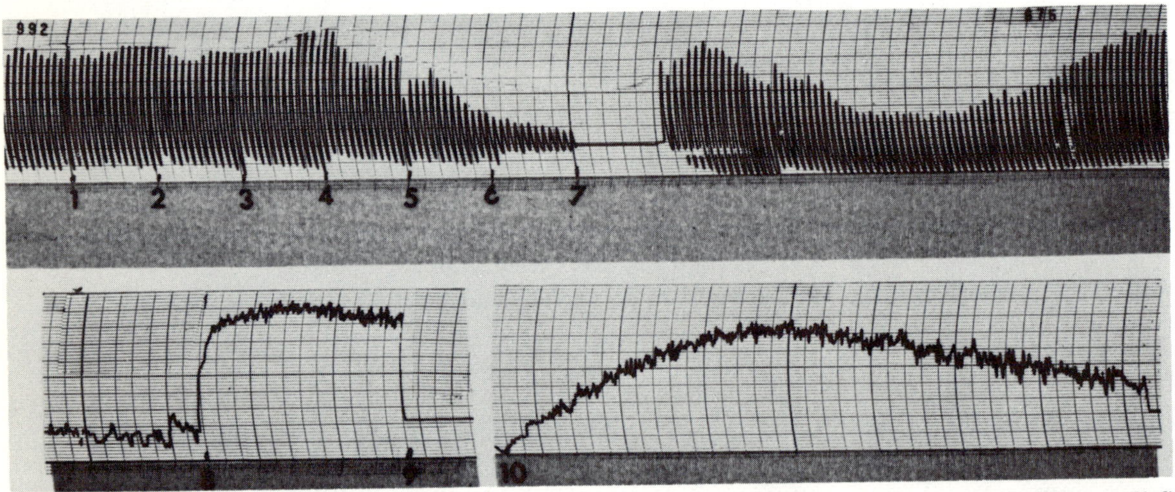

FIGURE 4. Dissociation of naloxone-induced contracture from recovery of contractions after morphine exposure. (1-6) Morphine, final concentrations 4 ng/ml, 8 ng/ml, 16 ng/ml, 32 ng/ml, 72 ng/ml, 152 ng/ml. (7) Wash 15 min. Note complete recovery of contractions. (8) Naloxone, 40 ng/ml. Note marked contracture of tissue. (9) Wash 5 min. (10) Naloxone, 40 ng/ml. Contracture still occurs but is much reduced as compared with (8).

An important example of the distinction between morphine action on "T" and on "I" receptors was demonstrated with tissues removed from animals injected chronically with morphine (100 mg/kg) for one week. These tissues responded to electrical stimulation in a normal or exaggerated way (Figure 6). Therefore, the "T" receptors were not blocked by the injected morphine. However, as shown in Figure 7, addition of naloxone to such preparations resulted in a marked contracture. As shown in Figure 8, contracture was completely abolished by atropine and thus reflected the action of ACh. Similarly, naloxone-induced contracture following addition

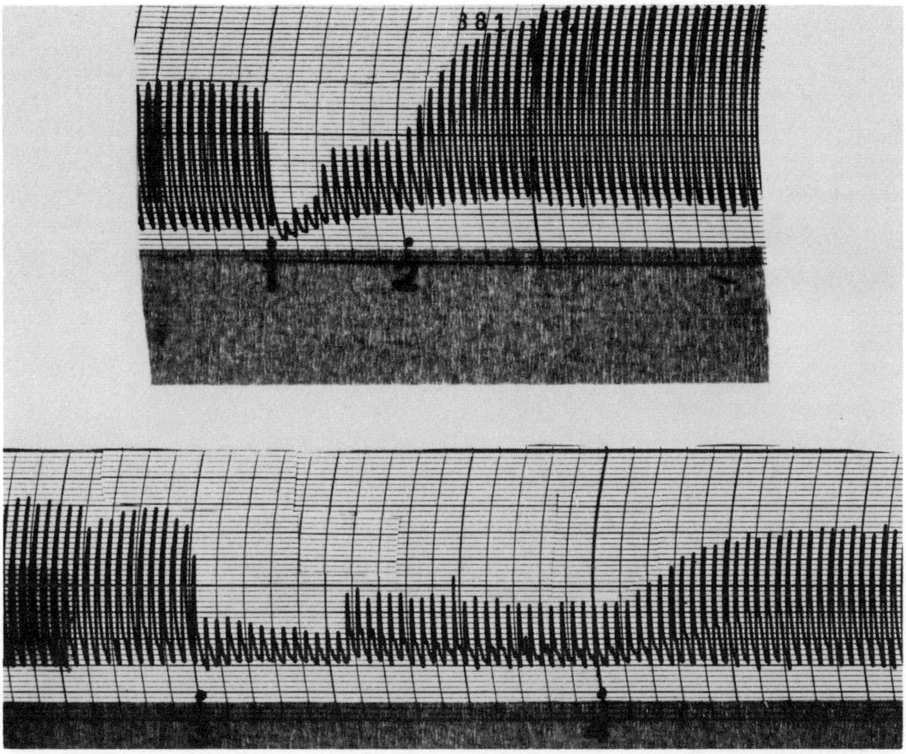

FIGURE 5. Contracture by naloxone: dependence on time given after morphine. (1) Morphine, 12 ng/ml applied for 2 min. (2) Naloxone, 2 ng/ml. Note recovery of contractions without contracture. Wash 10 min. (3) Morphine, 12 ng/ml, 3 min. (4) Naloxone, 2 ng/ml. Again improvement of contractions is observed without contracture.

of morphine to normal tissues, was reversed by atropine.

We have considered that the "I" receptor may be localized on the synaptic vesicle containing ACh; binding of morphine to synaptic vesicles isolated from brain has been reported.[31,32] Binding of morphine to this site does not in itself result in an overt effect. However, if naloxone enters the nerve terminal and interacts at the same or adjacent (allosteric) site, the interaction results in rupture of the vesicle and liberation of its contents directly to the outside medium. Massive rupture of such vesicles causes the observed contracture. If the tissue is stimulated tetanically to partially deplete its store of ACh, naloxone contracture is greatly reduced. Many other aspects of the naloxone-morphine interaction have been described in detail elsewhere.[6]

The two specific morphine sites in this tissue have also been demonstrated by studies on kinetics of binding of radioactive drug by the tissue.[33] The binding curve at 20 ng/ml morphine exhibits a distinct break after exposure for one minute. This morphine concentration blocks electrical stimulation by about 90% in one minute. The first portion of the curve is considered to reflect binding to the "T" receptors. The second part of the binding curve indicates a slower rate (first order rate constant about 1/3 that of the rapid phase) as well as a much greater capacity to bind morphine. This is considered to represent "I" site occupation by the drug. Only a single site of binding is observed at very low morphine concentrations (6 ng/ml). Specificity of binding at the lower concentration was shown by the fact that naloxone at 10 times the initial morphine concentration inhibited binding by 30 to 60%. Our interpretation of these data for the development of a concept of morphine tolerance will be discussed later.

The morphine receptor involved in controlling ACh release by electrical stimulation might be involved with calcium. Mulé[19] summarized evidence implicating Ca^{++} in morphine action,

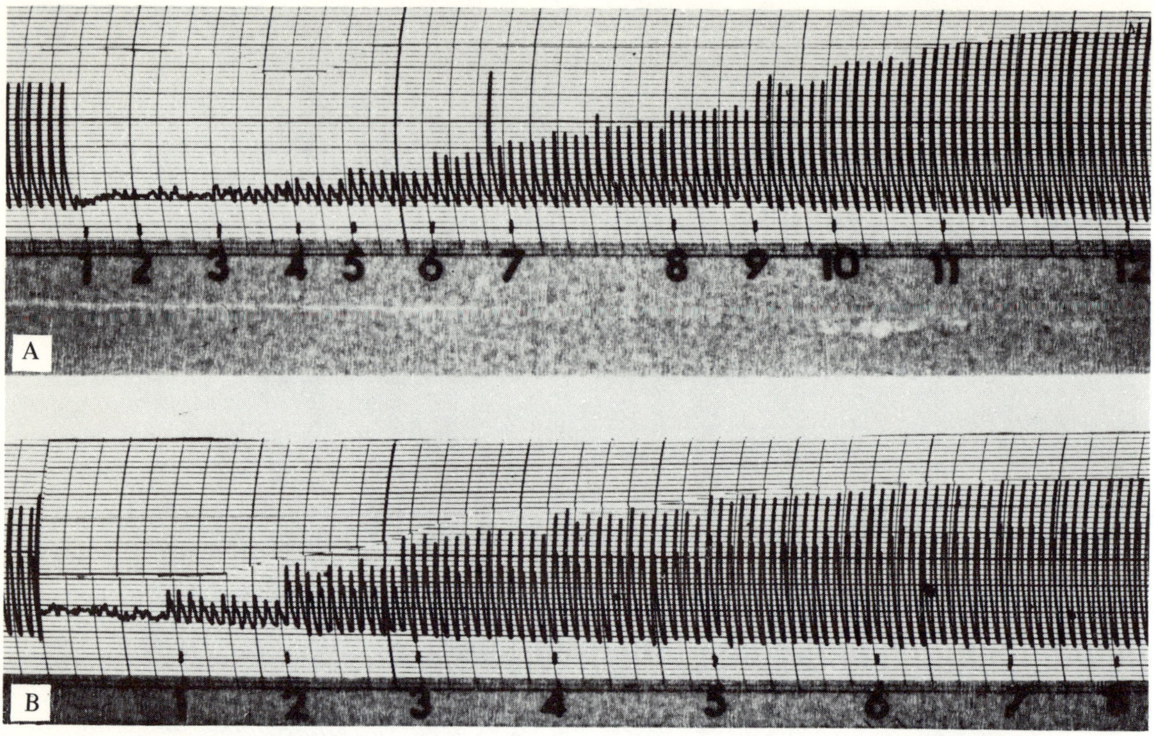

FIGURE 6. Current duration-contraction height for ileum removed from normal and morphinized guinea pig. Panel A. Normal guinea pig ileum. Current duration times, msec.: (1) 0.02 (2) 0.03 (3) 0.04 (4) 0.05 (5) 0.06 (6) 0.08 (7) 0.12 (8) 0.15 (9) 0.2 (10) 0.3 (11) 0.4 (12) 1.0. Panel B: Ileum from tolerant guinea pig (100 mg/kg morphine/day, one week) (1) 0.03 (2) 0.04 (3) 0.05 (4) 0.06 (5) 0.08 (6) 0.12 (7) 0.15 (8) 0.2. Note that not only does the ileum removed from the morphinized guinea pig respond to electrical stimulation, but the threshold and midpoint of current strength for maximum contraction are much lower than in the control. This indicates supersensitivity of the experimental ileum to ACh released during nerve stimulation. Enchanced sensitivity of this ileum to exogenous acetylcholine could also be demonstrated.

including the fact that Ca^{++} antagonized the blockade of electrically-stimulated guinea pig ileum.[34]

In a morphine-treated tissue, it is possible that naloxone might displace ACh from its presynaptic binding. This does not occur in untreated tissue. If this were the case, it would indicate an allosteric effect upon the presynaptic ACh binding site by morphine. Smythies et al.[2] considered that ACh was stored in association with phosphorylated polynucleosides. They found that morphine bound very well to poly-C, the suggested storage site for ACh. Neither morphine nor naloxone liberated ACh. However, it would be of interest to determine whether these drugs alter the stacking of poly-C, thereby causing the unbinding of ACh.

Effects of morphine on ACh in the CNS are somewhat similar to those in guinea pig ileum. Morphine increases the level of CNS ACh[35] which may be attributed to accumulation of the transmitter due to blockade of its release. Blockade of ACh release in the CNS is highly specific. This has been demonstrated conclusively by Jhamandas et al.,[36] who showed that naloxone completely reverses inhibition of ACh release in cat cortex.

Morphine has similar effects on neuromuscular junctions of striated muscles. Extremely high concentrations are required as compared to ileum; 0.1 mg/ml morphine blocks release of ACh from electrically-stimulated sartorius muscles of *Rana pipiens.*[24] Despite this blockade of ACh release, morphine initially facilitates the action of ACh on postsynaptic receptors. Apparently this also occurs in frog rectus abdominis muscle and cat superior cervical ganglion.[37] This facilitation was not due to inhibition of AChE since it occurred even in the presence of large concentrations of inhibitors of the enzyme.

Morphine and nalorphine also block indirect stimulation of the isolated rat phrenic nerve-diaphragm preparation.[38] However, $10^{-3}M$ morphine was required. The effect again was attributed primarily to blockade of ACh release.

In view of the extremely high concentrations

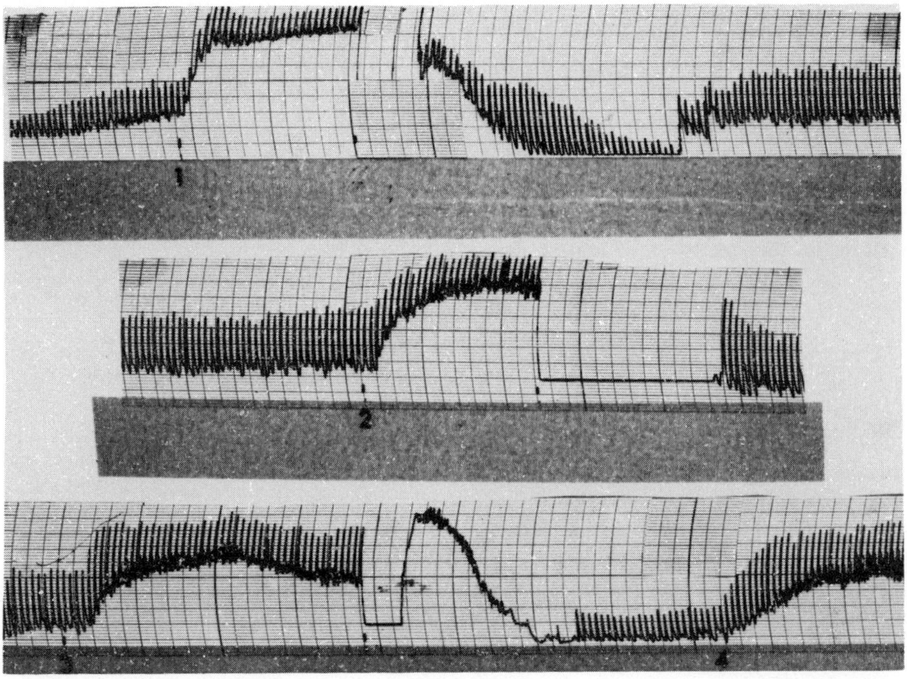

FIGURE 7. Naxolone contracture of ileum removed from morphinized guinea pig. Ileum was the same as that used in experiment shown in Figure 6. (1) Naloxone, 40 ng/ml. Note the marked contracture; no improvement of contraction height is observed. Following wash, the same amount of naloxone is added at (2); another contracture is observed, but of lesser extent than in (1). Subsequent additions of naloxone (at 3 and 4) result in diminishing contractures. This experiment clearly shows that a large amount of morphine is present within the ileum but does not inhibit contractions elicited by electrical stimulation.

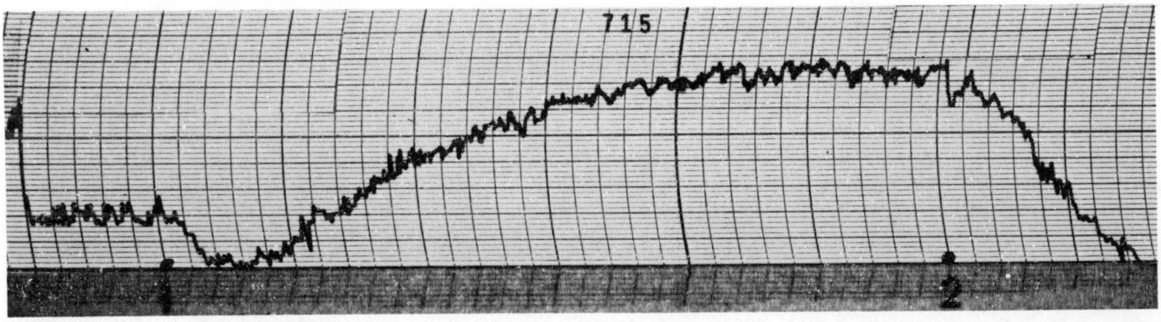

FIGURE 8. Reversal of naloxone contracture by atropine in ileum from morphinized guinea pig. (1) Naloxone, 2 ng/ml. Note marked contracture. (2) Atropine, 8 ng/ml causes a rapid return of tension to the base line.

required, and the fact that morphine is relatively devoid of blocking action of striated muscle in doses well above those required to produce complete analgesia, it is unlikely that use of such preparations provides an adequate model for determining the mechanism of action of the drug as an analgesic. However, the "receptor" for morphine appears to be functionally similar in smooth and striated muscle. The reason for the great difference in sensitivity is an important unsolved problem and may be related to the neural organization in these tissues.

Adrenergic Neurone Receptors

The NE-depleting action of morphine in various species (rat, cat, etc.) has been well documented[17,21,39-41] and also has been suggested as the mechanism of analgetic action.[40,42] The exact localization of the receptors through which the adrenergic effects are produced is not known.

These may be on the storage sites themselves or sites involved with catecholamine transport to the vesicles. Morphine and other potent analgesics have been shown to block active transport at various sites.[43] Morphine is taken up by synaptosomes by a transport mechanism.[32] These findings, taken together, suggest that inhibition of NE transport into the nerve terminal is the mechanism by which depletion occurs. On the other hand, direct displacement from binding sites, as suggested by Smythies et al.[2] is another possiblility.* A third possibility is suggested by results previously described with naloxone which, at high morphine levels, apparently causes a release of ACh from its storage site. If a molecule of morphine on an adrenergic vesicle causes an allosteric change sufficient to permit a second molecule of morphine to act in a manner similar to naloxone (i.e., by causing release of transmitter) this allosteric effect might explain the fact that catecholamine depletion requires very high doses of morphine and exhibits tachyphylaxis.

These interactions should result in an initial release of NE together with an increased turnover since the amine is no longer protected from monoamine oxidase. An increased turnover of catecholamines following morphine was reported by Heinrich et al.[44] although this was not confirmed by Costa and Algeri.[45] In any event, some specific receptors are almost certainly involved in these effects as shown by the fact that naloxone given before morphine prevents the catecholamine action of the drug.[41]

The possible involvement of an adrenergic neuronal receptor in the analgesic effects of morphine is certainly not clear cut. Important studies by Lee and Fennessy[40] correlating analgesia with both Ne and 5-HT levels, indicate that the type of pain stimulus used in the assay is of utmost importance. Thus, analgesia in the naphthaquinone writhing test was not accompanied by changes in NE levels, whereas inhibiting pain produced with the hot plate required higher doses of morphine and was accompanied by changes in NE and 5-HT levels. It would be of interest to examine the changes in free and bound ACh in the CNS using these two tests.

Because morphine has various effects on catecholamine levels in different species, the involvement of an adrenergic receptor for the development of analgesia by potent narcotics has been questioned.[21] The relationship between ACh and catecholamines is complex and the degree of dominance of one type of neurotransmitter when the other is affected by morphine may explain the variation seen in different test systems and species. In this respect, determination of biogenic amine levels in whole brain, or even in select parts, may be of little use in understanding the basic mode of action of a drug. Possibly only a few neuronal pathways are involved in the true analgetic and other actions of morphine. This contention is supported by recent findings that only about 2% of the total morphine bound to CNS components constitutes specific binding.[46] A similar conclusion has been reached in the case of morphine binding to intact guinea pig ileum.[33] Furthermore, if it is conceded that there may be several classes of receptors within a population of adrenergic neurones, a small percentage of these may be involved with the analgesic effect, whereas the large fraction remaining is involved with other actions of the drug, including effects on gross levels of NE. Thus, the conclusions of Way and Shen[21] that NE "does not play a primary role in mediating morphine effects" – either acute or chronic – may be correct, but cannot be directly inferred from evidence based solely on levels of this biogenic amine.

On the other hand, it would have seemed possible to affirm or deny the role of central adrenergic transmitter in morphine action by depleting the brain of its NE store with reserpine, which has effects on morphine analgesia. However, as pointed out by Way and Shen, results of such studies are contradictory from laboratory to laboratory – and even in reports from the same laboratory.[21] Species differences, dose of resperine, extent of NE depletion, and differing methods for assessing analgesia could account for some of these results. Furthermore, reserpine depletes the brain of dopamine and 5-HT which further complicates the experimental system. Therefore, although the consensus is that reserpine antagonizes morphine analgesia, use of this drug has not permitted a definitive statement to be made as to how each neurotransmitter is involved with analgesia.

One prominent effect of reserpine is parasympathetic (ACh) predominance. As our experiments on guinea pig ileum indicate, an

***Dr. Isabel Wajda is currently investigating this problem (personal communication).**

increase in cholinergic activity (e.g., by increasing the rate or duration of neuronal stimulation) results in antagonism of morphine action and this indirect action of reserpine may account for its effect on morphine analgesia.[16] Cholinesterase inhibitors will also antagonize morphine action.[47] This has not always been reported to be the case; as Weinstock[27] has pointed out, the ChE inhibitor must reach the CNS in sufficiently high concentration to be effective. Conversely, MAO inhibitors increase adrenergic activity and concomitantly reduce cholinergic. By the same reasoning, this would be expected to enhance morphine analgesia, as has actually been shown to occur. The same is true for amphetamines which are central adrenergic stimulants.

Serotonergic Neurone Receptors

Evidence for morphine action at 5-HT pathways in the CNS has been accumulating for a number of years,[48] and more recently through the studies of Way and Shen.[21] While it is well known that morphine is a rather potent inhibitor of serotonin receptors at peripheral sites,[49] such a mechanism has rarely been invoked to explain morphine action in the CNS. Perhaps one of the reasons for this is that even more potent inhibitors of 5-HT receptors, such as LSD and BOL, are devoid of analgesic activity.

One of the problems in implicating serotonergic pathways in morphine action is the clear demonstration that the level of 5-HT in different species is scarcely altered by massive doses of the drug.[21] A recent study, however, did reveal a significant increase in mouse brain 5-HT following methadone.[48] Way and Shen[21] and others[50] have reported an increased rate of turnover of 5-HT during chronic administration of morphine. This was prevented or reversed by naloxone and other antagonists, suggesting that a receptor mechanism is involved. However, it should be noted that the entire question of 5-HT involvement in morphine effects has now been disputed by findings from several groups who could not confirm the increased turnover of this amine after acute or chronic administration of morphine.[45,51,52]

Interaction with Brain Components

Perhaps the first step in understanding the mode of action of morphine and other potent analgesics would be to determine precisely where their receptors are localized in the CNS. Methods used for this purpose have included measuring the distribution of morphine in various discrete brain regions by simple extraction of the radioactive drug or by use of autoradiography and subcellular fractionation. Proper controls are essential and should include use of stereoisomeric compounds, one of which is pharmacologically inert, as well as specific antagonists. In addition, a comparison of tolerant and nontolerant animals is important.

Mulé and Woods showed that morphine was distributed in gray matter of cerebral and cerebellar tissue (dog) at a concentration about twice that in white matter.[53] Enhanced binding to gray matter as compared with white could also be demonstrated by autoradiography.[54] Bound morphine was evenly distributed throughout nine different regions of the brain and was approximately 0.2 μg/g tissue, or 5×10^{-10} mol drug/g gray matter.[53] Assuming that the weight of dog brain is about 500 g (2% of the weight of the dogs used in these experiments), the amount "bound" in the total gray matter was approximately 10^{-7} mol, or 6×10^{16} molecules. The number of true receptors may constitute only about 2% of the total binding sites.[46] Therefore, the value obtained by Mulé and Woods in the dog was identical with that expected on the basis of studies by Goldstein et al.[46] for the number of specific sites which, in mouse brain, was 6×10^{14}.* However, these numbers may be coincidental because of the differences in dose used (5 x the ED_{50} in the mouse, about ED_{25} for the dog) and fortuitously compensated for by the vast differences in brain mass.

One major complication which arises when considering that tissue fixation reflects binding to specific receptors is the distinct possibility that more than one receptor type exists. From our studies on the pharmacological effects of morphine on guinea pig ileum, and in particular its antagonism by naloxone, we concluded that there are at least two very important binding sites or receptors for morphine. Both sites show specificity; morphine is displaced from them by naloxone. However, the binding capacity as well as affinities of the sites are very different, one having a much greater binding capacity and lower affinity than the other. Therefore, a much higher drug

*This calculation is performed as follows: $0.02 \times 6 \times 10^{16} \times 0.5$ (gray matter constituting about 50% of total brain mass).

concentration is required for its saturation. This finding may explain the results of Goldstein et al. who reported that stereospecific binding appeared to be nonsaturable, increasing progressively with the dose given. Their interpretation of this observation is that "pharmacological action of an opiate must require only a very low fractional occupancy of the receptors" as Schild[55] postulated for other systems. However, there is the possibility that Goldstein et al. may have actually isolated two or more populations of binding components or receptors and that the different affinities and capacities account for the binding data obtained.

The studies of Goldstein et al.[46] are notable because they provide the means for distinguishing between the small amount of binding to specific receptors and the much larger "pharmacologically irrelevant" binding. This was accomplished by (1) utilizing subcellular fractionation to concentrate the receptor population in synaptosomes, (2) studying binding of levorphanol in the presence of dextrorphan in order to saturate nonspecific sites with the latter, and (3) accounting for drug physically trapped within particles or dissolved within membranes. The salient feature of the study is that although virtually all of the levorphanol was nonspecifically bound or trapped, a small, but significant fraction, amounting to about 2% was bound specifically when 0.5 μg/ml levorphanol was added to the homogenate. When the particulate fraction was subfractionated by standard techniques, the bulk of the stereospecific binding was confined to "floated membranes" of the crude nuclear fraction. Surprisingly, in view of the established localization of morphine receptors in nerve terminals, little if any specific binding was found in synaptosomal membranes. The precise role of such nuclear receptors in morphine effects on transmission is difficult to understand in view of the rapidity of action of the drug. This conclusion is also arrived at in another way. Synaptosomes are typed according to their content of a particular transmitter.[56] It is unlikely that the site(s) of binding at these different terminals would be identical. In view of the very different effects which morphine and other potent analgesics have on the various neurotransmitters, the Goldstein preparation of synaptosomes undoubtedly contained a spectrum of levorphanol receptors. On the other hand, the nuclear membrane composition might be uniform regardless of the type of neuron; therefore, it is suggested that the Goldstein "receptor" is not directly related to synaptic transmission. This binding site might be related to secondary metabolic events as well as addiction development through alteration of protein synthesis.

Despite these conclusions, there is little doubt that this important study must be taken into account in interpreting other work on binding of analgesic drugs by CNS components. In this context, the lack of specificity of localization in the CNS of *d*- and *l*-methadone[57] or of the optical isomers of pentazocine[58] becomes quite understandable. The number of stereospecific sites is so much smaller than the nonspecific ones that quantitation of pharmacologically active receptors becomes virtually impossible in an intact brain preparation.

Other workers have reported that nuclei, mitochondria, and various mitochondrial subfractionations do bind morphine and dihydromorphine.[31,32] In these studies, uptake of radioactive morphine was significantly reduced in the presence of another unlabeled narcotic or by an antagonist. Thus, at least some element of specificity in binding was demonstrated. It should be noted that these results differ from those of Goldstein et al. who reported that levorphanol does not bind to the synaptic vesicle or mitochondrial fractions.[46]

Receptors and Morphine Tolerance

Many mechanisms of tolerance to potent analgesics have been proposed through the years; these have been summarized in excellent articles by Cochin[59] and by Seevers and Deneau.[16] Our discussion will be confined to the possible role of receptors with regard to tolerance to the analgesic action.

In view of the evident multiplicity of putative CNS receptor sites for these drugs, and general lack of agreement as to which neuronal pathway is involved with the most readily accepted action of these drugs, analgesia, it is clearly hazardous to specify that a particular interaction is involved with tolerance, dependence, etc. Fortunately, the relatively simple receptor system of the guinea pig ileum shows many properties in common with receptors for these drugs in the CNS. The following discussion will utilize results obtained with the ileum to provide insight into tolerance development.

That the ileum can develop acute tolerance to morphine and related drugs was first shown by Paton,[23] by Gyang and Kosterlitz,[60] and more recently by Fennessey et al.[28] This was a good indication that some alteration in receptor structure might be involved with morphine action. Desensitization of receptors by these drugs may be the simplest mechanism to explain tolerance. On the other hand, if one considers the mechanism of action of the drug, namely block of ACh release, then it follows that a long-term effect of these drugs is *supersensitivity* of the effectors subserved by the particular nerve ending.[22] Such supersensitivity may work to counteract the blocking action of the drug thereby restoring the status quo ante.

Our studies on the ileum have revealed a new type of tolerance, manifested toward *injected morphine* rather than exogenously applied drug, as shown in Figure 9. Injection of an extremely large dose of morphine (750 mg/kg) into a tolerant animal does not at all influence electrical stimulation of the guinea pig ileum, whereas contractions of the ileum from a nontolerant animal similarly injected are completely abolished. Ileum from the tolerant animal contains large amounts of morphine as revealed by naloxone contracture (Figure 7). However, it was shown that the "T" receptors in ileum of the tolerant animals responded normally to exogenous morphine. We suggest that morphine tolerance and addiction are primarily functions of the "I" receptors. This could come about in the following way. The "I" receptors have a very large capacity to bind morphine. With continuing morphine administration, the number of such receptors, their affinity, or capacity to bind morphine increase rapidly. We have already indicated the possibility that morphine binding to the "I" receptor induces an allosteric change in binding sites for additional morphine or naloxone. Thus, with prolonged administration, the "I" receptors compete more effectively with the "T" receptors where the pharmacological effect of the drug is

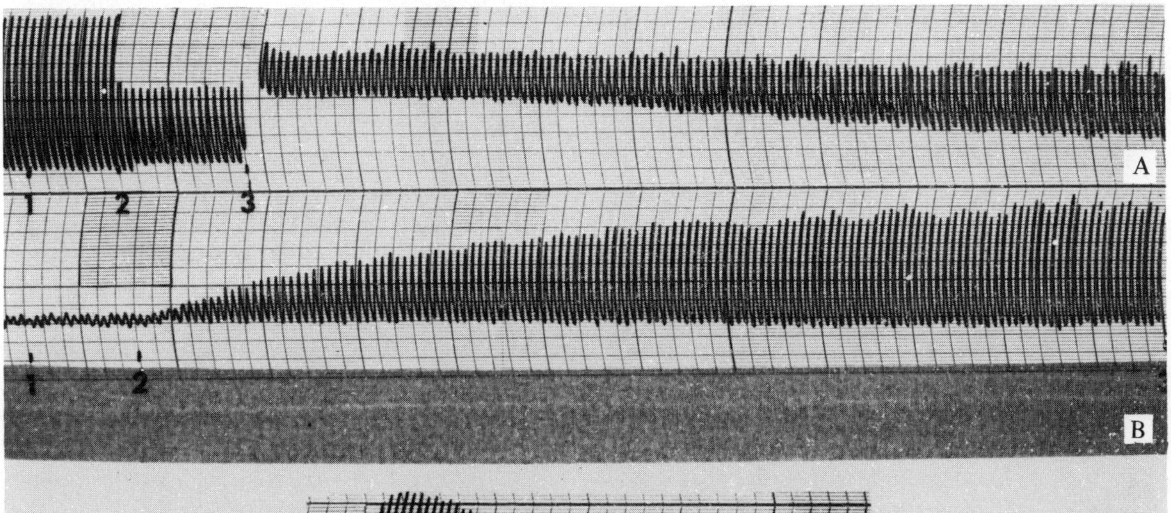

FIGURE 9. Effect of a very large dose of morphine (150 mg) injected into a normal and a tolerant guinea pig on the electrical stimulation of the ileum in vitro. The ileum was removed from the control and tolerant animals 2 hours following injection. A. Ileum from tolerant guinea pig. This responds with such a large contraction to electrical stimulation that the sensitivity was reduced at (2, . At (3), naloxone, 40 ng/ml was added. A very marked contracture results with no increase of contraction amplitude. B. Normal ileum. Note that this ileum does not respond at all to electrical stimulation. At (1), naloxone, 40 ng/ml, produced an immediate increase in contraction amplitude but did not cause contracture. Following wash, the contractions gradually fail, indicating that a large amount of morphine is still present within the tissue. Unlike the tolerant animal, this morphine can block electrically-induced contractions.

mediated, i.e., block of transmission. Thus, greater and greater amounts of the drug must be administered to achieve the initial blocking action. Concomitant with these events, supersensitivity develops and thus each quantum of transmitter released becomes more effective. Even though release is diminished, the supersensitivity restores the physiological response to a passably normal level; in some systems, hyperactivity may result.

Based on these studies, it should be possible to predict which drugs would or would not be highly addictive, the assumption being that ability to interact with "I" receptors would correlate with addiction. This contention is supported by the finding that naloxone causes a more reduced contracture after nalorphine than after morphine.[29] This is consistent with the reduced addiction liability of nalorphine as compared with morphine and serves to overcome one of the major objections of Seevers and Deneau[16] to using the guinea pig ileum as a model for explaining the mode of action of these drugs in the CNS. Seevers is perhaps correct in this criticism if one simply considers the effects of drugs on the "T" receptors alone, but when the entire spectrum of interaction is examined, then the correlation between addiction and "I" receptor interaction might well be sustained.

These concepts have a distinct bearing on the initiation of withdrawal symptoms that are observed when a narcotic antagonist is given. Two factors may be noted in this regard. The first is competition by the antagonist for the "T" receptors which immediately reverses the block of ACh release, resulting in improved transmission across the synapse. However, if the dose of antagonist is sufficiently high, the narcotic will also be displaced from the "I" sites with the liberation of larger amounts of ACh. This outpouring of ACh at a partially inhibited synapse, together with the supersensitive postsynaptic sites, result in parasympathetic activity with intense physiological consequences.

Use of a narcotic antagonist could even create a problem in an addicted, asymptomatic individual. It should be recognized that in such individuals large amounts of the narcotic may still be bound to the "I" sites. Administration of an antagonist or other drug which effectively competes with binding at the "I" site could still produce drastic parasympathetic dominance and withdrawal symptoms. This may explain some of the "paradoxical reactions" observed in the early stages of methadone maintenance treatment.

HALLUCINOGENS

Reviews of hallucinogenic substances suggest that pharmacological receptors for this class of drugs exist in CNS synapses. Lajtha[61] reviewed some of the older tissue and cell experiments with hallucinogens, mainly mescaline, LSD, and bufotenin. At that time, the main emphasis was on the effects of these drugs on transport of amino acids and carbohydrate metabolism. The comprehensive review of the hallucinogenic substances by Hoffer and Osmond[62] has references through 1964 and includes adrenochromes, taraxein, indoles, anesthetics, and cholinergic agents. An early review of the metabolism of the hallucinogenic substances appeared in 1963 by Gillette.

Other recent reviews of conformation *vs.* potency or effect for this series include a noncritical, excellent, comprehensive, and clear compilation on the phenylethylamine derivatives by Nieforth,[64] and indole derivatives, with particular reference to serotonin by McIsaac et al.[65] This review includes suggestions for experimental approaches to the question of the role of this neurohormone in hallucinogenesis. Chothia and Pauling[66] critically discuss the earlier steric conformation calculations of the hallucinogens by Snyder and Richelson.[67] A later approach by Kang and Green[68] for computing and predicting pharmacological effect based upon bond angle, ring orientation, and flexibility of analogs in relation to a basic LSD-like structure has helped resolve some of the discrepancies arising from the work of Snyder and Richelson.

LSD

Interaction with Physiological Receptors

Research leading to our present understanding of LSD action has undergone several phases: serotonin antagonism, adrenergic agonist activity, and presynaptic effects. Each concept will be reviewed with typical supporting results.

Woolley and Campbell first linked LSD action with 5-HT by demonstrating that contractions of uterine muscle preparations in vitro were blocked at extremely low concentrations of the drug.[69] Indeed, the action of this drug and its congeners on many tissues seems to be directed toward the specific antagonism of 5-HT. In view of the behavioral effects accompanying altered serotonin levels, it was only natural to interpret at least some of the actions of LSD to inhibition of 5-HT physiological receptors in the CNS. The finding that LSD reverses the sedation produced by intraventricular injection of 5-HT seemed to suggest that the same type of antagonism occurred in the CNS that was seen in the peripheral nervous system. The entire subject of LSD-5-HT interaction has been reviewed by Hoffer and Osmond.[62]

Attractive as this hypothesis may be, lack of acceptance stemmed from the important finding that the bromo derivative of LSD, a more potent peripheral serotonin antagonist than LSD itself, is not hallucinogenic. Moreover, 5-HT does not block the central effects of LSD.[62] Because of these and other discrepancies, as well as the evident sympathomimetic actions of the drug, many investigators attempted to explain its central actions via adrenergic stimulation.

Cerletti and Doepfner[70] attempted to set the anti-5-HT vs. adrenergic agonist role of LSD in perspective by pointing out that the early claims of the dissociation of adrenergic from anti-5-HT activity could not be confirmed. Reports that LSD might potentiate 5-HT[71] were also in error. Among 20 amide derivatives, none were as potent as LSD in antagonizing the effects of 5-HT. The three stereoisomers other than d-LSD were ineffective as 5-HT antagonists or as psychotomimetics. However, in the natural ergot derivative series, only moderate anti-5-HT activity was observed, with the exception of methyl ergonovine, which was very potent and specific. By chemical modification of the ring structure of LSD, a whole group of substances were produced with anti-5-HT activity much greater than that of LSD, the most potent being 1-methyl, 2-bromo-LSD. Anti-5-HT activity and psychotomimetic potency appeared to correlate well for those compounds of the series which have been tested clinically.

Dixon[72] examined the effects of adrenergic and serotonergic agents on two LSD-induced effects in rats, locomotor activity and aberrant behavior. The latter was considered to be the analog of psychotomimetic activity. It was necessary to attempt to obtain selective effects since the aberrant behavior resembled increased locomotor activity in some respects. Effects of various drugs on these two actions of LSD are summarized in Table 2. α-adrenergic blocking agents were quite effective in antagonizing both effects, whereas β-receptor blockers showed greater specificity, blocking the aberrant behavior but not locomotor activity. On the other hand, drugs blocking serotonin receptors (BOL-148 or Deseril) were ineffective in abolishing aberrant behavior, except possibly at extremely high doses (15 mg/kg for BOL). Depletion of serotonin by

TABLE 2

Effects of Adrenergic and Serotonergic Agents on LSD Activity

Compound	Type of Agent	Dose mg/kg	Effect on aberrant behavior	Effect on locomotor excitation
Dibenamine	adrenergic	30	decreases	decreases
Phenoxybenzamine	blocking	7.5 to 30	decreases	decreases
Pronethalol	β-adrenergic	15 to 30	decreases	no effect
Propanolol	blocking	15 to 30	decreases	no effect
Deseril	5-HT blocking	10 to 15	decreases	no effect
BOL-148	5-HT blocking	5 to 10	decreases	no effect
p-chlorophenyl-alanine	depletes 5-HT	3 x 100	no effect	no effect
alpha-methyl *p*-tyrosine	depletes catecholamines	120	decreases	decreases
Disulfiram	depletes catecholamines	300	decreases	no effect

Adapted from Dixon[72]

p-chlorophenylalanine had no effect on either parameter, whereas α-methyltyrosine, a catecholamine depleter, blocked both actions of LSD. Chloropromazine and perphenazine, central adrenergic blocking agents, also blocked both effects. From this study Dixon concluded that "the action of LSD is subserved by an adrenergic component", possibly through β-adrenergic receptors. In view of the fact that LSD releases NE, these results still do not indicate whether LSD is an adrenergic receptor activator or acts indirectly.

One important finding was that reserpine potentiated the behavioral effects of LSD. Such a result might suggest direct receptor activation by LSD, since under the conditions used (1.5 to 6 mg/kg reserpine 20 hours before testing) most of the catecholamine store would have been depleted. With interruption of adrenergic transmission, the postsynaptic receptors might show supersensitivity to any agonist, including LSD.

Interaction with Presynaptic Nerve Terminal Sites

Indirect evidence for the existence of pharmacologically important presynaptic binding of LSD is derived from the profound effect the drug has on metabolism of serotonin and catecholamines. With the use of potent inhibitors of monoamine oxidase, it could be shown that the psychotropic agents cause a release of neurohormones. Thus, nialimide given before LSD causes an accumulation of 5-HT, after which neither LSD nor psilocybin have an effect.[73] Tonge and Leonard[74] have developed a pattern of LSD effects on 5-HT and NE levels, metabolites, and turnover, for comparison with those of other hallucinogens or CNS-active agents. The pattern for LSD is increased brain 5-HT, tryptophan and tyrosine; decreased brain norepinephrine, blood tryptophan and tyrosine; and little or no increase in brain dopamine. These changes are not matched by, and are probably more specific for LSD than for other hallucinogenic agents. At the present time, their results suggest that the 5-HT presynaptic vesicle may be one locus for the CNS effects of LSD. Interaction at this site results in a blockade of the release of 5-HT, concomitant use and release of NE, and possibly a stimulation of dopaminergic pathways in the absence of the normal release patterns of 5-HT and NE.

We suggest that the receptor-associated effects produced by LSD occur in the following sequence:

a. Postsynaptic binding to the physiological 5-HT receptor.

b. Blockade of the release of 5-HT, possibly mediated at the level of the 5-HT storage site (vesicle).

c. Release and depletion of NE stores.

d. Stimulation of dopaminergic pathways due to disinhibition resulting from depression of adrenergic outflow.

Interaction with Subcellular Fractions and Other Brain Components

Snyder and Reivich[75] were the first to obtain data for subcellular localization of LSD in brain using fluorometric and radioactive tracer methods. Their data show that 75 to 80% of the drug was present in the "soluble supernatant", 15 to 20% in the microsomal-myelin band, and 3 to 8% in the synaptosomes and mitochondria. Such results cannot be used as an argument[75] that the drug does not have an important membranous site of action in the CNS, i.e., the small binding to the fraction containing formed elements could be highly specific. Unfortunately, there is no direct way to check the specificity of interaction of a drug such as LSD except perhaps to determine the effect on its binding of the closely-related lysergic acid, which is devoid of psychomimetic activity. The LSD receptors contribute very minimally to the total LSD-binding capacity of any cell fraction, since the hallucinogen is known to interact strongly with many types of macromolecules. Its presence to a great extent in the soluble fraction could reflect complex formation with the large amounts of protein, nucleic acids, etc., present. Thus, just as in the case of many other drugs, subcellular distribution, unaccompanied by tests of specificity of binding, cannot shed light on the locus of action in vivo.

A further complication in interpreting the results of Snyder and Reivich, is that this work was carried out on a single monkey receiving an enormous dose of LSD, 2 mg/kg. This is about 1,000 times the pharmacologically active dose in humans. At the high dose used, grey frontal cortex contained 1 μg/g tissue. This represents 0.05 μg/g tissue (per mg injected/100 g body wt). After a 2 μg/kg dose in man, if the same relative distribution to the brain occurs as in the monkey, only 3 to 8% of the amount per gram of brain would appear to saturate the receptors. This is deduced from the fact that higher doses do not intensify the behavioral effects of LSD, but merely prolong the effect or cause toxic reactions. At the dose producing maximum effects in a 70 kg man, only 0.1 ng/g would be contained in grey matter, and the comparable level in the synaptosomal–mitrochondrial fraction would be 1 to 10 pg. If this amount could cause a behavioral effect, then certainly the large amounts found in the supernatant by Snyder and Reivich may simply reflect that which has spilled over from the synaptosomal fraction and represents essentially nonpharmacologically active material.

In addition, no values were given for the total mass of the drug in the starting material before separation, or for the protein concentrations of the cell fractions in the density gradient bands. Therefore, the specific activity or relative specificity of the localization could not be determined. The separation procedure was an unusual one, and the amount of LSD in the nuclear fraction and unbroken tissue pellet was not reported. Thus, these data do not provide information about LSD binding sites in the brain.

There is no doubt that LSD can bind to specific membrane sites. For example, Alivisatos et al.[76] reported that LSD displaces 5-HT from a subsynaptosomal macromolecule considered to be a receptor for serotonin. A similar displacement of 5-HT by mescaline could not be determined. In addition, De Robertis showed that LSD can bind to subcellular particles in vitro.[77,78] He reported that LSD bound tightly to the postsynaptic junctional complex after digestion of the presynaptic components of the synaptosomal fraction. In addition, isolated proteolipid from the postjunctional complex bound LSD in nonaqueous solvents. This proteolipid probably lost much of its pharmacological specificity during preparation with organic solvent extraction and might have been only a model of the type of drug-receptor interaction that could occur in a nonpolar membrane region. It was reported that the LSD binding capacity of human serum albumin was 8 μg/mg protein.[79] This in vitro binding capacity indicates that the normal human dose of LSD is probably travelling within the blood in a bound form prior to the time that it is taken in rapidly to the CNS. Once the drug enters the CNS, it reaches a peak within 5 minutes and declines to undetectable levels in 2 to 4 hours.[80] This may be of extreme importance because, in common with mescaline, effects in the CNS outlast its presence in the brain.[5,81] There is the possibility that nonneuronal binding sites in the brain area may serve as LSD depots. For example, both pineal and pituitary accumulate greater concentrations than do the brain tissues. This is also true for mescaline.

Interaction with Soluble Macromolecules

Several investigators have studied soluble macromolecules as receptor models for LSD. Studies of nucleic acid binding were stimulated by reports that LSD caused chromosome damage and was teratogenic. Smit and Borst[82] and Brady et al.[83] recently reviewed these studies. They have shown that although LSD does bind with DNA, it neither intercalates nor induces conformational changes. However, when the drug is photoirradiated, it causes changes in DNA structure. Smythies et al.[2] reported that LSD fluorescence at 1 μg/ml is quenched best by polyuridine (poly-U), whereas no quenching occurs with uridine monophosphate alone or with other nucleotides. Quenching the LSD fluorescence by 50% required 50 μg/ml of poly-U. Binding was usually promoted by allowing the polynucleotides to stack at pH 3, in water at 4°. Since poly-U does not stack well at pH 7.5 in saline solution, there may be some question of the relevance of this binding for the pharmacological effects of the drug. In the medium used by Smythies, LSD fluorescence was quenched fivefold more by the stacked polycytidine than by the random coil configuration.

The relevance of these studies to LSD is speculative, but let us consider the following:

a. LSD reaches very high levels in the eye after injection.

b. Material moves from the eye, via axoplasmic flow, to the optic cortex.

c. Photoirradiated and polynucleotide-bound LSD might reach the optic tract of the brain much later than the drug given in the original dose.

d. There are reports of "delayed-psychotic," pharmacologically inexplicable episodes after some LSD experiences.

The LSD-polynucleotide complex, whether altered in conformation or not, reaches the cortical optic center after much of the free drug has disappeared, and after neurotransmitters in the CNS have reverted to their normal levels.[84]

Dissociation of the drug from its complex may produce a second episode. It has been suggested that ambient light levels have some effect on potentiating the LSD "trip" for new users, while tolerant individuals may seek psychedelic displays to intensify the drug experience.[85] We wonder if the current vogue employing fluorescent paints ("Day-Glo") illuminated by long wave UV (LSD absorbs at 330 nm to fluoresce at 430 to 450 nm in the deep blue) may not be an intuitive attempt on the part of the drug-abuser to maximize the photoirradiation of LSD to prolong or intensify certain effects.

Another approach to the study of the LSD receptor site is the pioneering work of Van Vunakis et al.[86] who developed antibodies to *d*-lysergic acid (LSA) in rabbits and guinea pigs. LSD and related ergot derivatives compete effectively with LSA for binding to this antibody, whereas *N,N*-dimethyl derivatives of tryptamine, 5-HT, 4-HT, 5-methyl tyrosine, and mescaline are 10 times less active than LSA. They suggest that the aromatic nuclei and dimethylated amino groups may assume a conformation resembling ring A of LSD, and that the methylated nitrogen in ring C may be mimicked by conformational bends. This tends to support predictions described before based on steric relationships.

Receptor Interactions, Tolerance, Dependence, and Addiction

There is no evidence for induction of receptors for LSD which might explain tolerance. This includes physiological receptors as well as sites normally involved with 5-HT metabolism, transport and storage.[87] Tolerance to LSD and cross-tolerance to mescaline are not accompanied by changes in the amount or concentration of the drug in brain or liver. However, such findings may not be significant because of the small amount of drug present in the brain which may be bound to specific sites. Other results argue against any significant metabolic component for development of tolerance to LSD. According to Winter,[88] there are several alternative hypotheses to that of a common cellular receptor for LSD activity and tolerance. Perhaps, the attachment of LSD to polynucleotides in vivo may produce an immune response in key areas of the body. The resulting antibody binds the circulating drug and renders it inactive.

Chronic administration of LSD produces tolerance to mescaline, to amphetamines, and to psilocybin (and vice versa).[62] Kalant et al.[89] have thoroughly reviewed the proposed mechanisms of tolerance and dependence for most classes of drugs of abuse with the exception of the potent analgesics. Only a few aspects will be discussed subsequently because conclusive data are lacking to substantiate the concept that acute tolerance does develop to hallucinogenic drugs, cannabis, amphetamines, or minor tranquilizers.

LSD and tetrahydrocannabinol produce indistinguishable subjective effects,[90] but whereas LSD has rather profound autonomic effects (increased body temperature and blood pressure, pupil dilation and hyperthermia, and tachycardia), with the exception of tachycardia, none of these are shown by THC. However, subjects who are tolerant to LSD are still highly reactive to THC. On the basis of these findings, it was concluded that the central effects of both drugs are mediated by two different (receptor) mechanisms.

Indoleamine Derivatives

Dimethyl-, diethyl-, α-methyl-, α-ethyltryptamine, harmine, psilocybin, and ibogaine are included in this group of hallucinogenic amines. Freedman et al.[91] showed that the indoleamine psychotomimetics exert LSD-like effects on 5-HT which differ from those of the phenylethylamines, e.g., mescaline and amphetamine. The indoleamines increase central 5-HT and at higher doses also increase 5-HIAA, a metabolite of 5-HT. Meek and Fuxe[73] reported that after nialimide, dimethyl- and α-methyltryptamine reduce 5-HT accumulation. LSD and psilocybin are then without psychotomimetic effect. They suggested that the tryptamine derivatives may directly stimulate central 5-HT receptors, e.g., those involved in the hind limb extensor reflex. This action is shared by some substituted amphetamines. Therefore, a gradation of activity with respect to 5-HT receptors is shown by indoleamines, LSD producing a blockade of the physiological receptors, while DMT and α-MT produce stimulation.

In a recent study of indoleamine drug effects on CNS serotonin and NE, Andén et al.[92] attempted to reconcile the various effects of LSD on 5-HT receptors, turnover of serotonin, etc. This work shows the complex interrelationship among various CNS pathways and illustrates some of the problems that arise when drug effects are studied.

LSD produces a brief rise in the brain level of 5-HT by decreasing the activity of serotonergic neurons. This drug combines with and stimulates 5-HT receptors postsynaptically, which depresses presynaptic outflow of 5-HT. (The hind-limb extensor reflex is considered to reflect CNS serotonergic activity in a rat with a spinal section, and LSD stimulates this system.) Other LSD-like and indolealkylamine hallucinogens share some of these effects:

a. Psilocybin can prevent depletion of 5-HT by H 22/54, while dimethyltryptamine is less effective.

b. This effect of psilocybin is similar to that of pargyline, an MAO inhibitor. However, none of the indolealkylamines are themselves MAO inhibitors.

c. The indolealkylamines enhance the NE depletion by H 22/54.

d. LSD produces a decrease in 5-HIAA as it increases 5-HT.

Andén et al. suggest that LSD and the other indolealkylamines, psilocybin and DMT, which stimulate spinal reflexes in the same way as 5-HT, are distinguishable in the test from tryptamine and bufotenin. These tests are carried out on animals depleted of NE by reserpine; additionally 5-HT synthesis has been blocked. The extension of the hind limb results from stimulation of CNS 5-HT-receptors by LSD, psilocybin, DMT and 5-HT. DMT and tryptamine cause a release of 5-HT presynaptically, while LSD does not.

McIsaac et al.[65] reviewed the gradation in activity for the substituted tryptamines, β-carbolines (harmaline), yohimbine, etc. McIsaac et al. note that "unlike marijuana, mescaline and STP, most of the indolic hallucinogenic agents do not seem to be abused frequently" with the exception of LSD.

Using physicochemical methods, it has been shown that slight modifications of the psychotomimetic tryptamine derivatives produce ring systems which are similar to LSD, bufotenin, or psilocybin.[66-68,93,94] In particular, attempts have been made by Kang and Green[68] to relate potency of these drugs to their electronic configuration using molecular orbital calculations. Although it is true that at times such correlations are extremely good, this might simply be coincidence. This is inevitable when a series of drugs is examined in animal experiments in which chemical modification can give rise to variable effects on activity, and these effects are modified by such factors as distribution, excretion, metabolism, binding to serum proteins, binding to nonreceptor macromolecules, and ability to penetrate into the CNS. Furthermore, in such complex systems, there is no direct evidence that the drugs are all acting by a common mechanism; this is even true when one is dealing with series of drugs acting on an isolated tissue.[95] Such SAR studies carried out in whole animals may have only limited value in defining the configuration of the receptor site which is involved with their effects. A useful test for the ideas which emerged from these various SAR studies would be the antibodies to LSA prepared by Van Vunakis et al.[86] Moreover, it was shown that various tryptamine derivatives have graded affinities for this antibody.

Mescaline

Interaction with Subcellular Fractions and Other Brain Components

Studies on the interaction of phenethylamines and mescaline with tissues were reported by Block in 1958,[96-99] and thus these compounds are among the first for which attempts were made to learn something about receptors in vitro. Subsequently, Denber and associates reported very extensive results of the distribution of mescaline in various organs, brain regions, and cortical subcellular fractions.[100,101] The overall conclusion of these studies is that the primary site of mescaline action is the presynaptic membrane.[5,102] These studies, together with some concepts of the mechanism of action of this drug, will constitute the bulk of the discussion to follow.

It should be noted that the analysis of mescaline's activity in these studies was conducted from a clinical and biological point of view. Although this led to the development of hypotheses regarding mescaline's receptor effects, classical pharmacological approaches were not used.

Early results of extended clinical trials convinced Denber and his associates[103] that examination of the biochemical effects of mescaline in humans was interesting but not rewarding since the localization of the drug was unknown at that time. Therefore, Denber undertook the first comprehensive investigation of the subcellular localization of radioactive mescaline.[100] The background and protocols of the animal studies on subcellular localization were those of the early clinical trials with mescaline-blocking agents.[103] Denber[100] and Denber and Teller[101] reported that none of the potent blocking agents used clinically prevented entry of mescaline into the brain, although the behavioral effects were completely blocked. Various in vivo and in vitro experiments employing the same drugs as had been used 10 years previously in patients[103] and *at the same dose per kg* (with the exception of d-amphetamine, which was given at a reduced dose in the rat) demonstrated the following with reference to mescaline's pharmacology:

1. For changes to be observed in the animal's behavior within 30 minutes, 10 to 20 mg/kg of mescaline was required.
2. The concentration of mescaline in brain and all organs studied was directly proportional to the dose from 5 to 40 mg/kg.
3. The brain accumulated very little of the i.v. or i.p. dose, 0.0014 to 0.002%. The concentration of mescaline that produced behavioral disturbances in the rats was 2 to 3 μM (0.6 to 1 μg/g). Based on various doses, this was equivalent to uptake of 1.4 to 1.5 μg/g of brain for each mg injected per 100 g body weight.
4. The peak brain mescaline concentration occurred between 20 to 40 minutes after injection, unlike LSD which shows a maximum brain concentration within 5 minutes.[101]
5. One hour after injection, the mescaline concentration was slightly decreased. Not only was there a decrease in total radioactivity, but the inactive metabolite, 3,4,5-trimethoxyphenylacetic acid, accounted for 35% of the total counts. Two hours after injection, the brain level of radioactivity (60% of which was composed of inactive metabolites of mescaline) was below that found 5 minutes after injection when no symptoms occurred. However, at this 2-hour point the animals still showed effects of mescaline and continued to do so for several hours.

The analysis of subcellular fractions revealed that mescaline moved rapidly into the NEPs and was loosely bound. The drug was metabolized in that fraction by mitochondria to trimethoxyphenylacetic acid. Mescaline is also bound by the microsomal and nuclear fractions in a nonsaturable manner.[100,104] Mescaline causes the rupture of NEPs with the release of NE and vesicles into the gradient during the preparation of brain subcellular particles from treated animals (Figure 10). The released NE appears not only in the upper sample layer of the gradient from which the NEPs are removed by centrifugation, but also in the interspersed bands through which particles sediment to their isopycnic resting point further down the tube (Table 3). It is of some interest that

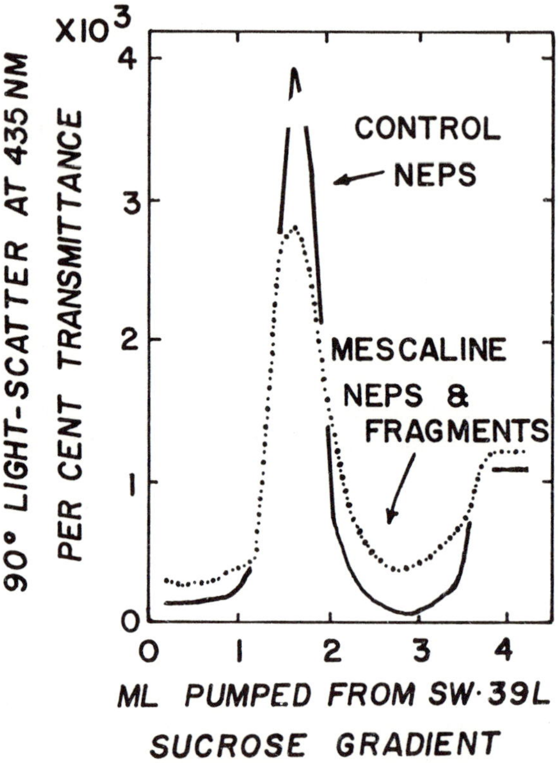

FIGURE 10. Destabilizing effects of mescaline on nerve ending particles isolated from rat cerebral cortical grey matter. Principles, design, and operation of the equipment used to obtain these data have been described elsewhere,[105,106] A preliminary account of these experiments has been presented.[102] Briefly, the light-scattering profile of a centrifuged sucrose gradient was recorded, using an Aminco-Bowman spectrophotofluorometer, a micro flow cuvet and a high pressure pump. As shown by the solid line, the profile of NEPs in the gradient from control animals indicated a loss of material at the top of the gradient, at the 0.8/0.32 *M* sucrose interface. However, as the NEPs from rats treated with 20 mg/kg mescaline for 30 minutes sediment through the sucrose, they leave fragments behind (dotted line). The analyses for protein, acetylcholine esterase, NE, etc., indicate that these NEPs are fragmenting during the separation. If the mescaline-treated rats' NEPs are mixed with 5μg chlorpromazine (CPZ) per ml suspension before this centrifugation, no fragmentation occurs.

TABLE 3

Recovery of Protein, NE, Acetylcholine Esterase in the Soluble (Supernatant), and Particulate (Pellet) Components of NEP Fractions from Mescaline and CPZ-Mescaline Treated Rats

		CPZ + Mescaline			Mescaline Only		
Gradient Fraction	iso-pycnic sucrose *M*	NE ng S/P	Protein mg S/P	AChE * S/P	NE ng S/P	Protein mg S/P	AChE * S/P
Supernatant	0.32	9.5/0	1.73/1.05	0.041/0.071	44/12	1.86/0.86	0.042/0.108
Myelin + Vesicles	0.32/0.4	32/0	0.83/0.47	0.067/0.112	9.6/0	1.06/0.55	0.050/0.119
Membrane	0.4/0.6	0/0	0.20/0.56	0.267/0.494	0/0	0.70/0.78	0.221/0.228
Fragments	0.6/0.8	0/12	0.20/2.44	0.534/0.314	0/22	0.39/3,18	0.307/0.214
NEPs	0.8/1.0	0/25	0.15/1.58	0.742/0.326	0/0	0.39/1.95	0.397/0.378
NEPs	1.0/1.2	0/11.1	0.18/3.14	0.289/0.219	0/0	0.24/3.05	0.202/0.176
NEPs + Mits	1.2 pellet	0/23	0.06/6.70	0.133/0.410	0/11	0.16/6.26	0.032/0.040
Original NEPs	0.8/1.2	44/84.5	3.84/15.68	0.070/0.750	52.8/48.6	4.22/14.6	0.091./0.420
Recovery, % in Original NEPs		94/96	87/99		102/93	87/100	

Thirty minutes before sacrifice, 200 g Wistar rats received 20 mg/kg mescaline, i.p. A second group received 5 mg/kg CPZ, i.p., 30 minutes before the mescaline. Cortical grey matter NEPs were prepared by a standard method.[104,107] The NEP band at the 0.8/1.2 *M* sucrose interface was layered over a compound gradient which normally is used to isolate the fragments from hypoosomotically-shocked NEPs.[108] After centrifugation each band was reconstituted to 0.3 *M* sucrose and centrifugation at 16,000 rcf x g, av., for 5 minutes at 4° in micro tubes separated the particulate, pelletable (P) and soluble, supernatant (S) of each band. Note that the mescaline-treated animals produced NEPs with less NE than controls or the CPZ-mescaline treatment. The NEPs fragmented and released membrane material, particulate NE (vesicles) and soluble NE into the layers of this second gradient after mescaline treatment. However, after treatment with CPZ and mescaline, there was no unusual loss of protein or NE from the NEPs during the gradient fractionation. NE was determined by increasing the sensitivity of the method of Maickel et al.;[109] acetylcholine esterase by radioisotopic assay;[110] other methods were as previously described.[104,107,111]

S = in supernatant after reconstitution to 0.3M sucrose and centrifugation at 80,000 g-min.
P = in pellet
*μmol acetylcholine hydrolyzed per minute, per mg protein. The estimated standard errors for the determinations from nine gradients were less than 12% of the values reported. Three cortices were trimmed of white matter and were used for each preparative 0.8/1.2 *M* sucrose gradient in SW 41 tubes.

prior treatment of the animal with chlorpromazine prevents release of vesicles and NE as well as loss of protein from the NEPs.

These findings suggested a theoretical basis for mescaline activity[5] involving the ability of the drug to destabilize membranes during its passage through the CNS. The ability of chlorpromazine to block the psychotomimetic effects of mescaline is attributed to the powerful membrane-stabilizing effects of the neuroleptic at low doses.[4,5,83]

Since these studies appeared, additional evidence for mescaline's destabilizing effects on various organized macromolecules in vivo was obtained by Datta and Ghosh.[112,113] They found that mescaline caused the release of protein, RNA, acid-soluble nucleotides, and ninhydrin-positive materials, as well as the loss of enzymatic activity from ribosomes isolated from goat brain cortex slices incubated with the drug. However, they used 10μg mescaline hemisulfate/mg protein; this is much greater than occurs in vivo in brain after 20 mg/kg. In a subsequent paper,[114] they report that respiring cortex slices treated with 5 to 10 μg/g wet weight (which might occur in vivo after 250 to 500 mg/kg) show marked decreases in the amino acid incorporating ability of their ribosomes. However, Lajtha and Toth earlier showed in rat and mouse brain that amino acid transport into slices was unaffected when mescaline or LSD was in the medium.[115] The inhibition of amino acid incorporation was both time and concentration dependent, and was partially blocked by spermidine. These latter findings agree with some of Denber's earlier results,[103] while Cohen and Vogel have confirmed his uptake data in vivo.[116] De Robertis[78] reported that mescaline binds weakly to synaptic vesicles in contradistinction to the strong binding of LSD in the subcellular fraction of nerve-ending membranes, confirming the ease of translocation of mescaline observed in vitro by Denber.[100] In cooperation with Pelligrino de Iraldi and De Robertis, the following changes after mescaline treatment in vivo were observed by electron microscopy:

1. The number of electron-dense vesicles was decreased in rat pineal and cortical neurons one hour after treating rats with up to 40 mg of mescaline per kg.
2. The number of vesicles was increased in the upper, myelin and cytosol-containing sample band of the sucrose gradients containing the NEPs from those animals.
3. The number of empty vesicles was increased in the synaptosomes prepared from mescaline-treated animals.
4. The morphology and particle recovery was essentially normal in the gradients from animals treated with 2 mg/kg of chlorpromazine 30 minutes prior to injection of 20 mg/kg mescaline.

These results were confirmed in later experiments using animals that showed behavior changes at 10 mg/kg mescaline, i.p.[107,117]

Results from a number of studies have suggested that although mescaline may have a single type of receptor interaction, nevertheless it produces multiple effects. This is apparent from the variety of agents which block its pharmacological effects, such as atropine, azacyclonol, phenothiazines, and amytal.[62] This relative nonspecificity is unfortunate since mescaline often is used as the reference compound in studies of other psychotomimetic drugs. If mescaline has several different areas in which it is acting pharmacologically, it would probably be more advantageous when studying SAR to relate potency to the brain concentrations of the drugs rather than to their dosages. This point will be discussed further in the section on amphetamines, where STP is compared with mescaline.

Mescaline does not seem to have a significant effect when it is tested in various systems in vitro, e.g., brain slices, whereas the effective CNS concentration is in the micromolar range. This is often the case with other drugs, particularly when a specific receptor exists.

The following molecular mechanism has been proposed to account for some of these effects of mescaline on formed elements of nerves.[5] Mescaline is taken into the surface of the presynaptic neuronal terminal by carriers that normally transport aromatic amines; the amine end of the molecule penetrates first. The methoxy groups of mescaline represent a rigid hydrophobic area which prevents the membrane from enclosing the molecule; thus at this point the membrane remains open, providing a channel for ionic movement. As the bulky portion of the aromatic ring combines with the membrane's hydrophobic interior, there is a simultaneous leakage of ions and the delocalization of membrane-bound water that is also accompanied by a release of NE. The released NE, not being coordinated with synaptic activity, causes random bursts of transmission that are interpreted as sensory or proprioceptor signals of distorted strength. The organism responds to these strange signals in terms of its individual experience with uninterpreted input, i.e., anxiety, fear, release of an escape or sublimation reaction.

Receptor Interactions and Tolerance

There is neither evidence that mescaline causes dependence nor have withdrawal symptoms after chronic usage been reported. On the other hand, tolerance develops rapidly and may be attributed to effects of drug interactions with tissue sites.

Repeated doses of 10 mg/kg i.v., once daily for three to four days, usually produce tolerance in humans to most CNS and peripheral nervous system effects of mescaline. Similar results have been obtained in almost all species. One possible explanation for tolerance is induction of MAO (mescaline being rapidly metabolized), but this has not been established using pharmacologically meaningful doses (5 to 40 mg/kg). In addition, there is no evidence that raising or lowering of blood levels of mescaline alters the behavioral effects.[118] Alternatively, in view of the suggested mechanical effects of mescaline, NE stores may be very rapidly replenished, thereby restoring transmission in those pathways initially disrupted by mescaline. This suggests examination of NE turnover and vesicle synthesis, perhaps using inhibitors of protein synthesis. The investigations of Datta and Ghosh[112-114] indicate that recovery from mescaline treatment may involve a reordering of microsomal structure, and perhaps the synthesis of new ribonucleoprotein. This seems to be an interesting system for studying tolerance development. Furthermore, if the mescaline-induced state is a model of an active schizophrenic state, then their conclusions as to the effect of mescaline are entirely in accord with the hypothesis proposed by Teller and Denber[5] for mescaline's action and the nature of the molecular changes that may produce the schizophrenic symptoms.

The question is open whether the rapid development of tolerance may be attributed to some effect of the drug on its receptor (or receptors) present in the nerve terminal. It is possible that only a limited number of such sites are actually available for mescaline action at a given dosage. These disrupted sites may require a long period of time for recovery to receive a second dose of the drug.* In order to achieve a comparable psychotomimetic effect, a higher dose of the drug must be administered. Still another possibility for tolerance is suggested by the appearance of the electron photomicrographs of rat brains two hours after mescaline. Increased numbers of empty vesicles were observed which may provide inactive receptor sites for the subsequent doses of the drug.

Compounds that block release of NE and in general stabilize membranes against hyposmotic shock generally block mescaline's effects on peripheral tissues, while others, such as azacyclonol, must be injected directly into the CNS in order to do so.[119] Amphetamine is potentiated by mescaline and vice versa.[103] Although chlorpromazine (CPZ) antagonizes mescaline, if the dose of the tranquilizer is reduced, a prolongation and intensification of the mescaline-induced state occurs; the same is true with amphetamine-CPZ.[103,120,121] This may indicate that the phenothiazine tranquilizers are acting on the same site as mescaline. However, in patients there was no direct evidence for mescaline potentiation by chlorpromazine because the neuroleptic dose may have been too high for this to occur.[103] A very definite phenothiazine structure, diethylaminopropyl, does potentiate mescaline in man.[103] Cross tolerance to other hallucinogens has been reviewed by Appel and Freedman[122] and by Winter.[88]

AMPHETAMINES

Some investigators consider amphetamines in the same category as psychotomimetics due to their common EEG (and sometimes motor) arousal effects. Amphetamines at high doses produce an aberrant behavior in man that appears either as a toxic and confusional, or as a schizophreniform psychosis with delusional, paranoid, and hostile overtones. Hallucinations have been reported. In addition, after chronic usage, withdrawal of the drug frequently causes anxiety and depression.

The basic structure of the amphetamines, phenylisopropylamine, immediately suggests comparison with mescaline and other phenylethylamines. Compounds derived from and related to phenylisopropylamines were the subject of a recent volume edited by Costa and Garrattini.[123] Sulser and Sanders-Bush[124,125] reviewed the effects on amines in the CNS. Ho et al.[126] described effects of analogs and derivatives on animal behavior and barbiturate sleeping time. Specific derivatives such as 2,5-dimethoxy-4-methylamphetamine (STP, DOM) have received much attention from Idänpään-Heikkilä, et al.,[127,128] Tacker et al.,[129] Joffe,[130] Snyder and Richelson,[94] and Snyder et al.[131] Innumerable SAR studies have been carried out to define receptors for the various activities of amphetamines. Many of these studies have been reviewed by Kang and Green,[68] Appel and Freedman,[132] Ho et al.,[126] Snyder et al.,[131] Antun et al.,[133] and Everett and Yellin.[134]

Antun et al.,[133] suggest that the highest molecular orbital of amphetamine derivatives is involved with hallucinogenic potency, since the fluorescence yield, due in part to π electron delocalization, correlates well with the psychotomimetic effects (exceptions are mescaline, 3, 4; 2,4,6-and 2,3,4,5-methoxyamphetamines). Snyder et al.[131] have shown that unlike STP, the 2,5 dimethoxy-4-ethyl amphetamine, DOET is not hallucinogenic. Chothia and Pauling[66] describe 2,4,5-trimethoxyamphetamine as having planar methoxy groups, with the ethylene perpendicular to the phenyl ring and the nitrogen normal to the

*Alternatively, a subsequent dose may find all or most of the receptors in a state in which they are not oriented to combine with the drug.

ring, giving a τ-shaped structure. This is in accord with the model for mescaline proposed by Teller and Denber,[5] rather than the stressed or bent form suggested by the models of Snyder and Richelson.[67,94] Despite these elegant studies, it is clearly too early to relate electronic or steric measurements to hallucinogenic potency since there are multiple sites of action (receptors) in the CNS for this class of compounds, possibly with differing affinities for the various drugs.

In addition, variation in the concentration of STP in different brain areas was suggested by Idänpään-Heikkilä et al.[127,128] to be partly responsible for its spectrum of activity in cats.* Fujimori et al.[135] noted that the psychotomimetic amphetamine derivatives, 2,5 dimethoxy- and 3,4,5,-trimethoxyamphetamine synchronized EEG arousal patterns arising in the medullary region, giving a net inhibitory effect. The non-psychotomimetic, 2,3, dimethoxy-, and 2,3,4 trimethoxyamphetamine stimulated arousal EEG patterns from the midbrain, a net activation effect. These findings suggest that the drug-evoked behavior pattern may be a function of the brain regions in which the drugs reach a critical concentration for a particular pharmacological effect. Lack of a change in catecholamine turnover or uptake in brain slices or in the whole organ may obscure more localized effects. Recent findings with unrelated compounds such as L-DOPA, and studies on the drug sensitivity of the raphe neurons, indicate that it may soon become possible to plot a physiological receptor and activity map of the CNS which will allow localization of the pharmacological effects of various compounds within a specific region. Ott et al.[136] have just completed a comprehensive survey along these lines.

Two additional anatomical sites for actions of amphetamine, the midbrain reticular formation and medial septal nucleus were proposed by Izquierdo and Izquierdo.[42] They showed the former to be involved with the alerting or arousal EEG, while the hippocampus showed increased RNA concentrations due to stimulation of the medial septal nucleus. These deep brain center effects are also found after nicotine. Thus, it is apparent that discrete regional effects by this class of compounds greatly complicate description of receptor interactions.

Interactions with Physiological Receptors

Amphetamine has been considered to combine with α-adrenergic receptors in the CNS, mimicking the action of NE. In recent years, more and more doubt has been cast on this mechanism and today the major site of action of the drug is considered to be presynaptic. However, Hendley and Snyder[11] presented fairly conclusive, but perhaps indirect, evidence for the interaction of various psychotomimetic methoxyamphetamines with central adrenergic receptors. These studies were based on the observation that normetanephrine is taken up in peripheral tissues by an extraneuronal mechanism, presumably through the postsynaptic membrane. Hendley and Snyder determined the effectiveness with which a series of these methoxyamphetamines inhibit normetanephrine uptake in brain slices. In this fashion, the methoxyamphetamines may be acting similarly to adrenergic blocking agents. Indeed, a close correlation existed between potency to block uptake of normetanephrine and psychotropic activity of these drugs in man and monkey. They concluded that the site of inhibition of normetanephrine uptake "might be the postsynaptic receptors for norepinephrine in the brain."

Hill and Horita[137] have shown that amphetamine hyperthermia is due to the CNS activity of amphetamine, particularly a central dopaminergic system. The fact that spinal section blocks or reduces amphetamine hyperthermia is direct support for a central mechanism. Similarly, blockade of peripheral α- or β-adrenergic receptors has no effect on amphetamine hyperthermia. Several neuroleptic drugs antagonize amphetamine hyperthermia in rats; these neuroleptics are potent inhibitors of dopaminergic function. Low doses of amphetamine can elevate both body temperature and the turnover rate of brain dopamine without altering the turnover rate of brain NE in the rat. These effects are primarily presynaptic. However, the effects of other compounds support the concept that amphetamine also increases the postsynaptic dopamine receptor activity. Andén et al.[138] have shown that pimozide exerts an in-

*It should be noted that STP reaches much higher brain levels (ca. 1% or 6.3 ug/g/mg injected/100g body weight) and remains in the brain much longer than mescaline in mice, rats and cats. Rather than estimating it to be 100-fold more potent than mescaline, on the basis of the brain content STP appears to be three to tenfold more potent. This relationship is supported by Shulgin's data on the behavioral effects of STP compared to mescaline.[93]

hibitory effect on central dopaminergic neurons in rabbits at the receptor level. This compound blocks the hyperthermic effects of amphetamine, suggesting that dopamine receptors are necessary for the production of the hyperthermia by amphetamine.

Interaction with Presynaptic Binding Sites

Perhaps the most important action of amphetamine is to release catecholamines from nerve terminals and prevent their reuptake. It also prevents the reuptake of dopamine and thus dopaminergic effects may be very important for some actions of the drug.[139] Brodie et al.[140] reviewed early evidence linking amphetamine actions to release of NE. They noted that hyperactivity due to amphetamine was no longer considered to be a result of a direct effect on adrenergic receptors. NE release was now considered to be the primary means by which amphetamines act even after the catecholamine stores were depleted by reserpine. Brodie and co-workers[140] suggested that tolerance to the central effects of amphetamine might actually have been a result of exhaustion of those central stores of NE that could be released by the drug.

That amphetamine has several important presynaptic receptor sites has been demonstrated in several ways. For example, Taylor and Snyder[141,142] were able to differentiate *d*- from *l*-amphetamine. The *d*-form is a much more potent inhibitor of NE uptake than is *l*-amphetamine. However, both isomers inhibit catecholamine uptake by dopaminergic neurons in the corpus striatum. In producing locomotor excitation, *d*-amphetamine is ten times more potent than *l*-amphetamine. However, the *d*-form is only twice as potent in eliciting a compulsive gnawing syndrome. They suggest that locomotor stimulation by amphetamine involves central norepinephrine, while dopaminergic neurones are important in drug induced compulsive gnawing behavior.

Simpson and Iversen[143,144] distinguished between amphetamine receptors involved in locomotor effects and those responsible for the stimulation of stereotyped behavior. Rats received bilateral lesions in the substantia nigra. Two weeks postoperatively, the lesioned animals and a sham-operated group were injected with *d, l*-amphetamine sulfate at 3, 5, and 10 mg/kg. The sham-operated animals showed a marked increase in spontaneous activity which lasted about two hours after 3 and 5 mg/kg. After 5 mg/kg the sham-operated animals also demonstrated stereotyped head movements, as well as sniffing and gnawing. At the highest dose, 10 mg/kg, these animals showed ataxia during the first hour and stereotyped responses somewhat later. However, in the animals where the substantia nigra (zona compacta) was destroyed, the usual excitation responses to amphetamine were abolished. In contrast, the larger dose of amphetamine still produced the stereotyped behavior. The results of this study appear to contradict the conclusions expressed by Taylor and Snyder,[141,142] noted previously. Taylor and Snyder[142] suggest that brain NE is selectively involved in mediating amphetamine-induced locomotor stimulation, while stimulation of a dopaminergic component may produce the compulsive gnawing syndrome. However, the study by Simpson and Iverson[143,144] indicates that only a small portion of the (dopaminergic) substantia nigra may be responsible for the compulsive gnawing and locomotor excitation, while the dopaminergic system of the substantia nigra itself is responsible for the stereotyped behavior.

At *low* doses, α-methyltyrosine blocks most of the CNS activity of amphetamine, although amphetamine transport to, and metabolism in, the CNS are unaffected. By causing a release of newly synthesized and freshly stored NE, amphetamine may increase NE and DA turnover and alter the catecholamine "pool" equilibrium in the CNS. This would produce increased locomotor activity (NE) and stereotyped behavior (DA). The locomotor activity is blocked by disulfiram and diethyldithiocarbamate which inhibit dopamine β-hydroxylase. The amphetamine-induced stereotyped activity may be further stimulated by the inhibition of dopamine β-hydroxylase. Therefore, the overall activity of amphetamine, including dopaminergic stimulation, is considered to be indirect.[124,125] According to Sulser and Sanders-Bush:[125] "Locomotor stimulation, stereotyped behavior, anorexigenic effects and stimulation of nondiscriminated avoidance behavior evoked by amphetamine are blocked by low doses of α-methyl tyrosine (α-MT) which do not alter the locomotor activity of control animals and do not exert central adrenergic blocking properties."

The phenothiazine tranquilizers block amphetamine's hallucinogenic effects, although at low doses potentiation occurs. Chlorpromazine produces a dose-dependent elevation of brain amphetamine levels, but at high doses the phenothiazine blocks the effects arising from the increased amphetamine concentration.[120] Potentiation by chlorpromazine can be explained on the basis that the phenothiazine blocks p-hydroxylation of amphetamine, catecholamine uptake, and adrenergic receptors.[121]

In the near future, it may be possible to study the effect of a drug such as amphetamine on different terminal receptors in a clear fashion. Synaptosomes could be separated by transmitter type and tested for their responses to the various actions of amphetamines. Gfeller, el al.,[56] prepared various types of NEPs by varying the K^+ concentration in a density gradient. The synaptosomes in the denser regions of the gradient contain many presynaptic elements and intraterminal mitochondria with vesicular NE, dopamine, 5-HT, and ACh. Synaptosomes in the lighter sections of the gradient were rich in γ-aminobutyric acid and other amino acids. The authors suggest that significant morphological variations may exist among different neurotransmitter-specific nerve terminals in the brain.

An interesting approach to amphetamine action was provided by a report of Doggett and Spencer[145] who found that amphetamine antagonizes the marked fall in esophogeal temperature caused when ouabain is injected into cerebral ventricles. Injection of amphetamine (10 mg/kg) into such a ouabain-treated animal produces a return to normal temperature and even an overshoot above control levels within 30 minutes. Presumably, the mechanism of ouabain effect is to block Na-K ATPase at sensitive temperature-controlling sites. The antagonistic action of amphetamine suggests a competition for ATPase. This might account for the amphetamine inhibition of NE reuptake which may be mediated by membrane ATPase. Waser and Schaub[146] showed that guinea pig cortex synaptosomal Na-K ATPase is stimulated in vitro (~10%) by amphetamine, while other psychotomimetics either inhibited or had no effects on this ouabain-sensitive enzyme. These studies are mentioned to indicate that the "receptor" for one of amphetamine actions in the CNS may well be the pump mechanism by which NE, DA, and 5-HT are taken up into nerve endings after their initial release from the vesicle.

We consider amphetamine to have not only a spectrum of effects via dosage increment (from arousal-physiological stimulation-psychotomimetic activity), but also multiple effects within a single neuron: a)release of NE and b)blockade of reuptake of NE or DA. It may be that release of NE occurs at the vesicle, while the blockade of NE or DA reuptake may be the effect at the presynaptic membrane. It would then be possible to explain many of amphetamine's actions as follows:

(a) Release of NE at the vesicle produces arousal; this is accompanied by a decrease in MAO activity.

(b) Blockade of NE and DA uptake in the nerve ending yields altered sympathetic nervous system activity.

(c) Increased release or subsequent blockade of DA uptake in the nigrostriatal region or ventral mesencephalic neurons produces a high level of DA and hallucinogenic effects.[147,148]

No doubt this is an oversimplification, but the recent reviews by Sulser and Sanders-Bush[124,125] support this schema.

Receptors and Tolerance

Synthesis of p-hydroxynorephedrine (pHE) in peripheral neuronal elements has been shown to occur following amphetamine administration. The blockade of amphetamine's actions by this false-transmitter might explain some aspects of the tolerance that develops in the peripheral nervous system. Although pHE is reported to occur in brain,[140] the question of whether *acute* tolerance occurs to the CNS effects of amphetamine is moot. What has been termed "tolerance" to the central effects of amphetamines is probably the exhaustion of those NE stores which the drug is capable of releasing.[89,140] Acute tolerance to amphetamines is difficult to study, because unlike hallucinogens in general, they are retained in the body for up to 48 hours. Despite this, development of tolerance to *chronic* amphetamine does occur; tolerance is slow in onset as compared with other hallucinogens. Cross-tolerance occurs with some other psychotomimetic drugs.

Except for the possible increase in microsomal hydroxylase, reported only in peripheral adrenergic neurons (synthesis of pHE), there is no evidence that acute usage of amphetamine induces enzyme formation. Therefore, it is possible that tolerance to amphetamines may be considered entirely due to receptor mechanisms. However, chronic amphetamine dosage changes almost all CNS and liver enzyme systems, and this has been the basis for innumerable studies from 1930 to 1960 on the biochemical effects of amphetamines. These have been reviewed by Utena[149,150] and by Costa and Garattini.[123]

It appears that the unravelling of direct and indirect amphetamine effects on CNS receptors is still in the future. However, the existence of a multiplicity of anatomical sites, as well as a variety of receptor sites, may provide a better theoretical framework for understanding the drug's wide spectrum of activity.

BARBITURATES

Interaction with Physiological Receptors

By far the greatest number of studies with these drugs has been concerned with their effects on CNS metabolism. Until recently little attention has been paid to the question of whether metabolic or other CNS actions, e.g., sedation, are brought about by receptor mechanisms. Although the ability of these drugs to depress polysynaptic reflexes has long been known, the precise localization of the receptor sites, whether pre or postsynaptic, has not been determined. One aspect of their action in the CNS, namely, the speed with which an intravenous injection of a barbiturate can produce coma or sleep, strongly suggests interaction with a receptor. The ability of these drugs to block neuromuscular transmission has been known for some time,[151,152] although only recently has the effect been analyzed by means of micro-electrodes. With this technique, evidence has been presented for a distinct postsynaptic effect of at least some barbiturates. Galindo[153] has shown that pentobarbital produces depolarization of the postsynaptic membrane, presumably by some mechanism involving interaction with receptors located there. A similar depolarizing action for methohexital was discerned by Westmoreland et al.[154] in the rat phrenic nerve-diaphragm preparation. Single end plates were used for this study, which for the first time revealed a definite effect of a barbiturate on miniature end plate potentials (MEPP). This was a rather complex effect; the frequency of MEPPs was increased, but at the same time, the amplitude progressively decreased. The latter probably resulted from the postsynaptic action of the drug, whereas the former arose from a presynaptic effect.

The inhibitory actions of barbiturates on smooth muscle are also well established. Recently, we have shown that various barbiturates not only block contractions of electrically-stimulated guinea pig ileum but also contractions elicited by ACh,[29] suggesting barbiturate combination with muscarinic receptors in this tissue, as well as a pre-synaptic site of action. Specificity was shown by the fact that barbituric acid failed to have an effect.

Interaction with Prejunctional Receptors

Although, as indicated above, barbiturates combine with nicotinic and muscarinic receptors, their more prominent effects at cholinergic synapses are pre-synaptic. Riker et al.[155] demonstrated that pentobarbital depresses repetitive antidromic firing induced by electric stimulation or by drugs. The studies of Galindo[153] showed that the primary effect of pentobarbital on the phrenic nerve-diaphragm preparation is to depress activity in prejunctional structures. The mechanism is prolongation of the absolute refractory period of the nerve terminals. This could come about by combination with nerve terminal receptors resulting in block of Na^+ conductance; such an effect on squid axonal membrane has recently been shown.[156,157] Westmoreland et al.[154] have suggested another effect of barbiturates, a hemicholinium type of action which prevents uptake of choline. This depletes ACh and causes failure of transmission.

Studies of electrically-stimulated ileum have revealed that the presynaptic receptor site most likely has a higher affinity for various barbiturates than the postsynaptic ACh receptor, since blockade of transmission preceeded inhibition of exogenous ACh. Biochemical evidence for rather important presynaptic effects of barbiturates was obtained by Balfour and Gilbert[158] who reported that 0.1 to 2 mM phenobarbital caused permeability changes in isolated NEPs on transfer from 0.2 to 0.05 *M*NaCl.

Büch et al.[159] recently demonstrated that many of the barbiturate interactions are stereospecific. In spite of the generally accepted concept of a diffuse nature of barbiturate interaction with tissue components,[160,161] there appears to be evidence for site specificity in the same manner as other CNS-active compounds. Working with diphenylhydantoin, a compound related structurally to barbiturates, Nielsen and Cotman[162] showed a very specific binding to brain subcellular membrane components at $10^{-8} M$ and lower concentrations. Diphenylhydantoin was not appreciably bound to myelin or to lipid, despite its lipid solubility.

Work by Duggan[163] has shown a direct interaction of barbiturates with muscle sarcoplasmic reticulum membranes of rabbit and frog, the drugs stimulating the uptake of calcium. However, when 100 mM potassium was incorporated into the medium, barbiturates reduced the rate of calcium uptake. Barbituric acid was without effect. It was suggested that these compounds act on nerve tissue by reducing calcium dissociation from stimulated membranes and in this way render the tissue inexcitable. Moreover, it should be noted that the phenothiazines produce a similar effect, the potencies being in the same order as their potency as CNS depressants.

Receptor Interactions and Tolerance

Long-term (addiction) dosage with barbiturates may produce suppression of RNA synthesis,[164] but the depressant effect of phenobarbital (for example) is not of importance for the induction of tolerance via microsomal enzymes.[165] Thus, the endoplasmic reticulum contains a dual receptor site for barbiturate action after prolonged treatment: induction of enzymes for drug metabolism and suppression of RNA synthesis. We suggest that the former is only responsible for tolerance, while the latter may be involved with addiction.* Kalant et al.[89] have recently reviewed tolerance development to barbiturates and related drugs.

ALCOHOL

Alcohol (ethanol) is undoubtedly one of the most addicting drugs, yet perhaps the least is known about the mechanism of this effect. One of the major problems in this field is the fact that alcohol most likely does not act via a specific receptor mechanism, but rather influences all sensitive areas of the body indiscriminately.[89,167]

Thus, whereas ethanol has profound effects on protein, RNA, and amino acid metabolism,[168,169] these are probably secondary to its action on the cell membrane. These secondary effects may produce addiction and withdrawal symptoms.[170] That the drug can have primary effects on the neuronal membrane has been indicated in experiments on axonal conduction and on synaptic transmission. At low concentrations ethanol stimulates neural activity, while at high concentrations conduction is blocked.[12,171] This may be interpreted on the basis that alcohol promotes binding of ions, particularly Ca^{++} and Mg^{++}, to various negative sites on membranes.[13,14] Evidence has been obtained that ethanol greatly increases affinity of divalent cations to soluble macromolecules extracted from nerve tissue.[13] At low ethanol concentration, promotion of binding destabilizes the membrane and nerve firing ensues; with increased binding to the membrane of both calcium and magnesium a stabilization occurs with block of conduction. The course of events is analogous to increasing the Ca^{++} ion concentration bathing a nerve. (See also Seeman et al.[172])

At terminals, ethanol could promote binding of Ca^{++} to the system involved with excitation-transmitter release, thereby producing excessive release of transmitter. Such a presynaptic effect of the drug has been noted.[173]

At postsynaptic sites, ethanol could promote binding of transmitter to its receptor; the net effect of the pre- and postsynaptic activity would serve to enhance synaptic transmission, possibly accounting for the initial excitement observed. With higher concentrations, depression of neuronal activity occurs. Secondarily to these effects, transport across all neuronal membranes would be impeded,[172] giving rise to the profound metabolic effects noted. Ethanol probably acts in a similar manner at every locus where it penetrates, promoting ion binding to nucleic acids, proteins, polysaccharides, etc. Such effects add to those already operating at cell membranes, membranes of mitochondria,[174] microsomes, etc.

Possible presynaptic receptor sites for ethanol are the catecholamine uptake and storage sites. It has been suggested that ethanol produces alkaloid-like compounds during its metabolism by condensation of acetaldehyde and catecholamines.[175-178] Heikkilä et al.[179] have shown that tetrahydroisoquinoline alkaloids (TIQ), produced by condensation of dopamine and

*Essig[166] has suggested that other sedative drugs may produce a barbiturate-like dependence including paraldehyde, chloral hydrate, meprobamate, glutethimide, methyprylon, ethinamate, ethchlorvynol, chlordiazepoxide, and diazepam. These may all be acting at the subcellular level as described above.

acetaldehylde, are taken up and concentrated in the presynaptic region, and that the catecholamine uptake mechanism is inhibited by salsolinol, a TIQ condensation product of dopamine and acetaldehyde.

Therefore, at least part of the same transport and binding sites for catecholamines is shared by TIQ. "By sharing uptake and storage mechanisms with the catecholamines, the TIQ alkaloids would be in a unique position to interfere with catecholaminergic mechanisms in brain."[179] These alkaloids might release catecholamines, interfere with their reuptake, or act as false transmitters. There is evidence that TIQ alkaloids block uptake and cause neurohormone release.

Somjen[180] has reported that ether and phenylpentol act by reducing the presynaptic output of spinal neurones. He concluded that the presynaptic terminals in spinal reflex pathways conduct normal impulses at a level of depression where the reflex is reduced to less than 10% of its normal height. The most probable explanation according to Somjen is a nonspecific stabilization of the subsynaptic membrane. Decreasing the amount of transmitter released per impulse cannot be ruled out as an alternative explanation.

CONCLUDING REMARKS

We have presented various types of evidence which suggest that drugs of abuse interact with a number of different neuronal components. For the most part, the sites of interaction are presynaptic. In some instances, these interactions have proved to be specific enough to consider the target site to contain a receptor for the particular drug. These interactions, whether receptor- or nonreceptor-mediated, produce a multitude of physiological, biochemical, and pharmacological sequelae, the most important of which are summarized in Table 4. Although at the present time it cannot be stated with certainty which of these interactions is directly responsible for the major pharmacological actions of these drugs, i.e., analgesia, tolerance, addiction, or hallucinations, there is little doubt that the clues provided by these studies will go a long way toward elucidating the fundamental mechanisms involved.

Acknowledgments

We wish to thank Mrs. Louise Mussolini for her expert secretarial assistance. This work was supported in part by USPHS Grants NS 03226 and 04360.

TABLE 4

Interactions of Drugs of Abuse at Various Neuronal Sites and The Effect Produced

Compound	Site(s) of interaction	Effect(s) produced
Morphine, other potent analgesics	Cholinergic nerve terminal membrane (presynaptic)	Block acetylcholine release: sympathetic predominance
	Acetylcholine storage vesicle(?)	Temporary storage of drug (?)' site for tolerance development(?)
	Adrenergic nerve terminal (presynaptic)	Release NE
LSD	Physiological 5-HT receptor (postsynaptic):peripheral NS	Blocks, followed by feedback to presynaptic endings
	Physiological 5-HT receptor (postsynaptic): CNS	Stimulates (?); feedback to presynaptic endings causing block of 5-HT release
	5-HT storage vesicle	Blocks 5-HT release
	Catecholamine storage vesicle	Stimulates NE release, depletes NE stores; this results in activation of dopaminergic pathways
	Dopaminergic receptors (postsynaptic)	Stimulates(?)
	Cytoplasmic polynucleotides	Tolerance(?); metabolic effects(?)
Other indoleamines	Physiological 5-HT receptors (postsynaptic)	Stimulate (tryptamines)
	Catecholamine storage vesicle	Release NE; deplete NE stores (psilocybin)
Mescaline	Nerve ending membranes (presynaptic)	Disrupts ionic integrity
	Catecholamine storage vesicle	Releases NE
	Ribosomal system	Stimulates synthesis of vesicles(?) site of tolerance development(?)
Amphetamines	Catecholamine storage vesicle (midbrain)	Release NE: arousal and locomotor excitation
	Membrane Na–K ATPase	Block NE reuptake resulting in depletion
	Dopaminergic receptor(?) (postsynaptic)	Stimulates, resulting in hyperthermia
	Dopaminergic nerve terminal (presynaptic)	Block dopamine reuptake; responsible for stereotyped behavior, hallucinogenesis
Barbiturates	Cholinergic nerve terminals (muscarinic, nicotinic)	Block acetylcholine release
	Cholinergic receptors (muscarinic, nicotinic)	Inhibit: block transimission
Alcohol	Nerve axon	Stimulates, then blocks conduction
	Adrenergic nerve terminal	Synthesis of TIQ derivatives: blocks NE uptake

REFERENCES

1. Ehrenpreis, S., Fleisch, J. H., and Mittag, T. W., Approaches to the molecular nature of pharmacological receptors, *Pharmacol. Rev.*, 21, 131, 1969.

2. Smythies, J. R., Antun, F., Yank, G., and Yorke, C., Molecular mechanisms of storage of transmitters in synaptic terminals, *Nature*, 231, 185, 1971.

3. Shanes, A. M., Electrochemical aspects of physiological and pharmacological action in excitable cells. I. The resting cell and its alteration by extrinsic factors, *Pharmacol. Rev.*, 10, 59, 1958.

4. Seeman, P. M., Membrane stabilization by drugs: tranquilizers, steroids and anesthetics, *Int. Rev. Neurobiol.*, 9, 145, 1966.

5. Teller, D. N. and Denber, H. C. B., Defining schizophrenia with the techniques of molecular biology, *Dis. Nerv. Syst.*, 29, 93, 1968.

6. Ehrenpreis, S., Light, I., and Schonbuch, G., Use of electrically stimulated guinea pig ileum to study potent analgesics, in *Drug Addiction: Experimental Approaches*, Singh, J. M., Miller, L. H., and Lal, H., Eds., Symposium Specialists, Miami, Fla., in press.

7. Michaelson, I. A., The subcellular distribution of acetylcholine, choline acetyltransferase and acetylcholinesterase in nerve tissue, *Ann. N.Y. Acad. Sci.*, 144, 383, 1967.

8. Appel, S. M., Festoff, B. W., Autilio, L., and Escueta, A. V., Biochemical approaches to the study of synaptic function, *Biol. Psych.*, 2, 219, 1970.

9. Standaert, F. G. and Riker, W. F., The consequences of cholinergic drug actions on motor nerve terminals, *Ann. N.Y. Acad. Sci.*, 144, 517, 1967.

10. Koelle, G. B., A new general concept of the neurohumoral functions of acetylcholine and acetylcholinesterase, *J. Pharm. Pharmacol.*, 14, 65, 1962.

11. Hendley, E. and Snyder, S. H., Correlation between psychotropic potency of psychotomimetic methoxyamphetamines and their inhibition of ^{3}H-normetanephrine uptake in rat cerebral cortex, *Nature*, 229, 264, 1971.

12. Mardones, J., The alcohols, in *Physiological Pharmacology*, Vol. 1, Root, W. S. and Hofmann, F. G., Eds., Academic Press, New York, 1963, 100.

13. Ehrenpreis, S., An approach to the molecular basis of nerve activity, *J. Cell. Comp. Physiol.*, 66, 159, 1965.

14. Ehrenpreis, S., Acetylcholine and nerve activity, *Nature*, 201, 887, 1964.

15. Martin, W. R., Strong analgesics, in *Physiological Pharmacology*, Vol. 1, Root, W. S. and Hofmann, F. G., Eds., Academic Press, New York, 1963, 275.

16. Seevers, M. H. and Deneau, G. A., Physiological aspects of tolerance and physical dependence, in *Physiological Pharmacology*, Vol. 1, Root, W. S. and Hofmann, F. G., Eds., Academic Press, New York, 1963, 565.

17. Clouet, D. H., Biochemical responses to narcotic drugs in the nervous system and in other tissues, *Int. Rev. Neurobiol.*, 11, 99, 1968.

18. Clouet, D. H., Protein and nucleic acid metabolism, in *Narcotic Drugs: Biochemical Pharmacology*, Clouet, D. H., Ed., Plenum Press, New York, 1971, 216.

19. Mulé, S. J., Phospholipid metabolism, in *Narcotic Drugs: Biochemical Pharmacology*, Clouet, D. H., Ed., Plenum Press, N.Y. 1971, 190.

20. Takemori, A. E., Intermediary and energy metabolism, in *Narcotic Drugs: Biochemical Pharmacology*, Clouet, D. H., Ed., Plenum Press, New York, 1971, 159.

21. Way, E. L. and Shen, F., Catecholamines and 5-Hydroxytryptamine, in *Narcotic Drugs: Biochemical Pharmacology*, Clouet, D. H., Ed., Plenum Press, New York, 1971, 229.

22. Collier, H. O. J., Tolerance, physical dependence and receptors. A theory of the genesis of tolerance and physical dependence through drug-induced changes in the number of receptors, *Advances Drug Res.*, 3, 171, 1966.

23. Paton, W. D. M., The action of morphine and related substances on contraction and on acetylcholine output of coaxially stimulated guinea pig ileum, *Brit. J. Pharmacol.*, 11, 119, 1957.

24. Frederickson, R. C. A. and Pinsky, G., Morphine impairs acetylcholine release but facilitates acetylcholine action at a skeletal neuromuscular junction, *Nature,* 231, 93, 1971.

25a. Satoh, M. and Takagi, H., Enhancement by morphine of the central descending inhibitory influence on spinal sensory transmission, *Europ. J. Pharmacol.*, 14, 60, 1971.

25b. Satoh, M. and Takagi, H., Effect of morphine on the pre- and postsynaptic inhibitions in the spinal cord, *Europ. J. Pharmacol.*, 14, 150, 1971.

26. Schaumann, W., Inhibition by morphine of the release of acetylcholine from the intestine of the guinea pig, *Brit. J. Pharmacol.*, 12, 115, 1957.

27. Weinstock, M., Acetylcholine and cholinesterase, in *Narcotic Drugs: Biochemical Pharmacology*, Clouet, D. H., Ed., Plenum Press, New York, 1971, 254.

28. Fennessy, M. R., Heimans, R. L. H., and Rand, M. J., Comparison of effect of morphine-like analgesics on transmurally stimulated guinea pig ileum, *Brit. J. Pharmacol.*, 37, 436, 1969.

29. Ehrenpreis, S. and Light, I., unpublished data.

30. Ehrenpreis, S. and Light, I., Morphine-naloxone antagonism in electrically stimulated guinea pig ileum: evidence for two morphine receptors, *Fed. Proc.*, in press.

31. Hug, C. C., Jr. and Oka, T., Uptake of dihydromorphine-^{3}H by synaptosomes, *Life Sci.*, 10, 201, 1971.

32. Navon, S. and Lajtha, A., Uptake of morphine in particulate fractions from rat brain, *Brain Res.*, 24, 534, 1970.

33. Schonbuch, G. and Ehrenpreis, S., Uptake of radioactive morphine by isolated guinea pig intestine, *Fed. Proc.*, in press.

34. Nutt, J. G., Inhibition of the action of morphine by calcium, *Fed. Proc.*, 27, 753, 1968.

35. Richter, J. and Goldstein, A., Effects of morphine and levorphanol on brain acetylcholine content in mice. *J. Pharmacol. Exp. Ther.*, 175, 685, 1970.

36. Jhamandas, K., Pinsky, C., and Phillis, J. W., Effects of morphine and its antagonists on release of cerebral cortical acetylcholine, *Nature*, 228, 176, 1970.

37. Hebb, C. O. and Konzett, H., Difference between morphine and synthetic analgesics in their actions on ganglionic transmission, *Nature*, 163, 720, 1949.

38. Pinsky, C. and Frederickson, R. C. A., Morphine and nalorphine impair neuromuscular transmission, *Nature*, 231, 94, 1971.

39. Vogt, M., The concentration of "sympathin" in different parts of the CNS under normal conditions and after administration of drugs, *J. Physiol.*, 123, 451, 1954.

40. Lee, J. R. and Fennessy, M. R., The relationship between morphine analgesia and the levels of biogenic amines in the mouse brain, *Europ. J. Pharmacol.*, 12, 65, 1970.

41. Rethy, C. R., Smith, C. B., and Villareal, J. E., Effects of narcotic analgesics upon the locomotor activity and brain catecholamine content of the mouse, *J. Pharmacol. Exp. Ther.*, 176, 472, 1971.

42. Izquierdo, I. and Izquierdo, J. A., Effects of drugs on deep brain centers, *Ann. Rev. Pharmacol.*, 11, 189, 1971.

43. Teller, D. N., De Guzman, T., and Lajtha, A., Effects of morphine and phenobarbital on uptake of some amino acids into mouse cortex slices, *Trans. Amer. Soc. Neurochem.*, 2, 114, 1971.

44. Heinrich, U., Lichtensteiger, W., and Langemann, H., Effect of morphine on the catecholamine content of midbrain nerve cell groups in rat and mouse, *J. Pharmacol. Exp. Ther.*, 179, 259, 1971.

45. Costa, E. and Algeri, S., Physical dependence on morphine fails to increase serotonin turnover rate in rat brain, *Biochem. Pharmacol.*, 20, 877, 1971.

46. Goldstein, A., Lowney, L. E., and Pal. B. K., Stereospecific and nonspecific interactions of the morphine congener levorphanol in subcellular fractions of mouse brain, *Proc. Nat. Acad. Sci. (USA)*, 68, 1742, 1971.

47. Sharkawi, M. and Goldstein, A., Antagonism by physostigmine of the "running fit" caused by levorphanol, a morphine congener, in mice, *Brit. J. Pharmacol.*, 37, 123, 1969.

48. Bowers, M. B., Jr. and Kleber, H. D., Methadone increases mouse brain 5-hydroxyindoleacetic acid, *Nature*, 229, 134, 1971.

49. Gaddum, J. H. and Vogt, M., Some central actions of 5-hydroxytryptamine and various antagonists, *Brit. J. Pharmacol.*, 11, 175, 1956.

50. Yarbrough, G. G., Buxbaum, D. M., and Sanders-Bush, E., Increased serotonin turnover in the acutely morphine treated rat, *Life Sci.*, 10, 977, 1971.

51. Cheney, D. L. and Goldstein, A., The effect of β-chlorphenylalanine on opiate-induced running, analgesia, tolerance and physical dependence in mice, *J. Pharmacol. Exp. Ther.*, 177, 309, 1971.

52. Marshall, I. and Grahame-Smith, D. G., Unchanged rate of brain serotonin synthesis during chronic morphine treatment and failure of parachlorophenylalanine to attenuate withdrawal syndrome in mice, *Nature*, 228, 1206, 1970.

53. Mulé, S. J. and Woods, L. A., Distribution of N-C^{14}-methyl labeled morphine: I. In central nervous system of nontolerant and tolerant dogs, *J. Pharmacol. Exp. Ther.*, 135, 232, 1962.

54. Schubert, P., Teschemacher, H., Kreutzberg, G. W., and Herz, A., Intracerebral distribution pattern of radioactive morphine and morphine-like drugs after intraventricular and intrathecal injection, *Histochemie*, 22, 277, 1970.

55. Schild, H. O., "pA", a new scale for the measurement of drug antagonism, *Brit. J. Pharmacol.*, 2, 189, 1947.

56. Gfeller, E., Kubar, M. J., and Snyder, S. H. Neurotransmitter-specific synaptosomes in rat corpus striatum: morphological variations, *Proc. Nat. Acad. Sci. (U.S.A.)*, 68, 155, 1971.

57. Ingoglia, N. A. and Dole, V. P., Localization of *d*- and *l*-methadone after intraventricular injection into rat brains, *J. Pharmacol. Exp. Ther.*, 175, 84, 1970.

58. Berkowitz, B. A. and May, L. L., Analgesic activity and central nervous system distribution of the optical isomers of pentazocine in the rat, *J. Pharmacol. Exp. Ther.*, 177, 500, 1971.

59. Cochin, J., Biochemical aspects of tolerance, *Univ. Mich. Med. Cent. J.*, 36, 225, 1970.

60. Gyang, E. A. and Kosterlitz, H. W., Agonist and antagonist actions of morphine-like drugs on the guinea pig isolated ileum, *Brit. J. Pharmacol.*, 27, 514, 1966.

61. Lajtha, A., The biochemistry of hallucinogens, in *Progress in Neurobiology*, Vol. 3, Pennes, H., Ed., Paul B. Hoeber, Inc., New York, 1958, 126.

62. Hoffer, A. and Osmond, H., *The Hallucinogens*, Academic Press, New York, 1967.

63. Gillette, J. R., Metabolism of drugs and other foreign compounds by enzymatic mechanisms, *Progr. Drug Res.*, 6, 13, 1963.

64. Nieforth, K. A., Psychotomimetic phenylethylamines, *J. Pharm. Sci.*, 60, 655, 1971.

65. McIsaac, W. M., Harris, R. T., and Ho, B. T., The indole hallucinogens in *Drug Dependence, Advances in Mental Science*, Vol. 2, Harris, R. T., McIsaac, W. M., and Schuster, C. R., Eds., University of Texas Press, Austin, Texas, 1970, 41.

66. Chothia, C. and Pauling, P., On the conformations of hallucinogenic molecules and their correlation, *Proc. Nat. Acad. Sci. (U.S.A.)*, 63, 1063, 1969.

67. Snyder, S. H. and Richelson, E., Psychedelic drugs: steric factors that predict psychotropic activity, *Proc. Nat. Acad. Sci. (U.S.A.)*, 60, 206, 1968.

68. Kang, S. and Green, J. P., Steric and electronic relationships among some hallucinogenic compounds, *Proc. Nat. Acad. Sci. (U.S.A.)*, 67, 62, 1970.

69. Woolley, D. W. and Campbell, N. K., Exploration of the central nervous system serotonin in humans, *Ann. N. Y. Acad. Sci.*, 96, 108, 1962.

70. Cerletti, A. and Doepfner, W., Comparative study on the serotonin antagonism of amide derivatives of lysergic acid and of ergot alkaloids, *J. Pharmacol. Exp. Ther.*, 122, 124, 1968.

71. Cohen, S., The hallucinogens, in *Principles of Psychopharmacology*, Clarke, W. G. and del Giudice, J., Eds., Academic Press, New York, 1970, 489.

72. Dixon, A. K., Evidence of catecholamine mediation in the aberrant behavior induced by lysergic acid diethylamide (LSD) in the rat, *Experientia*, 24, 743, 1968.

73. Meek, L. and Fuxe, K., Serotonin accumulation after monoamine oxidase inhibition, *Biochem. Pharmacol.*, 20, 693, 1971.

74. Tonge, S. R. and Leonard, B. E., Hallucinogens and non-hallucinogens: a comparison of the effects on 5-hydroxytryptamine and noradrenaline, *Life Sci.*, 10, 161, 1971.

75. Snyder, S. H. and Reivich, M., Regional localization of lysergic acid diethylamide in monkey brain, *Nature*, 209, 1093, 1966.

76. Alivisatos, S. G. A., Ungar, F., Seth, P. K., Georgiu, D. C., and Geroulis, A. J., Subcellular localization and specificity of binding of serotonergic receptors in the CNS, *Trans. Amer. Soc. Neurochem.*, 2, 55, 1971.

77. De Robertis, E., Molecular biology of synaptic receptors, *Science*, 171, 963, 1971.

78. De Robertis, E., Ultrastructure and cytochemistry of the synapse: isolation and nature of the receptors in the central nervous system, in *Advances Cytopharmacol.*, Vol. 1, 1st Int. Symp. Cell Biol. and Cytopharmacology, Clementi, F. and Ceccarelli, B., Eds., Raven Press, New York, 1971, 291.

79. Teller, D. N. and Denber, H. C. B., Binding of psychotropic drugs to soluble proteins, *Excerpta Medica I.C.S. Congr. Ser.*, 129, 1177, 1966.

80. Idänpään-Heikkilä, J. E., Schoolar, J. C., and Allen, A., Total body kinetics and placental transfer of labelled LSD in mice, in *Drug Dependence, Advances in Mental Science*, Vol. 2., Harris, R. T., McIsaac, W. M., and Schuster, C. R., Eds., University of Texas Press, Austin, Texas, 1970, 55.

81. DeLaTorre, J. C., Effect of LSD-25 on the septal region of the rat brain, *Nature*, 219, 954, 1968.

82. Smit, E. M. and Borst, P., LSD-25 does not intercalate in DNA, *Nature*, 232, 191, 1971.

83. Brady, A. H., Brady, E. M., and Boncek, F. C., Optical activity of LSD-DNA mixtures, *Nature*, 232, 189, 1971.

84. Schanberg, S. M. and Giarman, N., Drug-induced alterations in the subcellular distribution of 5-hydroxytryptamine in rat's brain, *Biochem. Pharmacol.*, 11, 187, 1962.

85. Szara, S., DMT, (N, *n*-dimethyl tryptamine) and homologues, clinical and pharmacological considerations, in *Psychotomimetic Drugs*, Efron, D. H., Ed., Raven Press, New York, 1970, 275.

86. Van Vunakis, H., Farrow, J. T., Gjika, H. B., and Levine, L., Specificity of the antibody receptor site to D-lysergamide: model of a physiological receptor for lysergic acid diethylamide, *Proc. Nat. Acad. Sci. (U.S.A.)*, 68, 1483, 1971.

87. Diaz, J-L. and Huttunen, M. O., Persistent increase in brain serotonin turnover after chronic administration of LSD in the rat, *Science*, 174, 62, 1971.

88. Winter, J. C., Tolerance to a behavioral effect of lysergic acid diethylamide and cross-tolerance to mescaline in the rat: absence of a metabolic component, *J. Pharmacol. Exp. Ther.*, 178, 625, 1971.

89. Kalant, H., LeBlanc, A. E., and Gibbons, R. J., Tolerance to, and dependence on, some non-opiate psychotropic drugs, *Pharmacol. Rev.*, 23, 135, 1971.

90. Isbell, H. and Jasinski, D. R., A comparison of LSD-25 with (-) Δ^9 transtetrahydrocannabinol (THC) and attempted cross tolerance between LSD and THC, *Psychopharmacologia*, 14, 115, 1969.

91. Freedman, D. X., Gottlieb, R., and Lovell, R. A., Psychotomimetic drugs and brain 5-hydroxytryptamine metabolism, *Biochem. Pharmacol.*, 19, 1181, 1963.

92. Anden, N. -E., Corrodi, H., and Fuxe, K., Hallucinogenic drugs of the indolealkylamine type and central monoamine neurons, *J. Pharmacol. Exp. Ther.*, 17, 236, 1971.

93. Shulgin, A. T., Chemistry and structure activity relationships of the psychotomimetics, in *Phychotomimetic Drugs*, Efron, D. H., Ed., Raven Press, New York, 1970, 21.

94. Snyder, S. H. and Richelson, E., Steric models predicting psychedelic activity, in, *Psychotomimetic Drugs*, Efron, D. H., Ed., Raven Press, New York, 1970, 43.

95. Ariens, E. J., Simonis, A. M., and van Rossum, J. M., Drug-receptor interaction: Interaction of one or more drugs with one receptor system, *Molecular Pharmacology*, Vol. 1, Ariens, E. J., Ed., Academic Press, New York, 1964, 119.

96. Block, W., Zur physiologie des ^{14}C radioaktiven mescaline im tierversuch. IV Mitt., *Z. Naturforsch.*, 86, 440, 1953.

97. Block, W., In-vitro versuche zum einbau von ^{14}C-mescalin und ^{14}C-β-phenyläthylamin in proteine. III. Mitt., *Hoppe Seyler Z. Physiol. Chem.*, 296, 1, 1954.

98. Block, W., The mescaline psychosis, in *Chemical Concepts of Psychosis*, Rinkel, M. and Denber, H. C. B., Eds., McDowell, Obolensky, New York, 1958, 106.

99. Block, W., Block, K., and Patzig, B., Zur physiologie des ^{14}C-radioaktiven mescalins im tierversuch. II Mitt. Verteilung der radioaktivitat in dem organen in abhangigkelt von der zeit, *Hoppe Seyler Z. Physiol. Chem.*, 290, 230, 1952.

100. Denber, H. C. B., Intracellular localization of psychotomimetic and psychotropic drugs, Ph.D. Thesis, New York University, New York, 1967.

101. Denber, H. C. B. and Teller, D. N., Mescaline. XVIII. Effect of phenothiazines, amphetamine, and amobarbital sodium on uptake into brain and viscera, *Agressologie*, 9, 127, 1968.

102. Teller, D. N. and Denber, H. C. B., Mescaline and phenothiazine tranquilizers: Recent studies on subcellular localization and effects upon membranes, in *Protein Metabolism of the Nervous System*, Lajtha, A., Ed., Plenum Press, New York, 1970, 685.

103. Denber, H. C. B., Teller, D. N., Rajotte, P. R., and Kauffman, D., Studies on mescaline. XIII: The effect of prior administration of various psychotropic drugs on different biochemical parameters: a preliminary report, *Ann. N.Y. Acad. Sci.*, 96, 14, 1962.

104. Denber, H. C. B. and Teller, D. N., Subcellular localization of mescaline at the synapse, *Arzneimittel-Forschung*, 20, 903, 1970.

105. Teller, D. N., Scattered light measurement for molecular pharmacology, in, *Methods in Pharmacology, Physical Methods*, Vol. 2, Schwartz, A. and Chignell, C. F., Eds., Appleton-Century-Crofts, New York, 1972, Chapt. 8.

106. Teller, D. N. and Denber, H. C. B., Increasing the utility of spectrophotofluorometers with inexpensive accessories. II. Macro and micro-flow cuvettes (cells), *Fluoresc. News*, 4, 4, 1969.

107. Denber, H. C. B. and Teller, D. N., Mescaline. XXI: Subcellular localization in adult rats, *Pharmacologist*, 11, 291, 1969.

108. Whittaker, V. P., Subcellular localization of neurotransmitters, in, *Advances in Cytopharmacology*, Vol. 1, First Intl. Sympos. Cell Biol. and Cytopharmacol., Clementi, F. and Ceccarelli, B., Eds., Raven Press, New York, 1971, 319.

109. Maickel, P., Cox, H., Jr., Saillant, J., and Miller, E. P., A method for the determination of serotonin and norepinephrine in discrete areas of rat brain, *Int. J. Neuropharmacol.*, 7, 275, 1968.

110. Siakotos, A. N., Filbert, M., and Hester, R., A specific radioisotopic assay for acetylcholinesterase and pseudocholinesterase in brain and plasma, *Biochem. Med.*, 3, 1, 1969.

111. Teller, D. N., Orenstein, S., Horn, B., and Denber, M. J. A., The effects of various prior treatments upon the transport of chlorpromazine and trifluoperazine into rat brain, *Dis. Nerv. Syst.*, 31, 20, 1970.

112. Datta, R. K. and Ghosh, J. J., Mescaline-induced changes of brain-cortex ribosomes: Effect of mescaline on the stability of brain-cortex ribosomes, *Biochem. J.*, 117, 961, 1970.

113. Datta, R. K. and Ghosh, J. J., Mescaline-induced changes of brain-cortex ribosomes: Effect of mescaline on the hydrogen-bonded structure of ribonucleic acid of brain-cortex ribosomes, *Biochem. J.*, 117, 969, 1970.

114. Datta, R. K. and Ghosh, J. J., Mescaline-induced changes of brain cortex ribosomes: Effect of mescaline on amino acid incorporating ability of ribosomes, *Brain Res.*, 33, 193, 1971.

115. Lajtha, A. and Toth, J., The effects of drugs on uptake and exit of cerebral amino acids, *Biochem. Pharmacol.*, 14, 729, 1965.

116. Cohen, I. and Vogel, W. H., An assay procedure for mescaline and its determination in rat brain, liver and plasma, *Experientia*, 26, 1231, 1970.

117. Denber, H. C. B. and Teller, D. N., Experimental observations on the problem of schizophrenia, in *Schizophrenia: Current Concepts and Research*, Siva Sankar, D. V., Ed., P.J.D. Publications, Hicksville, N.Y., 1969, 477.

118. Mokrasch, L. C. and Stevenson, I., The metabolism of mescaline with a note on correlations between metabolism and psychological effects, *J. Nerv. Ment. Dis.*, 129, 177, 1959.

119. *Psychopharmacology Handbook*, Vol. 1., Rev. P.H.S. 1297. Animal Research in Pharmacology 1954-9, U.S. Govt. Printing Office, Washington, D.C., 1965.

120. Halasz, M. F., Formanek, J., and Marrazzi, A. S., Hallucinogen tranquilizer interaction: its nature, *Science*, 164, 569, 1969.

121. Borella, L. E., Pinski, J., and Herr, F., Effect of chlorpromazine on the disposition and excretion of amphetamine in the rat, *Res. Comm. Chem. Pathol. Pharmacol.*, 1, 667, 1970.

122. Appel, J. B. and Freedman, D. X., Tolerance and cross-tolerance among psychotomimetic drugs, *Psychopharmacologia*, 13, 267, 1968.

123. Costa, E. and Garattini, S., *International Symposium on Amphetamines and Related Compounds*, Raven Press, New York, 1970.

124. Sulser, F., and Sanders-Bush, E., Biochemical and metabolic considerations concerning the mechanism of action of amphetamine and related compounds, in, *Psychotomimetic Drugs*, Efron, D. H., Ed., Raven Press, New York, 1970, 83.

125. Sulser, F. and Sanders-Bush, E., Effects of drugs on amines in the CNS, *Ann. Rev. Pharmacol.*, 11, 209, 1971.

126. Ho, B. T., McIsaac, W. M., An, R., Tansey, L. W., and Walker, K. E., Effect of amphetamine analogs on disruption of animal behavior and barbiturate sleeping time, in *Drug Dependence, Advances in Mental Science*, Vol. 2, Harris, R. T., McIsaac, W. M. and Schuster, C. R., Eds., University of Texas Press, Austin, Texas, 1970, 13.

127. Idänpään-Heikkilä, J. E., McIsaac, W. M., Ho, B. T., Fritchie, G. E., and Tansey, L. W., Relation of pharmacological and behavioral effects of a hallucinogenic amphetamine to distribution in cat brain, *Science*, 164, 1085, 1969.

128. Idänpään-Heikkilä, J. E., Fritchie, G. E., and McIsaac, W. M., Pharmacological and behavioral studies of STP: relationship to tissue distribution, in, *Drug Dependence, Advances in Mental Science*, Vol. 2, Harris, R. T., McIsaac, W. M., and Schuster, C. R., Eds., University of Texas Press, Austin, Texas, 1970, 24.

129. Tacker, M., Creaven, P. J., and McIsaac, W. M., Preliminary observations on the metabolism of ^{3}H-2, 5-dimethoxy-4-methyl-amphetamine (STP, DOM), in *Drug Dependence, Advances in Mental Science*, Vol. 2, Harris, R. T., McIsaac, W. M., and Schuster, C. R., Eds., University of Texas Press, Austin, Texas, 1970, 21.

130. Joffe, M., Behavioral effects of STP, in *Drug Dependence, Advances in Mental Science*, Vol. 2, Harris, R. T., McIsaac, W. M., and Schuster, C. R., Eds., University of Texas Press, Austin, Texas, 1970, 36.

131. Snyder, S. H., Weingartner, H., and Faillace, L. A., DOET (2, 5-dimethoxy-4-ethylamphetamine) and DOM (STP) (2, 5-dimethoxy-4-methylamphetamine), new psychotropic agents: Their effects in man, in *Psychotomimetic Drugs*, Efron, D. H., Ed., Raven Press, New York, 1970, 247.

132. Appel, J. B., and Freedman D. X., The relative potencies of psychotomimetic drugs, *Life Sci.*, 4, 2181, 1965.

133. Antun, F., Smythies, J. R., Benington, F., Morin, R. D., Barfkencht, C. F., and Nichols, D. E., Native fluorescence and hallucinogenic potency of some amphetamines, *Experientia*, 27, 62, 1971.

134. Everett, G. M. and Yellin, T. O., Effect of 4-chlorophenoxyamphetamine (A-6587), α-amphetamine and 4-chloroamphetamine on brain biogenic amines and behavior in mice, *Res. Comm. Chem. Pathol. Pharmacol.*, 2, 407, 1971.

135. Fujimori, M., Bost, K. L., and Himwich, H. E., E. E. G. arousal sites of amphetamine and its psychotomimetic methoxy derivatives in rabbit brain, *Biol. Psychiat.*, 3, 367, 1969.

136. Ott, T., Schmitt, M., Pohle, W., and Matthies, M., The effect of methamphetamine on the norepinephrine and 5-hydroxytryptamine contents in eleven rat brain regions, *Brain Res.*, 25, 171, 1971.

137. Hill, A. F. and Horita, A., Inhibition of (+)-amphetamine hyperthermia by blockade of dopamine receptors in rabbits, *J. Pharm. Pharmacol.*, 23, 715, 1971.

138. Andén, N. -E., Butcher, S. G., Corrodi, H., Fuxe, K., and Ungerstedt, U., Receptor activity and turnover of dopamine and noradrenaline after neuroleptics, *Europ. J. Pharmacol.*, 11, 303, 1970.

139. Porter, C. C., *Chemical Mechanisms of Drug Action,* C C Thomas, Springfield, Ill., 1970, 165.

140. Brodie, B. B., Cho, A. K., Stefano, F. J. E., and Gessa, G. L., On mechanisms of norepinephrine release by amphetamine and tyramine and tolerance to their effects, in *Advances in Biochemical Psychopharmacology*, Vol. 1., Costa, E. and Greengard, P., Eds., Raven Press, New York, 1969, 219.

141. Taylor, K. M. and Snyder, S. H., Amphetamine: differentiation by *d* and *l* isomers of behavior involving brain norepinephrine or dopamine, *Science*, 168, 1487, 1970.

142. Taylor, K. M. and Snyder, S. H., Differential effects of D- and L-amphetamine on behavior and catecholamine dispositions in dopamine and norepinephrine containing neurons of rat brain, *Brain Res.*, 28, 295, 1971.

143. Simpson, B. A. and Iversen, S. D., Effects of substantia nigra lesions on the locomotor and stereotypy responses to amphetamine, *Nature,* (New Biol.) 230, 30, 1971.

144. Iversen, S. D., The effect of surgical lesions to frontal cortex and substantia nigra on amphetamine response in rats, *Brain Res.*, 31, 295, 1971.

145. Doggett, N. S. and Spencer, P. S-J., Pharmacological, properties of centrally administered ouabain and their modification by other drugs, *Brit. J. Pharmacol.*, 42, 242, 1971.

146. Waser, P. G. and Schaub, E., The action of some neuro- and psychopharmacological agents on the membrane ATPase of cortical synaptosomes, in *Advances in Cytopharmacology,* Clementi, F. and Ceccarelli, B., Eds., Raven Press, New York, 1971, 397.

147. Anlezark, G. M., Arbuthnott, G. W., Christie, J. E., and Crow, T. J., Role of cerebral dopamine in the action of psychotropic drugs, *Brit. J. Pharmacol.*, 41, 406, 1971.

148. Angrist, B. M., Shopin, B., and Gershon, S., Comparative psychotomimetic effects of stereoisomers of amphetamine, *Nature*, 234, 152, 1971.

149. Utena, H., Behavioral aberrations in methamphetamine-intoxicated animals and chemical correlates in the brain, *Prog. Brain Res.*, 21, 192, 1966.

150. Utena, H., Ezoe, T., Kato, N., and Hada, H., Effects of chronic administration of methamphetamine in enzymic patterns in brain tissue, *J. Neurochem.*, 4, 161, 1959.

151. Quilliam, J. P., The action of hypnotic drugs on a frog skeletal muscle, *Brit. J. Pharmacol.*, 10, 133, 1950.

152. Thesleff, S., The effect of anesthetic agents on skeletal muscle membrane, *Acta Physiol. Scand.*, 37, 3, 1956.

153. Galindo, A., Procaine, pentobarbital and halothane: effects on the mammalian myoneural junction, *J. Pharmacol. Exp. Ther.*, 177, 360, 1971.

154. Westmoreland, B. F., Ward, D., and Johns, T. R., The effect of methohexital on the neuromuscular junction, *Brain Res.*, 26, 365, 1971.

155. Riker, W. F., Fr., Werner, G., Roberts, J., and Kuperman, A., Pharmacologic evidence for the existence of a pre-synaptic event in neuromuscular transmission, *J. Pharmacol. Exp. Ther.*, 125, 150, 1959.

156. Narahashi, T., Frazier, D. T., Deguchi, T., Cleaves, C. A., and Ernau, M. C., The active form of pentobarbital in squid giant axons, *J. Pharmacol. Exp. Ther.*, 177, 25, 1971.

157. Narahashi, T., Moore, J. W., and Poston, R. N., Anesthetic blocking of nerve membrane conductances by internal and external applications, *Neurobiol.*, 1, 3, 1969.

158. Balfour, D. J. and Gilbert, J. C., Some effects of phenobarbitone on the properties of synaptosomes, *Brit. J. Pharmacol.*, 41, 400P, 1971.

159. Büch, H., Knabe, J., Buzello, W., and Rummel, W., Stereospecificity of anesthetic activity, distribution, inactivation and protein binding of the optical antipodes of two N-methylated barbiturates, *J. Pharm. Exp. Ther.*, 175, 709, 1970.

160. Gey, K. F., Rutishauser, M., and Pletscher, A., Suppression of glycolysis in rat brain *in vivo* by chlorpromazine reserpine and phenobarbital, *Biochem. Pharmacol.*, 14, 5020, 1965.

161. Doggett, N. S., Spencer, P. S. J., Waite, R., Hypnotic activity of centrally-administered barbiturate and uncouplers of oxidative phosphorylation, *Europ. J. Pharmacol.*, 13, 23, 1970.

162. Nielsen, T. and Cotman, C., The binding of diphenylhydantoin to brain and subcellular fractions, *Europ. J. Pharmacol.*, 14, 344, 1971.

163. Duggan, P. F., Stimulation of calcium uptake of muscle microsomes by phenothiazines and barbiturates, *Europ. J. Pharmacol.*, 13, 381, 1971.

164. Seifert, J. and Remmer, H., Suppression of synthesis of RNA present in microsomal membranes after administration of phenobarbital, *Biochem. Pharmacol.*, 20, 553, 1971.

165. Kato, R., Chiesara, E., and Vassanelli, P., Factors influencing induction of hepatic microsomal drug-metabolizing enzymes, *Biochem. Pharmacol.*, 11, 211, 1962.

166. Essig, C., Barbiturate dependence, in *Drug Dependence, Advances in Mental Science*, Vol. 2, Harris, R. T., McIsaac, W. M., and Schuster, C. R., Eds., University of Texas Press, Austin, Texas, 1970, 129.

167. Rubin, E. and Lieber, C. S., Alcoholism, alcohol, and drugs, *Science*, 172, 1097, 1971.

168. Tewari, S. and Noble, E. P., Ethanol and brain protein synthesis, *Brain Res.*, 26, 469, 1971.

169. Kuriyama, K., Sze, P. Y., and Rauscher, G. E., Effects of acute and chronic ethanol administration on ribosomal protein synthesis in mouse brain and liver, *Life Sci.*, 10, 181, 1971.

170. Goldstein, D. B. and Pal, N., Alcohol dependence produced in mice by inhalation of ethanol: grading the withdrawal reaction, *Science*, 172, 288, 1971.

171. Gallego, A., On the effect of ethyl alcohol upon frog nerve, *J. Cell. Comp. Physiol.*, 31, 97, 1948.

172. Seeman, P., Kwant, W. O., Goldberg, M., and Chau-Wong, M., The effects of ethanol and chlorpromazine on the passive membrane permeability to Na^+, *Biochim. Biophys. Acta*, 241, 349, 1971.

173. Radouco-Thomas, S., Cellular and molecular aspects of transmitter release: Calcium/monoamine dynamics, *Advances in Cytopharmacology*, 1st Intl. Sympos. Cell Biol. and Cytopharmacol., Clementi, F. and Ceccarelli, B., Eds., Raven Press, New York, 1971, 457.

174. Israel, A. and Kuriyama, K., Effect of *in vivo* ethanol administration on adenosinetriphosphatase activity of subcellular fractions of mouse brain and liver, *Life Sci.*, 10, 591, 1971.

175. Davis, E., Walsh, M. J., and Yamanaka, Y., Augmentation of alkaloid formation from dopamine by alcohol and acetaldehyde *in vitro, J. Pharmacol. Exp. Ther.*, 174, 401, 1970.

176. Seevers, M. H., Morphine and ethanol physical dependence: A critique of a hypothesis, *Science*, 170, 1113, 1970.

177. Davis, V. E. and Walsh, M. J., Morphine and ethanol physical dependence: A critique of a hypothesis, *Science*, 170, 1114, 1970.

178. Goldstein, A. and Judson, B., Alcohol dependence and opiate dependence: Lack of relationship in mice, *Science*, 172, 290, 1971.

179. Heikkilä, R., Cohen, G., and Dembiec, D., Tetrahydroisoquinoline alkaloids: Uptake by rat brain homogenate and inhibition of catecholamine uptake, *J. Pharmacol. Exp. Ther.*, 179, 250, 1971.

180. Somjen, G. G., Effects of ether and thiopental on spinal presynaptic terminals, *J. Pharmacol. Exp. Ther.*, 140, 396, 1963.

DISPOSITION AND METABOLISM OF DRUGS OF DEPENDENCE

A. L. Misra

TABLE OF CONTENTS

INTRODUCTION

In the last 15 years considerable work has been done on the basic principles underlying the absorption, distribution, and fate of drugs in the body. Developments in this area of investigation have underscored the importance of lipid solubility, ionization constant, and protein binding as important determinants of drug dynamics.[1-11] Penetration into and the exit of drugs from the central nervous system are also governed by these factors and filtration and active transport are important in preventing the accumulation of drugs within the central nervous system.[12-14] Factors other than the distribution coefficient and ionization constant, notably solubility in water, rate of dissolution, physical form, and state of subdivision of drugs administered as crystalline solids may be important, if not actually rate-determining in the oral absorption process.[9,15] Excretion of many drugs from the body may occur via alimentary tract, lungs, or kidney. Glomerular filtration, passive tubular reabsorption of the lipid-soluble unionized form of drugs, and active tubular secretion of the ionized moiety are the main processes involved in the renal excretion of drugs. The passage of drugs across the lipid-like placental barrier has come into sharp focus due to the recent recognition of teratogenic effect of some drugs ingested by the mother on the fetus.[16-18] The rate and/or the course of metabolism of many drugs[19] can be influenced by route of administration,[20] species,[21,22] strain,[23-25] age,[26] sex,[21,27] nutritional state, state of health,[26] hormones,[28] and various other chemicals. The marked induction of liver microsomal enzymes with certain drugs, hormones, insecticides, and carcinogens has important pharmacological consequences, for it leads to an accelerated biotransformation of drugs in vivo and can be an important factor in altering the duration and intensity of drug action in animals and man.[29,30]

Development of highly sensitive analytical techniques (gas and thin layer chromatography, spectrophotofluorometry, mass spectrometry, nuclear magnetic resonance, and radioisotope methodology) for the estimation of submicrogram quantities of drugs and their metabolites in biological materials has considerably extended the scope of many studies on drug dynamics and aided in the accumulation of important information on the biological disposition of drugs of dependence. The purpose of this chapter is to review the present status of our knowledge on the biological disposition and metabolism of narcotic agonists and antagonists, barbiturates, some nonbarbiturate sedative-hypnotics, tranquilizers, and ethanol. Some information on physicochemical characteristics and dosage of drugs pertinent to this presentation has also been included. The older literature on morphine and its surrogates and barbiturates which has been covered in excellent detail in earlier reviews cited in the text, has been incorporated in a condensed form for the sake of continuity of discussion.

DISPOSITION AND METABOLISM OF NARCOTIC AGONISTS AND ANTAGONISTS

Morphine

Chemical Properties and Dosage

Morphine was first isolated by Sertürner in 1803. It constitutes approximately 8 to 12% by weight of opium depending on the geographical source. Its structural formula was proposed in 1925[31] and confirmed by total synthesis in 1952 and 1956.[32a,b] The levo isomer D(-) is responsible for the pharmacological activity, the *d*-isomer L(+) being inactive (Figure 1). The crystalline morphine monohydrate base m. 254 to 256°C has a pK_a 8.02 to 8.05. Morphine sulfate is a fine crystalline odorless solid with a bitter taste. It is easily soluble in water and the pH of aqueous saturated solutions is 4.3 to 5.0. The olive oil/buffer (pH 7.4) partition coefficient of morphine is 0.4. A recent report[33] describes an interaction of morphine and sodium bisulfite in aqueous solution to form a sulfonic acid derivative of dihydromorphinone. The usual analgesic dose of morphine by subcutaneous injection is 8 to 15 mg, 8 to 20 mg orally, and 2.5 to 15 mg by slow intravenous injection.

The structural features[34] common to potent morphine group of analgesics were (1) a tertiary basic function in which at least one of the groups linked to nitrogen is relatively small, (2) a central carbon atom with none of its valency bonds linked to hydrogen, (3) a phenyl group or a group isosteric with phenyl connected to the central carbon atom, and (4) a two carbon chain separating the central carbon atom from nitrogen

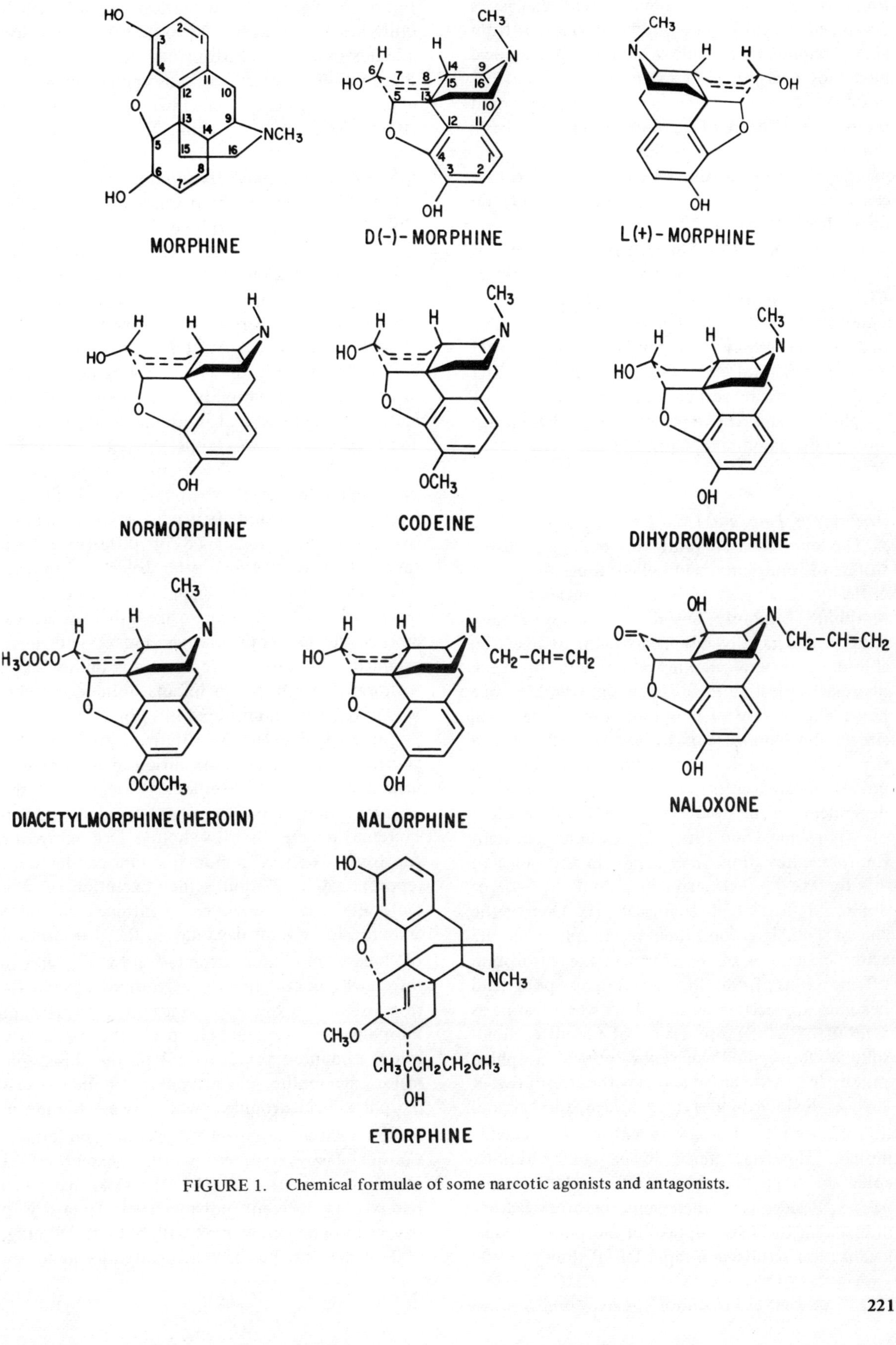

FIGURE 1. Chemical formulae of some narcotic agonists and antagonists.

for maximum activity. Some potent analgesics developed recently have shown deviations from above requirements and work on topographical model of analgesic drug-receptor interaction has emphasized the stereochemical aspects and presence of hydrophobic groups containing a basic center with an overall optimum spatial arrangement.[35,36] The substitutions in the basic center can confer agonistic or antagonistic properties on the molecule.

A close correlation between lipid solubility of morphine-like analgesics and their rate of onset of effect (tooth-pulp test) following intraventricular administration has recently been reported.[37] The analgesic efficiency was found to be a good approximation for the "receptor-activities." The evidence underscored the importance of lipophilicity and passive penetration of these drugs through the blood-brain barrier.[37]

Absorption, Fate, and Excretion

The enormous literature on biological disposition of morphine and allied drugs has been critically analyzed in classical reviews.[38-44] Morphine is poorly absorbed on oral administration and rapidly disappears from its injection site on parenteral administration with the peak pharmacological effects appearing within one hour. The passage of morphine from its injection site to the blood occurs by passive diffusion and the base penetrates the tissue as lipid-soluble unionized molecules. The absorption rate is dependent on the lipid-water partition coefficient of morphine and its dissociation constant (morphine-like drugs have a pK_a in the range of 7.5 to 9.0,[45a,b] corresponding to 2 to 14% of unionized drug at physiological pH). Due to the almost complete ionization of morphine in the acidic conditions of the stomach, the absorption of morphine from the stomach is poor and becomes appreciable only in the lower intestine as a result of greater proportion of unionized lipid-soluble form. Following absorption, morphine rapidly leaves the blood and penetrates into tissues such as the kidney, liver, lung, spleen, adrenals and thyroid, and to a lesser extent in the skeletal muscle. However, much lower concentrations enter the brain due to a significant blood-brain barrier. Besides pK_a, there must be other factors influencing the tissue uptake of morphine. Tissue localization results in a rapid fall of drug concentration in plasma and tissue levels of drug fall to quite low values within 24 to 48 hours after drug administration. In experimental animals the gross distribution pattern of morphine was not appreciably altered by treatment with vasopressin, ACTH,[46,47] or neostigmine,[48,49] but adrenalectomy which affected the sensitivity of response to morphine in animals, resulted in increased tissue levels of morphine without impairing the animals' ability to conjugate morphine.[50]

Neonatal rats showed increased brain permeability and consequently increased susceptibility to morphine compared to the adult animals.[51] The blood-brain barrier to morphine developed approximately 16 days after birth in rats.[52] In contrast to the rat, the guinea pig exhibited little difference in susceptibility to morphine with age and the brain uptake of morphine in neonate and adult guinea pig was approximately the same, possibly due to the development at birth of a blood-brain barrier to morphine as a result of a long gestation period. It was concluded that the susceptibility or resistance of different animal species to narcotics may often be related to drug dynamics rather than changes in sensitivity of receptor sites.[53] Morphine, like other analgesics, crosses the placental barrier and is known to produce respiratory depression, miosis, and withdrawal syndrome in infants born to mothers who have been administered this drug.[16]

Although detailed quantitative information on absorption and tissue distribution of morphine in man is not available, studies[54,55] show that the major portion of morphine and its metabolites is excreted in the first 24 hours; free morphine constitutes only a minor fraction of the dose (approximately 7%) in urine. Excretion of free morphine may, however, continue in trace amounts for several days due to the reabsorption of biliary morphine excreted into the gastrointestinal tract. Biliary excretion is chiefly responsible for the appearance of 7 to 10% of morphine in feces. Excretion via the pulmonary route accounted for 3 to 6% of the dose. The major metabolite of morphine in humans is morphine-3-glucuronide, which was found in highest concentration in gall bladder and kidney. Considerable variation in the excretion of morphine-3-glucuronide (11 to 45%) has been observed in different individuals and from day to day in the same individual. With ^{14}C-labeled drug, 70% of the dose has been accounted for in human urine as morphine and morphine-3-glucuronide. Species and sex differences in the metabolism of morphine have been reported earlier.[42]

A relatively good correlation between analgesia and peak concentration of morphine has been reported in the rat. Autoradiographic studies of brain sections of rats injected with ^{14}C-labeled morphine showed concentrations of radioactivity in vascular choroid plexus and ventricles, rather than in the neural elements of the brain.[56] Following intraventricular and intracerebral injections of ^{14}C-morphine (10 to 50 μg) in rat brain, the autoradiographic distribution pattern of drug was found to depend both on the diffusion and binding of drug with neuronal elements.[57] Duration of analgesia and drug levels, however, did not correlate very well in guinea pigs.[58] Intracellular distribution studies[59] with ^{3}H-morphine in nontolerant and tolerant guinea pigs showed that the major portion of the drug was localized in the microsomal supernatant fraction of both brain and liver and not bound significantly to brain nerve endings or synaptic vesicles. Neither the antagonism of pharmacologic effects of morphine nor the precipitated abstinence by nalorphine and tolerance development to morphine, altered the intracellular localization of ^{3}H-morphine in brain and liver. The study[59,60] on regional distribution of morphine-*N*-methyl ^{14}C in the central nervous system of nontolerant and tolerant dogs showed somewhat lower levels of drug in the CNS of tolerant animals compared to those in nontolerant animals at time intervals higher than four hours. The administration of nalorphine after morphine resulted in a significant increase (25 to 42%) in the CNS levels of morphine in nontolerant dogs. In tolerant dogs, nalorphine-precipitated abstinence resulted in a significant decrease (42 to 56%) in the CNS levels of morphine at one hour and no change at three or four hours after administration. No evidence for the existence of any radioactive metabolite of morphine in the CNS of nontolerant and tolerant dogs was provided by these studies.[61,62] These regional distribution studies in nontolerant and tolerant dogs using sensitive isotopic techniques and earlier studies in dogs,[63,64] monkeys,[65] rabbits,[66] rats,[67] and guinea pigs have not demonstrated marked differences of sufficient magnitude to explain the high degree of tolerance observed in animals. Unfortunately, no definitive information on specific sites of localization of morphine within the matrix of the central nervous system or events occurring at these sites during antagonism with nalorphine and development of central receptor tolerance has been obtained from these comprehensive regional distribution studies. A comparison of the regional distribution of morphine in cat brain with that in dog apparently did not show any consistent differences which could account for the delirious excitement and mania commonly observed in cats, in contrast to the depressant effect in dogs after morphine administration.[68]

More recent work[69] on the kinetics of distribution of morphine in the rat brain has provided evidence that at all periods of time up to 3 weeks or more after a single s.c. 10mg/kg injection of morphine-*N*-methyl-^{14}C, there was consistently higher radioactivity in the brain than could be accounted for on the basis of free morphine alone. Measurable and significant amounts of drug were present as polar "conjugated" drug, and part of the radioactivity due to this polar metabolite up to two hours after injection of drug could be acid-hydrolyzed to free morphine, but at later time periods, the "conjugate" was not hydrolyzed with dilute acid. Thin layer chromatographic study of pooled rat brain extracts reinforced the evidence of the presence of two polar metabolites. The postulated formation of a catechol (or quinonoid) type of polar metabolite of morphine in the CNS which could become an essential substrate in an alternative pathway of metabolism due to its close similarity to epinephrine, its covalent binding to target protein to bring about a biochemical alteration in specific neuronal structure in the CNS, and its implications in the development of tolerance to morphine has been outlined in this report. Development of sensitive methods for the estimation of morphine-*N*-methyl-^{14}C-oxide[70] and ^{3}H-pseudomorphine[71] from biological materials has provided evidence that these are not the metabolites of morphine in the CNS of rats and pseudomorphine is not responsible for or associated with the agonistic actions of morphine, the phenomena of tolerance, and/or physical dependence.

Choroid plexus[72,73] and rat brain slices[74] have been shown to take up morphine by an active transport mechanism. A similar type of process intricately linked to Na^{+}, K^{+}-active ATPase system has also been shown to be involved in the removal of morphine from the rabbit cerebral ventricles.[75] Such a transport by choroid plexus could serve to remove morphine and allied drugs from the brain and the çerebrospinal fluid.

The in vitro active uptake and tissue binding of morphine have been shown to occur in the specific CNS structures of rat such as nuclei, mitochondria, and synaptosomes and this accumulation and heterogenous distribution depended on the metabolic state of the particular area or structure.[76] Recent study on the failure to saturate the transport system in rat cerebral cortical slices in concentration ranges likely to be encountered in vivo and the inability of glucose-substrate and metabolic inhibitors to depress the uptake has furnished evidence that an active transport mechanism of analgesics in rat cerebral cortical slices is not involved.[77] Lipophilicity, passive diffusion, and physicochemical binding of drug to brain tissue protein or intracellular constituent could explain its accumulation without the need for invoking the concept of active transport.[69]

Morphine and allied drugs have been recently reported to be preferentially localized in the synaptosomal fraction of rat brain in vitro and in vivo and the extent of binding and exact localization depended upon the pH and the presence of divalent ions. Neither this localization nor its loss on particle rupture was reversed by the administration of antagonists or by tolerance development.[78]

Although the exact site of analgesic action of morphine is not known, the studies by intracerebral microinjection technique showed the central gray matter surrounding the third ventricle to be an area most sensitive to morphine in respect of painthreshold to thermal stimulus.[79] The anterior thalamus appeared to be the site essential for hyperactivity induced by morphine in the rat.[80]

Biotransformation of Morphine

The different pathways for the metabolism of morphine are as follows:

Conjugation with glucuronic acid – Glucuronide conjugation of morphine at position 3 is the major route for the detoxication of morphine in several mammalian species[42] with the exception of the cat and chicken. The synthesis of morphine-3-glucuronide requires uridine diphosphate (UDPG), a liver supernatant dehydrogenase, DPN, and microsomal transferase to transfer glucuronic acid moiety from UDPGA to morphine. Minor glucuronide conjugation at position 6 (0.3% of the dose) has recently been reported in the rabbit,[81] in the dog,[82] (2 to 4% of the dose) and in the rat and mice.[83,84] Morphine 3- and 6-glucuronides have also been synthesized.[85] The glucuronyl transferase activity of the liver microsomes has been shown to decrease on chronic morphine treatment and tolerance development in male rats.[86-88] Treatment with chloroquine has been reported to produce higher levels of morphine-3-glucuronide in rat liver.[89] Pargyline was capable of both decreasing and increasing morphine glucuronide formation in vitro.[90] No significant difference was observed in in vitro conjugation of morphine by liver microsomes of adult Wistar rats and Gunn rats, a mutant strain lacking UDP-glucuronyl transferase activity towards bilirubin. It was concluded that for substances forming ether type of glucuronides, there were a number of UDP-glucuronyl transferase enzymes of relatively high substrate specificity.[91]

Ethereal sulfate conjugation – This conjugation has been shown to be a major metabolic pathway for the metabolism of morphine in the cat and the chicken.[92-95]

***N*-demethylation** – Oxidative *N*-demethylation of morphine has been demonstrated in vitro[96,97] and in vivo[98-102] in the rat and the cat.[95,103] *N*-dealkylation of morphine in vitro has been studied in kinetic analysis of substrate competition[104] and diminished capacity of liver enzymes of tolerant rats to *N*-demethylate morphine has been shown to be due to the reduced availability of microsomal enzymes rather than to an alteration in enzyme structure.[105] Tolerance development did not seem to make any difference in the *N*-demethylation of labeled morphine in whole animals as measured by the rate of pulmonary excretion of $^{14}CO_2$ [106] Chronic morphine treatment produced a substantial decrease in liver microsomal drug metabolizing enzymes in male rats,[107] and an increase in the activity of liver microsomal enzymes catalyzing the *N*-demethylation of morphine and other analgesics has been reported by treatment with inducer drugs such as phenobarbital.[108-112] The significance of *N*-dealkylation of narcotic analgesics to the mechanism of analgesia or the development of tolerance has been critically analyzed in a recent review[43] and several lines of evidence have suggested that *N*-dealkylation of narcotic analgesics need not necessarily be involved in initiation of analgesia.

***O*-methylation** – The conversion of morphine to codeine has been reported[113] in a strain of rats deficient in liver microsomal glucuronide conjugation ability. Incubation of morphine with rat liver homogenates in the presence of *S*-adenosylmethionine did not lead to the formation of codeine indicating that some other methyl donor must presumably be involved in in vivo conversion of morphine to codeine.

Catechol-type biotransformation – In vitro conversion of some phenolic compounds including morphine to catechol type of derivatives has been reported by rat liver microsomes in the presence of NADP, glucose-6-phosphate, catechol *O*-methyl transferase, and *S*-adenosylmethionine.[114] These derivatives were subsequently methylated. The reported yield with morphine as substrate was much lower compared to other phenols. Conversion of morphine to a catechol (or quinonoid) type of derivative has recently been postulated to occur in rat brain in vivo.[69]

***N*-oxide formation** – The biotransformation of morphine to its *N*-oxide has not been reported in normal circumstances. However, *N*-oxide has been shown to be a urinary metabolite in cancer patients treated with combinations of morphine, 2,4-diamino-5-phenyl thiazole or 1,2,3,4-tetrahydro-9-aminoacridine,[115] possibly through the inhibition of major metabolic pathway or the inhibition of breakdown of *N*-oxide by the thiazole or acridine derivative. Formation of *N*-oxides of tertiary amines as intermediates or as an alternative pathway in oxidative *N*-dealkylation of drugs has previously been postulated.[116,117] *N*-oxide was not detected as a metabolite of morphine in the rat brain.[70]

Oxidation of morphine to pseudomorphine – In vitro oxidation of morphine under aerobic conditions by rat liver homogenates fortified with cytochrome C to a compound chromatographically indistinguishable from pseudomorphine has been reported,[118] but attempts to establish its presence in vivo after morphine administration have not been successful. A recent study has shown that pseudomorphine is not a metabolite of morphine in rat brain.[71]

Trans-*N*-methylation – Trans-*N*-methylation apparently does not play a significant role in the metabolism of morphine.[119]

Normorphine

Chemical Properties and Dosage

Normorphine was first synthesized[120] in 1914. The colorless crystalline base, a hemihydrate, and its water-soluble hydrochloride melt at 273°C and 305°C (decomp.), respectively. It is a weaker agonist than morphine in analgesic potency and addiction liability[121,122] and approximately twice as toxic as morphine on intraperitoneal injection in mouse.[123,124] Normorphine gained prominence due to its implication in the initiation of analgesia and tolerance development to morphine.[96,125]

Absorption, Fate, and Excretion

The biotransformation of morphine to normorphine in vitro and in vivo[99-101] in the rat has also been shown to occur in the brain of rats. Following administration of a 2 mg/kg subcutaneous dose of ^{3}H-normorphine to dogs and monkeys, about 70% of the dose was accounted for in urine, 34 to 40% as free drug, and the rest as a conjugate.[126] A peak plasma level of 1 to 3 μg/ml was attained 15 to 30 minutes after injection and levels of conjugate peaked at 1 to 3 hours in both species. In monkeys, less free drug was found in urine and physical activity of the monkey determined to some extent the conjugation of drug appearing in the urine and also the duration of pharmacological response.[126,127] In monkeys, 22 to 39% of the dose was excreted in feces as free drug.

The concentration of normorphine in brain has been reported to be four to five times higher than the concentration of morphine when two drugs were administered in equianalgesic doses to the rats.[128,129]

The methylation of normorphine to morphine has been shown to occur in rat liver and brain in vitro[130,131] and in vivo[130,132] after intracisternal injection of normorphine and ^{14}C-methyl labeled methionine. Since no evidence for transmethylation or *N*-methylation as a metabolic pathway has been forthcoming, the significance of the above findings on very low conversion of normorphine to morphine (0.053%) would appear to be in doubt. The preparation of a partially purified *N*-methyl transferase from rat brain and liver requiring *S*-adenosyl methionine as a methyl donor has been reported[130,131] and a similar enzyme from rabbit lung has been shown to catalyze the transfer of methyl group of

S-adenosyl methionine to a variety of amines including normorphine in vitro.[132-134]

Codeine

Chemical Properties and Dosage

Codeine is prepared from morphine by methylation. It is present in opium from 0.7 to 2.5% depending on geographical source. The monohydrate base, a crystalline compound m. 154 to 156°C (pK_a 8.22, 8.55) is sparingly soluble in water, but readily in organic solvents. The olive oil/buffer pH 7.4 partition coefficient of codeine is 0.8. Codeine is much less potent than morphine on a weight basis as an analgesic and a respiratory depressant. Tolerance, physical dependence and cross-tolerance with other narcotic analgesics have been known to develop to codeine. In contrast to morphine, codeine is effective orally as an analgesic and antitussive presumably due to better absorption. Analgesic dose range of codeine phosphate is 15 to 60 mg, orally or subcutaneously (120 mg s.c. is equianalgesic to 10 mg morphine).

Absorption, Fate, and Excretion

The earlier work on the biological disposition of codeine has been exhaustively covered in previous reviews.[39,42] Following s.c. administration of 2 mg/kg dose of *N*-$^{14}CH_3$-codeine to the rat, 82% of the injected dose was recovered in urine, bile, feces, or by pulmonary route as $^{14}CO_2$.[135] Maximum levels of codeine and its metabolites in plasma and of free codeine in brain appeared 15 to 30 minutes after injection of the drug. Brain to plasma ratio of free codeine was 2:1.[135] The sex difference in the drug metabolizing enzymes of rat liver was shown by the excretion of 7.6% and 18.5% of injected radioactivity by female and male rats as $^{14}CO_2$ in expired air.[107,135] Approximately 2% of radioactivity was retained in the body of the rat 24 hours after injection. Peak concentrations of 0.68 μg/g of codeine in rat brain were achieved 40 minutes after the administration and declined to 0.08 μg/g at 2 hours. Peak concentrations of free drug in plasma at 15 minutes rapidly fell to 0.050 μg/ml at 2 hours. Free morphine derived from codeine in plasma appeared to maintain a sustained level of about 0.02 μg/ml through 2 hours; the conjugated morphine, however, declined from 0.09 μg/ml to 0.04 μg/ml at 2 hours. Neither free nor conjugated morphine was detected in the rat brain.

Most of the drug was excreted as morphine and morphine-3-glucuronide[136] with minor amounts of norcodeine and normorphine as reported earlier in rats and guinea pigs.[137] No evidence for the formation of codeine-6-glucuronide was obtained in the rat although this was isolated and characterized as a major metabolite of codeine in the dog[138] and presumably in man and other species.

Codeine required doses 100 times greater than that for morphine to elicit tail flick response to thermal stimulus after intraventricular injection in mice. It was concluded that morphine or normorphine must be the active compound responsible for the pharmacologic effect of codeine.[123] A similar conclusion was reached in studies in which brain levels of morphine and codeine were measured after the systemic administration of codeine to rats.[129] Evidence that codeine itself was the active drug was, however, provided by studies in which nalorphine provoked (a) withdrawal in codeine users and (b) pupil diameter change in codeine-treated dogs, a species in which biotransformation of codeine to morphine is not significant.[139]

Earlier findings[106] that *N*-demethylation of ^{14}C-labeled codeine as measured by pulmonary $^{14}CO_2$ increased in tolerant rats in contrast to that of morphine following morphine administration could not be confirmed.[140] *N*-demethylation of codeine in rats made tolerant to morphine by pellet implantation was reported to decrease significantly compared to nontolerant male rats, whereas in nontolerant female rats and mice and tolerant male mice it was unchanged.[140]

Codeine acted similarly to morphine as an inhibitor of liver drug metabolizing activity.[141] The kinetic study of *O*- and *N*-demethylation of codeine by liver microsomal enzymes requiring TPNH and molecular oxygen led to the postulate that different enzymes may be involved in demethylation at the *N*- and *O*- positions.[113]

Tolerance development to codeine did not appear to be related to an alteration of drug levels of codeine in rat brain.[67] The observed decrease in hepatic drug metabolizing enzyme activity in chronic codeine treated rats was nonspecific in nature. It was concluded that reduced conversion of codeine to morphine in codeine tolerant rats is probably a result rather than the cause of tolerance development.[109]

Dihydromorphine

Chemical Properties and Dosage

Dihydromorphine is prepared by the catalytic hydrogenation of morphine. The monohydrate colorless, crystalline base and the water-soluble hydrochloride (pK_a 8.55) melt at 157°C (decomp.) and 280°C, respectively. It is considered equipotent to morphine in analgesic activity.[142]

Absorption, Fate, and Excretion

The pattern of absorption, metabolism and excretion of dihydromorphine is very similar to that of morphine. Following a 5 mg/kg subcutaneous dose of ^{3}H-dihydromorphine in the rat, 85% of the dose could be accounted for in urine as free and conjugated drug after 92 hours with a minute fraction of dihydronormorphine in feces.[143] In a study by stop-flow analysis on the active excretion of free and conjugated drug by proximal portions of renal tubules of dog and monkey, the excretion pattern was not appreciably altered in tolerant monkeys or on administration of nalorphine.[144] A sex related difference was observed in the amount of conjugated dihydromorphine excreted in the rat; the females excreted twice as much conjugate as the males. Enzymic hydrolysis of conjugate with β-glucuronidase provided evidence of existence of other conjugates besides glucuronides. Pulmonary excretion studies with *N*-$^{14}CH_3$-dihydromorphine confirmed *N*-demethylation as a route of biotransformation in rats.[145] Male rats showed eightfold greater *N*-demethylation (3.7%) compared to female rats (0.5%) and chronic treatment of rats with dihydromorphine decreased *N*-demethylation, which returned to control values 9 days after withdrawal of the drug.[145]

The pattern of regional distribution of ^{3}H-dihydromorphine[146] in the CNS of dogs was similar to that of morphine and rats injected subcutaneously with drug showed peak concentration in CNS, one hour after administration[147] and the drug level within the rat brain increased with increasing dosage. The differences in methods and techniques could account for the discrepancy[146,147] in quantitative distribution in CNS of dihydromorphine and morphine in dog and rat. Dihydromorphine crosses the placental barrier.[148]

The study on the maternal and fetal distribution of ^{3}H-dihydromorphine in tolerant and nontolerant rats[149] showed that the movement of dihydromorphine across the placental barrier is more rapid in tolerant than in control rats. The mobilization of drug from injection site in tolerant animals was also more rapid compared to nontolerant animals and the distribution of drug into maternal brain, fetal plasma, and fetal brain was more prompt compared to control rats, although the latter showed somewhat higher maternal plasma levels. A significant reduction in reproduction in rats was observed with chronic administration of dihydromorphine in high doses.[149]

Following administration of a sufficient dose of ^{3}H-dihydromorphine to block neuro effector transmission in vivo, the concentration of dihydromorphine in autonomic nervous tissue was similar to the concentration of morphine causing block in vitro.[150] The general pattern of uptake of ^{3}H-dihydromorphine (10 mg/kg, s.c.) in vivo in rat eye tissue was similar to that for brain and plasma levels; the peak values of total radioactivity (1.45 μg/g) at 1 hour declined to 168 ng/g 12 hours after injection. Evidence for biotransformation of dihydromorphine in eye tissue was not obtained in this study.[77]

Study on the intracellular distribution[151] of radioactivity in the brain and liver of rats injected intraperitoneally with 100 mg/kg dose of ^{3}H-dihydromorphine revealed the major portion of the drug (70%) in soluble supernatant fraction and 15 to 20% of radioactivity of the homogenate in brain nuclear fraction. Nalorphine did not affect the tissue levels, intracellular distribution, and binding of dihydromorphine to liver, brain homogenates and serum proteins. The degree of binding in different tissues of nontolerant and tolerant rats was similar suggesting that most, if not all, of the observed binding was nonspecific.[151]

Dihydromorphine has been shown to be accumulated by rabbit choroid plexus[73] and by rat, mouse, rabbit, and monkey cerebral cortical slices against an apparent concentration gradient at least in part by an active transport process.[74] A subsequent study showed that in concentration ranges likely to be encountered in vivo, active transport mechanism of dihydromorphine in cerebral cortical slices is not involved and lipophilicity, passive diffusion and physicochemical binding of the drug to brain tissue protein or intracellular constituent could explain its accumulation without the need for invoking the concept of active transport.[77] Recent work[37] has further underscored the importance of lipophilicity and passive penetration of morphine-like analgesics through the blood-brain barrier and no criteria were found which could be in accord with a special importance of an active transport through this barrier. Furthermore, the active transport of narcotic analgesics into nervous tissue is not the determining factor in the action of these drugs.[152]

Further extension of subcellular fractionation studies revealed that ^{3}H-dihydromorphine was accumulated in vitro primarily by rat brain synaptosomal fraction (nerve endings) of homogenates of cerebral cortex by a metabolically dependent process[153,154] and it was speculated that the norepinephrine transport system of synaptosomes may be involved since dihydromorphine inhibited the uptake of norepinephrine by synaptosomes. The particles derived from osmotic shock exhibited a higher concentration of ^{3}H-dihydromorphine than did the other subcellular fractions of the brain in vitro.[155] Nalorphine in large concentration reduced the uptake of drug by all fractions to the same degree. Subcellular fractions from brains of nontolerant and tolerant rats showed no significant difference in the uptake of drug. This uptake by nerve endings was attributed to a binding phenomenon with active transport process providing the drug an access to the binding sites in intact tissue. It was concluded that the biological significance of uptake of analgesics by nerve endings is not yet clear since the observations do not throw light on the basis of analgesia, tolerance, and physical dependence to this drug.[155]

Heroin (3,6-Diacetyl Morphine)

Chemical Properties and Dosage

Heroin was first prepared in 1874 by acetylation of morphine. The colorless crystalline compound m. 173°C (pK_a, 7.83) has a characteristic bitter taste. It is sparingly soluble in water, but readily in organic solvents. On prolonged exposure to air, it turns light pink and emits odor of acetic acid due to hydrolysis. The water-soluble hydrochloride melts at 243 to 244°C. Heroin has been estimated to be two to ten times as potent as morphine depending on experimental measurement technique for analgesia or euphoria[156,157] and has very high addiction liability. A subcutaneous dose of 3 mg is equianalgesic to 10 mg of morphine.

Absorption, Fate, and Excretion

In all species including the human, heroin is promptly absorbed by parenteral routes producing systemic effects within a couple of minutes. Oral and sublingual administration, however, produces erratic and irregular absorption with a delayed onset of action. Heroin is rapidly hydrolyzed to 6-monoacetylmorphine and to a lesser extent to morphine by homogenates of liver, kidney, brain, and blood of rats, mice, dogs, rabbits, and man in vitro and in vivo.[158–160]

Following intrapoplital injection of 75 mg/kg in the rat, the peak level of drug (0.9 μg/g) was attained in brain 15 minutes after injection which declined to barely detectable levels in 60 minutes. The peak level of its deacetylation product, 6-monoacetylmorphine in brain was 6.3 μg/g 15 minutes after injection, which declined to 1.9 μg/g at 2 hour period. The peak levels of morphine derived from heroin (1.8 μg/g) were, however, sustained for about 2 hours. In mouse, following an intravenous injection of 37.5 mg/kg, the levels of heroin, 6-monoacetylmorphine and morphine in brain at 2.5 minutes were 8.2, 23, and less than 2 μg/g, respectively. At 7.5 minutes heroin was barely detectable in brain, but morphine concentrations reached a peak (5 μg/g) at 15 to 30 minutes after injection and a drop in level of 6-monoacetylmorphine to morphine levels was also noticed during this time. It was concluded that the pharmacologic effects of heroin are mediated primarily by 6-monoacetylmorphine and morphine.[53,162]

Early studies[163] on metabolic fate of heroin in addicts showed free morphine (6%) and morphine conjugate (47.2%) as urinary metabolites. More sensitive methods have also shown the presence in urine of small amounts of 6-monoacetylmorphine.[160]

Etorphine [Tetrahydro-7 α-(1-hydroxy-1-methyl butyl)-6,14,endo-etheno oripavine]

Chemical Properties and Dosage

Etorphine, one of the more active of a number of derivatives of 6,14-endo-etheno tetrahydro oripavine, was synthesized in 1963.[164] The free base and the hydrochloride melt at 215° and 266 to 267°C, respectively. It is one of the most potent analgesics described to date. Given subcutaneously it was 1000 to 80,000 times more potent than morphine, depending on test situation and species studied.[165] Its ability to cause catatonia at very low dose levels has resulted in its use for immobilizing wild and domestic animals.[166] The analgesic potency as measured by the minimal analgesic dose is 2 μg/kg i.v., 2.5 μg/kg i.m., and 5 to 10 μg/kg sublingually.

Absorption, Fate and Excretion

Etorphine rapidly passed from intramuscular injection sites and across the buccal mucosa into systemic circulation and was relatively much more effective than morphine after sublingual administration.[167] Etorphine was taken up selectively by rat brain tissue and against the brain-blood concentration gradient. Following intramuscular administration (12 μg/kg), etorphine was taken up by maternal and fetal rat brain tissue with such avidity that the concentration found was above that of circulating blood even ten minutes after the administration of drug. The concentration of etorphine ten minutes after the administration in maternal blood had almost reached a maximum with a plateau maintained for one hour after which clearance from the blood appeared to be fairly rapid. The level of etorphine in fetal rat brain reached a peak 30 minutes after injection into mothers. The lipophilic character of etorphine (partition coefficient carbon tetrachlororide/buffer pH 7.3 of 20 compared to dihydromorphine 7) undoubtedly favored some degree of selective uptake into the CNS and contributed in part to its very high potency. The rate of transfer of etorphine across the placental barrier and its accumulation in fetal brain were shown to be much faster than those of dihydromorphine.[168]

The ED_{50} for analgesia with etorphine in rats by subcutaneous route was found to be 1.7 μg/kg. Etorphine was approximately 5000 times more potent than morphine as a depressant of respiratory rate in rabbits.[169] Nalorphine readily antagonized the central depression due to etorphine.[165]

Nalorphine (*N*-allyl normorphine)

Chemical Properties and Dosage

Nalorphine was synthesized in 1941.[170,171] The colorless crystalline base and its water-soluble hydrochloride (pK_a, 7.83) melt at 208 to 209°C, and 269°C (decomp.), respectively. It is an effective antagonist against a wide variety of potent analgesics structurally related to morphine. It also has a weak agonist activity[172] and produces a type of physical dependence not characterized by drug-seeking behavior.[173] Dose of hydrochloride i.v., i.m., or s.c. as antagonist is 5 to 10 mg and approximately 3 mg in diagnostic test for physical dependence.

Absorption, Fate, and Excretion

The pharmacology of nalorphine has been adequately reviewed.[174-176] Nalorphine is much more rapidly absorbed from subcutaneous sites[177] compared to morphine. Following administration of a 30 mg/kg subcutaneous dose to dogs, the levels of free and conjugated nalorphine in plasma 20 minutes after injection were 11 to 12 μg/ml compared to 6 to 7 μg/ml at the same time with same dose of morphine. The maximum plasma levels of free and conjugated drug amounted to 5 μg/ml and 20 μg/ml, respectively, at 20 to 60 minutes after injection. The biologic halflife of free drug in plasma was 1.5 to 2 hours, that of conjugated drug, 2.5 hours. The concentrations of free and conjugated drug in most tissues were lower than for morphine at the same dose. Nalorphine penetrated the brain tissue more rapidly and in three to fourfold greater concentration as compared to morphine at 90 minutes after injection. Likewise, the rate of egress of nalorphine from dog brain was much faster than morphine.[178] When administered together with morphine, nalorphine did not affect the gross concentrations of morphine in the brain.[178]

The conjugation of nalorphine took place more completely and quickly than that for morphine in the dog. Following administration of 2 mg/kg of ^{3}H-nalorphine[179] to dogs, the values for plasma halflife were similar to those reported earlier.[177] Eighty-one to ninety percent of the dose could be accounted for in urine of which 2 to 6% was free drug and 79 to 84% the conjugated drug. Peak levels of 1.12 and 1.15 μg/g were attained in cerebral cortical gray matter at 30 and 60 minutes, respectively, which declined to 0.062 μg/g at 2 hours. The corresponding levels of drug in cerebral white matter at 30 and 60 minutes were 0.80 and 0.99 μg/g which declined to 0.131 μg/g at 2 hours.[179]

Nalorphine is dealkylated to normorphine in vitro by rat liver microsomes[180] and in the brain of living rats.[101] Conjugation in vitro by liver slices has been reported.[181] Nalorphine did not modify in vitro the capacity of mouse brain homogenates to take up or retain morphine.[182]

Nalorphine-3-ethereal sulfate and 3-glucuronide have been isolated and characterized as chief metabolites of nalorphine in cat and rabbit.[183] The major metabolite in dog was nalorphine-3-glucuronide with minor amounts of 6-glucuronide, and in cat small amounts of nalorphine-3-glucuronide were also present along with 3-ethereal sulfate.[184] Synthesis of nalorphine 3- and 6-glucuronides has also been reported recently.[185]

Intracisternally administered nalorphine was found to be much less effective in mice in antagonizing morphine than when given systemically.[186] In mice made tolerant to morphine by pellet implantation, intraventricularly administered nalorphine produced minimal signs of withdrawal providing suggestive evidence that nalorphine itself may not be the "active" antagonist.[187]

Naloxone (*N*-allyl-7,8-dihydro-14-hydroxy normorphine)

Chemical Properties and Dosage

Naloxone is a potent antagonist with little or no agonist activity.[188,189] It is approximately 10 to 30 times as potent as nalorphine and has been proposed in treatment of opiate dependence.[190] The colorless crystalline compound and its water-soluble hydrochloride melt at 184°C and 200 to 205°C, respectively.

Absorption, Fate, and Excretion

Quantitative information on absorption and metabolic fate of naloxone is not available but studies on human pharmacology and abuse potential[191] have shown that it does not produce physical dependence. Naloxone-3-glucuronide has been shown to be a major urinary metabolite in rabbits and humans. In addition to this metabolite, *N*-allyl-14-hydroxy-7,8-dihydro-normorphine-3-glucuronide was isolated and characterized as a metabolite in chicken.[192,193] Cats, however, metabolize it principally to naloxone-3-ethereal sulfate.[194]

Levorphanol (*l*-3-hydroxy-*N*-methyl morphinan)

Chemical Properties and Dosage

The racemic compound, Racemorphan (*dl*-Dromoran), was synthesized in 1949[195a] and its *l*-isomer in 1951.[195b] The *l*-isomer D(-) (Figure 2) is a potent analgesic having twice the activity of the racemate.[196] The *d*-isomer lacks analgesic activity and addiction liability. Levorphanol tartrate is a water-soluble, colorless crystalline compound m. 113 to 115° (anhydrous 206 to 208°C). The free base m. 198 to 199°C has a pK_a, 8.18. Oral or s.c. analgesic dose is 2 to 3 mg; intravenous 1.0 to 1.5 mg.

Absorption, Fate, and Excretion

Studies on biological disposition[197-200] in different species including humans, showed that levorphanol is rapidly absorbed, producing peak effects within one hour after subcutaneous and within 2 hours after oral administration. Following absorption, it rapidly leaves blood and localizes in the lung, spleen, kidney, liver, and heart and to a small extent in muscle and brain.[199] The biological halflife in dog was less than one hour. Slightly higher value (75 to 90 minutes) was reported for free levorphanol in dog and monkey in a subsequent study[200] using ^{14}C-labeled drug. Levorphanol is metabolized at a fairly rapid rate in dog and monkey, chiefly to a glucuronide conjugate.[198-200] In dog, 4.4% of the dose appeared as free drug and 42% as free and bound drug. In monkey, 2.5% appeared as free drug and 35% as conjugated drug. In both species, less than 0.1% of the dose was found in feces. In monkey, rat, and dog, 20, 5, and 1.5% of the dose, respectively, could be accounted for as $^{14}CO_2$ by pulmonary excretion.[200] Suggestive evidence for *N*-dealkylation[107] has also been obtained in vitro with liver microsomal enzymes of mice and rat, but not of dog. The *d* and *l*-isomers were metabolized with equal facility with hepatic enzymes in vitro.[201]

No statistical difference in levels of levorphanol was observed in cerebral cortical gray and white matter of nontolerant and tolerant monkey at 1 hour after s.c. injection of 2 mg/kg.[202] The simultaneous administration of levallorphan or nalorphine with levorphanol resulted in a reduction of cerebral cortical gray levels from 2.0 μg/g to 1.35 μg/g and cerebral cortical white levels from 1.3 μg/g to 0.66 μg/g.[203] This contrasted with the earlier results on rats where no difference in CNS

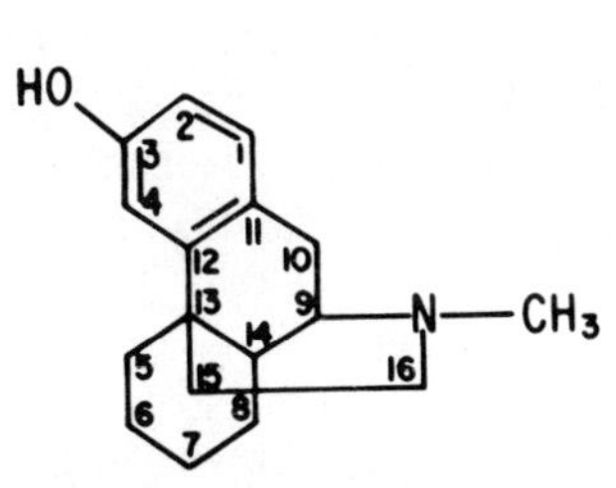

RACEMORPHAN
(planar structure)

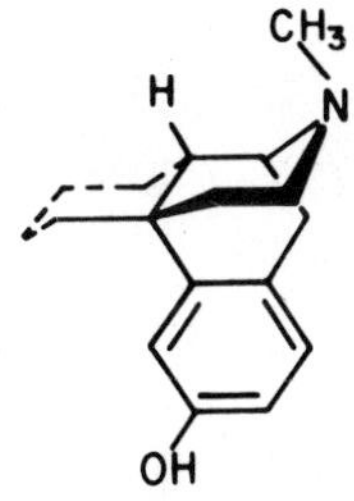

D(-)-LEVORPHANOL

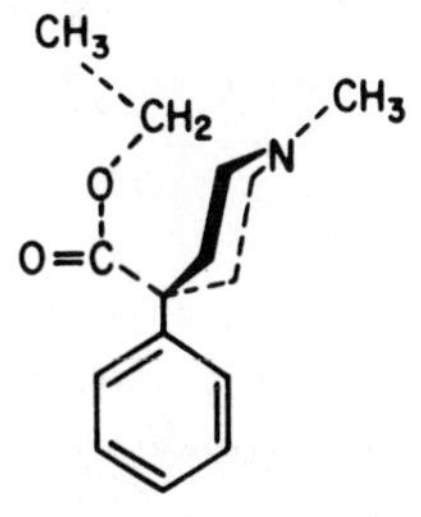

D(–)-MEPERIDINE

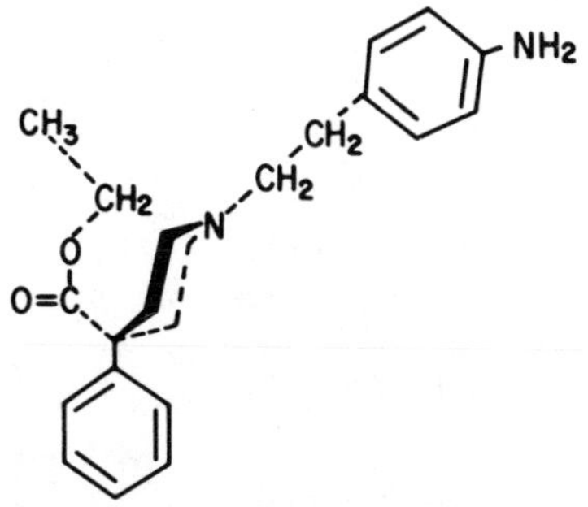

ANILERIDINE

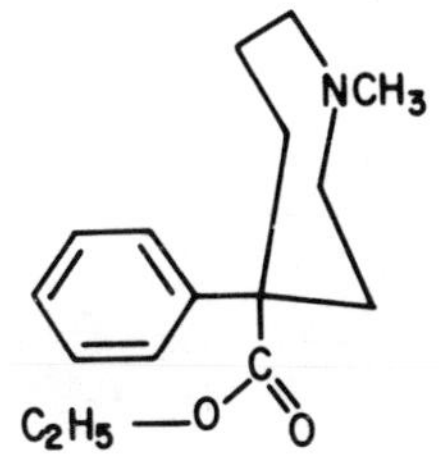

ETHOHEPTAZINE

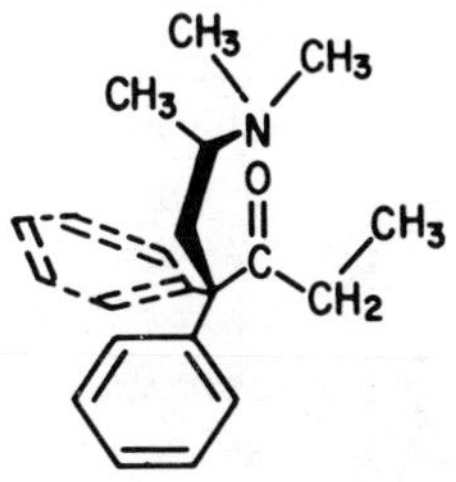

D(-)-METHADONE

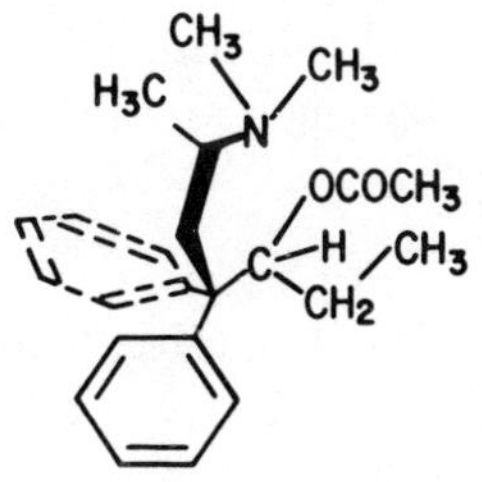

ACETYLMETHADOL

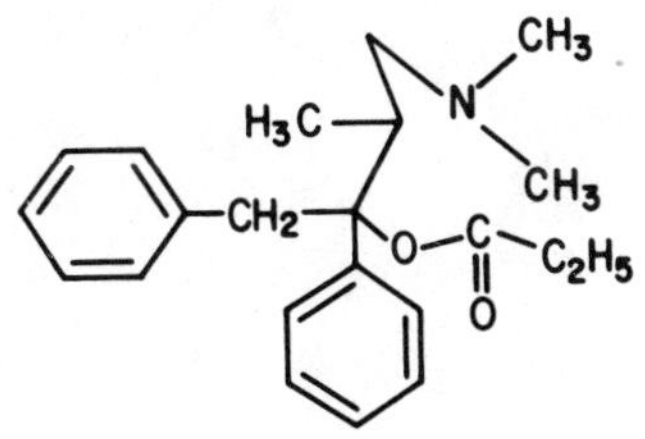

PROPOXYPHENE

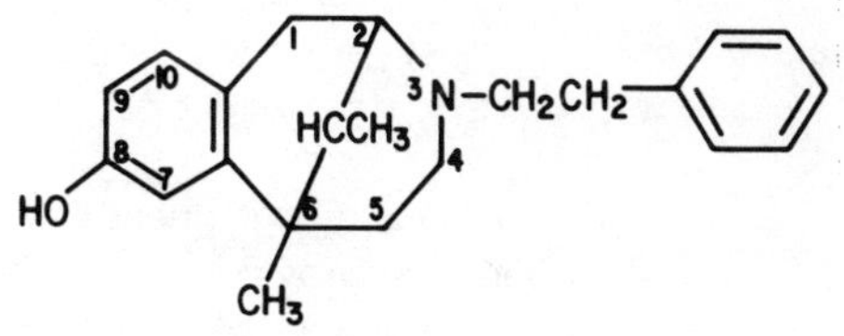

PHENAZOCINE

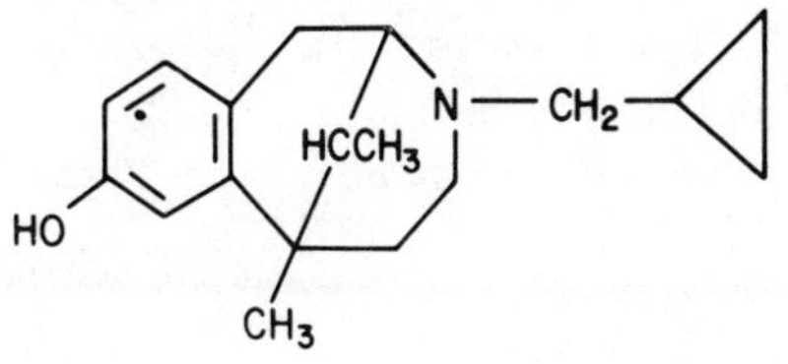

CYCLAZOCINE

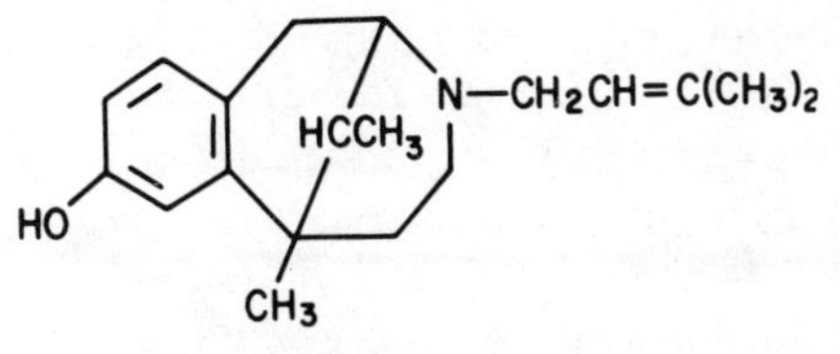

PENTAZOCINE

FIGURE 2. Chemical formulae of some narcotic agonists and antagonists.

levels of levorphanol were observed upon nalorphine administration.[204]

Study on the distribution of ^{14}C-levorphanol in subcellular fractions[205] of rat brain, liver, and kidney showed the highest concentration (69 to 82%) of the drug in soluble and microsomal fraction, intermediate in nuclear, and lowest in mitochondrial fraction. The first nuclear fraction from all three organs showed greater uptake in vivo than in vitro and bound levorphanol to a greater extent compared to those from liver and kidney. Autoradiography of liver and kidney sections showed uniform distribution throughout the liver, but decreasing amounts from cortex towards collecting ducts in kidneys.

Qualitatively similar excretion of free and bound drug (42 to 62%) was noticed for *dextro* and *levo* isomers. The two isomers were also excreted as conjugates at the same rate and the development of tolerance in dogs did not affect the excretion of free drug and its conjugate.[198,199]

In view of the fact that a large proportion of the drug has not been accounted for as known metabolites in biological species, the possibility exists that it must be metabolized by other metabolic pathways, e.g., oxidation.

The uptake of labeled levorphanol into the eye lenses and brains of mice was found to be similar to that in controls. It was concluded that tolerance to the lenticular effects of levorphanol actually may represent resistance or insensitivity to catechol cofactor (norepinephrine) rather than primarily to the narcotic drug.[206]

A typical pharmacologic effect in mice induced by the morphinan group of analgesics is the "running fit" which has been found to be a sensitive measure of analgesia.[207] A high degree of stereospecificity in the measurement of this parameter was observed for *d*- and *l*-isomers of racemorphan. Levorphanol, but not dextrorphan, increased the content of "bound" acetyl choline in pooled cerebral cortex, cerebellum, and the rest of the brains of mice.[208] Tolerance development to levorphanol caused only a small increase in brain acetyl choline content. In ultrafiltrates of brain homogenates of mice made tolerant to levorphanol, there was a high enough concentration of unchanged free drug to produce intense pharmacological effects on nontolerant mice and it was concluded that brain tolerance to opioid narcotics represented a decreased sensitivity to drug at the cellular or subcellular level.[209] In a recent investigation[210a,b] stereospecific binding of levorphanol-^{3}H was reported to be localized in certain membrane fractions separated by floatation from crude nuclear fractions of mouse brain homogenates and represented only 2% of the total association of this drug with tissue. Major regions of brain did not differ significantly in stereospecific binding capacity which was retained even after extraction with dilute solutions of Triton X-100 or sodium dodecyl sulfate. The binding had a pH optimum in the neutral region, was greatly inhibited by Ca^{2+}, Mg^{2+} ions, stimulated by EDTA, and not affected by iodoacetic acid and *p*-chloromercuribenzoate. Neuraminidase or pronase, but not trypsin, abolished this binding. The binding material had properties characteristics of proteolipids and it was implied that this stereospecific binding material might be the opiate receptor. Further extension of these interesting findings to the stereoisomers of other narcotic drugs and the effect of narcotic antagonists and development of tolerance on the stereospecific binding would throw more light on the true native state of receptor molecules.

Phenazocine (1,2,3,4,5,6-hexahydro-6,11-dimethyl-3-phenethyl-2,6-methano-3-benzazocin-8-ol)

Chemical Properties and Dosage

Phenazocine was the first compound of the benzomorphan series to be introduced into medicine. It was synthesized in 1959.[211] The free base (pK_a,8.50) and the hydrobromide melt at 181 to 182°C and 166 to 170°C, respectively. The analgesic potency of phenazocine is three to four times as great as morphine.[212,213] The average analgesic dose i.m. or i.v. is 2 to 3 mg.

Absorption, Fate, and Excretion

Quantitative information on the metabolism and biological disposition of phenazocine is not available. The pharmacology[214] and clinical evaluation and addiction liability[215-217] have, however, been reported. Orally administered, it is one fourth as effective as by intramuscular route. It is primarily metabolized in the liver presumably by conjugation and *N*-dealkylation.

Cyclazocine [3-(cyclopropylmethyl)-1,2,3,4,5,6-hexahydro-6,11-dimethyl-2,6-methano-3-benzazocin-8-ol]

Chemical Properties and Dosage

Cyclazocine, a member of benzomorphan group, is a potent narcotic antagonist with agonist activity and was synthesized in 1962.[218] A colorless cystalline compound m. 201 to 204°C, it produces physical dependence not characterized by drug-seeking behavior[219] and atypical abstinence syndrome. A number of clinical studies with cyclazocine in the treatment of drug dependence have been reported.[220-222] Unlike nalorphine, it is effective by oral route.

Absorption, Fate, and Excretion

Following 1.25 mg/kg s.c. dose of ^{3}H-cyclazocine in dogs,[223] 4% of the dose was excreted as free drug and 29 to 36% as a conjugate in urine. Peak plasma concentration of 0.156 μg/ml occurred at 30 minutes after administration and declined to barely detectable levels in 6 hours in nontolerant and tolerant dogs. The pattern of excretion of drug was similar in nontolerant, cyclazocine-tolerant, and abstinent dogs.[223] Forty-seven to sixty-six percent of the drug and its metabolites were eliminated in urine in five days following a s.c. dose of 1.25 mg/kg in dog. The amount of free cyclazocine in feces of tolerant dogs (16%) was higher than that in nontolerant (4%) or abstinent dogs (7%). In peripheral tissues, high levels were observed in lung, kidney, spleen, liver, and adrenals. The maximum concentration of cyclazocine in cerebral cortical gray and white matter of nontolerant dogs was 1.215 μg/g and 0.895 μg/g, respectively, 1 hour after administration which declined to 0.036 and 0.056 μg/g, respectively, at 6 hours. The values in tolerant dogs were not markedly different from non-tolerant dogs. No drug was detectable at 24 hours in CNS of abstinent dog.[223] Cyclazocine-8-glucuronide, norcyclazocine, and norcyclazocine glucuronide were shown to be the urinary metabolites of cyclazocine.[224] Approximately 2.5% of norcyclazocine and an equal amount as its glucuronide were found in the urine. Free norcyclazocine (2%) and bound product (0.36%) were also found in feces. No norcompound was detected in the brain of dogs.[224] These metabolic disposition studies did not reveal marked differences in gross distribution pattern of ^{3}H-cyclazocine in nontolerant and tolerant dogs and minor *N*-dealkylation pathway apparently did not account either for antagonistic action nor its atypical abstinence syndrome.

Pentazocine [3-(3-methyl-2-butenyl)-1,2,3,4,5,6-hexahydro-6,11-dimethyl-2,6-methano-3-benzazocin-8-ol)

Chemical Properties and Dosage

Pentazocine (Talwin®) was synthesized[225] in 1962 and introduced into medicine in 1967. The colorless crystalline compound m. 145 to 147°C (pK_a, 8.76) has 3 asymmetric carbon atoms and only the *l*-isomer possesses most of the analgesic activity. The partition coefficient in chloroform and buffer pH 7.4 is 25.4, in contrast to that for morphine, 0.0879.[226] It has both strong agonist and weak antagonist activity. The analgesic potency is approximately one fourth that of morphine.[227] Physical dependence and tolerance have been shown to develop to pentazocine after chronic administration.[228] The usual analgesic dose parenterally administered is 30 mg.

Absorption, Fate, and Excretion

Pentazocine is poorly absorbed from the gastrointestinal tract and is one fourth to one third as potent by oral route as by parenteral route.[216] Following intramuscular (45 mg) and oral administration (75 mg) in man, peak plasma levels of 0.14 μg/ml and 0.16 μg/ml coincided closely with onset, duration and intensity of analgesia, and other pharmacological effects. The plasma halflife after intramuscular and intravenous administration was about two hours.[229] Less than 13% of the dose in man appeared as free drug, and 12 to 30% as a glucuronide conjugate and another unidentified polar metabolite. Although the major portion of the drug and its metabolites was excreted within 12 hours, trace amounts of these could still be detected in urine for several days.[230] Pentazocine has been shown to pass the placental barrier.[231]

Following a 1 mg/kg intramuscular dose of ^{3}H-labeled pentazocine in cat, gastrointestinal tract and liver showed relatively high percentages of absorbed drug amounting to 27 and 23%, respectively. Bile contained 6% of the dose 2 hours after injection; and other fluids, urine, blood and tissues and kidney, adrenals, spleen, pancreas, heart, lung, thyroid, and brain contained less than 5% of the drug with the exception of muscle, which had

13% of the dose 2 hours after administration. The peak concentration in sensory motor cerebral gray matter at 30 minutes was 1.52 μg/g which declined to 0.62 μg/g at 2 hours. The corresponding values for cerebral white matter were 1.30 μg/g and 0.54 μg/g, respectively. The cortical and subcortical areas of brain did not show any preferential localization of the drug.[226]

A recent study[232] on the biologic disposition of pentazocine in rats showed rapid, but erratic absorption after oral administration. Peak organ levels were reached at 15 minutes with highest drug concentration in liver; the lungs, kidneys, and spleen contributed low, but appreciable levels which were not detected after 2 hours. Following intravenous administration, the peak levels of 11.7 μg/ml at 1 minute declined to 2.8 μg/ml at 15 minutes, after which the rate of decay slowed down considerably. Rapid metabolism of drug was indicated by low drug levels in liver. Lungs and kidney had high drug levels. Brain levels were appreciable one minute after injection and were still detectable after two hours. Pentazocine persisted in gastrointestinal tract after disappearance from other organs. Only minor amounts of free drug were excreted in urine and feces. The major metabolic pathway was glucuronide conjugation and to a minor extent, conjugation with ethereal sulfate and formation of phenolic metabolites (less than 0.6%). *N*-dealkylation was not detected in the rat. Extensive metabolism of drug also occurred in vitro by liver homogenates.[232]

Liver preparations from monkey, mice, and rats in vitro oxidized the methyl group of the dimethyl allyl side chain to isomeric alcohol derivatives. Quantitative species differences were noticed in the amounts of each isomeric alcohol derivative and the liver of the monkey oxidized one of the alcohols to a carboxylic acid.[233] In vivo, 70% of the dose could be recovered in monkey urine in 48 hours following administration of 0.3 to 34 mg/kg. The unchanged drug, the alcohols, and carboxylic acid derivatives found in vitro were also detected in urine along with conjugated drug. The overall recovery of drug in human urine was 61.5% of the dose of which free pentazocine, "*cis*-alcohol" and "*trans*-acid" averaged 9.5, 11.4, and 40.6%, respectively.[234] These values for overall recovery agreed with those reported previously.[235]

In another study[236] the concentration in blood and urinary excretion rate of pentazocine in humans were found to be much lower after oral administration (88.7 mg as base) than after intravenous administration (24 mg). The concentration in blood after intravenous administration declined exponentially, but fluctuated with time after oral administration indicating erratic absorption of drug. Following intravenous and oral administration, 8 to 24% and 3 to 15% of unchanged drug were recovered in urine in 32 hours under conditions of maintained acidic urinary pH.

A study[237] on the CNS distribution of isomers of pentazocine showed that most of the analgesic activity resided in the *l*-isomer and *d*-isomer was at least eight times less potent than *l*-isomer. Plasma halflife of two isomers did not appear to differ much. Maximum levels of drug were attained in plasma and CNS within 30 minutes after a subcutaneous dose of 15 mg/kg and levels of *d*-isomer in cortex, medullapons, midbrain, hypothalamus, hippocampus, striatum, and cord tended to be slightly higher and declined more rapidly than those of *dl*- and *l*-isomer. Differences in the regional CNS localization of optical isomers of pentazocine failed to account for the differences in their pharmacological activity.[237]

Meperidine (1-methyl-4-phenyl-ethyl isonipecotate)

Chemical Properties and Dosage

Meperidine was introduced into medicine in 1939 as a spasmolytic agent with analgesic properties.[238a,b] It is a colorless crystalline compound m. 186 to 189°C (pK_a, 8.72) with a slightly bitter taste. It has no asymmetric carbon atom and hence no stereo isomers. Oral, intramuscular, or subcutaneous analgesic dose is 25 to 150 mg.

Absorption, Fate, and Excretion

Unlike morphine, meperidine is well absorbed by oral route. Following administration of a single dose of 150 mg in 3 patients, peak plasma levels were observed between the first and second hour after administration.[239] Absorption by oral and intraperitoneal routes in rats and mice was also rapid,[240] but mobilization from subcutaneous injection sites was prolonged with 12.3% drug still persisting at site of injection.[241]

In dog, after intravenous administration, and in rats after intraperitoneal administration, high levels of drug were found in kidney, liver, lung, spleen, brain, and adrenals.[239-241] Meperidine has been shown to cross the placental barrier.[242]

Liver is an important site for biotransformation of meperidine in vitro[243] and in vivo and the main metabolic pathways[241] are (1) hydrolysis to the corresponding acid (meperidinic acid), (2) partial conjugation of this acid, (3) *N*-demethylation to normeperidine, and (4) hydrolysis of normeperidine to normeperidinic acid and partial conjugation.

Liver microsomal enzymes have been shown to *N*-demethylate meperidine, but not meperidinic acid,[243] and the latter is not *N*-demethylated in vivo to any significant degree. It was concluded that normeperidinic acid arises primarily from hydrolysis of normeperidine in liver. Normeperidine can penetrate the central nervous system and was shown to be more toxic than meperidine.[124] None of the other metabolites had any significant analgesic activity.

The average overall recovery of meperidine and its identifiable metabolites in human volunteers and hospital patients[244] was reported to be 53% with the mean value for meperidine 5%, normeperidine 7%, meperidinic acid 22%, bound meperidinic acid 5%, normeperidinic acid 11%, and bound normeperidinic acid 12%. Total urinary recovery of ^{14}C-labeled drug in rats ranged between 18 to 40%, the free drug 2 to 7%, meperidinic acid 4 to 12%, normeperidine 9 to 35%; bound forms of meperidine and normeperidine were not found in the rat. In dog, 5% of the dose appeared as unchanged drug and 50% as normeperidine in urine and feces. The gastrointestinal tract still retained radioactivity 24 hours after administration.[241]

The nature of excretion products depended to a great extent on the pH of urine.[245] In acid urine, meperidine and normeperidine were found as such while in alkaline urine, meperidinic acid and normeperidine were found as free acids and as conjugates. The excretion of normeperidine was slow and it could be detected in urine for at least three days after the last dose.[245]

There was no significant difference in the metabolism of meperidine in normal subjects and those addicted to this drug.[239] Increased capacity for inactivation of meperidine was not considered to be an important factor in development of tolerance to this drug.

The administration of inducer drugs such as phenobarbital to rats resulted in an increase in the activity of liver microsomal enzymes catalyzing the *N*-demethylation of meperidine.[111]

Ethoheptazine (hexahydro-1-methyl-4-phenyl-4-azepine ethyl carboxylate)

Chemical Properties and Dosage

Ethoheptazine (Zactirin®) was synthesized in 1954.[246a,b] It is a mild analgesic possessing an addiction liability less than that of codeine. It is a meperidine congener having a seven membered azepine ring instead of an aromatic ring structure. The base, b. 133 to 134°C/1 mm Hg forms a crystalline hydrochloride m. 151 to 153°C, pK_a, 8.45. Oral analgesic dose is 50 to 100 mg.

Absorption, Fate, and Excretion

Study on the metabolic fate[247] of ethoheptazine showed that it is rapidly absorbed. Following intraperitoneal administration of 73.5 mg/kg in the rat, a peak plasma level of 7.7 μg/ml was attained within 1 hour with no detectable amounts in plasma at 8 hours. Liver showed the highest radioactivity, followed by levels in kidney 30 minutes after intraperitoneal administration. These and other tissue levels declined from one third to one half at 90 minutes. The activity in intestines, however, increased several fold, indicating that this was the excretory route for the drug. Very little drug was excreted unchanged in the dog. Following an intraperitoneal dose of 35 mg/kg, less than 4% of the dose could be accounted for in 24 hours in urine, with most of the drug appearing in the first four hours after injection. In the rat and rabbit, 2 and 1.5%, respectively, of the dose was recovered unchanged. The metabolic pathways for ethoheptazine in dog, rat, and rabbit were (1) hydrolysis to corresponding acid, (2) oxidation to a hydroxy derivative in an undetermined position on the hexamethyleneimine ring, and (3) tentative *N*-demethylation to a norcompound.

Approximately 7 to 8% of the respective doses in dog and rat and less than 5% of the dose in rabbit were recovered as deesterified compound and hydroxyethoheptazine. In dogs, 9% of the dose could be accounted for as hydroxy metabolite while in rabbit, evidence for a secondary amine metabolite and another unidentified compound was obtained.

There were quantitative differences in the urinary excretion of *d*- and *l*-isomers of this drug in the dog. The excretion of unchanged drug, deesterified and hydroxymetabolite, was approximately three times greater after injection of *d*-isomer compared to the *l*-isomer.

Anileridine [ethyl (1-4-aminophenethyl)-4-phenyl isonipecotate]

Chemical Properties and Dosage

Anileridine was synthesized in 1956.[248] It is a congener of meperidine and is a potent analgesic drug. The crystalline hydrochloride, m. 280 to 287°C of the base m. 83°C, is freely soluble in water and sparingly so in alcohols. The pH of aqueous solutions ranges between 2.0 to 2.5. The aqueous solutions are stable at pH 3.5 and below, and the free base is precipitated from solutions at higher pH. The distribution coefficient in water (at pH 3.6) and *n*-butanol is 0.9. The oral analgesic dose is 25 to 60 mg.

Absorption, Fate, and Excretion

Anileridine is rapidly absorbed in rats producing a peak analgesia 20 to 30 minutes after oral or subcutaneous administration.[249] Peak effects were produced within one hour in the dog.[250] Following subcutaneous administration (8 mg/kg) in rats, the drug concentrated in the lungs, brain, kidney, liver, and muscle, in that order. *N*-acetyl anileridine appeared in high concentration in tissues within one hour. In brain this metabolite appeared somewhat slowly and to a lesser extent. Detectable amounts were only present in liver 24 hours after administration. After intravenous administration, the peak levels of drug were reached in brain two to four minutes after injection and declined to 11% of the peak value 30 minutes later. The metabolic pathways for biotransformation of anileridine in rat, guinea pig, and man have been shown[249] to be (1) hydrolysis to anileridinic acid, (2) acetylation of anileridinic acid, (3) acetylation of anileridine and excretion as such or as acetyl anileridinic acid, and (4) acetylaminophenyl acetic acid excreted free in humans and in a bound form in rats and guinea pigs.

In human subjects, rats and guinea pigs 5, 0.2 to 0.5%, respectively, of an oral dose was excreted unchanged in urine. All three species excreted 0.5 to 2% of dose as acetyl anileridine and approximately 10 to 19% of the dose was identified in urine of man, rats and guinea pigs as either free or acetylated anileridinic acid. Rats and guinea pigs excreted only 2% of dose as free anileridinic acid and 17% as conjugated anileridinic acid in urine. In man about 20% of dose could be accounted for as metabolites of anileridine, 7 to 14% as free anileridinic acid, and only 1 to 2% as conjugated derivatives. In addition, 15 to 35% of dose could be accounted for as *p*-acetylaminophenylacetic acid.[251] Normeperidine and *p*-aminophenylacetic acid have also been reported as urinary metabolites of anileridine.[251]

Methadone (6-dimethylamino-4,4-diphenyl-3-heptanone)

Chemical Properties and Dosage

Methadone was synthesized[252] in 1949. Racemic methadone hydrochloride, a colorless crystalline compound m. 235°C (pK_a, 8.25, 8.99) with a bitter taste, is soluble in water and chloroform. The free base m. 78°C is precipitated from aqueous solution at pH higher than 6. The three dimensional models of methadone reveal spatial structural similarity to morphine molecule. The racemic compound has been resolved into its stereo isomers and the pharmacology of these isomers extensively investigated.[253] The *levo* isomer is approximately 20 times as potent as *dextro* isomer, depending on animal species and test employed. It is an effective analgesic, efficacious by oral route and is being used in maintenance programs with ex-heroin addicts[254] and treatment of narcotic abstinence syndrome. Oral, subcutaneous, or intramuscular analgesic dose is 2.5 to 10 mg.

Absorption, Fate, and Excretion

Methadone is rapidly absorbed from injection site and on oral administration.[255-257] Following absorption, the drug rapidly leaves blood and localizes in lungs, liver, kidney, and spleen but the concentrations in brain, muscle, and heart are low.[255-257] Adrenals and thyroid also contain drug,[56,255,258] but a large part is present in carcass. Following a subcutaneous injection of 3 mg/kg in rat, peak levels ranging between 0.6 to 0.9 μg/g occurred in various areas of CNS at 30 minutes and declined to 0.20 to 0.40 μg/g at 3 hours after administration. Highest levels of 8 μg/g were found in adrenal gland 30 minutes after injection. The peak levels in CNS correlated well with intensity and duration of analgesia.[56] Methadone was firmly bound to tissue proteins, but repeated doses for several days in rats did not show cumulation of drug in tissue.[259,260]

The rate of metabolism in vitro of *d*- and *l*-isomers by liver slices and the pattern of distribution and excretion were similar.[261] In a recent study, no significant differences were noticed in the concentrations or halflives of two isomers in the rat blood.[262] Brain levels of *d*-methadone were consistently higher than blood levels in rats regardless of route of administration of analgesically equivalent doses. The differences in the analgesic activity and in the p.o./s.c. potency ratios of the methadone isomers did not appear to be due to differences in their accumulation in the blood or the brain. It was speculated that the observed differences were due to an active analgesic metabolite of *d*-methadone.[262] Excretion and distribution of methadone in various tissues of tolerant rats did not significantly differ from that in normal rats.[256,259,260] Tolerant rats, however, showed a slightly lower rate of liver metabolism and a greater amount of urinary metabolites compared to normal rats.

Study on the regional distribution of *d*- and *l*-isomers after stereotaxic injection of 10 μg of ^{14}C-labeled drug with mannitol as an inert marker into the lateral cerebral ventricle of rats showed no significant difference in the accumulation and diffusion of the two isomers in different regions of the brain, although analgesia was produced only in those animals injected with *l*-isomer.[263]

Approximately 4% of methadone is excreted free in urine and 5% in feces of man given 20 mg orally and in the rat.[264] Biliary excretion is an important route for the elimination of methadone and its metabolites.[264] *N*-demethylation is an important metabolic pathway for methadone in vitro[107] and in vivo.[265] Evidence has also been produced for the formation of primary and secondary amine metabolites[266] and for *N*-methylation to a quaternary ammonium compound in vitro to the extent of 15% by guinea pig liver slices.[267] *N*-demethylation of methadone to a secondary amine which spontaneously rearranged to form 1,5-dimethyl-3,3-diphenyl-2-ethylidene pyrrolidine (A) as a major metabolite in man has been reported.[268] This metabolite was found particularly in bile. Lung tissue localized methadone to the greatest extent. Approximately 60% of the dose in man could be accounted for as methadone and pyrrolidine metabolite. Chromatographic evidence for three other unidentified metabolites has also been obtained.[269] Evidence for further metabolism of the above pyrrolidine metabolite to 2-ethyl-5-methyl-3,3′-diphenyl-1-pyrroline (B) has recently been produced.[270] These two metabolites have been isolated, characterized and synthesized and found to be pharmacologically inactive.[270] In vitro conversion of methadone to its *N*-oxide has been shown to occur on incubation of methadone with 10,000 x g microsomal supernatant of male guinea pig liver homogenates.[271]

dl-α-Acetyl Methadol (6-dimethylamino-4,4-diphenyl-3-acetoxy heptane)

Chemical Properties and Dosage

dl-α-Acetyl methadol was synthesized[252,272] in 1948 to 1949. The presence of two asymmetric carbon atoms in the molecule results in two pairs, α and β of diastereoisomers. The *levo* isomer is derived from *d*-methadone and *dextro* isomer from

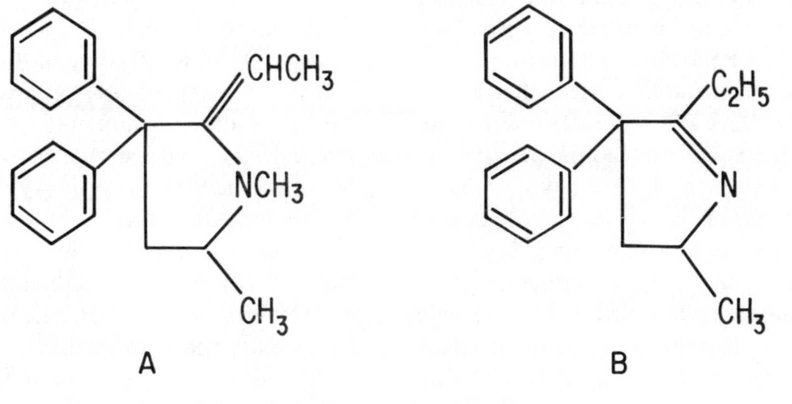

FIGURE 3. Methadone metabolites.

l-methadone. The α-*l*-acetyl methadol hydrochloride m. 215°C is soluble in water and is a potent analgesic structurally related to methadone with a prolonged duration of action providing practical therapeutic advantages over methadone in treatment of heroin addicts;[273] thus a patient on a 50 mg daily methadone regimen could be maintained on 40 to 60 mg of *dl*-α-acetyl methadol three times a week. The oral analgesic dose is 7.5 to 10 mg.

Absorption, Fate, and Excretion

Following parenteral administration of this drug in man, morphine-like effects appeared four to six hours later and lasted two to three days. The onset of effects was faster after oral administration and lasted for two days.[274] Following a 20 mg/kg subcutaneous dose of *l*-isomer in rats, the drug was found in highest concentration in lungs, to a lesser extent in muscle, and in much smaller concentrations in kidney, spleen, liver, fat, heart, blood, and brain.[275] The *l*-isomer persisted in most tissues after 24 hours. The *d*-isomer which resembled *l*-isomer in its tissue distribution, disappeared faster from the tissues compared to *l*-isomer. Both isomers were bound firmly to brain and tissue proteins and gave low recoveries (10 to 25%) of drug in vitro. The slow rate of metabolism of *l*-isomer could presumably account for its longer duration of action.

Liver microsomal enzymes in vitro and in vivo catalyzed the *N*-demethylation of the first methyl group with a halflife of two hours. The second methyl group was removed much more slowly.[276] The active metabolite was suggested to be ℓ-α-noracetylmethadol and methadol was reported to be much less active.[277] The acetyl groups are removed from acetylmethadol much more slowly compared to methyl groups and the resulting carbinols have not been identified in tissues nor excreted in bile. Following administration of N-$^{14}CH_3$-noracetylmethadol to rats, half the dose was eliminated in feces and very little in urine. An unidentified ^{14}C-labeled metabolite persisted in the body with a halflife of 15.5 days, probably related to the 1-carbon pool which the oxidized methyl group enters via formaldehyde.[276]

The postulation of ℓ-α-noracetylmethadol as the active metabolite does not, however, explain why the *d*-isomer with a shorter duration of action does not undergo similar *N*-dealkylation with resulting cumulative effects.

d-Propoxyphene (α-dextro-4-dimethylamino-3-methyl-1,2-diphenyl-2-butanol propionate)

Chemical Properties and Dosage

d-Propoxyphene (Darvon®) was synthesized[278] in 1953. It is a crystalline compound m. 170 to 171°C, pK_a, 6.30. Of the four stereoisomers of propoxyphene, only the α-dextroisomer has marked analgesic properties and low addiction liability.[279,280] Oral analgesic dose is 32.5 to 65 mg.

Absorption, Fate, and Excretion

d-Propoxyphene is rapidly absorbed on parenteral administration producing peak analgesic effects at 60 to 90 minutes following a 5 to 10 mg/kg dose in rats.[281] Like codeine, it is considerably less effective by oral route. Following a 4 mg/kg i.v. dose of ^{14}C-labeled drug in rats, 38% of the radioactivity was eliminated as $^{14}CO_2$ via pulmonary route within 24 hours and very little after this time. The halflife for elimination of $^{14}CO_2$ was approximately 130 minutes. Kidney tissue exhibited *N*-demethylation to a much smaller extent, compared to liver slices, while other tissues and whole blood did not show *N*-demethylation capacity. Most of the radioactivity (about 13%) in urine appeared during first 22 hours in rats and approximately 35% of the dose appeared in feces in 48 hours. Following administration of 100 mg orally every 4 hours for 16 hours in man, the amount of dose recovered in 24-hour urine in 3 subjects ranged between 3 to 10%. *N*-demethylation to des-*N*-methyl propoxyphene is an important metabolic pathway for this drug in rat, dog, and humans[282-284] and this metabolite has been isolated and characterized. Approximately 25% of a 65 mg dose in humans was recovered in urine as a mixture of unchanged drug and this metabolite in 48 hours. Norpropoxyphene concentrations in human plasma were higher than those of propoxyphene and the halflife of the norcompound was also substantially longer than that of the latter.[284] The mean biological halflife for propoxyphene administered i.v. in normal human volunteers was 1.85 hours which was much shorter than that for i.m. and oral route.[285] A sensitive method for the determination of propoxyphene and its metabolites in man has recently been reported.[286]

In addition to *N*-demethylation, propoxyphene was also metabolized in the rat via ester hydrolysis to its conjugates which were mainly excreted in the bile.[284]

DISPOSITION AND METABOLISM OF BARBITURATES

Chemical Properties and Dosage

The first barbiturate hypnotic, barbital (5,5-diethyl barbituric acid) was introduced into medicine in 1903. The pharmacologically active derivatives of barbituric acid (Figure 4) have alkyl or aryl radicals on C(5), substitution on N(1), or N(3) atoms. The thiobarbiturates possess a S atom in place of oxygen at C(2). Barbiturates are weakly acidic in nature due to the ionization of hydrogen atom of their enol-form, allowing the formation of water-soluble sodium salts with alkali. Free acids are colorless, odorless, crystalline solids with a bitter taste; sparingly soluble in water, but easily soluble in common organic solvents. Barbiturates form strong specific hydrogen bonds with adenine derivatives.[287]

Studies on structure-activity relationship in barbiturates have provided some generalizations: (a) substitution of both hydrogen atoms on C(5) was an essential requisite for activity; (b) substitution with phenyl group on C(5) conferred anticonvulsant properties in compounds; (c) increase in length of alkyl side chains on C(5) to five or six carbon atoms increased depressant action and larger carbon chains produced stimulant activity; (d) branched chains on C(5) produced long-acting barbiturates and substitution of cyclopentenyl or cyclohexenyl groups on C(5) resulted in short-acting compounds; (e) unsaturation in side chains on C(5) enhanced depressant properties; and (f) substitution of S atom in place of 0 at 2-position produced short-acting barbiturates. The names and chemical structures of different barbiturates are given in Table 1.

It has been customary to classify barbiturates into long, intermediate, short, and ultrashort-acting types on the basis of their duration of action in experimental animals. This classification can be highly misleading[288] as species differences[289-291] in response to barbiturates prevent indiscriminate application to man of data received from experimental animals. The rates of metabolism of clinically available barbiturates fall into two groups, one ranging from 10 to 70% per day (long and medium-acting ones) and the other 0.5 to 20% per hour (anesthetic and short-acting ones). On the basis of clinical experience, the original classification could be supplanted by a simple more accurate designation of sedative-hypnotic drugs and anesthetic barbiturates and the drug, dosage, and route of administration could be left to the physician based on familiarity and experience.[288] Phenobarbital, mephobarbital, and metharbital (long-acting barbiturates) are usually

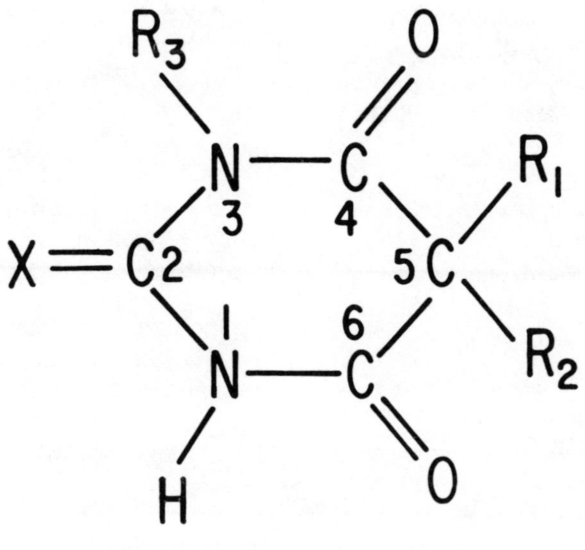

FIGURE 4. General formula of barbiturates.

TABLE 1

Names, Structural Features, and Hypnotic Doses of Some Barbiturates

Barbiturate	Trade name	R_1	R_2	R_3	X	Hypnotic dose (g)
Allobarbital	Dial®	allyl	allyl	H	O	0.1 – 0.3
Amobarbital	Amytal®	ethyl	isopentyl	H	O	0.1 – 0.3
Aprobarbital	Alurate®	allyl	isopropyl	H	O	0.06 – 0.13
Barbital	Veronal®	ethyl	ethyl	H	O	0.3 – 0.5
Butabarbital	Butisol®	ethyl	sec-butyl	H	O	0.1 – 0.2
Hexethal	Ortal®	ethyl	*n*-hexyl	H	O	0.2 – 0.4
Hexobarbital	Evipal®	methyl	1-cyclohexen-1-yl	CH_3	O	0.25 – 0.5
Mephobarbital	Mebaral®	ethyl	phenyl	CH_3	O	0.03 – 0.06
Metharbital	Gemonil®	ethyl	ethyl	CH_3	O	0.1
Methitural	Neraval®	2-methyl thioethyl	1-methylbutyl	H	S	0.5 – 2.5 g i.v.
Methohexital	Brevital®	allyl	1-methyl-2-pentynyl	CH_3	O	2.5% solution i.v.
Pentobarbital	Nembutal®	ethyl	1-methylbutyl	H	O	0.05 – 0.2
Phenobarbital	Luminal®	ethyl	phenyl	H	O	0.1 – 0.2
Secobarbital	Seconal®	allyl	1-methylbutyl	H	O	0.1 – 0.2
Thiamylal	Surital®	allyl	1-methylbutyl	H	S	0.075 – 0.15 (as 2.5% sol. i.v.)
Thiopental	Pentothal®	ethyl	1-methylbutyl	H	S	0.075 – 0.15 (as 2.5% sol. i.v.)
Vinbarbital	Delvinal®	ethyl	1-methyl-1-butenyl	H	O	0.1 – 0.2

employed as sedative-hypnotics and antiepileptic agents; amobarbital, aprobarbital, butabarbital, pentobarbital, secobarbital, and vinbarbital (short to intermediate-acting barbiturates) as sedative-hypnotics and methohexital, thiopental, and thiamylal (ultrashort-acting types) as intravenous anesthetic agents.

Barbiturates are usually administered orally, rectally, intramuscularly, or by slow i.v. injection in an emergency. The hypnotic doses of various clinically useful barbiturates are listed in Table 1. Physical dependence on barbiturates does not develop on therapeutic doses and in this respect the barbiturates differ from opiate narcotic drugs. Excessive use of barbiturates causes physical dependence, which has been amply demonstrated.[292-296]

Physicochemical Factors Affecting the Distribution and Metabolic Fate of Barbiturates

Lipid solubility – Most barbiturates with sustained hypnotic activity had a low, and those with short activity and rapid onset of action a high, distribution coefficient in lipid-water systems.[297-299] The barbiturates with high lipid-water partition coefficients entered the brain rapidly due to the lipoidal nature of blood-brain barrier and likewise were completely reabsorbed by lipoidal renal tubular epithelium and were sequestered in depot fats and more rapidly metabolized.

Protein-binding – In general, the barbiturates with high lipid-water partition coefficient were bound to plasma proteins to a higher extent compared with those having a lower partition coefficient;[300,301] e.g., barbital, phenobarbital, pentobarbital, secobarbital, and thiopental were bound to the extent of 5, 20, 35, 44, and 65%, respectively. A similar affinity was seen with brain and other tissue proteins.

Ionization – The degree of ionization of barbiturates which are weak acids can be computed from Henderson-Hasselbalch equation. The barbiturates with phenyl groups on C(5) had a pK_a of approximately 7.2 and those with alkyl or alkenyl groups on C(5) in the range of 7.6 to 8.0.[297,302] Increase in plasma pH, therefore, can affect duration of anesthesia,[303] tubular reabsorption, and excretion of barbiturates.

Absorption and Distribution of Barbiturates

The barbiturates are rapidly absorbed from the gastrointestinal tract by passive diffusion. The particle size and dissolution rate of barbiturates play an important role in gastrointestinal absorption and dissolution and dispersal of drug in the gastrointestinal contents appears to be the rate-determining step in this absorption.[304] Little or no difference in the rates of absorption of various short and intermediate-acting barbiturates was indicated with encapsulated free acid forms of such barbiturates. The water-soluble sodium salts of barbiturates were more efficiently absorbed compared to sparingly soluble free acids. The gastrointestinal absorption,[305] pharmacological action, and brain levels of barbital and phenobarbital have been reported to increase after ingestion of ethanol in the rat.[306] It was concluded from a study on the pharmacokinetics of this interaction that ethanol increased phenobarbital transport across the peritoneum and acute administration of ethanol temporarily delayed renal excretion of barbiturates.[307] No correlation between buccal absorption of barbiturates and chloroform/0.1 N hydrochloric acid partition coefficients was observed, indicating that the absorption power of buffer-buccal membrane interface may represent more exactly the real affinity of the membrane for barbiturates than do the solvent-water partition coefficients.[308]

Following absorption, barbiturates distribute in body tissues and fluids. Barbiturates readily cross the placental barrier and become widely distributed in the fetal tissue. The distribution and rate of entry of barbiturates[309] into the brain are governed by the lipid solubility of these drugs. Barbiturates with high lipid-water partition coefficients cross the blood-brain barrier within 30 seconds and attain maximum concentrations in regions which have the greatest blood flow. Phenobarbital penetrates the brain more slowly compared to thiopental as it has a much lower partition coefficient though it is less ionized than thiopental at plasma pH. Similarly barbital, although ionized to approximately the same extent as thiopental and much less bound to plasma protein, penetrates the brain very slowly due to a very low lipid-water partition coefficient. Even after i.v. administration of barbital in anesthetic doses to experimental animals, many minutes elapse before the onset of pharmacologic effects.

The redistribution of thiopental within the body has been studied in great detail.[310-313] Following i.v. administration of thiopental, the maximum concentrations of drug were reached in brain, liver, kidney, and heart in 30 seconds and redistribution amounting to approximately 80% of the initial peak level of thiopental from brain to muscle and skin occurred in the first 15 to 30 minutes. Subsequent uptake by fat and metabolic degradation was responsible for the decline in drug plasma levels. The slow release of drug from fat depots, where it gets sequestered, may be a determining factor in the rate of metabolism of thiopental and other thiobarbiturates. The biotransformation of thiopental is a slower process occurring at the rate of 10 to 15% per hour[314] compared to other ultrashort-acting thiobarbiturates like thiohexital[315] (25% per hour) and thiamylal. It was concluded that prompt recovery from anesthesia following i.v. thiopental is not due to the swift metabolic degradation, but primarily due to the redistribution of drug from plasma to the tissues. The post anesthetic somnolence or "hangover" after larger doses or prolonged administration is due to the persistence of drug in plasma in appreciable concentrations which are maintained for a long time by the extensive tissue reservoir of this drug.[316]

Metabolic Fate and Biotransformation of Barbiturates

A considerable amount of work has been done on the metabolic fate of different barbiturates[309,317-324] and this subject has been thoroughly covered in comprehensive reviews.[297,309,316-318,325] In many cases the complete elucidation of metabolic fate of barbiturates has not been done and all metabolites have not been identified or accounted for. These metabolites have been shown to be pharmacologically inactive except in the case of amobarbital,[326] where the principal metabolite hydroxy amobarbital had half the activity of the parent drug in mice.

The primary site of metabolic degradation of barbiturates is the liver,[327-334] though brain and kidney can metabolize some barbiturates to a small extent.[335]

Metabolism of Barbiturates

Barbiturates are metabolized by the following pathways.[317,336,337]

Oxidation of substituents at C(5) – This is the most important pathway for the metabolism of barbiturates. Oxidation usually occurs at the larger of the two C(5) substituents primarily in the penultimate or (ω- 1) position of the alkyl side chain producing polar alcohols,[317,318,338,339] phenols,[340] ketones,[341-343] (oxidation of S-atom of methyl thio ethyl side chain produces sulfoxide) or carboxylic acids[314] by ω-oxidation. Ethyl groups resist oxidation and alicyclic groups like 1-cyclohexenyl or 1-cycloheptenyl are oxidized in 3-position to form alcohols and ketones. The allyl groups either escape metabolism or are transformed to 2,3-dihydroxypropyl groups. The hydroxylation of phenyl groups takes place in the para position. The hydroxy metabolites are excreted in the urine either as free or as glucuronide conjugates and are generally pharmacologically inactive.

Biotransformation of barbiturates is mediated primarily by the liver microsomal enzymes which, in the presence of reduced triphosphopyridine nucleotide and molecular oxygen, hydroxylate a wide variety of barbiturates. These microsomal enzymes possess very low substrate specificity.[21] Studies on biotransformation of barbiturates in vitro or in vivo by liver microsomes have only been done in experimental animals, not in humans.

***N*-dealkylation**[341,342,344] – Oxidative *N*-dealkylation accounts for a very small fraction of metabolic degradation of ultrashort-acting barbiturates such as hexobarbital and methohexital; however, metharbital and mephobarbital are *N*-dealkylated to barbital. Such a pathway has not been demonstrated in man and is not considered an important detoxication mechanism.

***S*-demethylation**[345] – This new type of enzymatic mechanism has also been shown to occur with rat liver microsomes in the case of 5-(*S*-methyl thio ethyl)-5-(1′-methyl butyl)-2-thiobarbituric acid (methitural). The demethylating system was not stimulated by phenobarbital nor inhibited by SKF-525A. It has recently been proposed that microsomal *S*-dealkylation may actually be microsomal sulfoxidation coupled to the metabolism of alkylsulfoxides to aldehydes by an enzyme or enzymes in the soluble fraction.[346]

Desulfuration of thiobarbiturates to barbiturates[347] – Although variable in extent, this appears to be a general, but minor, reaction of thiobarbiturates and accounts for only a small fraction of the administered dose.

Fission of the barbiturate ring[348-350] – Although occurring in vivo, this is a very minor route and has not been demonstrated in man. The ring appears to be relatively stable in vivo.

Dealkylation[351,352] **of substituents at C(5)** – Dealkylation of either group at C(5) has been shown as a minor pathway for inactivation of barbital and vinyl analogue of barbital. 1.5% of the dose of barbital was eliminated as 5-ethyl barbituric acid. Evidence for C(5) dealkylation has also been presented for secobarbital. The previously reported minor metabolites have recently been shown to be impurities present in commercial samples of barbiturates.[353]

***N*-methylation**[354,355] – Methylation of N(1) or N(3) was demonstrated only in experimental animals but could not be confirmed by subsequent experiments.[356] No conclusive evidence for such a pathway has been obtained in man. However, such a route could lead to the formation of pharmacologically active products.

Excretion of Barbiturates

The barbiturates and their metabolites are primarily eliminated by renal excretion[317,357] and to a small extent in the feces. The renal excretion of barbiturates involves glomerular filtration and tubular back diffusion of the undissociated form of the drugs due to the lipid-like barrier of tubular epithelium. Barbiturates with high lipid-water partition coefficients generally appeared only in traces in urine, but the polar metabolites escape tubular resorption and are readily excreted. Binding of barbiturates to plasma proteins reduced glomerular filtration. Barbiturates like barbital, which are not metabolized significantly, are eliminated very slowly, approximately 8% of a single hypnotic dose in 12 hours, 20% in 24 hours, 35 to 65% in 48 hours with traces of drug still detectable in urine for as long as 8 to 12 days.[317] Phenobarbital, allobarbital, and aprobarbital are partly metabolized and 15 to 30% of the dose appeared in urine. Over 50% of the dose of probarbital was excreted unchanged and slowly eliminated in urine in the course of many days. Daily consumption of therapeutic doses of such drugs may therefore lead to cumulation. Pento and secobarbital, which are more thoroughly metabolized, appear in urine only in traces and their administration in usual doses does not lead to cumulation.

Enzyme Stimulation and Inhibition of Metabolism of Barbiturates

As mentioned earlier, the liver microsomal enzymes are responsible for oxidative metabolism of barbiturates. Studies[358-361] on the more precise localization of the activity of these enzymes by subfractionation technique furnished microsomes of "rough" and "smooth" variety. The latter was reported to have about four times greater activity than the former in metabolizing hexobarbital. Recently it has been demonstrated[362,363] that the rat liver microsomal enzymes were more labile than the similar rabbit and mouse preparations and the rate of many enzymatic reactions with rat liver microsomes was constant only during the first 30 minutes or so. The times at which deviations from linearity occurred differed for each substrate studied. These studies emphasized the importance of incubation time in experiments on interspecies comparison of drug metabolism. Rabbit liver microsomes were shown to be more active for *N*-demethylation of certain barbiturates.

A variety of factors[365] such as stress, state of health, nutritional deficiency, liver disease, and certain chemicals influenced the activity of liver microsomal enzymes in experimental animals. Inhibition of these enzymes with β-diethylaminoethyl diphenyl propyl acetate (SKF-525A) potentiated and prolonged the duration of action of barbiturates. Chronic pretreatment of rats with codeine inhibited the in vitro metabolism of hexobarbital by rat liver microsomes.[109] Barbiturates stimulate the enzymes responsible for their own metabolism and that of other drugs; thus barbital, which is metabolized to a very small extent by liver microsomal enzymes, has been shown to enhance the enzyme activity responsible for metabolizing other barbiturates.[22,29,366,367] Subchronic administration of phenobarbital in rats may increase by as much as 700% the in vitro rate of metabolism of hexobarbital.[368,369] Drugs which induce the synthesis of drug metabolizing enzymes in liver microsomes also stimulated the ascorbic acid synthesis in rats.[370]

The phenomenon of the increase in the amount of drug metabolizing enzymes in liver microsomes (enzyme induction) has clinical implications as well.[371-373] Patients treated with phenobarbital became less responsive to the anticoagulant action of the coumarins and administration of griseofulvin to patients treated with phenobarbital produced significantly lower plasma levels of griseofulvin compared to controls.[374]

The ability of stress situations to stimulate drug metabolism of hexobarbital and pentobarbital and its dependence upon an intact pituitary-adrenal axis is suggestive of a regulatory function of the endocrine system in mediating a rapid induction of liver microsomal enzymes responsible for drug metabolism.[375,376] The stimulation of metabolism of pentobarbital can be blocked by protein synthesis inhibitors like actinomycin-D.[377]

Enzyme Induction and Tolerance to Barbiturates

Following administration of one or two doses of barbiturates, resistance to the hypnotic action has been shown in dogs, rats, and rabbits.[378] Acute tolerance to barbiturates,[379-381] which is dose-related, may develop quickly even after a single administration and the tolerance developed to one barbiturate can be transferred to other barbiturates (cross-tolerance). Acute changes in rat serum proteins after a single dose of barbital have also been reported.[382]

In the case of barbiturates whose duration of action in animals is determined by the rate of metabolic degradation, enzyme induction can lead to increased rate of detoxication and produce drug-disposition tolerance in animals.[368,369,383-385] Part of the tolerance observed with many barbiturates could be explained by the accelerated rate of their metabolism; however, chronic administration of barbital which undergoes very little metabolic alteration[386] (approximately 6% in tolerant rats and 4% in nontolerant rats) has also been shown to produce a gradual decrease in hypnotic action without any decrease in tissue concentration, indicating that mechanisms other than accelerated metabolism of drugs must also be involved. This pharmacodynamic tolerance due to barbiturates appears to be an adaptation of the tissue of central nervous system to the presence of the drug which changes the sensitivity of the tissue to the drug. Such an acquired tolerance has been shown to disappear almost completely during one to two weeks of abstinence with elimination of barbiturates.[383-385]

A recent study[387] with hypnotic and nonhypnotic isomers of methylphenobarbital showed that induction of barbiturate tolerance was not stereospecific. It was possible, however, that induction observed in this study was due to the principal metabolite, phenobarbital, and not to methylphenobarbital. As the (+) isomer of methylphenobarbital is more readily taken up by brain tissue than its more active (−) isomer and the demethylation of (+) isomer is preferentially enhanced by induction with phenobarbital, it has been concluded[388] that the differences in their anesthetic effectiveness could not be necessarily related to their different patterns of distribution and metabolic inactivation. Different rates of oxidative metabolism for *l*- and *d*-isomers of hexobarbital have been reported in a recent study,[389] that of *l*-isomer occurring for only five minutes, whereas that of *d*-isomer continued for much longer periods. Pretreatment with phenobarbital or 3-methyl cholanthrene decreased the apparent K_m for *l*-isomer but not the *d*-isomer, suggesting that the inducing agent brings about the synthesis of a qualitatively different hexobarbital oxidase system.

DISPOSITION AND METABOLISM OF NONBARBITURATE SEDATIVE-HYPNOTICS

Meprobamate (2-methyl-2-propyl-1,3-propanediol dicarbamate)

Chemical Properties and Dosage

Meprobamate (Miltown®, Equanil) was synthesized[390] in 1950. It is a colorless crystalline substance m. 104 to 106°C with a characteristic bitter taste. It is sparingly soluble in water and freely soluble in most organic solvents. The average oral sedative dose for adults is 200 to 400 mg three times daily, total daily dose not exceeding 2.4 g. It is a widely used tranquilizer for control of anxiety, tension, and muscle spasm.

Absorption, Fate, and Excretion

Meprobamate is readily absorbed from the gastrointestinal tract and does not cause nausea or emesis.[391] Following oral and intraabdominal administration of ^{14}C-labeled meprobamate (label in both carbamate groups) in rats and dogs, significant amounts of the radioactivity appeared in urine within 30 minutes after administration and most of the dose was excreted within 24 hours.[392] The feces contained less than 10% of the dose. Blood levels of ^{14}C reached a peak 2 hours after oral administration and 50% of the drug present in blood was unchanged meprobamate. After administration of drug to the rat, highest levels were found in lungs, kidney, and liver. The major metabolite accounting for about 60% of dose in dogs was isolated and identified as 2-hydroxymethyl-2-propyl-1,3-propanediol dicarbamate. This metabolite was devoid of meprobamate-like activity in dogs. About 10 to 12% of dose is excreted unchanged in urine; the rest consisted of metabolite conjugated with glucuronic acid.

The distribution of ^{14}C-meprobamate[393] (100 mg/kg i.p.) in rats was uniform in all areas of the central nervous system (cerebrum, cerebellum, midbrain, and hindbrain) and reached the peak within one hour after injection. Using a dose of 250 mg/kg in nephrectomized rats (30 μCi/rat), three compounds, meprobamate, hydroxy meprobamate, and a glucuronide, were found in the blood, but only unchanged meprobamate in the brain.

Autoradiographic studies with tritium labeled meprobamate[394] (sp. act. 2.3 mCi/mg) administered orally and intravenously to pregnant and nonpregnant mice at levels of 460 to 675 μCi per mouse, one minute after injecting the drug showed radioactivity in most of the body tissues. Thereafter, up to 24 hours, minor changes were observed in ^{3}H-levels of different tissues but there tended to be a very even distribution of ^{3}H with passage of time. No specific localization of ^{3}H in brain was observed. Most of the meprobamate was excreted within 24 hours.

Meprobamate penetrated placental barrier more rapidly in later stages of pregnancy.[395]

Subsequent studies[396] established β-hydroxypropyl meprobamate and its glucuronide, not the hydroxymethyl derivative reported earlier,[392] as the major metabolites of meprobamate. A number of other minor metabolites, including an *N*-glucuronide (at one of the carbamate groups) not hydrolysable by β-glucuronidase, have been reported in rabbits' urine.[397] Stress by ligation of hind leg stimulated drug metabolism of meprobamate, but this increased metabolism was not observed in livers of adrenalectomized, hypophysectomized, or actinomycin-D treated animals, indicating that stress-drug interaction is dependent upon intact pituitary-adrenal axis.[398]

In patients with liver cirrhosis and chronic hepatitis, the halflife of meprobamate[399] in blood following i.v. injection of 8 mg/kg was reported to

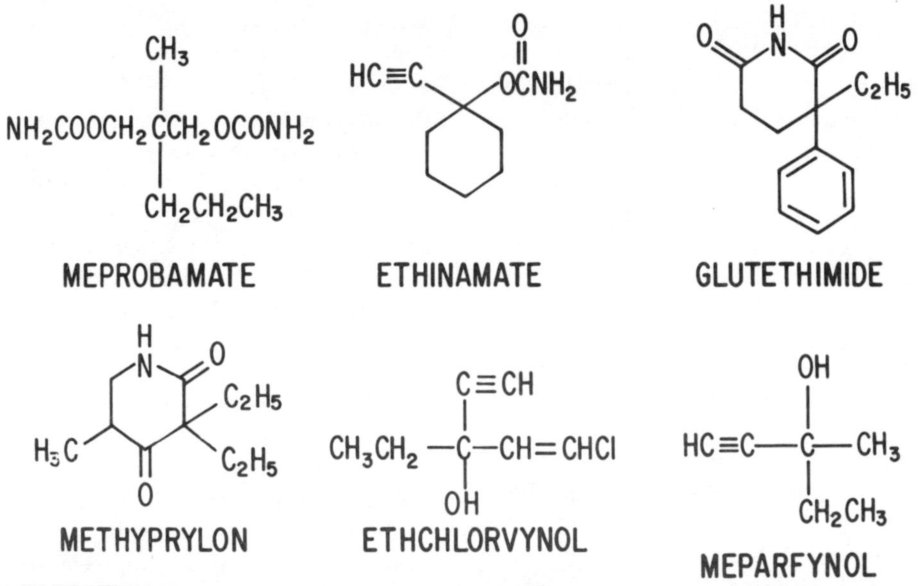

FIGURE 5. Chemical formulae of some nonbarbiturate sedative-hypnotics.

be 24.3 hours, compared to 12.6 hours in patients without liver disease. In two patients with severe drug addiction, the halflife was shortened to 4.5 and 7.0 hours, respectively. The average halflife for elimination of meprobamate in 12 healthy adults was 11.3 hours. Elimination of meprobamate by subjects receiving larger doses for prolonged periods was considerably lower than in those receiving a single dose.

Meprobamate was capable of inducing hepatic microsomal enzymes involved in drug metabolism and accelerated the metabolic disposition of a large number of drugs that were affected by such degradation.[400] Chronic daily feeding of 0.04 to 0.10 mg of DDT to male and female rats significantly enhanced hepatic drug-metabolizing enzyme activity and shortened the duration of action of meprobamate.[401]

Following fatal meprobamate poisoning in man, the concentrations of meprobamate[402] in blood were reported in the range of 142 to 342 μg/ml (mean 226 μg/ml). In the case of poisoning with meprobamate-alcohol combination, the blood levels of meprobamate were 43 to 155 μg/ml (mean 117 μg/ml), in meprobamate-barbiturate poisoning 30 to 276 μg/ml (mean 117 μg/ml), and in meprobamate-barbiturate-alcohol poisoning 33 to 460 μg/ml (mean 133 μg/ml).

Ethinamate (ethynylcyclohexyl carbamate)

Chemical Properties and Dosage

Ethinamate (Valmid®), a potent sedative hypnotic,[403] was introduced into medicine in 1953. It is a stable, colorless, odorless crystalline solid with a slightly bitter taste, m. 96 to 98°C. It is slightly soluble in water, but readily soluble in alcohol and other organic solvents. The partition coefficient in oil/water is 1.48. The sedative hypnotic oral dose is 500 mg to 1 g 20 minutes before retiring.

Absorption, Fate, and Excretion

Ethinamate is readily absorbed from the gastrointestinal tract and when administered in hypnotic doses[404] to normal human subjects does not produce specific effects on respiration, pulse, and blood pressure. Metabolic studies in rats[405] with ethinamate labeled with ^{14}C in the carboxy group revealed that the major route is the hydroxylation in the para position of the cyclohexane ring, approximately half the amount being eliminated in the urine in the free form and the remainder as a glucuronide. Hydrolytic cleavage of ester grouping is a minor pathway. The major hydroxylated metabolite has been isolated from urine of human subjects and characterized.[406] The identity of glucuronide has also been established by synthesis.[407] Liver plays an important role in the degradation of this compound. Rats with liver damage induced from carbon tetrachloride showed prolonged sleeping time and longer duration of action. Ethinamate has also been shown to inhibit respiration of KCl-stimulated rat brain cortical slices in vitro.[407]

N-glucuronide formation has been shown to take place in rabbits.[408] The conformation of hydroxyl groups in hydroxylated metabolites of ethinamate in human subjects has been investigated by proton resonance spectra.[409] In addition to *trans*- and *cis*-isomers of 1-ethynyl-1,4-cyclohexane diol and 1-ethynyl-1,3-cyclohexane diol and their glucuronides, evidence for the formation of 1-a-ethynyl-4e-acetoxy cyclohexylcarbamate, 1-e-ethynyl-4e-acetoxy cyclohexylcarbamate and 1-a-ethynyl-3e-acetoxy cyclohexylcarbamate in human subjects has also been obtained.[410]

Glutethimide (3-ethyl-3-phenyl-2,6-piperidine dione)

Chemical Properties and Dosage

Glutethimide (Doriden®) was introduced[411,412] into medicine in 1954. It is a colorless, odorless, tasteless crystalline powder m. 84 to 87°C, insoluble in water and soluble in nonpolar solvents. It has a high lipid-water partition coefficient. Oral hypnotic dose is 500 mg and daytime sedation dose is 125 to 250 mg three times daily after meals.

Absorption, Fate, and Excretion

Due to the poor solubility of glutethimide in water, the absorption from gastrointestinal tract is irregular. Distribution studies[413,414] have shown that glutethimide is adequately absorbed from the gastrointestinal tract of experimental animals. High lipid-water partition coefficient of this drug facilitates penetration through diffusion barriers. After absorption the drug is widely distributed and reaches a somewhat higher concentration in fat than in other tissues. The halflife of the drug in the rat is about 6 1/2 hours, apparently much shorter in dogs and probably also in man. It is almost completely metabolized in the body and less than 0.2% of a therapeutic dose appears unchanged in urine. The metabolites tend to be captured in hepatic circulation and excretion of metabolites is therefore quite slow. Fecal excretion amounts to only 1 or 2% of the dose in the form of metabolites. When injected intravenously, the concentration in brain and other highly vascular tissue rises rapidly and then falls as the drug is redistributed to poorly perfused tissues.

The two optical antipodes are biotransformed by different pathways.[415,416] The *d*-form is hydroxylated in 5-position of the piperidine ring; most of the alcohol is then conjugated with glucuronic acid, but a small portion is dehydrated to form approximately 2% α-ethyl-α-phenyl glutaconimide. The *l*-form is hydroxylated at the α-carbon of the ethyl group, most of which is also conjugated with glucuronic acid, but a small portion suffers the loss of ethyl group to form 3 phenyl 2,6-piperidine dione. The halflife of a therapeutic dose has been estimated to be about 10 hours.

N-dealkylation products of both *d, l* antipodes and one metabolite of each of the *d*- and *l*- form conjugated at *N*-hydroxymethyl group with glucuronic acid were also detected.

Except for glutaconimide, none of the metabolic products of glutethimide have hypnotic activity. The small yield of glutaconimide (about 2%) is insufficient to contribute significantly to the hypnotic action of this drug.

Glutethimide enhances the ability of rat hepatic microsomes to metabolize other drugs and patients recovering from glutethimide poisoning have been shown to demethylate certain drugs at an accelerated rate.[417]

A marked acceleration of metabolic inactivation of glutethimide has been reported in humans habituated to 250 mg daily dose compared to nonhabituated subjects and this metabolism of drug returned to normal levels following a 20-day withdrawal period.

In vivo and in vitro experiments[419] with racemic drug containing different radioactive labels in two enantiomorphs showed that liver enzymes responsible for degradation of these hypnotics were stereospecific. The difference in biological activity of investigated antipodes was attributed largely to the different rates of metabolism which gave rise to different blood and tissue concentration of drug and its metabolites.

In patients intoxicated with glutethimide and those treated with hemodialysis the serum halflife was 40.1 hours and 14.6 hours, respectively. Renal failure did not prolong the serum halflife nor did diuresis shorten it. The positive correlation between serum level and serum halflife was attributed to rate-limited enzymatic degradation of glutethimide. Impaired perfusion of liver which normally degrades glutethimide may account for the prolonged elevation of serum level in some instances of glutethimide intoxication.[420]

Methyprylon (3,3-diethyl-5-methyl-2,4-piperidine dione)

Chemical Properties and Dosage

Methyprylon (Noludar®) was introduced into medicine[421] in 1955. It is a colorless powder m. 74 to 77°C with a slight odor and bitter taste. It is soluble in water and organic solvents. The oral sedation dose is 50 to 100 mg and the oral hypnotic dose 200 to 400 mg.

Absorption, Fate, and Excretion

Metabolic disposition studies[422] in rats given an oral dose of 40 mg/kg of methyprylon labeled with ^{14}C in 6-position of the ring showed that about half the radioactivity was excreted in the urine and very little $^{14}CO_2$ appeared in expired air. Considerable amount of drug passed into the bile in altered form. Very little radioactivity was found in liver, kidney, brain, and spinal cord 15 hours after administration. Approximately 90.4% of dose could be accounted for in urine. The biologic halflife of this drug by subcutaneous route was 20 to 28 hours.

The drug was adequately absorbed from the gastrointestinal tract of dogs and man. In 144 hours, dogs excreted 92.7% of administered dose of which 50% was accounted for as conjugates. In the dog, reabsorption from the intestines was more efficient. The drug was partly dehydrogenated between C-5 and C-6, possibly by hydroxylation and subsequent dehydration. Two to ten percent of dehydrogenated compound and approximately a similar amount of unchanged drug appeared in the urine. In dog, most of the dehydrogenated product was further metabolized by oxidation of methyl group to hydroxy methyl and carboxylic acid derivatives. Traces of dehydrogenated decarboxylated metabolite have also been found in urine along with intermediate biotransformation products. These metabolites were excreted unchanged and partly as glucuronides. The latter were secreted into the bile and reabsorbed.[423,424]

After oral administration 2,4-dioxo-3,3′-diethyl-5-methyl-1,2,3,4-tetrahydropyridine, 2,4,6-trioxo-3,3′-diethyl-5-methyl piperidine, 2,4-dioxo-3,3′-diethyl-5-hydroxy methyl tetrahydropyridine and 2,4-dioxo-3,3′-diethyl-5-carboxy tetrahydropyridine have been isolated and characterized as metabolites of methyprylon in humans.[425-427]

Ethchlorvynol (1-chloro-3-ethyl-1-penten-4-yn-3-ol)

Chemical Properties and Dosage

Ethchlorvynol (Placidyl®) was introduced[428] into medicine in 1955. It is a colorless liquid b. 173 to 174°C with pungent aromatic odor and is sensitive to light and air. It is immiscible with water, but miscible with most organic solvents. It is an effective hypnotic with short latency to the onset and a short duration of effect. The oral hypnotic dose is 500 mg, 100 to 200 mg for sedation (2 to 3 times daily).

Absorption, Fate, and Excretion

Methods for the determination of ethchlorvynol in urine and serum by gas chromatography[429] and ultraviolet spectrophotometry[430] have been described. The rapid onset of hypnotic effect on administration of oral doses in animals indicates that it is efficiently absorbed from the gastrointestinal tract. In human subjects after oral ingestion, the maximum blood level was attained in one to one and a half hours, then declined to undetectable levels in blood three hours after administration.[431] Ethchlorvynol does not induce or inhibit hepatic drug metabolizing enzymes.[432] Recent study[433] on serum and urine levels of ethchlorvynol in man (500 mg dose) using a gas chromatographic technique showed very rapid absorption with an absorptive halflife of 0.3 hour. In 25 hours, 0.025% of the total dose is excreted unchanged or as glucuronide. Peak serum levels of 2.5, 6.5, or 8.0 μg/ml were seen at 1 hour after administration of 200, 500, and 750 mg capsules, respectively. The decline of serum levels was biphasic with disappearance constants of 0.5 and 0.03 $hour^{-1}$ and the rate constant for elimination was calculated to be 0.13 $hour^{-1}$. There was also evidence for extensive tissue localization of ethchlorvynol.

Meparfynol (3-methyl-1-pentyn-3-ol)

Chemical Properties and Dosage

Meparfynol (Dormison) is a mobile colorless liquid b. 121 to 122°C with acrid odor and burning taste. It is fairly soluble in water and miscible with organic solvents. The recommended hypnotic dose for adults is 500 mg to 1 g and the sedative dose 250 to 500 mg in soft gelatine capsules or as elixirs.

Absorption, Fate, and Excretion

A method for the estimation of this drug in biological materials has been described and studies with isolated tissues have shown that liver, kidney, and to a smaller extent, brain can inactivate this drug.[434] Studies on its metabolic disposition[435] in dog and man have suggested that in the dog, 17 to 29% of the drug is metabolized to a glucuronide conjugate lacking the acetylenic group. Fate of the remaining drug was unknown. Orally administered meparfynol appears to be adequately absorbed from the gastrointestinal tract; however, the metabolism[436] in human patients is slow and the drug can be detected in patients 48 hours after its administration. It is distributed in total body water and reaches somewhat higher concentrations in liver and depot fats than in other tissues. Small amounts of unchanged drug are eliminated in breath and in urine.[437]

DISPOSITION AND METABOLISM OF TRANQUILIZERS

Chlordiazepoxide (7-chloro-2-methylamino-5-phenyl-3H-1,4-benzodiazepine-4-oxide)

Chemical Properties and Dosage

Chlordiazepoxide (Librium®) was synthesized in 1957. It is a light yellow crystalline solid m. 236.5°C, soluble in water as its hydrochloride. It is sensitive to light[438] and β-radiation and somewhat unstable in solution. NMR spectral studies[439] have shown that 1,4-benzodiazepine has a chair type of configuration. It is an important tranquilizer in various psychoneuroses. The single oral dose as a tranquilizer ranges from 5 to 25 mg.

Absorption, Fate, and Excretion

The psychosedative and pharmacological properties of chlordiazepoxide have been the subject of a number of studies.[440-443] Studies on the metabolism[444,445] of ^{14}C-labeled chlordiazepoxide in rat, dog, and man showed it to be rapidly absorbed from the gastrointestinal tract. After oral administration in the rat, the drug appears in blood in a few minutes and peak levels were produced in about two hours. In rat the plasma halflife of orally administered drug was estimated to be four to six hours. In man several hours were required for peak blood levels to be reached. Effects persisted for about 48 hours in the rat, but longer in man. The drug is extensively metabolized in both species. None of the ^{14}C-labeled drug appears as $^{14}CO_2$ via the pulmonary route. In rats four metabolic products have been separated and characterized[446] by high resolution mass spectrometry: (1) 7-chloro-1,3-dihydro-5-(4-hydroxy phenyl)-2H-1,4-benzodiazepine-2-one-4-oxide; (2) 2-amino-7-chloro-5-(4-hydroxy phenyl)-3H-1,4-benzodiazepine-4-oxide; (3) 7-chloro-5-(4-hydroxy phenyl)-2 methylamino-3H-1, 4-benzodiazepine-4-oxide; (4) 7-chloro-1,3-dihydro-5-(4-hydroxy phenyl)-2H-1,4-benzodiazepine-2-one. In man the halflife of orally administered drug was 20 to 24 hours. On discontinuation of drug, plasma drug levels decline slowly over a period of several days. Excretion of drug was also very slow with 1 to 2% of drug eliminated as free and 3 to 6% as a conjugate in urine. Maximum urinary excretion of drug occurred 24 to 30 hours after administration, but small amounts of drug and its metabolites appeared to be excreted over a long period. Slow excretion of drug in the human in contrast to experimental animals may lead to cumulative effects which may be responsible for its side-reactions. The primary metabolic product in man was

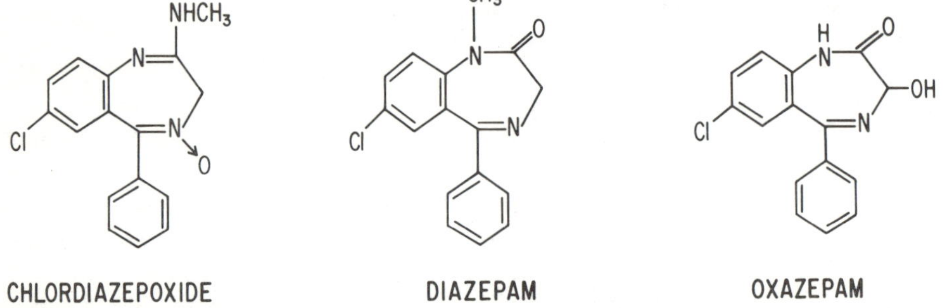

FIGURE 6. Chemical formulae of some tranquilizers.

7-chloro-1,3-dihydro-5-phenyl-2H-1,4-benzodiazepine-2-one-4-oxide excreted as such or further metabolized.

Administration of large doses (approximately ten times the therapeutic dose) to psychiatric patients increased the plasma halflife to approximately 48 hours.

In dogs a single oral dose of drug resulted in high plasma levels for 24 hours and measurable amounts were still present after 48 hours. Peak levels were reached in about 8 hours and the drug was slowly excreted in urine with 12% of the dose accounted for in 96 hours. The plasma halflife on oral administration was 14 to 20 hours. Oxazepam was identified as a metabolite in urine and feces. Chronic administration of chlordiazepoxide at a daily dose of 5 mg/kg for 9 weeks had no significant effect in amount converted to oxazepam.

In mice quick metabolic degradation and rapid elimination resulted in its low toxicity towards this species.[447]

Increased rate of tissue disappearance and excretion of ^{14}C-labeled chlordiazepoxide in tolerant rats suggested[448] that tolerance development involved stimulation of hepatic microsomal enzymes responsible for drug metabolism.

Metabolic *N*-demethylation of chlordiazepoxide has also been reported[449] by rat and dog liver microsomal preparations and pretreatment of rats with phenobarbital resulted in approximately threefold increase in metabolism of chlordiazepoxide to oxazepam after a two hour incubation with liver microsomal preparation.

Diazepam (7-chloro-1,3-dihydro-1-methyl-5-phenyl-2H-1,4-benzodiazepine-2-one)

Chemical Properties and Dosage

Diazepam (Valium®) was synthesized in 1959. It is a crystalline solid m. 125 to 126°C. Its hydrochloride salt is soluble in water. It is used as a tranquilizer and skeletal muscle relaxant. Oral dose as a tranquilizer ranges from 2 mg to 10 mg per day with wide variation in dosage depending on the patient.

Absorption, Fate, and Excretion

In syrup or tablet form, diazepam was equally well absorbed in children, but peak blood levels were reached later following administration as tablets.[450] In adults, the absorption of diazepam from suppositories was more gradual and to a lesser extent than in tablet form.

Studies on metabolism and disposition of diazepam[451-454] in experimental animals and man have shown that following single oral dose of 10 mg in man, 71% of the drug was excreted in urine, and 10% in the feces. Peak plasma levels of 0.07 μg/ml of diazepam were reached in 2 to 4 hours after administration. A portion of the drug is excreted rapidly with a halflife of 7 to 10 hours, while the remainder is excreted slowly with a halflife of 2 to 8 days. Oxazepam accounted for 33% of the metabolites, while *N*-demethylated derivative and 3-hydroxy compound each accounted for over 10%.

Repeated daily doses of diazepam (30 mg) caused a progressive increase in drug levels in man. *N*-demethylated diazepam appeared 24 to 36 hours after the first dose, and therafter these levels increased rapidly approaching those of diazepam. Upon discontinuing diazepam after repeated dosing, *N*-demethylated compound disappeared from blood very slowly and persisted longer than diazepam. Oxazepam and 3-hydroxy diazepam were found only in traces in blood.

Rats given 0.6 mg/kg of labeled drug intraperitoneally showed highest radioactivity in liver and perirenal fat and lowest in brain one hour after injection. Over 50% of an oral or i.p. dose of 0.6 mg/kg was excreted in the feces.[452]

Following an i.v. dose of 1 mg/kg, dogs excreted 61% of the dose in urine, 34% in feces. After a 10 mg/kg dose, the urinary excretion decreased to 40% and average fecal excretion was 35%. Ether-extractable metabolites of dog's blood consisted of a mixture of diazepam, *N*-demethylated diazepam and small amounts of oxazepam. *N*-demethylated diazepam was excreted free and major metabolite was oxazepam glucuronide.[453]

In rats following an i.p. dose of 25 mg, four metabolites of diazepam in the intestinal tract of animals were separated and characterized[455] by NMR and high resolution mass spectrometry. These were glucuronide or sulfate conjugates of 3-hydroxy diazepam, conjugate of 5-hydroxy phenyl analogue of diazepam, 3-hydroxy diazepam, and *N*-demethylated diazepam. The phenolic group was in para position in phenolic metabolite.

Studies on metabolism of diazepam in rabbits showed three identified metabolites representing less than 10% of the injected dose.[456] Also

2-methyl-amino-4-chloro benzophenone, 2-methylamino-5-chloro-4′-hydroxy benzophenone, 2-amino-5-chlorobenzophenone, and 2-amino-5-chloro-4′-hydroxy benzophenone (tentative) were isolated and identified as the products of hydrolysis of conjugated precursors from rabbit urine.

Pretreatment of dogs with phenobarbital resulted in an increased conversion of diazepam to its *N*-demethylated derivative and oxazepam.[457] No metabolite of ^3H-diazepam was detected on incubation of drug with 9000 xg supernatant of dog brain homogenate. Species differences have been noticed in diazepam metabolism.[458]

Oxazepam (7-chloro-1,3-dihydro-3-hydroxy-5-phenyl-2H-1,4-benzodiazepine-2-one)

Chemical Properties and Dosage

Oxazepam (Serax®) was introduced into medicine in 1962. It is a crystalline solid m. 205 to 206°C, practically insoluble in water and soluble in common organic solvents. Its hydrochloride salt is soluble in water. The usual oral dose as a tranquilizer is 10 to 30 mg.

Absorption, Fate, and Excretion

Disposition and metabolism studies[459] of oxazepam and its succinate half-ester showed that after oral administration to dog, rat, and pig, the drug is well absorbed and single doses were largely eliminated in two days in urine of dog and pig and in feces in the rat. In dog and pig, the glucuronide metabolite accounted for 95% of the drug, but in rat at least seven metabolites were observed. After i.m. injection oxazepam disappeared rapidly from the injection site in rats, uniformly distributed with somewhat higher concentration in gastrointestinal tract, liver, and kidney. In dogs after i.v. injection, peak blood levels occurred in 15 minutes, but declined so slowly that at four hours the blood levels were approximately the same as after oral administration. After 48 hours appreciable levels of drug were still present. Chromatography of the urine of dog and pig showed unchanged half-ester, oxazepam, and glucuronide of oxazepam. The fate of drug in humans presumably is similar to that in dog and pig.

A report on metabolism of oxazepam in organs isolated in situ[460] indicated that brain could partly conjugate oxazepam to its glucuronide.

Studies on tissue distribution[461] of oxazepam (20 mg/kg i.m.) in pregnant and fetal guinea pig and rat showed that concentration of oxazepam and its glucuronide was higher in guinea pig than in the rat. In both species, maternal levels were maximum at 30 and 60 minutes for oxazepam and its glucuronide, respectively. The drug and its conjugate were also present in fetus, though in lower concentration than those in maternal animals. At the end of pregnancy, fetal tissue could metabolize oxazepam in vitro; however, the activity was much lower than that in maternal organs.

DISPOSITION AND METABOLISM OF ETHANOL

Ethanol is a clear, colorless, mobile, flammable liquid b. 78.5°C, with pleasant odor and a burning taste. It is miscible with water and organic liquids. The level of blood alcohol associated with coma is usually between 0.45 to 0.55% by weight, the fatal level being 0.60 to 0.90%, which is further lowered to 0.35% in the presence of barbiturates.

Absorption, Fate, and Excretion

The metabolism of alcohol has been covered in excellent reviews.[462-466] Ethanol is rapidly absorbed from gastrointestinal tract, subcutaneous sites, and on inhalation from the lungs, but the absorption through the human skin is negligible. Following administration in fasting dogs through a stomach tube, approximately 95% was absorbed within 60 minutes. The brain to arterial blood ratio, 10 minutes after oral administration was 1:1.18 which remained practically constant during complete absorption of ethanol.[467] After absorption, ethanol was uniformly distributed throughout all tissues and body fluids. Although subject to dietary and hormonal factors, the average rate at which ethanol can be metabolized in adults is about 10 ml per hour.

In rats receiving a 1 g/kg oral dose of ^{14}C-ethanol, 75% of the dose is oxidized to $^{14}CO_2$ in 5 hours, 90% in 10 hours, and there was no difference between normal and ethanol-dependent rats with respect to this metabolism.[468] No significant differences were observed between the ability of tissue slices from normal and ethanol-habituated rats to oxidize ethanol in vitro. It was concluded that tolerance to ethanol may be a function of a developed insensitivity of neuronal receptor sites rather than an increased ability to dispose of the ethanol. With ^{14}C-label on first and second carbon atom of ethanol, it was shown[469] that both carbon atoms are converted to $^{14}CO_2$. Approximately 2.10% of the dose of ethanol is excreted unchanged in urine and expired air. In rabbits 0.5 to 2% of dose is excreted in urine as ethyl glucuronide.

The initial oxidation of ethanol to acetaldehyde which has been detected in in vitro metabolic studies, in blood of intact animals and in man given alcohol,[462] occurs chiefly in the liver and to a lesser extent in the kidney and lung. Other tissues including brain apparently do not oxidize alcohol. This oxidation is accomplished by alcohol dehydrogenase which utilizes NAD as hydrogen acceptor and is dependent upon free sulphydryl groups in protein for its activity.[464]

$$CH_3CH_2OH + NAD \xrightarrow[\text{dehydrogenase}]{\text{alcohol}} CH_3CHO + NADH + H^+$$

Using ethanol containing deuterium, it has been demonstrated that the hydrogen atom transferred to NAD comes directly from the α-carbon of ethanol.[465] Acetaldehyde dehydrogenase catalyzes the oxidation of acetaldehyde to acetic acid.[470,471]

$$CH_3CHO + NAD^+ + H_2O \longrightarrow CH_3COOH + NADH + H^+$$

$$\downarrow$$

$$\text{metabolic pool} \longrightarrow CO_2$$

$$\text{of 2 C atoms}$$

Other systems as catalase and the presence of hydrogen peroxide have also been implicated in ethanol oxidation.[462]

The rate of clearance of ethanol[463] in the dog was dose-dependent. At low doses giving a plasma concentration below 10 mg/100 ml, the rate of disappearance was proportional to the amount of ethanol present and the decline of plasma concentration followed an exponential curve. With larger doses, the rate of oxidation was not constant and varied in the same animal from hour to hour. Oxidation of ethanol was not sufficiently rapid to prevent its accumulation with larger doses of ethanol.

Ethanol given to animals pretreated with disulfiram[472] or cyanamide resulted in a two to ten times higher concentration of blood acetaldehyde than is found with same amount of ethanol in untreated animals. Disulfiram and cyanamide presumably inhibit or retard the metabolism of acetaldehyde, although the rate of disappearance of alcohol from blood is not changed from normal values.

Ethanol exhibited a dual effect of first decreasing and then increasing the activity of hepatic microsomal enzymes which may explain the seemingly less resistance of chronic alcoholics to barbiturates.[473a,b]

Recently liver microsomes have been reported[474,475] to contain an ethanol-oxidizing system distinct from alcohol dehydrogenase or catalase, that converts ethanol to acetaldehyde and NADPH and oxygen. The activity of this system has been reported[476] to increase with alcohol feeding which may explain the ability of chronic alcoholics to metabolize ethanol faster than normal subjects. Increased activity of other NADPH-dependent microsomal drug-detoxifying enzymes may explain the increased drug metabolism and resistance of alcoholics to various drugs.[477] It has recently been postulated that NADPH oxidase, in the presence of NADPH and oxygen leads to the production of NADP and hydrogen peroxide. NADP may then interact with ethanol and alcohol dehydrogenase to lead to acetaldehyde, and hydrogen peroxide may interact with ethanol via catalase to produce water and acetaldehyde.[478]

Physical dependence on ethanol could be demonstrated in mice within a very short time by maintenance of constant blood alcohol levels by housing them in an atmosphere of ethanol vapors. On removal from ethanol atmosphere, all animals developed withdrawal signs.[479] The ethanol-dependent mice did not show typical opiate-dependent behavior (withdrawal jumping syndrome) when challenged with opiate antagonist, naloxone.[480] It was concluded that alcohol dependence was not a manifestation of dependence upon any endogenous opiate as proposed earlier.[481]

THE IMPLICATIONS OF BIOLOGICAL DISPOSITION ON TOLERANCE AND PHYSICAL DEPENDENCE

Extensive research in the area of tolerance to and physical dependence[482-486] on opiates and barbiturates has led to the general belief that physical dependence on these agents does not develop outside the cerebrospinal axis, and the matrix of the central nervous system is critically involved in the genesis of these two parameters. Dependence varied from drug to drug even within the same chemical class, and the development of tolerance was a frequent but not invariable accompaniment of physical dependence. Compounds closely related to morphine, e.g., thebaine, and others such as cocaine and amphetamine with predominantly stimulant properties, did not produce physical dependence. Narcotic antagonists as cyclazocine and nalorphine produced tolerance and physical dependence without drug-seeking behavior.[175] Ethanol dependence was not a manifestation of dependence upon any endogenous opiate as proposed recently.[487-489]

The precise biochemical and physiological mechanisms involved in the development of tolerance and physical dependence are still not clear.[490,491] The concepts involving altered disposition, increased inactivation, more rapid disposal and metabolism of morphine, methadone, meperidine, and ethanol have not provided any insight into the mechanism of tolerance.[492,256,259,239,468] Enzymic studies[44] have actually shown less hepatic *N*-demethylating and glucuronyl transferase activity in morphine tolerant rats compared to nontolerant ones, and the decreased *N*-demethylation activity has been shown to be due to a decrease in the amount of enzyme, rather than to its inactivation as a result of alteration of receptor sites.[105] Several studies[43] do not support the hypothesis that *N*-dealkylation of analgesics[36] is an essential prerequisite for activation of these compounds and for initiation of analgesia. In spite of some resemblance of hepatic *N*-demethylating enzyme and narcotic drug receptor in respect of molecular specificity and antagonism to nalorphine, recent findings have challenged the suitability of this model.[493]

Diminished sensitivity of the receptor site in the central nervous system after chronic administration of narcotic analgesics and long-acting barbiturates has been attributed to cellular adaptation to an alien chemical environment.[368,494] Enzyme induction in the liver and accelerated oxidative breakdown to polar metabolites have been shown to be the principal causes of tolerance to short-acting barbiturates, tranquilizers (Librium®)[448] and sedative-hypnotics[400,418,476] (glutethimide, meprobamate, and ethanol) described in this chapter.

Although synthesis of new RNA and protein in brain of experimental animals has been shown to be an essential feature of the development of tolerance to morphine,[495] it is not yet certain whether the enzyme induction and synthesis of protein in the CNS is really involved in the development of physical dependence and tolerance in humans. Furthermore, protein synthesis inhibitors used in such studies on experimental animals are known to have many other direct and indirect effects on CNS, apart from the inhibition of protein synthesis.

Studies on the regional distribution[492] of labeled narcotic analgesics in the central nervous system and effects of antagonists thereon, have not provided any specific sites of localization of drug, and changes in drug concentrations in regional areas with antagonists were either small or not statistically significant. Similarly the studies with active and inactive isomers of levorphanol,[490] methadone,[263] and pentazocine[237] have not shown any meaningful differences in their regional distribution in the CNS which could explain the marked differences in biological activity of the isomers. Evidence that the induction of barbiturate tolerance was not stereospecific has also been produced recently.[387] No dramatic differences in the intracellular distribution[151,492] and uptake of narcotic drugs by nerve ending fractions have been shown in nontolerant and tolerant animals.[155]

Underlying most of these distribution studies in the CNS for the localization of primary sites of action of narcotics has been the assumption that cells particularly sensitive to morphine or other drugs will be concentrated in some discrete region of the brain. It is probable that such drugs do not act on specific regions of the brain, but rather on specific types of neurons or synapse. Cells situated in the same region may show different drug responses because of different chemical make-up and functional characteristics of neuronal membranes at different synaptic or axonal regions.[496] Future studies, no doubt, will be directed towards the elucidation of nature and mechanism of interaction of these centrally acting drugs on neuronal cell membranes with possible alteration of structure and organization of membranous proteins.

Recent studies[69,497,498] have furnished some information on the interrelationship of physical dependence and tolerance to morphine by the demonstration in the CNS of rats of a closely related morphine metabolite which could become an essential substrate in an alternative pathway of metabolism because of its close structural similarity to epinephrine. The covalent coupling of metabolite to specific neuronal proteins could result in biochemical alterations of neuronal structure and sensitivity due to prolonged occupation of essential target sites.

The ultimate goal of most of these biological disposition and intracellular distribution studies of narcotic analgesics has been the detection and isolation of the putative receptor for narcotics in the CNS which may exhibit molecular specificity and stereoselectivity. The topographical receptor model[499] and other variants involving different modes of interaction of practically all known analgesics with a hypothetical receptor region[500,501] have undoubtedly stimulated studies in the design of a large number of interesting compounds with a view to dissociate analgesia from physical dependence. The nature and character of narcotic receptor or its active site, however, have remained elusive so far.

There are many difficulties in the isolation of specific receptor substance free from tissue proteins producing nonspecific binding of drugs.[210a,b] Isolation procedures could bring about: (a) changes in structure, conformation, and function of macromolecules of which receptors may be an integral part, or (b) changes in spatial arrangement or charge distribution of receptors themselves which are the very basic elements of molecular specificity. A solution of some of these difficulties leading to a more precise knowledge of central receptor substance would indeed provide better understanding of the phenomena of tolerance and physical dependence.

REFERENCES

1. Brodie, B. B. and Hogben, C. A. M., Some physicochemical factors in drug action, *J. Pharm. Pharmacol.*, 9, 345, 1957.

2. Brodie, B. B., Distribution and fate of drugs; Therapeutic implications, in *Absorption and Distribution of Drugs*, Binns, T. B., Ed., Livingstone, Edinburgh, 1964, 199.

3. Schanker, L. S., Passage of drugs across body membranes, *Pharmacol. Rev.*, 14, 501, 1962.

4. Schanker, L. S., Pharmacologic implications of drug ionization, in *Uptake and Distribution of Anesthetic Agents*, Papper, E. M. and Kitz, R. J., Eds., McGraw-Hill, New York, 1963, 52.

5. Schanker, L. S., Physiological transport of drugs, *Advances Drug. Res.*, 1, 71, 1964.

6. Goldstein, A., The interaction of drugs and plasma proteins, *Pharmacol. Rev.*, 1, 102, 1949.

7. Wagner, J. G., Method for estimating rate constants for absorption, metabolism and elimination from urinary excretion data, *J. Pharm. Sci.*, 56, 489, 1967.

8. Gourley, D. R. H., Factors modifying drug action in the body, in *Modern Trends in Pharmacology and Therapeutics*, Fulton, W. F. M., Ed., Butterworths, London, 1967, 1.

9. Fincher, J. H., Particle size of drugs and its relationship to absorption and activity, *J. Pharm. Sci.*, 57, 1825, 1968.

10. Goldstein, A., Aronow, L., and Kalman, S. M., *Principles of Drug Action*, Hoeber Medical Division, Harper and Row, New York, 1968.

11. Gibaldi, M., Pharmacokinetic aspects of drug metabolism, *Ann. N. Y. Acad. Sci.*, 179, 19, 1971.

12. Roth, L. J. and Barlow, L. F., Drugs in the brain, *Science*, 134, 22, 1961.

13. Rall, D. P. and Zubrod, C. G., Mechanism of drug absorption and excretion - Passage of drugs in and out of the central nervous system, *Ann. Rev. Pharmacol.*, 2, 109, 1962.

14. Prockop, L. D., in *Uptake and Distribution of Anesthetic Agents*, Papper, E. M. and Kitz, R. J., Eds., McGraw-Hill, New York, 1963, 168.

15. Wagner, J. G., Biopharmaceutics - Absorption aspects, *J. Amer. Pharm. Ass.*, 50, 359, 1961.

16. Baker, J. B. E., The effect of drugs on the fetus, *Pharmacol. Rev.*, 12, 37, 1960.

17. Villee, C. A., Placental transfer of drugs, *Ann. N. Y. Acad. Sci.*, 123, 237, 1965.

18. Done, A. K., Perinatal pharmacology, *Ann. Rev. Pharmacol.*, 6, 189, 1966.

19. Gillette, J. R., Factors affecting drug metabolism, *Ann. N. Y. Acad. Sci.*, 179, 43, 1971.

20. Dollery, C. T., Davies, D. S., and Conolly, M. E., Differences in the metabolism of drugs depending upon their route of administration, *Ann. N. Y. Acad. Sci.*, 179, 108, 1971.

21. Brodie, B. B., Gillette, J. R., and La Du, B. N., Enzymatic metabolism of drugs and other foreign compounds, *Ann. Rev. Biochem.*, 27, 427, 1958.

22. Conney, A. H. and Burns, J. J., Factors influencing drug metabolism, *Advances Pharmacol.*, 1, 31, 1962.

23. Kalow, W., Dose-response relationships and genetic variation, *Ann. N. Y. Acad. Sci.*, 123, 212, 1965.

24. La Du, B. N., Pharmacogenetics, *Toxic. Appl. Pharmacol.*, 7, 27, 1965.

25. Motulsky, A. G., The genetics of abnormal drug responses, *Ann. N. Y. Acad. Sci.*, 123, 167, 1965.

26. Fouts, J. R. and Hart, L. G., Hepatic drug metabolism during perinatal period, *Ann. N. Y. Acad. Sci.*, 123, 245, 1965.

27. Gillette, J. R., Metabolism of drugs and other foreign compounds by enzymatic mechanisms, *Fortschr. Arzneimittelforschung*, 6, 11, 1963.

28. Kato, R. and Gillette, J. R., Sex differences in the effects of abnormal physiological states on the metabolism of drugs by rat liver microsomes, *J. Pharmacol. Exp. Ther.*, 150, 285, 1965.

29. Conney, A. H., Pharmacological implications of microsomal enzyme induction, *Pharmacol. Rev.*, 19, 317, 1967.

30. Breckenridge, A. and Orme, M., Clinical implications of enzyme induction, *Ann. N. Y. Acad. Sci.*, 179, 421, 1971.

31. Gulland, J. M. and Robinson, R., Constitution of codeine and thebaine, *Mem. Proc. Manchester Lit. Phil. Soc.*, 69, 79, 1925.

32a. Gates, M. and Tschudi, G., The synthesis of morphine, *J. Amer. Chem. Soc.*, 74, 1109, 1952.

32b. Gates, M. and Tschudi, G., Synthesis of morphine, *J. Amer. Chem. Soc.*, 78, 1380, 1956.

33. Yeh, S. Y. and Lach, J. L., Stability of morphine in aqueous solutions. IV. Isolation of morphine and sodium bisulfite interaction product, *J. Pharm. Sci.*, 60, 793, 1971.

34. Eddy, N. B., Chemical structure and action of morphine-like analgesics and related substances, *Chem. Industr.*, 1462, 1959.

35. Beckett, A. H., Analgesics: a general survey, *J. Pharm. Pharmacol.*, 4, 425, 1952.

36. Beckett, A. H., Analgesics and their antagonists: Some steric and chemical considerations I. Dissociation constants of some tertiary amines and synthetic analgesics: conformations of methadone type compounds, *J. Pharm. Pharmacol.*, 8, 848, 1956.

37. Kutter, E., Herz, A., Teschemacher, H. J., and Hess, R., Structure-activity correlations of morphine-like analgetics based on efficiencies following intravenous and intraventricular application, *J. Med. Chem.*, 13, 801, 1970.

38. Reynolds, A. K. and Randall, L. O., *Morphine and Allied Drugs*, University of Toronto Press, Toronto, 1957.

39. Mulé, S. J., Physiological disposition of narcotic agonists and antagonists, in *Narcotic Drugs – Biochemical Pharmacology*, Clouet, D. H., Ed., Plenum Press, New York, 1971, 99.

40. Scrafani, J. T. and Clouet, D. H., Biotransformations, in *Narcotic Drugs – Biochemical Pharmacology*, Clouet, D. H., Ed., Plenum Press, New York, 1971, 137.

41. Way, E. L. and Adler, T. K., The pharmacological implications of the fate of morphine and its surrogates, *Pharmacol. Rev.*, 12, 383, 1960.

42. Way, E. L. and Adler, T. K., The biological disposition of morphine and its surrogates, *World Health Organization*, Geneva, 1962.

43. Way, E. L., Distribution and metabolism of morphine and its surrogates, *Res. Publ. Ass. Nerv. Ment. Dis.*, 46, 13, 1968.

44. Takemori, A. E., The effects of morphine, other opioids and their derivatives on the metabolism of the cerebral cortex, *Res. Publ. Ass. Nerv. Ment. Dis.*, 46, 53, 1968.

45a. Farmilo, C. G., Oestreicher, P. M., and Levi, L., Common physical constants for identification of ninety-five narcotics and related compounds, *Bull. Narcotics, U.N. Dept. Social Affairs*, 6, 7, 1954.

45b. Martin, L., Genest, K., Cloutier, J. A. R., and Farmilo, C. G., Physicochemical methods for the identification of narcotics. VI. Common physical constants, ultraviolet, infrared and X-ray data for 12 narcotics and related compounds, *Bull. Narcotics, U.N. Dept. Social Affairs*, 15, 17, 1963.

46. Adler, T. K., Elliott, H. W., and George, R., Some factors affecting the biological disposition of small doses of morphine in rats, *J. Pharmacol. Exp. Ther.*, 120, 475, 1957.

47. Adler, T. K., George, R., and Elliott, H. W., Vasopressin potentiation of morphine action in rats, *Fed. Proc.*, 15, 393, 1956.

48. Szerb, J. C. and McCurdy, D. H., Concentration of morphine in blood and brain after intravenous injection of morphine in nontolerant, tolerant and neostigmine-treated rats, *J. Pharmacol. Exp. Ther.*, 118, 446, 1956.

49. Jóhannesson, T. and Schou, J., Analgesic activity and brain concentration of morphine in tolerant and nontolerant rats given morphine alone or with neostigmine, *Acta Pharmacol. Toxicol.*, 20, 213, 1963.

50. Way, E. L., Sung, C-Y., and Fujimoto, J. M., The effect of adrenalectomy on the development of tolerance to morphine and methadone, *J. Pharmacol. Exp. Ther.*, 110, 51, 1954.

51. Kupferberg, H. and Way, E. L., Pharmacological basis for the increased susceptibility of the newborn rat to morphine, *J. Pharmacol. Exp. Ther.*, 141, 105, 1963.

52. Way, E. L., Infantile drug distribution, *Rep. Ross. Pediat. Res. Conf.*, 58, 66, 1968.

53. Way, E. L., Brain uptake of morphine and its implications, *Fed. Proc.*, 26, 1115, 1967.

54. Elliott, H. W., Tolbert, B. M., Adler, T. K., and Anderson, H. H., Excretion of carbon-14 by man after administration of morphine-*N*-methyl-C^{14}, *Proc. Soc. Exp. Biol. Med.*, 85, 77, 1954.

55. Paerregaard, P., Excretion of morphine in the urine of addicts, *Acta Pharmacol. Toxicol.*, 14, 53, 1957.

56. Miller, J. W. and Elliott, H. W., Rat tissue levels of carbon-14 labeled analgesics as related to pharmacological activity, *J. Pharmacol. Exp. Ther.*, 113, 283, 1955.

57. Teschemacher, H. J., Schubert, P., Kreutzberg, G. W., and Herz, A., Autoradiographische Darstellung ^{14}C-markierten morphins nach intraventrikulärer und intracerebraler injection, *Arch. Exp. Path. Pharmak.*, 260, 211, 1968.

58. Mulé, S. J., Clements, T. H., Layson, R. C., and Haertzen, C. A., Analgesia in guinea pigs: A measure of tolerance development, *Arch. Int. Pharmacodyn.*, 173, 201, 1968.

59. Mulé, S. J., Redman, C. M., and Flesher, J. W., Intracellular disposition of H^3-morphine in the brain and liver of nontolerant and tolerant guinea pigs, *J. Pharmacol. Exp. Ther.*, 157, 459, 1967.

60. Mulé, S. J. and Woods, L. A., Distribution of N-^{14}C-methyl labeled morphine: I. in central nervous system of nontolerant and tolerant dogs, *J. Pharmacol. Exp. Ther.*, 136, 232, 1962.

61. Mulé, S. J., Woods, L. A., and Mellett, L. B., Distribution of N-^{14}C-methyl labeled morphine. II. Effect on nalorphine in the central nervous system of nontolerant dogs and observations on metabolism, *J. Pharmacol. Exp. Ther.*, 136, 242, 1962.

62. Mulé, S. J., Distribution of N-^{14}C-methyl labeled morphine, III. Effect of nalorphine in the central nervous system and other tissues of tolerant dogs, *J. Pharmacol. Exp. Ther.*, 148, 393, 1965.

63. Woods, L. A., Distribution and fate of morphine in nontolerant and tolerant dogs and rats, *J. Pharmacol. Exp. Ther.*, 112, 158, 1954.

64. Woods, L. A., Comparative distribution of morphine and nalorphine in dog brain, *J. Pharmacol. Exp. Ther.*, 120, 58, 1956.

65. Mellett, L. B. and Woods, L. A., The distribution and fate of morphine in the nontolerant and tolerant monkey, *J. Pharmacol. Exp. Ther.*, 116, 77, 1956.

66. Siminoff, R. and Saunders, P. R., Concentrations of free and conjugated morphine in brain and other tissues of tolerant and nontolerant rabbits, *J. Pharmacol. Exp. Ther.*, 124, 252, 1958.

67. Jóhannesson, T. and Woods, L. A., Analgesic action and brain and plasma levels of morphine and codeine in morphine tolerant, codeine tolerant and nontolerant rats, *Acta Pharmacol. Toxicol.*, 21, 381, 1964.

68. Chernov, H. I. and Woods, L. A., Central nervous system distribution and metabolism of ^{14}C-morphine during morphine induced feline mania, *J. Pharmacol. Exp. Ther.*, 149, 146, 1965.

69. Misra, A. L., Mitchell, C. L., and Woods, L. A., Persistence of morphine in the central nervous system of rats after a single injection and its bearing on tolerance, *Nature*, (London), 232, 48, 1971.

70. Misra, A. L. and Mitchell, C. L., Determination of morphine-*N*-methyl-^{14}C oxide in biological materials – its excretion and metabolites in the rat, *Biochem. Med.*, 5, 379, 1971.

71. Misra, A. L. and Mulé, S. J., Disposition and metabolism of ^{3}H-pseudomorphine in the rat, *Biochem. Pharmacol.*, 21, 103, 1972.

72. Takemori, A. E. and Stenwick, M. W., Studies on the uptake of morphine by choroid plexus *in vitro, J. Pharmacol. Exp. Ther.*, 154, 586, 1966.

73. Hug, C. C., Jr., Transport of narcotic analgesics by choroid plexus and kidney tissue *in vitro, Biochem. Pharmacol.*, 16, 345, 1967.

74. Scrafani, J. T. and Hug, C. C., Jr., Active uptake of dihydromorphine and other narcotic analgesics by cerebral cortical slices, *Biochem. Pharmacol.*, 17, 1557, 1968.

75. Asghar, K. and Way, E. L., Active removal of morphine from the cerebral ventricles, *J. Pharmacol. Exp. Ther.*, 175, 75, 1970.

76. Navon, S. and Lajtha, A., Uptake of morphine in particulate fractions from rat brain, *Brain Res.*, 24, 534, 1970.

77. Kayan, S., Misra, A. L., and Woods, L. A., Uptake of (7,8-^{3}H) dihydromorphine by rat cerebral cortical slices and eye tissue, *J. Pharm. Pharmacol.*, 22, 941, 1970.

78. Clouet, D. H. and Williams, N., The binding of narcotic analgesics in synaptosomal and other particulate fractions of rat brain, *Pharmacologist*, 13, 313, 1971.

79. Tsou, K. and Jang, C. S., Studies on the site of analgesic action of morphine by intracerebral micro-injection, *Sci. Sinica*, 7, 1099, 1964.

80. Buxbaum, D. M., Yarbrough, G. G., and Carter, M. E., Differentiation of possible sites of action of morphine and amphetamine in the rat, *Pharmacologist*, 13, 314, 1971.

81. Yoshimura, H., Oguri, K., and Tsukamoto, H., Metabolism of drugs – isolation and identification of morphine glucuronides in urine and bile of rabbits, *Biochem. Pharmacol.*, 18, 279, 1969.

82. Misra, A. L., Yeh, S. Y., and Woods, L. A., Morphine conjugates in the dog, *Biochem. Pharmacol.*, 19, 1536, 1970.

83. Yoshimura, H., Mori, M., Oguri, K., and Tsukamoto, H., Metabolism of drugs.LXV. Urinary conjugated metabolites of codeine, *Biochem. Pharmacol.*, 19, 2353, 1970.

84. Oguri, K., Ida, S., Yoshimura, H., and Tsukamoto, H., Metabolism of drugs. LXIX. Studies on urinary metabolites of morphine in several mammalian species, *Chem. Pharm. Bull.* (Tokyo), 18, 2414, 1970.

85. Yoshimura, H., Oguri, K., and Tsukamoto, H., Synthesis of codeine and morphine glucuronides, *Tetrahedron Lett.*, 483, 1968.

86. Takemori, A. E. and Glowacki, G. A., Studies on glucuronide synthesis in rats chronically treated with morphine and phenol, *Biochem. Pharmacol.*, 11, 867, 1962.

87. Kato, R. and Gillette, J. R., Sex differences in the effects of abnormal physiological states on the metabolism of drugs by rat liver microsomes, *J. Pharmacol. Exp. Ther.*, 150, 285, 1965.

88. Castro, J. A. and Gillette, J. R., Species and sex differences in the kinetic constants for the *N*-demethylation of ethyl morphine by liver microsomes, *Biochem. Biophys. Res. Comm.*, 28, 426, 1967.

89. Sanchez, E., Tampier, L., and Mardones, J., Effects of chloroquine pretreatment on lethal doses of morphine and on morphine metabolism in rats, *Europ. J. Pharmacol.*, 7, 106, 1969.

90. Yeh, S. Y. and Mitchell, C. L., Potentiation and reduction of analgesia and toxicity of morphine in the rat by pargyline, *Pharmacologist*, 13, 314, 1971.

91. Abrams, L. S. and Elliott, H. W., Morphine conjugation by the Gunn rats, *Pharmacologist*, 13, 194, 1971.

92. Woods, L. A. and Chernov, H. I., A new morphine metabolite from cat urine, *Pharmacologist*, 8, 206, 1966.

93. Fujimoto, J. M. and Haarstad, V. B., Isolation of 3-morphine ethereal sulfate from urine of chicken and cat, *J. Pharmacol. Exp. Ther.*, 165, 45, 1969.

94. May, D. G., Fujimoto, J. M., and Inturrisi, C. E., The tubular transport and metabolism of morphine-*N*-methyl-^{14}C by the chicken kidney, *J. Pharmacol. Exp. Ther.*, 157, 626, 1967.

95. Yeh, S. Y., Chernov, H. I., and Woods, L. A., Metabolism of morphine by cats, *J. Pharm. Sci.*, 60, 469, 1971.

96. Axelrod, J., Possible mechanism of tolerance to narcotic drugs, *Science*, 124, 263, 1956.

97. Cochin, J. and Axelrod, J., Biochemical and pharmacological changes in the rat following chronic administration of morphine, nalorphine and normorphine, *J. Pharmacol. Exp. Ther.*, 125, 105, 1959.

98. Misra, A. L., Mulé, S. J., and Woods, L. A., *In vivo* formation of normorphine in the rat as a metabolite of tritium nuclear labeled morphine, *Nature* (London), 190, 82, 1961.

99. Misra, A. L., Mule, S. J., and Woods, L. A., The preparation of tritium nuclear-labeled morphine and evidence for its *in vivo* biotransformation to normorphine in the rat, *J. Pharmacol. Exp. Ther.*, 132, 317, 1961.

100. Milthers, K., The *N*-demethylation of morphine in rats. Quantitative determination of normorphine and morphine in the urine and feces of rats given subcutaneous morphine, *Acta. Pharmacol. Toxicol.*, 19, 149, 1962.

101. Milthers, K., *N*-dealkylation of morphine and nalorphine in the brain of living rats, *Nature* (London), 195, 607, 1962.

102. Elison, C. and Elliott, H. W., *N*- and *O*-demethylation of some narcotic analgesics by brain slices from male and female Long-Evans rats, *Biochem. Pharmacol.*, 12, 1363, 1963.

103. Tampier, L. and Penna-Herreros, A., Normorphine – A metabolite of morphine and nalorphine in the cat, *Arch. Biol. Med. Exp.*, 3, 146, 1966.

104. Leadbeater, L. and Davies, D. R., The inhibition of the liver microsomal *N*-demethylation of morphine by *N*-allyl normorphine and its pharmacological implications, *Biochem. Pharmacol.*, 13, 1569, 1964.

105. Elison, C., Elliott, H. W., Look, M., and Rapoport, H., Some aspects of the fate and relationship of the *N*-methyl group of morphine to its pharmacological activity, *J. Med. Chem.*, 6, 237, 1963.

106. Adler, T. K., Studies on morphine tolerance in mice. I. *In vitro* *N*-demethylation of morphine and *N*- and *O*-demethylation of codeine, *J. Pharmacol. Exp. Ther.*, 156, 585, 1967.

107. Axelrod, J., The enzymatic *N*-demethylation of narcotic drugs, *J. Pharmacol. Exp. Ther.*, 117, 322, 1956.

108. Remmer, H. and Alsleben, B., Die Aktivierung der Entgiftung in den Lebermikrosomen während der Gewöhnung, *Klin. Wschr.*, 36, 332, 1958.

109. Jóhannesson, T., Rogers, L. A., Fouts, J. R., and Woods, L. A., The effects of codeine tolerance on hepatic microsomal drug metabolism in the rat, *Acta Pharmacol. Toxicol.*, 22, 107, 1965.

110. Mannering, G. J. and Takemori, A. E., The effect of repeated administration of levorphan, dextrorphan and morphine on the capacity of rat liver preparation to demethylate morphine and morphinan-type analgesics, *J. Pharmacol. Exp. Ther.*, 127, 187, 1959.

111. Clouet, D. H. and Ratner, M., The effect of altering liver microsomal *N*-demethylase activity on the development of tolerance to morphine in rats, *J. Pharmacol. Exp. Ther.*, 144, 362, 1964.

112. Schuster, L. and Hannan, R. V., Changes in morphine and chlorpromazine *N*-demethylase during the development of tolerance to chlorpromazine in mice, *Canad. J. Biochem.*, 43, 899, 1965.

113. Elison, C. and Elliott, H. W., Studies on the enzymatic *N*- and *O*-demethylation of narcotic analgesics and evidence for the formation of codeine from morphine in rats and dogs, *J. Pharmacol. Exp. Ther.*, 144, 265, 1964.

114. Daly, J., Inscoe, J. K., and Axelrod, J., The formation of *O*-methylated catechols by microsomal hydroxylation of phenols and subsequent enzymatic catechol *O*-methylation-substrate specificity, *J. Med. Chem.*, 8, 153, 1965.

115. Woo, J. T. C., Gaff, G. A., and Fennessy, M. R., A note on the effects of 2,4-diamino-5-phenyl thiazole and 1,2,3,4-tetrahydro-9-amino acridine on morphine metabolism, *J. Pharm. Pharmacol.*, 20, 763, 1968.

116. Fish, M. S., Johnson, N. M., Lawrence, E. P., and Horning, E. C., Oxidative *N*-dealkylation, *Biochim. Biophys. Acta*, 18, 564, 1955.

117. McMahon, R. E., Microsomal dealkylation of drugs-substrate specificity and mechanism, *J. Pharm. Sci.*, 55, 457, 1966.

118. Hosoya, E. and Brody, T. M., *In vitro* oxidation of morphine by rat tissue homogenates, *J. Pharmacol. Exp. Ther.*, 120, 504, 1957.

119. Mulé, S. J. and Mannering, G. J., Absence of trans-*N*-methylation of morphine in the rat, *Bull. Narcotics*, 17, 27, 1965.

120. Braun, J. V., Kruber, O., and Aust, E., Morphine alkaloids, *Ber. Dtsch. Chem. Ges.*, 47, 2312, 1914.

121. Lasagna, L. and Kornfield, T. J., Analgesic potency of normorphine in patients with post operative pain, *J. Pharmacol. Exp. Ther.*, 124, 260, 1958.

122. Orahovats, P. D. and Lehman, F. J., Studies with normorphine in animals, *J. Pharmacol. Exp. Ther.*, 122, 58, 1958.

123. Adler, T. K., The comparative potencies of codeine and demethylated metabolites after ventricular injection in the mouse, *J. Pharmacol. Exp. Ther.*, 140, 155, 1963.

124. Miller, J. W. and Anderson, H. H., The effect of *N*-demethylation on certain pharmacological actions of morphine, codeine and meperidine in the mouse, *J. Pharmacol. Exp. Ther.*, 112, 191, 1954.

125. Beckett, A. H., Casy, A. F., and Harper, N. J., Analgesics and their antagonists – steric and chemical considerations. III. Influence of the basic group on the biological response, *J. Pharm. Pharmacol.*, 8, 874, 1956.

126. Misra, A. L., Jacoby, H. I., and Woods, L. A., The preparation of tritium-labeled normorphine and its physiological disposition in dog and monkey, *J. Pharmacol. Exp. Ther.*, 132, 311, 1961.

127. Holtzmann, S. G. and Villarreal, J. E., Morphine dependence and body temperature in rhesus monkeys, *J. Pharmacol. Exp. Ther.*, 166, 125, 1969.

128. Jóhannesson, T. and Milthers, K., Morphine and normorphine in the brain of rats. A comparison of subcutaneous, intraperitoneal and intravenous adminstration, *Acta Pharmacol. Toxicol.*, 19, 241, 1962.

129. Jóhannesson, T. and Schou, J., Morphine and normorphine in the brain of rats given identically analgesic doses of morphine, codeine or normorphine, *Acta Pharmacol. Toxicol.*, 20, 165, 1963.

130. Clouet, D. H., The methylation of normorphine in rat brain and liver, *Life Sci.*, 1, 31, 1962.

131. Clouet, D. H., Ratner, M., and Kurzman, M., *N*-methylation of morphine by rat tissues *in vitro, Biochem. Pharmacol.*, 12, 957, 1963.

132. Clouet, D. H., The methylation of normorphine in rat brain *in vivo, Biochem. Pharmacol.*, 12, 967, 1963.

133. Axelrod, J., Enzymatic formation of morphine and nicotine in a mammal, *Life Sci.*, 1, 29, 1962.

134. Axelrod, J., The enzymatic *N*-methylation of serotonin and other amines, *J. Pharmacol. Exp. Ther.*, 138, 28, 1962.

135. Yeh, S. Y. and Woods, L. A., Physiologic disposition of N-^{14}C-methyl codeine in the rat, *J. Pharmacol. Exp. Ther.*, 166, 86, 1969.

136. Yeh, S. Y. and Woods, L. A., Isolation of morphine-3-glucuronide from urine and bile of rats injected with codeine, *J. Pharmacol. Exp. Ther.*, 175, 69, 1970.

137. Kuhn, H. F. and Friebel, H., Die Ausscheidung von Codein und Codein Metaboliten im Harn codeingewöhnter Ratten und Meerschweinchen, *Med. Exp.*, 7, 255, 1962.

138. Yeh, S. Y. and Woods, L. A., Isolation and characterization of codeine-6-glucuronide from dog urine, *J. Pharmacol. Exp. Ther.*, 173, 21, 1970.

139. Elliott, H. W., Nomof, N., and Parker, K. D., Correlation of the nalorphine test with concentration of metabolites of codeine in the urine after single and continuous administration, *Clin. Pharmacol. Ther.*, 8, 78, 1967.

140. Yeh, S. Y. and Woods, L. A., *N*-demethylation of N-^{14}C-methyl codeine in morphine tolerant and nontolerant rats and mice, *Proc. Soc. Exp. Biol. Med.*, 136, 782, 1971.

141. Rubin, A., Tephly, T. R., and Mannering, G. J., Inhibition of hexobarbital metabolism by ethyl morphine and codeine in the intact rat, *Biochem. Pharmacol.*, 13, 1053, 1964.

142. Eddy, N. B., Halbach, H., and Braenden, O. J., Synthetic substances with morphine-like effect – Relationship between analgesic action and addiction liabilities with a discussion of the chemical structure of addiction producing substances, *Bull. W.H.O.*, 14, 353, 1956.

143. Hug, C. C., Jr. and Mellett, L. B., Tritium-labeled dihydromorphine: its metabolic fate and excretion in the rat, *J. Pharmacol. Exp. Ther.*, 149, 446, 1965.

144. Hug, C. C., Jr., Mellett, L. B., and Cafruny, E. J., Stop-flow analysis of the renal excretion of tritium-labeled dihydromorphine, *J. Pharmacol. Exp. Ther.*, 150, 259, 1965.

145. Yeh, S. Y. and Woods, L. A., The effect of tolerance and withdrawal on *in vitro* metabolism of N-^{14}C methyl dihydromorphine in the rat, *J. Pharmacol. Exp. Ther.*, 169, 168, 1969.

146. Hug, C. C., Jr., Tritium-labeled dihydromorphine: A research tool for the investigation of the fate and distribution of narcotic analgesics, Ph.D. Thesis, The University of Michigan, Ann Arbor, Michigan, 1963.

147. Sanner, J. H. and Woods, L. A., Comparative distribution of tritium-labeled dihydromorphine between maternal and fetal rats, *J. Pharmacol. Exp. Ther.*, 148, 176, 1965.

148. Blane, G. F. and Dobbs, H. E., Distribution of tritium-labeled etorphine (M-99) and dihydromorphine in pregnant rats at term, *Brit. J. Pharmacol.*, 30, 166, 1967.

149. Yeh, S. Y. and Woods, L. A., Maternal and fetal distribution of ^{3}H-dihydromorphine in tolerant and nontolerant rats, *J. Pharmacol. Exp. Ther.*, 174, 9, 1970.

150. Kosterlitz, H. W., Thompson, J. W., and Wallis, D. I., Dihydromorphine in peripheral nervous tissue, *Nature* (London), 201, 719, 1964.

151. Van Praag, D. and Simon, E. J., Studies on the intracellular distribution and tissue binding of dihydromorphine-7,8^{3}H in the rat, *Proc. Soc. Exp. Biol. Med.*, 122, 6, 1966.

152. Hug, C. C., Jr., Transport in the central nervous system in *Narcotic Drugs – Biochemical Pharmacology*, Clouet, D. H., Ed., Plenum Press, New York, 1971, 132.

153. Scrafani, J. T., Williams, N., and Clouet, D. H., Binding of dihydromorphine to subcellular fractions of rat brain, *Pharmacologist*, 11, 256, 1969.

154. Oka, T., Scrafani, J. T., and Hug, C. C., Jr., Membrane transport and tissue binding of narcotic analgesics in brain, *Pharmacologist*, 11, 269, 1969.

155. Hug, C. C., Jr. and Oka, T., Uptake of dihydromorphine-^{3}H by synaptosomes, *Life Sci.*, Part I, 10, 201, 1971.

156. Seevers, M. H. and Pfeiffer, C. C., A study of analgesia, subjective depression, euphoria produced by morphine, heroin, dilaudid and codeine in normal human subjects, *J. Pharmacol. Exp. Ther.*, 56, 166, 1936.

157. Martin, W. R. and Fraser, H. F., A comparative study of physiological and subjective effects of heroin and morphine administered intravenously in addicts, *J. Pharmacol. Exp. Ther.*, 133, 388, 1961.

158. Kemp, J. W. and Way, E. L., *In vitro* studies on the metabolism of heroin, *Fed. Proc.*, 18, 409, 1959.

159. Way, E. L., Kemp, J. W., Young, J. M., and Grassetti, D. R., The pharmacologic effects of heroin in relationship to its rate of biotransformation, *J. Pharmacol. Exp. Ther.*, 129, 144, 1960.

160. Way, E. L., Young, J. M., and Kemp, J. W., Metabolism of heroin and its pharmacologic implications, *Bull. Narcotics*, 17, 25, 1965.

161. Nakamura, G. R. and Ukita, T., Paper chromatographic study *in vitro* and *in vivo* hydrolysis of heroin in blood, *J. Pharm. Sci.*, 56, 294, 1967.

162. Way, E. L., Pharmacologic implications of some factors in influencing the brain uptake of morphine, *Arch. Biol. Med. Exp.*, 4, 92, 1967.

163. Oberst, F. W., Studies on the fate of heroin, *J. Pharmacol. Exp. Ther.*, 79, 266, 1943.

164. Bentley, K. W. and Hardy, D. G., New potent analgesics in the morphine series, *Proc. Chem. Soc.*, 220, 1963.

165. Blane, G. F., Boura, A. L. A., Fitzgerald, A. E., and Lister, R. E., Actions of etorphine hydrochloride (M-99): a potent morphine-like agent, *Brit. J. Pharmacol.*, 30, 11, 1967.

166. Wallach, J. D., A new analgesic immobilizing agent and its antagonists, *Vet. Med.*, 64, 53, 1969.

167. Dobbs, H. E., Blane, G. F., and Boura, A. L. A., Uptake of etorphine and dihydromorphine after sublingual and intramuscular administration, *Europ. J. Pharmacol.*, 7, 328, 1969.

168. Blane, G. F. and Dobbs, H. E., Distribution of tritium-labeled etorphine (M-99) and dihydromorphine in pregnant rats at term, *Brit. J. Pharmacol.*, 30, 166, 1967.

169. Pleuvry, B. J. and Rees, J. M. H., The effects of etorphine and of morphine on respiration, blood carbon dioxide tension, and carbon dioxide sensitivity in the conscious rabbit, *J. Pharm. Pharmacol.*, 21, 814, 1969.

170. McCawley, E. L., Hart, E. R., and Marsh, D. F., The preparation of *N*-allyl-normorphine, *J. Amer. Chem. Soc.*, 63, 314, 1941.

171. Hart, E. R. and McCawley, E. L., The pharmacology of *N*-allyl normorphine as compared with morphine, *J. Pharmacol. Exp. Ther.*, 82, 339, 1944.

172. Eddy, N. B., Analgesic and dependence-producing properties of drugs, *Res. Publ. Ass. Nerv. Ment. Dis.*, 46, 1, 1968.

173. Martin, W. R. and Gorodetzky, C. W., Demonstration of tolerance to and physical dependence on *N*-allyl normorphine (nalorphine), *J. Pharmacol. Exp. Ther.*, 150, 437, 1965.

174. Woods, L. A., The pharmacology of nalorphine (*N*-allyl normorphine), *Pharmacol. Rev.*, 84, 175, 1956.

175. Martin, W. R., Opioid antagonists, *Pharmacol. Rev.*, 19, 464, 1967.

176. Archer, S. and Harris, L. S., in *Progress in Drug Research*, Jucker, E. J., Ed., Birkhaüser Verlag, Basel, 1965, 261.

177. Woods, L. A. and Muehlenbeck, H. E., Distribution and fate of nalorphine in the dog and cat, *J. Pharmacol. Exp. Ther.*, 120, 52, 1957.

178. Woods, L. A., Comparative distribution of morphine and nalorphine in dog brain, *J. Pharmacol. Exp. Ther.*, 120, 58, 1957.

179. Hug, C. C., Jr. and Woods, L. A., Tritium-labeled nalorphine – its CNS distribution and biological fate in dogs, *J. Pharmacol. Exp. Ther.*, 142, 248, 1963.

180. Axelrod, J. and Cochin, J., The inhibitory action of nalorphine on the enzymatic *N*-demethylation of narcotic drugs, *J. Pharmacol. Exp. Ther.*, 121, 107, 1957.

181. Seibert, R. A. and Huggins, R. A., Conjugation of *N*-allyl normorphine by liver slices, *Proc. Soc. Exp. Biol. Med.*, 82, 518, 1953.

182. Catalina, M. and Huidobro, F., Influence of nalorphine on morphine fixation by brain homogenates, *Arch. Biol. Med. Exp.*, 6, 53, 1969.

183. Fujimoto, J. M., Watrous, W. M., and Haarstad, V. B., Isolation of nalorphine ethereal sulfate and nalorphine glucuronide from urine of cat and rabbit, *Proc. Soc. Exp. Biol. Med.*, 130, 546, 1969.

184. Yeh, S. Y. and Woods, L. A., Isolation and characterization of urinary metabolites of nalorphine in dogs and cats, *J. Pharm. Sci.*, 60, 148, 1971.

185. Yoshimura, H., Mori, M., and Oguri, K., Synthesis of nalorphine 3- and 6-glucuronides and identification of urinary metabolites of nalorphine in rabbits, *Chem. Pharm. Bull.* (Tokyo), 18, 2548, 1970.

186. Lockett, M. F. and Davies, M. M., The analgesic action of normorphine administered intracisternally to mice, *J. Pharm. Pharmacol.*, 10, 80, 1958.

187. Maggiolo, C. and Huidobro, F., Intraventricular administration of nalorphine to mice implanted with pellets of morphine, *Nature* (London), 211, 540, 1966.

188. Blumberg, H., Dayton, H. B., George, M., and Rapoport, D. N., *N*-allyl noroxymorphone – a potent narcotic antagonist, *Fed. Proc.*, 20, 311, 1961.

189. Gordon, M., Lafferty, J. J., Tedeschi, D. H., Eddy, N. B., and May, E. L., A new potent analgesic antagonist, *Nature* (London), 192, 1089, 1961.

190. Zaks, A., Jones, T., Fink, M., and Freedman, A. M., Naloxone treatment of opiate dependence, *J.A.M.A.*, 215, 2108, 1971.

191. Jaisinski, D. R., Martin, W. R., and Haertzen, C. A., The human pharmacology and abuse potential of *N*-allyl noroxymorphone (naloxone), *J. Pharmacol. Exp. Ther.*, 157, 420, 1967.

192. Fujimoto, J. M., Isolation of two different glucuronide metabolites of naloxone from urine of rabbit and chicken, *J. Pharmacol. Exp. Ther.*, 168, 180, 1969.

193. Fujimoto, J. M., Isolation of naloxone-3-glucuronide from human urine, *Proc. Soc. Exp. Biol. Med.*, 133, 317, 1970.

194. Ober, K. F. and Fujimoto, J. M., Isolation of naloxone metabolite – naloxone 3-ethereal sulfate from the urine of the cat, *Pharmacologist*, 13, 263, 1971.

195a. Schnider, O. and Gruessner, A., Synthesis of hydroxymorphinans, *Helv. Chim. Acta*, 32, 821, 1949.

195b. Schnider, O. and Gruessner, A., Hydroxymorphinan – optically active-3-hydroxymorphinan, *Helv. Chim. Acta*, 34, 2211, 1951.

196. Randall, L. D. and Lehmann, G., Analgesic action of 3-hydroxy-*N*-methyl morphinan hydrobromide (dromoran), *J. Pharmacol. Exp. Ther.*, 99, 163, 1950.

197. Isbell, H. and Fraser, H. F., Actions and addiction liabilities of dromoran derivatives in man, *J. Pharmacol. Exp. Ther.*, 107, 524, 1953.

198. Fisher, H. and Long, J. P., The absorption and excretion of dromoran, *J. Pharmacol. Exp. Ther.*, 107, 241, 1953.

199. Shore, P. A., Axelrod, J., Hogben, C. A. M., and Brodie, B. B., Observations on the fate of dromoran in the dog and its excretion into the gastric juice, *J. Pharmacol. Exp. Ther.*, 113, 192, 1955.

200. Woods, L. A., Mellett, L. B., and Anderson, K. A., The synthesis and estimation of N-^{14}C-methyl labeled levorphanol and its biological disposition in the monkey, dog and rat, *J. Pharmacol. Exp. Ther.*, 124, 1, 1958.

201. Takemori, A. E. and Mannering, G. J., Metabolic *N* and *O*-demethylation of morphine and morphinan type of analgesics, *J. Pharmacol. Exp. Ther.*, 123, 171, 1958.

202. Wuepper, K. D. and Woods, L. A., The distribution of free N-^{14}C-methyl labeled levorphanol in the CNS of nontolerant and tolerant monkeys, *Fed. Proc.*, 19, 272, 1960.

203. Wuepper, K. D., Yeh, S. Y., and Woods, L. A., Effect of nalorphine and levallorphan on brain concentration of levorphanol in the dog, *Proc. Soc. Exp. Biol. Med.*, 124, 1146, 1967.

204. Heng, J. and Woods, L. A., Effect of nalorphine on concentration of N-^{14}C-methyl levorphanol in plasma and brain of rats, *Fed. Proc.*, 17, 376, 1958.

205. Mellett, L. B. and Woods, L. A., The intracellular distribution of N-^{14}C-methyl levorphanol in brain, liver, and kidney tissue of the rat, *J. Pharmacol. Exp. Ther.*, 125, 97, 1959.

206. Smith, A. A., Karmin, M., and Gavitt, J. A., Interaction of catecholamines with levorphanol and morphine in the mouse eye, *J. Pharmacol. Exp. Ther.*, 151, 103, 1966.

207. Goldstein, A. and Sheehan, P., Tolerance to opioid narcotics. I. Tolerance to the "running fit" caused by levorphanol in the mouse, *J. Pharmacol. Exp. Ther.*, 169, 175, 1969.

208. Richter, J. A. and Goldstein, A., Effects of morphine and levorphanol on brain acetyl choline content in mice, *J. Pharmacol. Exp. Ther.*, 175, 685, 1970.

209. Richter, J. A. and Goldstein, A., Tolerance to opioid narcotics. II. Cellular tolerance to levorphanol in mouse brain, *Proc. Nat. Acad. Sci.*, (Washington), 66, 944, 1970.

210a. Pal, B. K. and Goldstein, A., Stereospecific binding of morphine congener levorphanol by mouse brain preparations, *Fed. Proc.*, 30, 272, 1971.

210b. Goldstein, A., Lowney, L. I., and Pal, B. K., Stereospecific and nonspecific interactions of the morphine congener levorphanol in subcellular fractions of mouse brain, *Proc. Nat. Acad. Sci.*, (Washington), 68, 1742, 1971.

211. May, E. L. and Eddy, N. B., A new potent synthetic analgesic, *J. Org. Chem.*, 24, 295, 1959.

212. Eckenhoff, J. E., Phenazocine, a new benzomorphan narcotic analgesic, *Anesthesiology*, 20, 355, 1959.

213. Houde, R. W., Wallenstein, S. L., Bellville, J. W., Rogers, A., and Escarraga, L. A., The relative analgesic and respiratory effect of phenazocine and morphine, *J. Pharmacol. Exp. Ther.*, 144, 337, 1964.

214. Shemano, I., Wendell, H., and Ross, S. D., A pharmacological comparison of phenazocine hydrobromide and morphine sulfate as narcotic analgesics, *J. Pharmacol. Exp. Ther.*, 132, 258, 1961.

215. Lasagna, L., The clinical evaluation of morphine and its substitutes as analgesics, *Pharmacol. Rev.*, 16, 47, 1964.

216. Beaver, W. T., Wallenstein, S. L., Houde, R. W., and Rogers, A., A clinical comparison of the effects of oral and intramuscular administration of analgesics: Pentazocine and phenazocine, *Clin. Pharmacol. Ther.*, 9, 582, 1968.

217. Fraser, H. F. and Isbell, H., Human pharmacology and addiction liabilities of phenazocine and levophenacylmorphan, *Bull. Narcotics*, 12, 15, 1966.

218. Archer, S., Benzazocines, Belgian Patent 611000 (1962), *C.A.*, 58, 2440b, 1963.

219. Martin, W. R., Fraser, H. F., Gorodetzky, C. W., and Rosenberg, D. E., Studies of the dependence producing potential of the narcotic antagonist 2-cyclopropylmethyl-2-hydroxy-5,9-dimethyl-6,7-benzomorphan (cyclazocine, WIN-20, 740, ARC II-C-3), *J. Pharmacol. Exp. Ther.*, 150, 426, 1965.

220. Martin, W. R. and Gorodetzky, C. W., Cyclazocine, an adjunct in the treatment of narcotic addiction, *Int. J. Addict.*, 2, 1, 1967.

221. Freedman, A. M., Fink, M., Sharoff, R., and Zaks, A., Chemical studies of cyclazocine in the treatment of narcotic addiction, *Amer. J. Psychiat.*, 124, 1499, 1968.

222. Freedman, A. M. and Fink, M., Basic concepts and use of cyclazocine in the treatment of narcotic addiction, *Brit. J. Addict.*, 63, 59, 1968.

223. Mulé, S. J. and Gorodetzky, C. W., Physiological disposition of ^{3}H-cyclazocine in nontolerant, tolerant and abstinent dogs, *J. Pharmacol. Exp. Ther.*, 154, 632, 1966.

224. Mulé, S. J., Clements, T. H., and Gorodetzky, C. W., The metabolic fate of ^{3}H-cyclazocine in dogs, *J. Pharmacol. Exp. Ther.*, 160, 387, 1968.

225. Archer, S., Albertson, N. F., Harris, L. S., Pierson, A. K., Bird, J. G., Keats, A. S., Telford, J., and Papdopoulos, D. N., Narcotic antagonists, *Science*, 137, 541, 1962.

226. Ferrari, R. A., Differential distribution of pentazocine-^{3}H and *cis*-chloro-allylnorpentazocine-^{3}H in the cat, *Toxic. Appl. Pharmacol.*, 12, 404, 1968.

227. Keats, A. S. and Telford, J., Studies of analgesic drugs. VIII. A narcotic antagonist analgesic without psychotomimetic effects, *J. Pharmacol. Exp. Ther.*, 143, 157, 1964.

228. Sandoval, R. G. and Wang, R. I. H., Tolerance and physical dependence on pentazocine, *New Eng. J. Med.*, 280, 1391, 1969.

229. Berkowitz, B. A., Asling, J. H., Schnider, S. M., and Way, E. L., Relationship of pentazocine plasma levels to pharmacological activity in man, *Clin. Pharmacol. Ther.*, 10, 320, 1969.

230. Berkowitz, B. A. and Way, E. L., Metabolism and excretion of pentazocine in man, *Clin. Pharmacol. Ther.*, 10, 681, 1969.

231. Beckett, A. H. and Taylor, J. F., Blood concentration of pethidine and pentazocine in mother and infant at time of birth, *J. Pharm. Pharmacol.*, 19, 505, 1967.

232. El-Mazati, A. M. and Way, E. L., The pharmacologic disposition of pentazocine in the rat, *J. Pharmacol. Exp. Ther.*, 177, 332, 1971.

233. Pittmann, K. A., Rosi, D., Cherniak, R., Merola, A. J., and Conway, W. D., Metabolism *in vitro* and *in vivo* of pentazocine, *Biochem. Pharmacol.*, 18, 1673, 1969.

234. Pittmann, K. A., Human metabolism of orally administered pentazocine, *Biochem. Pharmacol.*, 19, 1833, 1970.

235. Matts, S. G. F., McCready, V. R., James, K. W., Gwyther, M. M., and Hammersley, P. A. G., Radioisotope studies of urinary excretion of pentazocine as an aid to its pharmacotherapeutic application, *Clin. Trials. J.*, 4, 842, 1967.

236. Beckett, A. H., Taylor, J. F., and Kourounakis, P., The absorption, distribution and excretion of pentazocine in man after oral and intravenous administration, *J. Pharm. Pharmacol.*, 22, 123, 1970.

237. Berkowitz, B. A. and Way, E. L., Analgesic activity and central nervous system distribution of the optical isomers of pentazocine in the rat, *J. Pharmacol. Exp. Ther.*, 177, 500, 1971.

238a. Eisleb, O. and Schaumann, O., Dolantin®, a new antispasmodic and analgesic, *Deutsch. Med. Wschr.*, 65, 967, 1939.

238b. Schaumann, O., A new class of compounds with spasmolytic and central analgesic action derived from 1-methyl-4-phenyl piperidine-4-carboxylic acid ethyl ester (Dolantin®), *Arch. Exp. Path. Pharmak.*, 196, 109, 1940.

239. Burns, J. J., Berger, B. L., Lief, P. A., Wollack, A., Papper, E. M., and Brodie, B. B., The physiological disposition and fate of meperidine (Demerol®) in man and a method for its estimation in plasma, *J. Pharmacol. Exp. Ther.*, 114, 289, 1955.

240. Way, E. L., Gimble, A. I., McKelway, W. P., Ross, H., Sung, C.-Y., and Ellsworth, H., The absorption, distribution and excretion of isonipecaine (Demerol®), *J. Pharmacol. Exp. Ther.*, 96, 477, 1949.

241. Plotnikoff, N. P., Elliott, H. W., and Way, E. L., The metabolism of *N*-$^{14}CH_3$ labeled meperidine, *J. Pharmacol. Exp. Ther.*, 104, 377, 1952.

242. Apgar, V., Burns, J. J., Brodie, B. B., and Papper, E. M., The transmission of meperidine across the human placenta, *Amer. J. Obstet. Gynec.*, 64, 1368, 1952.

243. Gaudette, L. E. and Brodie, B. B., The relation between the lipid solubility of drugs and their oxidation by liver microsomes, *Biochem. Pharmacol.*, 2, 89, 1959.

244. Plotnikoff, N. P., Way, E. L., and Elliott, H. W., Biotransformation products of meperidine excreted in the urine of man, *J. Pharmacol. Exp. Ther.*, 117, 414, 1956.

245. Asatoor, A. M., London, D. R., Milne, M. D., and Simenoff, M. L., The excretion of pethidine and its derivatives, *Brit. J. Pharmacol.*, 20, 285, 1963.

246a. Diamond, J. and Bruce, W., U.S. Patent 2666050, 1954.

246b. Diamond, J., Bruce, W. F., and Tyson, F. T., Synthesis of azacycloheptane derivatives related to piperidine analgesics, *J. Org. Chem.*, 22, 399, 1957.

247. Walkenstein, S. S., MacMullen, J. A., Knebel, C., and Seifter, J., The metabolic fate of a hexamethyleneimine analgesic, *J. Amer. Pharm. Ass.*, 47, 20, 1958.

248. Weijlard, J., Orahovats, P. D., Sullivan, A. P., Jr., Purdue, G., Heath, F. K., and Pfister, K., 3rd, A new synthetic analgesic, *J. Amer. Chem. Soc.*, 78, 2342, 1956.

249. Porter, C. C., The absorption and metabolism of anileridine, ethyl-1-(4-amino phenethyl)-4-phenyl-isonipecotate, *J. Pharmacol. Exp. Ther.*, 120, 447, 1957.

250. Orahovats, P. D., Lehman, E. G., and Chapin, E. W., Pharmacology of ethyl-1-(4-amino phenethyl)-4-phenyl isonipecotate, Anileridine, a new potent analgesic, *J. Pharmacol. Exp. Ther.*, 119, 26, 1957.

251. Lin, S.-C. C. and Way, E. L., *N*-dealkylation of anileridine to normeperidine, *J. Pharmacol. Exp. Ther.*, 150, 309, 1965.

252. Bockmühl, M. and Ehrhart, G., Spasmolytic and analgesic compounds, *Liebigs Ann. Chem.*, 561, 52, 1949.

253. Scott, C. C., Robbins, E. B., and Chen, K. K., Pharmacologic comparisons of the optical isomers of methadone, *J. Pharmacol. Exp. Ther.*, 93, 282, 1948.

254. Dole, V. P. and Nyswander, M. E., The use of methadone for narcotic blockade, *Brit. J. Addict.*, 63, 55, 1968.

255. Elliott, H. W., Chang, F. N. H., Abdou, I. A., and Anderson, H. H., The distribution of radioactivity in rats after administration of ^{14}C-labeled methadone, *J. Pharmacol. Exp. Ther.*, 94, 494, 1949.

256. Rickards, J. C., Boxer, G. E., and Smith, C. C., Studies on the distribution and metabolism of methadone in normal and tolerant rats by a new colorimetric method, *J. Pharmacol. Exp. Ther.*, 98, 380, 1950.

257. Way, E. L., Sung, C.-Y., and McKelway, W. P., The absorption, distribution and excretion of *dl*-methadone, *J. Pharmacol. Exp. Ther.*, 97, 222, 1949.

258. Adler, T. K. and Eisenbrandt, L. L., The initial uptake of ^{14}C-labeled methadone by rat tissues, *Proc. Soc. Exp. Biol. Med.*, 72, 347, 1949.

259. Sung, C.-Y., Way, E. L., and Scott, K. G., Studies on the relationship of metabolic fate and hormonal effects of *dl*-methadone to the development of drug tolerance, *J. Pharmacol. Exp. Ther.*, 107, 171, 1953.

260. Way, E. L., Sung, C.-Y., and Fujimoto, J. M., The effect of adrenalectomy on the development of tolerance to morphine and methadone, *J. Pharmacol. Exp. Ther.*, 110, 51, 1954.

261. Sung, C. -Y. and Way, E. L., The metabolic fate of the optical isomers of methadone, *J. Pharmacol. Exp. Ther.*, 109, 244, 1953.

262. Smits, S. E. and Sullivan, H. R., Optical isomers of methadone: analgesic activity and accumulation in blood and brain, *Pharmacologist*, 13, 262, 1971.

263. Ingoglia, N. A. and Dole, V. P., Localization of d- and l-methadone after intraventricular injection into rat brains, *J. Pharmacol. Exp. Ther.*, 175, 84, 1970.

264. Way, E. L., Signorotti, B. T., March, C. H., and Peng, C. T., Studies on the urinary, fecal and biliary excretion of *d,l*-methadone by counter-current distribution, *J. Pharmacol. Exp. Ther.*, 101, 249, 1951.

265. Sung, C. -Y. and Way, E. L., The effect of the liver on the metabolism of d,l-methadone *in vitro* and *in vivo, J. Pharmacol. Exp. Ther.*, 98, 72, 1950.

266. Vidic, E., Nachweis der renalen ausscheidungs Produkte toxicologisch wichtiger Arzneistoffe mit Hilfe der Papier Chromatographie, *Arzneimittelforschung*, 7, 314, 1957.

267. Schaumann, O., Determination of the quaternary ammonium base formed by *N*-methylation of methadone – fate of unchanged methadone, *Arch. Exp. Path. Pharmak.*, 239, 311 and 321, 1960.

268. Beckett, A. H., Taylor, J. F., Casy, A. F., and Hassan, M. M. A., The biotransformation of methadone in man – Synthesis and identification of major metabolite, *J. Pharm. Pharmacol.*, 20, 754, 1968.

269. Robinson, A. E. and Williams, F. M., The distribution of methadone in man, *J. Pharm. Pharmacol.*, 23, 353, 1971.

270. Pohland, A., Boaz, H. E., and Sullivan, H. R., Synthesis and identification of metabolites resulting from the biotransformation of *dl*-methadone in man and in the rat, *J. Med. Chem.*, 14, 194, 1971.

271. Beckett, A. H., Mitchard, M., and Shihab, A. A., Identification and quantitative determination of some metabolites of methadone, isomethadone and nórmethadone, *J. Pharm. Pharmacol.*, 23, 347, 1971.

272. Specter, M. E., Byrd, W. M., Cheney, L. C., and Binkley, S. B., Analgesic carbinols and esters related to Amidone (methadon), *J. Amer. Chem. Soc.*, 71, 57, 1949.

273. Jaffe, J. H., Schuster, C. R., Smith, B. B., and Blachley, B. B., Comparison of acetyl methadol and methadone in treatment of long-term heroin users, *J.A.M.A.*, 211, 1834, 1970.

274. Fraser, H. F. and Isbell, H., Actions and addiction liabilities of alpha acetyl methadols in man, *J. Pharmacol. Exp. Ther.*, 105, 458, 1952.

275. Sung, C. -Y. and Way, E. L., The fate of the optical isomers of alpha-acetyl methadol, *J. Pharmacol. Exp. Ther.*, 110, 260, 1954.

276. McMahon, R. E., Culp, H. W., and Marshall, F. J., The metabolism of α-dl-acetyl- methadol in the rat – the identification of the probable active metabolite, *J. Pharmacol. Exp. Ther.*, 149, 436, 1965.

277. Gruber, C. M. and Baptisti, A., Estimating the acceptability of morphine and noracylmethadol in post partum patients, *Clin. Pharmacol. Ther.*, 4, 172, 1963.

278. Pohland, A. and Sullivan, H. R., Analgesics - esters of 4-dialkylamino-1,2-diphenyl-2-butanols, *J. Amer. Chem. Soc.*, 75, 4458, 1953.

279. Fraser, H. F. and Isbell, H., Pharmacology and addiction liabilities of *dl*- and *l*-propoxyphene, *Bull. Narcotics*, 12, 9, 1960.

280. Salguerro, C. H., Villareal, J. E., Hug, C. C., Jr., and Domino, E. F., Propoxyphene dependence, *J.A.M.A.*, 210, 135, 1969.

281. Robbins, E. B., The pharmacologic effects of a new analgesic α-4-dimethyl-amino-1,2-diphenyl-3-methyl-4-propionyl oxybutane, *J. Amer. Pharm. Ass.*, 44, 497, 1955.

282. Lee, H. M., Scott, E. G., and Pohland, A., Studies on the metabolic degradation of propoxyphene, *J. Pharmacol. Exp. Ther.*, 125, 14, 1959.

283. Amundsen, M. E., Johnson, M. L., and Manthey, J. A., Urinary excretion of d-propoxyphene hydrochloride in man, *J. Pharm. Sci.*, 54, 684, 1965.

284. McMahon, R. E., Ridolfo, A. S., Culp, H. W., Wolen, R. L., and Marshall, F. J., Fate of radiocarbon-labeled propoxyphene in rat, dog and human, *Toxic. Appl. Pharmacol.*, 19, 427, 1971.

285. Wolen, R. L., Gruber, C. M., Jr., Kiplinger, G. F., and Scholz, N. E., Concentration of propoxyphene in human plasma following oral, intramuscular and intravenous administration, *Toxic. Appl. Pharmacol.*, 19, 480, 1971.

286. Althaus, J. R., Biemann, K., Biller, J., Donaghue, P. F., Evans, D. A., Förster, H. -J., Hertz, H. S., Hignite, C. E., Murphy, R. C., Preti, G., and Reinhold, V., Identification of drug darvon and its metabolites in urine of a comatose patient using a gas chromatographic-mass spectrometer-computer system, *Experientia*, 26, 714, 1970.

287. Kyoguku, Y., Lord, R. C., and Richi, A., Specific H-bonding of barbiturates to adenine derivatives, *Nature* (London), 218, 69, 1968.

288. Mark, L. C., The archaic classification of barbiturates, *Clin. Pharmacol. Ther.*, 10, 287, 1969.

289. Brodie, B. B., Pathways of drug metabolism, *J. Pharm. Pharmacol.*, 8, 1, 1956.

290. Mark, L. C., On species differences, *Anesthesiology*, 19, 799, 1958.

291. Quinn, G. P., Axelrod, J., and Brodie, B. B., Species, strain and sex differences in metabolism of hexobarbital , amido pyrine, antipyrine and aniline, *Biochem. Pharmacol.*, 1, 152, 1958.

292. Isbell, H., Altschul, S., Kornetsky, C. H., Eisenman, A. J., Flanary, H. G., and Fraser, H. F., Chronic barbiturate intoxication – an experimental study, *Arch. Neurol.* (Chicago), 64, 1, 1950.

293. Isbell, H. and White, W. M., Clinical characteristics of addiction, *Amer. J. Med.*, 14, 558, 1953.

294. Fraser, H. F., Isbell, H., Eisenman, A. H., Wikler, A., and Pescor, F. T., Chronic barbiturate intoxication, *Arch. Int. Med.*, 94, 34, 1954.

295. Essig, C. F., Addiction to barbiturates and nonbarbiturate sedative drugs, *Res. Publ. Ass. Nerv. Ment. Dis.*, 46, 180, 1968.

296. Yanagita, T. and Takahashi, S., Development of tolerance to and physical dependence on barbiturates in rhesus monkeys, *J. Pharmacol. Exp. Ther.*, 172, 163, 1970.

297. Bush, M. T., Sedatives and hypnotics. I. Absorption, fate and excretion in *Physiological Pharmacology*, Vol. 1, Root, W. S. and Hoffman, F. G., Eds., Academic Press, Inc., New York, 1963, 185.

298. Feltkamp, H., Distribution characteristics of barbiturates, *Arzneimittelforschung*, 15, 238, 1965.

299. Kakemi, K., Arita, T., Hori, R., and Konishi, R., Absorption and excretion of drugs – relation between partition coefficient and chemical structures of barbituric acid derivatives, *Chem. Pharm. Bull.* (Tokyo), 15, 1705, 1967.

300. Goldbaum, L. R. and Smith, P. K., The interaction of barbiturates with serum albumin and its possible relation to their disposition and pharmacological action, *J. Pharmacol. Exp. Ther.*, 111, 197, 1954.

301. Campion, D. S. and North, J. D. K., Effect of protein binding of barbiturates on the rate of removal during peritoneal dialysis, *J. Lab. Clin. Med.*, 66, 549, 1965.

302. Doornbos, D. A. and De Zeeuw, R. A., Determination of dissociation constants of barbiturates by pH measurements, *Pharm. Weekbl.*, 104, 233, 1969.

303. Waddell, W. J. and Butler, T. C., The distribution and excretion of phenobarbital, *J. Clin. Invest.*, 36, 1217, 1957.

304. Sjögren, J., Sölvell, L., and Karlsson, I., Studies on the absorption of barbiturates in man, *Acta Med. Scand.*, 178, 553, 1965.

305. Magnussen, M. P., The effect of ethanol on the gastrointestinal absorption of drugs in the rat, *Acta Pharmacol. Toxicol.*, 26, 130, 1968.

306. Coldwell, B. B., Wiberg, G. S., and Trenholm, H. L., Some effects of ethanol on toxicity and distribution of barbiturates in rats, *Canad. J. Physiol. Pharmacol.*, 48, 259, 1970.

307. Coldwell, B. B., Thomas, B. H., and Trenholm, H. L., Effect of ethanol on the distribution and excretion of barbiturates in the rat, *Pharmacologist*, 13, 220, 1971.

308. Beckett, A. H. and Moffat, A. C., The buccal absorption of some barbiturates, *J. Pharm. Pharmacol.*, 23, 15, 1971.

309. Richards, R. K. and Taylor, J. D., Some factors influencing distribution metabolism and action of barbiturates – a review, *Anesthesiology*, 17, 414, 1956.

310. Price, H. L., A dynamic concept of distribution of thiopental in human body, *Anesthesiology*, 21, 40, 1960.

311. Price, H. L., Kovnat, P. J., Safer, J. N., Conner, E. H., and Price, M. L., Uptake of thiopental by body tissues and its relation to duration of narcosis, *Clin. Pharmacol. Ther.*, 1, 16, 1960.

312. Mark, L. C., *Uptake and Distribution of Anesthetic Agents*, Papper, E. M. and Kitz, R. J., Eds., McGraw-Hill Book Co., New York, 1963.

313. Goldstein, A. and Aronow, L., The durations of action of thiopental and pentobarbital, *J. Pharmacol. Exp. Ther.*, 128, 1, 1960.

314. Brodie, B. B., Mark, L. C., Papper, E. M., Lief, P. A., Bernstein, E., and Roverstein, E. A., The fate of thiopental in man and a method for its estimation in biological materials, *J. Pharmacol. Exp. Ther.*, 98, 85, 1950.

315. Mark, L. C., Perel, J. M., Brand, L., and Dayton, P. G., Studies with thiohexital, an anesthetic barbiturate metabolized with unusual rapidity in man, *Anesthesiology*, 29, 1159, 1968.

316. Mark, L. C., Metabolism of barbiturates in man, *Clin. Pharmacol. Ther.*, 4, 504, 1963.

317. Maynert, E. W. and Van Dyke, H. B., The metabolism of barbiturates, *Pharmacol. Rev.*, 1, 217, 1949.

318. Palmer, K. H., Smith, D. J. S., Fowler, M. S., Martin, B. R., and Wall, M. E., Metabolism of optically active barbiturates. III. R(+) and S(-) secobarbital, *Pharmacologist*, 13, 220, 1971.

319. Maynert, E. W. and Dawson, J. M., Ethyl (3-hydroxy-1-methyl butyl) barbituric acid as metabolite of pentobarbital, *J. Biol. Chem.*, 195, 389, 1952.

320. Maynert, E. W., The distribution and fate of dialkylbarbiturates, *Fed. Proc.*, 11, 625, 1952.

321. Maynert, E. W. and Losin, L., The metabolism of butabarbital (butisol) in the dog, *J. Pharmacol. Exp. Ther.*, 115, 275, 1955.

322. Maynert, E. W., The alcoholic metabolites of pentobarbital and amobarbital in man, *J. Pharmacol. Exp. Ther.*, 150, 118, 1965.

323. Maynert, E. W., On the specificity of penultimate oxidation – the fate of 5-ethyl-5n-hexylbarbituric acid, *J. Pharmacol. Exp. Ther.*, 150, 476, 1965.

324. Waddell, W. J., The metabolic fate of 5-allyl-5-(1-methyl-butyl) barbituric acid (secobarbital), *J. Pharmacol. Exp. Ther.*, 149, 23, 1965.

325. Bush, M. T. and Sanders, E., Metabolic fate of drugs – barbiturates and closely related drugs, *Ann. Rev. Pharmacol.*, 7, 57, 1967.

326. Irrgang, K., Zur pharmakologie von 5-aethyl-5-(3-hydroxyisoamyl)-barbitur saüre einem Stoffwechsel produkte der 5-aethyl-5-isoamyl barbitursaüre, *Arzneimittelforschung*, 15, 688, 1965.

327. Dorfman, A. and Goldbaum, L. R., Detoxication of barbiturates, *J. Pharmacol. Exp. Ther.*, 90, 330, 1947.

328. Shideman, F. E., Kelly, A. R., and Adams, B. J., The role of liver in the detoxication of thiopental (pentothal) and other thiobarbiturates, *J. Pharmacol. Exp. Ther.*, 91, 331, 1947.

329. Shideman, F. E., The *in vitro* metabolism of barbiturates, *Fed. Proc.*, 11, 640, 1952.

330. Kelly, A. R. and Shideman, F. E., Liver as an organ in detoxication of thiobarbiturates by dogs, *Fed. Proc.*, 8, 306, 1949.

331. Gould, T. C. and Shideman, F. E., The *in vitro* metabolism of thiopentone by a fortified cell-free tissue preparation of the rat, *J. Pharmacol. Exp. Ther.*, 104, 427, 1952.

332. Messers, F. H. and Peoples, D., The possible role of liver in rapid metabolism of thiopental, *Anesthesiology*, 15, 146, 1954.

333. Brodie, B. B., Axelrod, J., Cooper, J. R., Gaudette, L., La Du, B. N., Mitoma, C., and Undenfriend, S., Detoxication of drugs and other foreign compounds by liver microsomes, *Science*, 121, 603, 1955.

334. Cooper, J. R. and Brodie, B. B., The enzymatic metabolism of hexobarbital (evipal), *J. Pharmacol. Exp. Ther.*, 114, 409, 1955.

335. Cooper, J. R. and Brodie, B. B., Enzymatic oxidation of pentobarbital and thiopental, *J. Pharmacol. Exp. Ther.*, 120, 75, 1957.

336. Raventos, J., The distribution in the body and the metabolic fate of barbiturates, *J. Pharmacol. Exp. Ther.*, 6, 217, 1954.

337. Williams, R. T., *Detoxication Mechanisms*, Chapman and Hall, Ltd., London, 1959, 593.

338. Brodie, B. B., Burns, J. J., Mark, L. C., Lief, P. A., Bernstein, E., and Papper, E. M., The fate of pentobarbital in man and dog and a method for its estimation in biological materials, *J. Pharmacol. Exp. Ther.*, 109, 26, 1953.

339. Niyogi, S. K., Detection of secobarbital metabolites in the urine of the rat, *Nature* (London), 202, 1225, 1964.

340. Butler, T. C., The metabolic hydroxylation of phenobarbital, *J. Amer. Pharm. Ass.*, 116, 326, 1956.

341. Bush, M. T., Butler, T. C., and Dickinson, H. L., The metabolic fate of 5-(1-cyclohexen-1-yl)-1-5-dimethyl barbituric acid (hexobarbital, evipal) and of 5-(1-cyclohexen-1-yl)-5-methyl barbituric acid (norevipal), *J. Pharmacol. Exp. Ther.*, 108, 104, 1953.

342. Tsukamoto, H., Yoshimura, H., and Toki, S., Metabolism of drugs. XVIII. The metabolic fate of methyl hexobarbital (5-cyclohexenyl-3,5-dimethyl barbituric acid) – the quantitative determination of main biotransformation products of methyl hexital in urine of rabbits by UV spectrophotometry, *Chem. Pharm. Bull.* (Tokyo), 6, 88, 1958.

343. Frey, H. H., Doenicke, A., and Jager, S., Qualitative bedeutung der Desulfurierung in Stoffwechsel von thiobarbituraten, *Med. Exp.*, 4, 243, 1961.

344. Butler, T. C., Quantitative studies of metabolic fate of mephobarbital (*N*-methyl barbital), *J. Pharmacol. Exp. Ther.*, 106, 235, 1952.

345. Mazel, P., Henderson, J. F., and Axelrod, J., *S*-demethylation by microsomal enzymes, *J. Pharmacol. Exp. Ther.*, 143, 1, 1964.

346. Farber, T. M., The mechanism of microsomal *S*-dealkylation, *Pharmacologist*, 13, 193, 1971.

347. Bush, M. T., Mazel, P., and Chambers, J., Metabolic fate of thiobarbiturates, *J. Pharmacol. Exp. Ther.*, 134, 110, 1961.

348. Maynert, E. W. and Van Dyke, H. B., The metabolic fate of pentobarbital – isotope dilution experiments with urine after administration of labeled pentobarbital, *J. Pharmacol. Exp. Ther.*, 98, 174, 1950.

349. Maynert, E. W. and Van Dyke, H. B., The metabolism of amytal labeled with ^{15}N in dog, *J. Pharmacol. Exp. Ther.*, 98, 180, 1950.

350. Titus, E. and Weiss, H., The use of metabolically prepared radioactive indicator in metabolic studies – metabolism of pentobarbital, *J. Biol. Chem.*, 214, 807, 1955.

351. Goldschmidt, S. and Wehr, R., Über barbiturat. III. Mitteilung Der metabolismus von Veronal, *Z. Physiol. Chem.*, 308, 9, 1957.

352. Cochin, J. and Daly, J. W., The use of thin layer chromatography for the analysis of drugs. Isolation and identification of barbiturates and nonbarbiturate hypnotics from urine, blood and tissues, *J. Pharmacol. Exp. Ther.*, 139, 154, 1963.

353. Bush, M. T., Smith, B., Suria, A., and Vore, M., The metabolic fate of 5-ethylbarbituric acid (EB) and 5-(2′-pentyl)-barbituric acid in the rat, *Pharmacologist*, 13, 220, 1971.

354. Deininger, R., Papier chromatographischer nachweis der methylierung von nor-evipan zu evipan, *Arch. Exp. Path. Pharmak.*, 225, 127, 1955.

355. Frey, H. H., Sudenday, F., and Krause, D., Vergleichende untersuchungen über stoffwechsel auscheidung und nachweis von schlafmitteln aus der Barbitursaüre reihe, *Arzneimittelforschung*, 9, 294, 1959.

356. Bush, M. T. and Parrish, H., Methylation of barbiturates *in vivo, Fed. Proc.*, 22, 480, 1963.

357. Giotti, A. and Maynert, E. W., The renal clearance of barbital and the mechanism of its reabsorption, *J. Pharmacol. Exp. Ther.*, 101, 296, 1951.

358. Remmer, H., Hydrolyse und oxydation von Pharmaka im verschidenen fraktionen der lebermikrosomen, *Arch. Exp. Path. Pharmak.*, 238, 36, 1960.

359. Rothschild, J. A., Subfractionation of rat liver microsomes, *Fed. Proc.*, 20, 145, 1961.

360. Fouts, J. R., The metabolism of drugs by subfractions of hepatic microsomes, *Biochem. Biophys. Res. Comm.*, 6, 373, 1961.

361. Fouts, J. R., Interaction of drugs and hepatic microsomes, *Fed. Proc.*, 21, 1107, 1962.

362. Leadbeater, L. and Davies, D. R., The stability of the drug metabolizing enzymes of liver microsomal preparations, *Biochem. Pharmacol.*, 13, 1607, 1964.

363. Gram, T. E. and Fouts, J. R., Time course differences in the metabolism of drugs by hepatic microsomes from rat, rabbits and mice, *J. Pharmacol. Exp. Ther.*, 152, 363, 1966.

364. McMahon, R. E., The demethylation *in vitro* of *N*-methyl barbiturates and related compounds by mammalian liver microsomes, *Biochem. Pharmacol.*, 12, 1225, 1963.

365. Kessel, J. F. E., The enzymic metabolism of barbiturates and influence of various factors on their metabolism, *Pharm. Weekbl.*, 99, 681, 1964.

336. Conney, A. H., Davison, C., Gastel, R., and Burns, J. J., Adaptive increases in drug metabolizing enzymes induced by phenobarbital and other drugs, *J. Pharmacol. Exp. Ther.*, 130, 1, 1960.

367. Burns, J. J. and Conney, A. H., Enzyme stimulation and inhibition of metabolism of drugs, *Proc. Roy. Soc. Med. (Part 2)*, 58, 955, 1965.

368. Remmer, H., Drug tolerance, in *Enzymes and Drug Action*, Ciba Foundation Symposium, Mongar, J. L. and de Reuck, A. V. S., Eds., Little Brown and Co., Boston, 1962, 276.

369. Remmer, H., Siegert, M., and Merkur, H. J., Acceleration of drug metabolism through enzyme induction, *Arch. Exp. Path. Pharmak.*, 246, 58, 1963.

370. Conney, A. H., Bray, G. A., Evans, C., and Burns, J. J., Metabolic interaction between *l*-ascorbic acid and drugs, *Ann. N. Y. Acad. Sci.*, 92, 115, 1961.

371. Dayton, P. G., Tarcon, Y., Chenkin, T., and Weiner, M., The influence of barbiturates on coumarin plasma levels and prothrombin response, *J. Clin. Invest.*, 40, 1797, 1961.

372. Cucinell, S. A., Conney, A. H., Sansur, M. S., and Burns, J. J., Drug interactions in man: lowering effect of phenobarbital on plasma levels of bis-hydroxy coumarin and diphenylhydantoin, *Clin. Pharmacol. Ther.*, 6, 420, 1965.

373. MacDonald, M. G. and Robinson, D., Anticoagulant antagonism of phenobarbital in man, *Pharmacologist*, 7, 146, 1965.

374. Busfield, D., Child, K. J., Atkinson, R. M., and Tomich, E. G., An effect of phenobarbitone on blood levels of griseofulvin in man, *Lancet*, 2, 1042, 1963.

375. Rupe, B. D., Bousquet, W. F., and Miya, T. S., Stress modification of drug response, *Science*, 141, 1186, 1963.

376. Bousquet, W. F., Rupe, B. D., and Miya, T. S., Endocrine modification of drug responses in the rat, *J. Pharmacol. Exp. Ther.*, 147, 376, 1965.

377. Driever, C. W. and Bousquet, W. F., Stress-drug interactions - evidence for rapid enzyme induction, *Life Sci.*, 4, 1449, 1965.

378. Gruber, C. M. and Keyser, G. F., A study on the development of tolerance and cross-tolerance to barbiturates in experimental animals, *J. Pharmacol. Exp. Ther.*, 86, 186, 1946.

379. Brodie, B. B., Mark, L. C., Lief, P. A., Bernstein, E., and Papper, E. M., Acute tolerance to thiopental, *J. Pharmacol. Exp. Ther.*, 102, 215, 1951.

380. Dundee, J. W., Price, H. L., and Dripps, R. D., Acute tolerance to thiopentone in man, *Brit. J. Anesth.*, 28, 344, 1956.

381. Maynert, E. W. and Klingman, G. I., Acute tolerance to intravenous anesthetics in dog, *J. Pharmacol. Exp. Ther.*, 128, 192, 1960.

382. Neubauer, J., Acute changes in rat serum proteins following administration of a single dose of barbital, *Z. Klin. Chem.*, 5, 74, 1967.

383. Remmer, H., Siegert, M., Nitze, H. R., and Kirsten, I., Development of tolerance to long-acting barbiturates, *Arch. Exp. Path. Pharmak.*, 243, 468, 1962.

384. Remmer, H., The cause of tolerance to oxidisable barbiturates, *Arch. Exp. Path. Pharmak.*, 244, 311, 1963.

385. Welch, R. M., Harrison, Y. E., and Burns, J. J., Role of enzyme induction in drug tolerance, in *Drug Abuse*, Cole, J. D. and Wittenborn, J. R., Eds., Charles C Thomas, Springfield, Illinois, 1969, 146.

386. Ebert, A. G., Yim, G. K. W., and Miya, T. S., Distribution and metabolism of barbital-^{14}C in tolerant and nontolerant rats, *Biochem. Pharmacol.*, 13, 1267, 1964.

387. Gordis, E., Tolerance to the hypnotic effect of *l*-methyl phenobarbital induced by its nonhypnotic stereoisomer, *Biochem. Pharmacol.*, 20, 246, 1971.

388. Buech, H., Buzello, W., Neurohr, O., and Rummel, W., Distribution and narcotic properties and metabolic characteristics of the optical antipodes of methyl phenobarbital, *Biochem. Pharmacol.*, 17, 2391, 1968.

389. McCarthy, J. S. and Stilzel, R. E., Kinetic differences in the microsomal metabolism of the isomers of hexobarbital, *J. Pharmacol. Exp. Ther.*, 176, 772, 1971.

390. Ludwig, B. J. and Piech, E. C., Some anticonvulsant agents derived from 1,3-propanediols, *J. Amer. Chem. Soc.*, 73, 5779, 1951.

391. Berger, F. M., The pharmacological properties of Miltown, a new interneuronal blocking agent, *J. Pharmacol. Exp. Ther.*, 112, 413, 1954.

392. Walkenstein, S. S., Knebel, C. W., MacMullen, J. A., and Seifter, J., Excretion and distribution of meprobamate and its metabolites, *J. Pharmacol. Exp. Ther.*, 123, 254, 1958.

393. Emmerson, J. L., Miya, T. S., and Yim, G. K. W., Distribution and metabolic fate of ^{14}C-meprobamate in the rat brain, *J. Pharmacol. Exp. Ther.*, 129, 89, 1960.

394. Ewaldsson, B., Autoradiographic studies on distribution of meprobamate-^{3}H in body of the mouse, *Arch. Int. Pharmacodyn.*, 142, 163, 1963.

395. Palmieri, A., Transplacental passage of 2-methyl-2-propyl-1,3-propanediol dicarbamate, *Arch. Ostet. Ginec.*, 69, 552, 1964.

396. Ludwig, B. J., Douglas, J. F., Powell, L. S., Meyer, M., and Berger, F. M., Structure of major metabolites of meprobamate, *J. Med. Pharm. Chem.*, 3, 53, 1961.

397. Tsukamoto, H., Yoshimura, H., and Tatsumi, K., Metabolic fate of meprobamate – a new metabolic pathway of carbamate group – the formation of *N*-glucuronide in the animal body, *Chem. Pharm. Bull.*, (Tokyo), 11, 421, 1963.

398. Driever, C. W., Bousquet, W. F., and Miya, T. S., Stress stimulation of drug metabolism in the rat, *Int. J. Neuropharmacol.*, 5, 199, 1966.

399. Held, H. and Von Olderhausen, H., Pharmacokinetics of meprobamate in chronic hepatopathy and drug addiction, *Klin. Wschr.*, 47, 78, 1969.

400. Kato, R., Chisara, E., and Vassanelli, P., The inhibition and stimulation of microsomal drug metabolizing enzymes of rat liver by various compounds, *Biochem. Pharmac.*, 13, 69, 1964.

401. Datta, P. R. and Nelson, M. J., Enhanced metabolism of methylprylon, meprobamate and chlordiazepoxide HCl after chronic feeding of a low dietary level of DDT to male and female rats, *Toxic. Appl. Pharmacol.*, 13, 346, 1968.

402. Felby, S., Concentrations of meprobamate in the blood and liver following fatal meprobamate poisoning, *Acta Pharmacol. Toxicol.*, 28, 334, 1970.

403. Langecker, H., Schüman, H. J., and Junkman, K., Chemische und pharmalogische Eigenschaften des Aethinyl cyclohexyl carbaminsaüre esters, *Arch. Exp. Path. Pharmak.*, 219, 130, 1953.

404. Gruber, C. M., Jr., Kohlstaedt, K. G., Moore, R. B., and Peck, F. B., Jr., Effect of Valmid® (ethinamate) – a nonbarbiturate central nervous system depressant in human subjects, *J. Pharmacol. Exp. Ther.*, 112, 480, 1954.

405. McMahon, R. E., The *in vivo* hydroxylation of 1-ethynylcyclohexyl carbamate, *J. Amer. Chem. Soc.*, 80, 411, 1958.

406. Murata, T., Metabolic fate of l-ethynyl cyclohexyl carbamate, *Chem. Pharm. Bull.* (Tokyo), 9, 146, 1961; 9, 335, 1961.

407. Tust, R. H., Hermann, R. G., and Chen, K. K., Comparison of effects of Valmid® (ethynylcyclohexylcarbamate) and other hypnotics on brain respiration *in vitro*, *Proc. Soc. Exp. Biol. Med.*, 92, 778, 1956.

408. Tsukamoto, H., Yoshimura, H., and Tatsumi, K., Carbamate *N*-glucuronide formation in animal body, *Life Sci.*, 382, 1963.

409. Preuss, Fr. R. and Mayer, E., Investigation of excretion products following administration of 1-ethynyl cyclohexyl carbamate, *Arch. Pharm.*, 298, 781, 1965.

410. Preuss, Fr. R. and Mayer, E., Demonstration of O-acetyl derivative after administration of 1-ethynyl cyclohexyl carbamate, *Arzneimittelforschung*, 15, 747, 1965.

411. Tagmann, E., Sury, E., and Hoffmann, K., Alkylenimine derivatives. I. Pyrrolidine, piperidine and hexamethylenimine derivatives with a basic substituent, *Helv. Chim. Acta*, 35, 1235, 1952.

412. Gross, F., Tripod, J., and Meier, R., Pharmacology of the hypnotic, Doriden®, *Schweiz. Med. Wschr.*, 85, 305, 1955.

413. Keberle, H., Hoffmann, K., and Bernhard, K., Metabolism of glutethimide (Doriden®), *Experientia*, 18, 105, 1962.

414. Butikofer, E., Cottier, P., Imhof, H., Keberle, H., Riess, W., and Schmid, K., Uber die eliminierung geschwindigkeit von Glutethimide (Doriden®) und die Nature der ausscheidungs produkte, *Arch. Exp. Path. Pharmak.*, 244, 97, 1962.

415. Keberle, H., Riess, W., and Hoffmann, K., The stereospecific metabolism of the optical antipodes of α-phenyl-α-ethyl glutarimide (Doriden®), *Arch. Int. Pharmacodyn.*, 142, 117, 1963.

416. Keberle, H., Riess, W., Schmid, K., and Hoffmann, K., The mechanism of the biological *N*-dealkylation (of doriden®), *Arch. Int. Pharmacodyn.*, 142, 125, 1963.

417. Remmer, H., Siegert, M., and Neuhaus, G., Die eliminierung von glutethimide und von langwirkenden Barbiturate nach toxisch und therapeutisch wirksamen Dosen, *Arch. Exp. Path. Pharmak.*, 245, 471, 1963.

418. Schmid, K., Cornu, F., Imhof, P., and Keberle, H., Biochemistry of the tolerance of hypnotics, *Schweiz. Med. Wschr.*, 94, 235, 1964.

419. Schmid, K., Riess, W., and Keberle, H., Racemic drugs containing different labels in the two enantiomorphs, *Isotop. Exp. Pharmacol.*, 383, 1965.

420. Maher, J. F., Determinants of serum half-life of glutethimide in intoxicated patients, *J. Pharmacol. Exp. Ther.*, 174, 450, 1970.

421. Pellmont, B., Studer, A., and Jurgen, R., 'Noludar' ein neues Schlafmittel der piperidine reihe, *Schweiz. Med. Wschr.*, 85, 350, 1955.

422. Bernhard, K., Brubacher, G., and Lutz, A., Investigation of distribution and excretion of sedative derivatives of hexa and tetrahydropyridines with the aid of ^{14}C labelling, *Helv. Physiol. Pharmak. Acta*, 12, C 12, 1954.

423. Randall, L. O., Iliev, V., and Brandman, O., Metabolism of methyprylon, *Arch. Int. Pharmacodyn.*, 106, 388, 1956.

424. Bernhard, K., Just, M., Lutz, A. H., and Vuilleumier, J. P., Behavior of 5-methyl substituted diethyl dioxo hydropyridine in metabolism, *Helv. Chim. Acta*, 40, 436, 1957.

425. Pribilla, O., A metabolic product of 2,4-dioxo-3,3-diethyl-5-methyl piperidine, *Arzneimittelforschung*, 6, 756, 1956.

426. Boesche, J. and Schmidt, G., 2,4,6-trioxo-3,3′-diethyl-5-methyl piperidine, a metabolite of methyprylon, *Arzneimittelforschung*, 16, 548, 1966.

427. Boesche, J., Concentration of methyprylon and its metabolites in urine after intoxication, *Arzneimittelforschung*, 19, 123, 1969.

428. P'an, S. Y., Kodet, M. J., Gardocki, J. F., McLamore, W. M., and Barley, A., Pharmacological studies on the hypnotic and anticonvulsant actions of ethyl β-chloro vinyl ethynyl carbinol, *J. Pharmacol. Exp. Ther.*, 114, 326, 1955.

429. Robinson, D. W., Method for determining ethchlorvynol in urine and serum by gas chromatography, *J. Pharm. Sci.*, 57, 185, 1968.

430. Wallace, J. E., Wilson, W. J., Jr., and Dahl, E. V., A rapid and specific method for determining ethchlorvynol, *J. Forensic Sci.*, 9, 342, 1964.

431. Algeri, E. J., Katsas, G. G., and Luongo, M. A., Determination of ethchlorvynol in biologic mediums and report of two fatal cases, *Amer. J. Clin. Path.*, 38, 125, 1962.

432. Martin, Y. C., The effect of ethchlorvynol on the drug metabolizing enzymes of rats and dogs, *Biochem. Pharmacol.*, 16, 2041, 1967.

433. Cummins, L. M., Martin, Y. C., and Scherfling, E. E., Serum and urine levels of ethchlorvynol in man, *J. Pharm. Sci.*, 60, 261, 1971.

434. Perlman, P. L. and Johnson, C. B., The metabolism of Dormison (3-methyl-1-pentyn-3-ol) and methods for estimation of drug in biological materials, *J. Amer. Pharm. Ass.*, 41, 13, 1952.

435. Perlman, P. L., Sutter, D., and Johnson, C. B., Further studies on metabolic disposition of Dormison (3-methyl-1-pentyn-3-ol) in dogs and man, *J. Amer. Pharm. Ass.*, 42, 750, 1953.

436. Bartholomew, A. A., Bourne, G. A., and Marley, E., Distribution of methyl pentynol and methyl pentynol carbamate in human body fluids, *Clin. Sci.*, 17, 629, 1958.

437. Marley, E. and Vane, J. R., The distribution of methyl pentynol and methyl pentynol carbamate in tissues and body fluids of cats, *Brit. J. Pharmacol.*, 13, 364, 1958.

438. Sternbach, L. H., Koechlin, B. A., and Reeder, E., Quinazolines and 1,4-benzodiazepins VIII. The photoisomerization of 7-chloro-2 methylamino-5-phenyl-3H-1,4-benzodiazepine-4-oxide, *Helv. Chim. Acta*, 45, 2226, 1962.

439. Nuhn, P. and Bley, W., NMR spectral studies on drug conformations of diazepine, netrazepam and chlordiazepoxide, *Pharmazie*, 22, 532, 1967.

440. Randall, L. O., Schalleck, W., Heise, G. A., Keith, E. F., and Bagdon, R. E., The psychosedative properties of methamine diazepoxide, *J. Pharmacol. Exp. Ther.*, 129, 163, 1960.

441. Randall, L. O., Pharmacology of chlordiazepoxide (Librium®), *Dis. Nerv. Syst.*,22, 7, 1961.

442. Zbinden, G., Bagdon, R. E., Keith, E. F., Phillips, R. D., and Randall, L. O., Experimental and clinical toxicology of chlordiazepoxide (Librium®), *Toxic. Appl. Pharmacol.*, 3, 619, 1961.

443. Zbinden, G. and Randall, L. O., Pharmacology of benzodiazepine - laboratory and clinical correlates, *Advances Pharmacol.*, 5, 213, 1967.

444. Smith, D. and Pennington, G. W., The detection and excretion of chlordiazepoxide (Librium®) in human plasma and urine, *Arch. Int. Pharmacodyn.*, 145, 154, 1963.

445. Koechlin, B. A., Schwartz, M. A., Krol, G., and Oberhausli, W., Metabolic fate of ^{14}C-labeled chlordiazepoxide in man, the dog and the rat, *J. Pharmacol. Exp. Ther.*, 148, 399, 1965.

446. Schwartz, M. A., Vane, F. M., and Postma, E., Chlordiazepoxide metabolites in the rat – characterization by high resolution mass spectrometry, *Biochem. Pharmacol.*, 17, 965, 1968.

447. Placidi, G. F. and Cassano, G. B., Distribution and metabolism of ^{14}C-labeled chlordiazepoxide in mice, *Int. J. Neuropharmacol.*, 7, 383, 1968.

448. Hoagland, D. R., Miya, T. S., and Bousquet, W. F., Metabolism and tolerance studies with chlordiazepoxide-$2^{14}C$ in the rat, *Toxic. Appl. Pharmacol.*, 9, 116, 1966.

449. Schwartz, M. A. and Postma, E., Oxazepam excreted by chlordiazepoxide-^{14}C dosed dogs, *J. Pharm. Sci.*, 55, 1358, 1966.

450. Schwartz, D. E., Veechi, M., Ronco, A., and Kaiser, K., Blood levels after administration of 7-chloro-1,3-dihydro-1-methyl-5-phenyl-2H-1,4-benzodiazepine-2-one (diazepam) in various forms, *Arzneimittelforschung*,16, 1109, 1966.

451. Randall, L. O., Heise, G. A., Schalleck, W., Bagdon, R. E., Banziger, R., Boris, A., Moe, R. A., and Abrams, W. B., Pharmacological and clinical studies on Valium® – a new psychotherapeutic agent of benzodiazepine class, *Curr. Ther. Res.*, 3, 405, 1961.

452. Schwartz, M. A., Koechlin, B. A., Postma, E., Palmer, S., and Krol, G., Metabolism of diazepam in rats, dogs and man, *J. Pharmacol. Exp. Ther.*, 149, 423, 1965.

453. Ruelius, H. W., Lee, J. M., and Album, H. E., Metabolism of diazepam in dogs – transformation to oxazepam, *Arch. Biochem. Biophys.*, 111, 376, 1965.

454. Arthur, J., DeSilva, F., Koechlin, B. A., and Bader, G., Blood level distribution patterns of diazepam and its major metabolites in man, *J. Pharm. Sci.*, 55, 692, 1966.

455. Schwartz, M. A., Bommer, P., and Vane, F. M., Diazepam metabolites in rat – characterization by high resolution mass spectrometry and nuclear magnetic resonance, *Arch. Biochem. Biophys.*, 121, 508, 1967.

456. Jommi, G., Manitto, P., and Silanos, M. A., Metabolism of diazepam in rabbits, *Arch. Biochem. Biophys.*, 108, 334, 1964.

457. Schwartz, M. A. and Postma, E., Metabolism of diazepam *in vitro*, *Biochem. Pharmacol.*, 17, 2443, 1968.

458. Marcucchi, F., Guaitani, A., Kvetina, J., Mussini, E., and Garattini, S., Species difference in diazepam metabolism and anticonvulsant effect, *Europ. J. Pharmacol.*, 4, 467, 1968.

459. Walkenstein, S. S., Wiser, R., Gudmundsen, C. H., Kummel, H. B., and Corradino, R. A., Absorption, metabolism, excretion of oxazepam and its succinate half-ester, *J. Pharm. Sci.*, 53, 1181, 1964.

460. Arrigoni, E., Manzo, L., and Sarti, P., Metabolism in organs isolated *in situ* – glucuronide conjugation of oxazepam in the brain, *Boll. Soc. Ital. Biol. Sper.*, 43, 1463, 1967.

461. Berte, F., Benzi, G., Manzo, L., and Horkari, S., Tissue distribution and metabolism of oxazepam in pregnant guinea pigs and rats, *Arch. Int. Pharmacodyn.*, 173, 377, 1968.

462. Jacobson, E., The metabolism of ethyl alcohol, *Pharmacol. Rev.*, 4, 107, 1952.

463. Marshall, E. K., Jr. and Fritz, W. F., The metabolism of ethyl alcohol, *J. Pharmacol. Exp. Ther.*, 109, 431, 1953.

464. Westerfield, W. W., The intermediary metabolism of alcohol, *Amer. J. Clin. Nutr.*, 9, 426, 1961.

465. Westheimer, F. H., Fisher, H. F., Conn, E. E., and Vennesland, B., The enzymatic transfer of H atom from alcohol to DPN, *J. Amer. Chem. Soc.*, 73, 2403, 1951.

466. Lieber, C. S. and Davidson, C. S., Some metabolic effects of ethyl alcohol, *Amer. J. Med.*, 33, 319, 1962.

467. Forney, R. B., Hughes, F. W., Harger, R. N., and Richards, A. B., Alcohol distribution in the vascular system. Concentration of orally administered alcohol in blood from various points in the vascular system and in rebreathed air during absorption, *Quart. J. Stud. Alcohol*, 25, 205, 1964.

468. Bartlett, G. R. and Barnet, H. R., Some observations on alcohol metabolism with radioactive ethyl alcohol, *Quart. J. Stud. Alcohol*, 10, 381, 1949.

469. Doncheff, L., E'tude de l'oxydation de l'alcool chez le rat au moyen d' ethanol marque au C^{14}, *C.R. Acad. Sci. (Paris)*, 231, 177, 1950.

470. Racker, E., Aldehyde dehydrogenase, a diphosphopyridine nucleotide-linked enzyme, *J. Biol. Chem.*, 177, 883, 1949.

471. Bartlett, G. R., Does catalase participate in physiological oxidation of alcohol?, *Quart. J. Stud. Alcohol*, 13, 583, 1952.

472. Hald, J., Jacobsen, E., and Larsen, V., The sensitizing effect of tetraethyl thiuram disulfide (antabuse) to ethyl alcohol, *Acta Pharmacol.*, 4, 285, 1948.

473a. Rubin, E. and Lieber, C. S., Hepatic microsomal enzymes in man and in the rat – induction and inhibition by ethanol, *Science*, 162, 690, 1968.

473b. Rubin, E. and Lieber, C. S., Alcohol induced hepatic injury in nonalcoholic volunteers, *New Eng. J. Med.*, 278, 869, 1968.

474. Orme-Johnson, W. H. and Ziegler, D. M., Alcohol mixed function oxidase activity of mammalian liver microsomes, *Biochem. Biophys. Res. Comm.*, 21, 78, 1965.

475. Lieber, C. S. and DeCarli, L. M., Hepatic microsomes, a new site for ethanol oxidation, *J. Clin. Invest.*, 47, 62a, 1968.

476. Lieber, C. S. and DeCarli, L. M., Ethanol oxidation by hepatic microsomes: adaptive increase after ethanol feeding, *Science*, 162, 917, 1968.

477. Lieber, C. S. and DeCarli, L. M., Hepatic microsomal ethanol-oxidizing system, *J. Biol. Chem.*, 245, 2505, 1970.

478. Carter, E. A. and Isselbacher, K. J., The role of microsomes in the hepatic metabolism of ethanol, *Ann. N. Y. Acad. Sci.*, 179, 282, 1971.

479. Goldstein, D. B. and Pal, N., Alcohol dependence produced in mice by inhalation of ethanol: grading the withdrawal reaction, *Science*, 172, 288, 1971.

480. Goldstein, A. and Judson, B. A., Alcohol dependence and opiate dependence – lack of relationship in mice, *Science*, 172, 290, 1971.

481. Davis, V. E. and Walsh, M. J., Alcohol, amines and alkaloids – a possible biochemical basis for alcohol addiction, *Science*, 167, 1005, 1970.

482. Seevers, M. H., Adaptation to narcotics, *Fed. Proc.*, 13, 672, 1954.

483. Seevers, M. H. and Woods, L. A., The phenomena of tolerance, *Amer. J. Med.*, 14, 546, 1953.

484. Seevers, M. H. and Deneau, G. A., Physiological aspects of tolerance and physical dependence, in *Physiological Pharmacology*, Vol. I, Root, W. S. and Hofmann, F. G., Eds., Academic Press, New York, 1953, 565.

485. Eddy, N. B., Halbach, H., Isbell, H., and Seevers, M. H., Drug dependence, its significance and characteristics, *Bull. W.H.O.*, 32, 721, 1965.

486. Seevers, M. H. and Deneau, G. A., A critique of the "dual action" hypothesis of morphine physical dependence, *Res. Publ. Ass. Nerv. Ment. Dis.*, 46, 199, 1968.

487. Halushka, P. V. and Hoffman, P. C., Alcohol addiction and tetrahydropapaveroline, *Science*, 169, 1104, 1970.

488. Seevers, M. H., Morphine and ethanol physical dependence – a critique of a hypothesis, *Science*, 170, 1113, 1970.

489. Goldstein, A. and Judson, B. A., Alcohol dependence and opiate dependence – lack of relationship in mice, *Science*, 172, 290, 1971.

490. Mellett, L. B. and Woods, L. A., Analgesia and addiction, *Fortschr. Arzneimittelforschung*, 5, 156, 1963.

491. Collier, H. O. J., Tolerance, physical dependence and receptors. A theory of the genesis of tolerance and physical dependence through drug-induced changes in the number of receptors, *Advances in Drug. Res.*, 3, 171, 1966.

492. Mule, S. J., The relationship of the disposition and metabolism of morphine in the CNS to tolerance, in *Scientific Basis of Drug Dependence*, Steinberg, H., Ed., J. A. Churchill Ltd., London, 1969, 97.

493. Axelrod, J., Cellular adaptation in the development of tolerance to drugs, *Res. Publ. Ass. Nerv. Ment. Dis.*, 46, 247, 1968.

494. Remmer, H., Tolerance to barbiturates by increased breakdown, in *Scientific Basis of Drug Dependence*, Steinberg, H., Ed., J. A. Churchill Ltd., London, 1969, 111.

495. Cox, B. M. and Osman, O. H., Inhibition of development of tolerance to morphine in rats by drugs which inhibit ribonucleic acid and protein synthesis, *Brit. J. Pharmacol.*, 38, 157, 1970.

496. Dews, P. B., in *Experimental Approaches to the Study of Drug Dependence*, Kalant, H. D. and Hawkins, R. D., Eds., University of Toronto Press, 1969, 104.

497. Misra, A. L. and Mitchell, C. L., Metal-ion catalyzed interaction of peroxidase with morphine and protein, *Experientia*, 27, 1442, 1971.

498. Misra, A. L. and Woods, L. A., Evidence for interaction *in vitro* of morphine with glutathione, *Nature*, (London), 228, 1226, 1970.

499. Beckett, A. H. and Casy, A. F., Synthetic analgesics: Stereochemical considerations, *J. Pharm. Pharmacol.*, 6, 986, 1954.

500. Portoghese, P. S., A new concept on the mode of interaction of narcotic analgesics with receptors, *J. Med. Chem.*, 8, 609, 1965.

501. Portoghese, P. S., Stereochemical factors and receptor interactions associated with narcotic analgesics, *J. Pharm. Sci.*, 55, 865, 1966.

DETECTION AND IDENTIFICATION OF DRUGS OF DEPENDENCE

S. J. Mulé

TABLE OF CONTENTS

INTRODUCTION

The methods used for the identification of drugs subject to abuse are essentially those utilized in analytical chemistry for the identification of chemical structures. These include: qualitative and quantitative color tests; microcrystal tests; physicochemical methods; ultraviolet, infrared, visible, mass and atomic absorption spectroscopy; x-ray diffraction; ion-exchange, thin-layer, gas and liquid-chromatography; spectrofluorometry, nuclear magnetic resonance, and isotope methods. Most of these techniques are quite effective for the identification of purified material, which, of course, is seldom the situation with drugs obtained from biological materials. Therefore, although many analytical methods are available, few are effective in the routine identification of psychoactive drugs obtained from biological materials. In this regard, certain minimal criteria must be met. These are: (a) *Specificity*. The psychoactive drugs should be separated from biological materials by chemical groups through differential pH extraction. Alternatively, it is possible to extract the drugs from biological materials nonspecifically and through the application of physical and chemical analysis identify each drug specifically; (b) *Sensitivity*. All drugs or metabolites must be detected and/or identified at the microgram-nanogram level; (c) *Time*. The entire procedure including documentation, extraction, analysis, and reporting the results should not exceed 24 hours following laboratory acquisition of the biological sample; (d) *Simplicity*. The analytical methods employed should not require skill or training beyond that normally achieved by a laboratory technician; (e) *Cost*. The analysis must be viewed economically, but ultimately assessed in terms of the effect upon society should the tests not be performed.

The purpose of this chapter is to review the more recent developments in the identification and detection of psychoactive drugs. The major emphasis will be upon identification from biological material, thus eliminating serious consideration of the hallucinogenic and cannabis class of compounds. Ethanol detection will not be discussed since this socially acceptable drug is not routinely screened for in an analysis of tissues and fluids for drugs subject to abuse.

EXTRACTION OF DRUGS FROM BIOLOGICAL MATERIAL

Narcotic Analgesics

A general method for the extraction of narcotic drugs from biological materials usually involves precipitation of the free base (pH 8 to 10) from aqueous solution and subsequent partitioning into an organic solvent. Several procedures[1-8] have been developed which are quite effective in extracting several chemical classes of narcotic analgesics. The following modification of the Mulé[1] procedure should provide reasonably good recoveries for narcotic drugs: transfer 10 ml sample (urine, plasma, 0.1 N HCl 10% tissue homogenate) to a 45 ml centrifuge tube, adjust the pH to 9 to 10 with 2.5 N NaOh, buffer with 3 ml of 1 M K_2HPO_4 (pH 9.6), saturate the sample with 1 to 2 g of NaCl, and add 15 ml of ethylene dichloride containing 25% isobutanol. Shake the sample for 10 minutes, centrifuge, and remove 12 to 14 ml of the upper organic phase. The organic extract may be evaporated to dryness for chromatographic detection or reextracted into acid for spectrophotometric detection.

Barbiturates

The general method for extracting organic acids from biological material or, in particular, the substituted cyclic ureides of malonic acid (pK_a 7.2 to 8.8) is to adjust the pH to 1 to 5 and extract the acidic solution with organic solvents such as: chloroform, ethylacetate, ether, or ethylene dichloride. Many specific methods for the extraction of barbiturates from biological materials have been reported.[2,3,8-12] The following method has proved to be effective in our laboratory for the extraction of barbiturates, as well as diphenylhydantoin and glutethimide: transfer 15 ml of urine or a suitable aliquot of plasma or a 10% tissue homogenate (0.1 N HCl) to a 45 ml centrifuge tube, add 0.3 ml of 9 N H_2SO_4, and 15 ml of chloroform. Shake the samples for 10 minutes on an Eberbach shaker, centrifuge, and remove the upper aqueous phase by aspiration. The organic phase may be filtered and evaporated to dryness on a steam bath at 85°C under a stream of air. The aqueous phase may be reextracted with an additional 15 ml of $CHCl_3$ and the organic phase may be washed with 2 ml of saturated $NaHCO_3$. The residue may be taken up in methanol (25 to 50 μl) and chromatographed (TLC or GLC).

Sympathomimetic Amines

A general method for the extraction of amphetamines from biological materials and related analogues involves adjustment of the pH of the solution to about 10 with alkali and subsequent extraction with an organic solvent (ether, chloroform, ethylene dichloride), evaporation of the solvent and application of analytical techniques.[2-4,6,8-16] The following procedure allows for the ready extraction of this class of drugs from biological materials: transfer a 15 to 25 ml aliquot of urine (suitable sample of plasma or tissue homogenate) to a 50 ml centrifuge tube, adjust the pH to 10 to 11 with 6 N NaOH, add 5 ml of potassium phosphate pH 10.3, and 12 ml of 25% ethanol in chloroform (v/v). Shake the sample for 10 minutes in an Eberbach shaker, remove organic phase, and reextract the aqueous phase with 10 ml of solvent. Add about 100 μl of 6 N HCl in ethanol to the organic extract and evaporate to dryness in a water bath at 75°C under a stream of air. Chromatographic techniques may be applied to the residue.

Psychosedatives

Many methods are available for the extraction and determination of phenothiazines,[2-4,6,8-20] benzodiazepines[2-4,6,21-23] carbamates,[2-4,6,24,25] glutethimide [2-4,6,26,27] and ethchlorvynol[28-30] from biological material. These compounds, except for glutethimide, (see barbiturates) may be extracted from biological materials as follows: transfer a 15 ml aliquot of urine (suitable aliquot of plasma or tissue homogenate) to a 45 ml centrifuge tube, adjust the pH to 9 to 10 with dilute NaOH, add 15 ml of chloroform, and shake for 10 minutes on an Eberbach shaker. Centrifuge, remove the organic phase, and reextract with 10 ml of 25% ethanol in chloroform. Combine the organic phases and evaporate to dryness under a stream of air at 75 to 80°C. The residue may be taken up in methanol (25 to 50 μl) and chromatographed.

Resin-Column Extraction of Drugs of Abuse

Although the solvent-solvent extraction techniques described above were quite effective in obtaining these drugs from biological material, they were still somewhat time consuming. Recently, we have developed and applied the XAD-2 resin column technique[31] to the routine analysis of psychoactive drugs from urine. A general description of the method is as follows: 25 ml of urine was applied to the polypropylene columns containing 1.1 g of Amberlite XAD-2 resin. The flow rate of the urine was controlled and the resin eluted with 15 ml of chloroform:isopropanol (3:1, v/v). The organic solvent extracts were shaken with 1 ml of saturated sodium bicarbonate and the separated organic phases evaporated to dryness in a water bath under a stream of air. The residues were dissolved in methanol and applied equally to silica gel plates and sheets. The effectiveness of this technique as compared to the extraction methods is shown in Table 1.

CHEMICAL DETECTION METHODS

Qualitative and Quantitative Color Tests

Narcotic Analgesics

The color reactions obtained with the opium alkaloids and synthetic analogues have been adequately reviewed.[5,7,32,33] It is, therefore, only necessary to emphasize certain important reactions (see Table 2) that have received wide application primarily in toxicological laboratories. These tests, however, are obviously limited, nonspecific, and usually conducted with the solid material, so that extracts of biological materials must be purified to be effective with these color tests.

Quantitative methods for the narcotic analgesics and, in particular, morphine were developed

TABLE 1

Comparison of the XAD-2 Resin Column Technique With Other Analytical Methods of Extracting Drugs[a]

		Percent recovery					
			Selective pH solvent[b] extraction at:				
Drug	Concentration μg/ml urine	XAD-resin method	pH 1	pH 9 (Mulé)	pH 10 – 11	Ethanol-K_2CO_3 extraction (Bastos)	Single Extraction at pH 9.5 (Davidow)
d-amphetamine-^{3}H	2.0	49.3			63.5	58.9	64.5
cocaine-^{14}C	1.0	91.6			86.0	73.8	93.1
meperidine-^{14}C	1.0	89.0			93.5	90.7	98.7
l-methadone-^{3}H	10.4	55.5			64.7	85.7	71.0
morphine-^{14}C	1.25	64.0		70.7	38.0	82.0	75.3
meprobamate-^{14}C	1.0	74.4	77.2		54.6	89.3	84.5
quinine[c]	10.0	78.4			90.4	92.8	98.0
pentobarbital-^{14}C	2.0	88.4	81.6			92.0	63.2
phenobarbital-^{14}C	1.0	83.1	89.5			72.2	39.3

[a]The labeled drugs were extracted by the XAD-2 resin technique[31] and by solvent extraction methods reported by Mulé,[3] Bastos et al.,[4] and Davidow et. al.[6]
[b]The data reported concerns primarily the narcotic analgesics which in general were more effectively extracted at pH 9. The pH 10-11 extraction was developed to obtain a large number of basic organic drugs including amphetamines, phenothiazines, and antihistamines.
[c]Quinine was determined spectrofluorometrically.[129]

TABLE 2

Color Tests for Narcotic Analgesics

Tests[a]	Color	Sensitivity (μg)	Specificity
Marquis	purple or violet	0.3	all phenolic and etheric opiates and other alkaloids
Flueckiger	orange-red	1.0	same, no reaction with codeine
Wassicky	orange-red	0.1	same
Froehde	purple-green	0.05	not specific
Mecke	bluish-green	0.1	phenolic group reagent
Folin-Ciocalteau	blue	0.5	same

[a]Composition of reagent as given by Farmilio and Genest.[7]

primarily for the colorimetric estimation of these drugs following extraction from biological materials. The organic extract was usually mixed with the dye which forms a complex with the basic compound. The dye was then extracted into acid in proportion to that complexing with the drug. The acidic dye method was used most successfully with narcotic drugs[34] by application of the dye methyl orange originally developed for organic bases.[35] Other dyes used in this manner are bromcresol green, bromcresol purple, and bromthymol blue. Coupling the drug with diazonium salts was used successfully with morphine[36] and organic bases.[37] In all cases, the final colored product was estimated by spectrophotometry. The major difficulties with these techniques were specificity and sensitivity. Some specificity may be imparted to the reaction by subjecting the extracts to column or thin-layer chromatography prior to preparation of the color complex.

Barbiturates

The use of color tests[38] for the detection of barbiturates has limited usefulness (except for thin-layer chromatography) in light of currently available analytical techniques. In any event, the Koppanyi test[39] involving cobalt acetate and isopropylamine to provide a red-violet color indicative of barbituric acid or one of its derivatives is still used, although normally modified by the addition of a chloroform extraction step.[40] However, this test,[39] in general, lacks specificity.

The 5,5 substituted barbiturates form insoluble white salts with mercury and silver.[41] Subsequent reaction with diphenylcarbazone yields purple-blue color with these compounds. Barbiturates with an unsaturated side chain will react with potassium permanganate[42] to provide a yellow color and the rate usually depends upon the site of the double bond. The bromobarbiturates react with fluorescein-casin solutions[43] to provide a pink color.

The mercuric-diphenylcarbazone, potassium permanganate, fluorescein reactions are capable of detecting 20 to 100 μg of the 5,5 substituted barbiturates. The effectiveness of any of these color producing reagents on biological materials requires purification of the extract prior to initiating the chemical reactions.

Sympathomimetic Amines

Color reactions for this group of compounds primarily concern reactions associated with primary, secondary, and tertiary amines. It is possible through reaction of sympathomimetic amines[44] with benzoyl chloride, *p*-nitrobenzoyl chloride, benzenesulphonyl chloride, picric acid, and ammonium reineckate to differentiate dexamphetamine, amphetamine, methamphetamine, and ephedrine by color and microcrystal tests. A dark red color may be obtained[45] when a sample solution in CCl_4 is treated with ethanolic quinhydrone, indicating a diamine. Primary amines give a gold color; secondary and tertiary amines do not react.

A colorimetric method for primary amines[46] was used to assay amphetamine by heating an acidic solution with 2,5-dimethoxytetrahydrofuran and subsequently with *p*-dimethylaminobenzaldehyde to provide a red color. Apparently, secondary and tertiary amines do not interfere.

It is, of course, a much more complicated matter to detect these amines extracted from biological materials. In all cases, the sympathomimetic amines obtained from urine must be subjected to countercurrent distribution or chromatography prior to reacting with a specific reagent.[47] Reagents[48] such as hexan-2:5-dione and *p*-dimethylaminobenzaldehyde were used in detecting primary amines following separation of the compounds on thin-layer chromatograms. Recently, it was shown[2-4,31] that ninhydrinacetone reagent was effective in detecting primary amines (i.e. *d*-amphetamine, phenylpropanalamine) and *p*-nitroaniline was quite effective in confirming the presence of primary amines. Ninhydrin acid[4,31] was capable of detecting secondary amines (i.e. methamphetamine).

Psychosedatives

Methods for the colorimetric detection of phenothiazines were developed by Forrest.[49] Although modifications exist, the basic technique employs the "FPN" universal test utilizing ferric chloride, perchloric acid, and nitric acid to provide a color reaction of different intensity depending upon concentration of the phenothiazine in urine.

A specific method for the estimation of phenothiazines in blood and urine was reported by Haux and Natelson[50] which required extraction into heptane, reextraction into HCl, and oxidation with arsenic acid to produce color. Absorptivities may then be determined with a spectrophotometer.

Chlordiazepoxide (Librium®) may be detected following extraction from serum[51] by hydrolytic cleavage and diazotization with *N*-(1-naphthyl)-ethylenediame to form a chromogen. Sulfanilamide and procainamide were found to interfere with the estimation of this drug.

Methods to determine carbamates (i.e. meprobamate) colorimetrically were developed for both blood[52] and urine.[53] These techniques provide color reactions either with Nessler's reagent or furfuraldehyde.

A procedure for the detection of ethchlorvynol (Placidyl®) in biological material was described[28] based on the production of an orange color when certain compounds containing an allyl group were treated with phlorglucinol and HCl.

Glutethimide (Doriden®)[26] was determined following isolation from biological material and was treated with *m*-dinitrobenzene in $CHCl_3$ containing 0.05 ml of dimethylsulphoxide and KOH. A deep violet color turning green following a reaction with benzoyl peroxide indicated a positive reaction. This drug may also be determined[54] by a reaction with diphenylamine in the presence of a mixture of sulfuric and acetic acids. Absorbance was determined at 510 mμ.

MICROCRYSTALLOGRAPHY

Microcrystal tests are extremely useful in the identification of organic compounds, in general, and organic bases in particular. Attempts have been made[55] to describe the colors and crystal aggregates with subsequent classification of the chemical reactions. Ultimately, however, experience is required to effectively utilize this technique. However, microcrystal tests still remain indispensable in distinguishing small quantities of optical isomers and racemic mixtures of the morphinans,[56] amphetamines,[57] and propoxyphene.[58]

Organic Bases

Anionic reagents are most important for the identification of basic compounds such as alkaloids, sympathomimetic amines, and other nitrogen-containing compounds.[59,60] These reagents are often halogen complexes of gold, platinum, or complexes of polyiodides, organic acid compounds, or common inorganic salts, i.e., AuCN, $HgCl_2$, $K_4Fe(CN)_6$, K_2CrO_4. The polyiodide complexes of Hg and Cd are quite selective precipitants of alkaloids and extremely useful for detection of the narcotic analgesics.[61] However, impurities affect the sensitivity and specificity of these reagents and, therefore, identification was more reliable following thin-layer chromatography (TLC) and subsequent extraction of the compounds from the TLC plate.[62] Platinic and gold reagents were effective even in the presence of impurities for the detection of sympathomimetic amines.[55]

Organic Acids

Organic base reagents: platinum polyiodide and K_2-KI may be used for precipitating barbiturates in phosphoric acid medium,[55] but selectivity of these reagents was poor. The usual barbiturate reagents were halogen-containing salts.[55,63] Microcrystal tests for barbiturates were not sensitive and not commonly used for the identification of these drugs from biological material.

Sensitivity

The minimal detection level for microcrystal tests usually was 20 to 200 μg/ml.[55] The most sensitive reactions were those that provided fine circular and rhomboidal crystals followed by dendrites and spherolites. From a practical viewpoint, the most reliable quantity of biological material available should provide about 50 μg of drug for the microcrystal test.

PHYSICAL DETECTION METHODS

Ultraviolet Spectrophotometry

Narcotic Analgesics

Quantitatively, this technique has limited value with the narcotic drugs as applied to biological materials because of the impurity of the extracted samples and the necessity for high concentrations of the material (20 to 500 μg/ml). However, much data has been obtained with the narcotic analgesics[1] (see Tables 3 and 4). It is obvious that within families the maximum and minimum wavelengths were similar, thus making it difficult to identify an individual analgesic drug. However, a shift in the spectra was observed in alkaline solution with those drugs that form the phenolate ion. Furthermore, it was quite easy to calculate maximim and minimum molar absorptivity values, peak ratio values and mμ values. This kind of data provide additional information for the identification of a given narcotic analgesic or chemical family.

Comprehensive reviews concerning the application of UV spectrophotometry to the analysis of narcotic analgesics[64,65] and, in particular, in relation to toxicological problems[66] are available. The most effective use of UV spectroscopy was following purification of the biological extract by chromatography or countercurrent distribution. However, some investigators have attempted to identify narcotic analgesics by application of UV spectroscopy directly to paper chromatograms,[67] thin-layer chromatograms,[19] or through conversion to reineckates[68,69] and tetraphenylborides.[70]

Barbiturates

The detection and/or determination of barbiturates in biological material by ultraviolet spectroscopy has been adequately demonstrated.[10,71,72] These techniques have usually utilized the difference in absorbance at pH 13/10 or pH 10/2 and have found wide application amongst toxicologists. The major difficulty with these methods was interference from other substances. Normally the biological materials were extracted at neutral or acidic pH into chloroform, with subsequent extraction in NaOH before UV spectrophotometry. Drugs[73] likely to interfere with this assay were weak acids or ampholytes possessing similar physical properties and absorbing within the UV spectrum.

Diphenylhydantoin often extracted at an acidic pH may be determined following hydrolysis in alkali and permanganate oxidation of the resulting amide to benzophenone. This compound, in contrast to diphenylhydantoin itself, has a well-defined absorption spectrum and exhibits a high molar absorptivity.[74]

Sympathomimetic Amines

Spectrophotometric methods for the analysis of phenethylamines were for the most part lacking in specificity and/or sensitivity.[75,76] However, Wallace developed a method[77] whereby a cerium oxidation product of amphetamine was produced that provided a sensitivity limit of about 0.5 μg/ml with a 10 ml sample. The specificity was limited to those compounds having a β-phenethylamine group as part of their structure. The specificity requirements were: a β-methylene carbon and no hydroxy, or methoxy substituent at the para position of the aromatic ring. Para-hydroxy amphetamine, 3-4-dimethoxy phenethylamine, and 3,4,5-trimethoxyphenethylamine did not react.

Ephedrine and related phenethanolamine compounds have a low order of molar absorptivity and are thus difficult to detect spectrophotometrically. Wallace, however, developed a method[78] utilizing the semicarbazone of ephedrine which reportedly provided sensitivity and specificity for ephedrine and related compounds.

TABLE 3

Ultraviolet Absorption Spectra Data for the Iminoethanophenanthrofurans[a]

Compound (free base)	Maximum wavelength, mu				Absorptivity molar, Σ max			
	0.1N HCl	0.2N NaOH	Abs. ETOH	Ib-[c] $ETCl_2$	0.1N HCl	0.2N NaOH	Abs. ETOH	Ib- $ETCl_2$
Morphine	285	297	287	287	1583	2421	1644	1514
Normorphine	285	297	287	287	1345	2233	1346	1245
Codeine[d]	285	285	286	287	1587	1479	1491	1494
Norcodeine[d]	285	285	285	286	1555	1478	1732	1478
Diacetylmorphine (heroin)	285	298	281	281	1950	3294	2190	1740
N-Allylnormorphine (nalorphine)	281	298	287	287	1466	2437	1635	1551
Methyldihydromorphinone (metapon)	281	291	285	285	1164	1982	1138	1121
Dihydromorphinone (dilaudid)	281	292	284	283	1331	2253	1250	1187
Ethylmorphine[d] (dionine)	285	285	285	285	1720	1501	1564	1551
Dihydrohydroxymorphinone (oxymorphone)	281	292	282	286	1270	2280	1392	1097
Dihydromorphine	284	297	285	287	1600	2556	1765	1582
Dihydrocodeinone[d] (hydrocodone)	280	280	282	283	1389	1302	1302	1344
Dihydrohydroxycodeinone[d] (oxycodone)	281	281	284	285	1375	1280	1309	1305
6-Monoacetylmorphine	285	297	287	287	1418	2498	1559	1513

[a]From Mulé[1] Courtesy of *Analytical Chemistry.*
[b]Difference between the maximum and minimum wavelengths.
[c]The free base was dissolved in ethylene dichloride containing 25% isobutanol (v./v.).
[d]The bathochromic shift was not observed in the 0.2N NaOH sample.

Psychosedatives

Utilization of ultraviolet spectrophotometry for the detection of psychosedatives was almost totally ineffective with regard to extracts of these compounds from biological material. There is little if any specificity and this technique is insensitive. However, a method[79] reported to be reliable although not extremely sensitive or fully specific allows for the determination of glutethimide in urine and blood at 235 mμ.

Gas-Liquid Chromatography (GLC)

Narcotic Analgesics

This technique, based upon partitioning the molecules between a gas phase and liquid support on the column has proven to be invaluable for the detection of a wide variety of chemical compounds. Lloyd, et al.[80] demonstrated the feasibility of using GLC for the separation of opium alkaloids and subsequently, a large number of the alkaloids were separated by gas chromatography,[81] confirming the speed, simplicity, and reproducibility of the method.

Application of GLC to solvent extracts from biological materials was reported by Kayzak and Knoblock[82] utilizing SE-30 and Qf-1 columns and an argon ionization detector. Retention data on 41 alkaloids separated on SE-30 and carbowax 20 M columns were obtained[83] with extracts from biological materials. One of the major difficulties encountered with biological material was the presence of GLC peaks due to the extraction of endogenous compounds from tissues, blood, and urine.

A relatively excellent approach to the GLC of narcotic drugs was the peak shift technique reported by Anders and Mannering[84] whereby derivatives of narcotic analgesics were prepared on the column by injecting anhydrides of acetate and propionate. The derivatives were formed with alcoholic or phenolic hydroxyl groups and with

TABLE 3 (continued)

Minimum wavelength, mu				Absorptivity molar Σ min						Δmμ[b]	
0.1N HCl	0.2N NaOH	Abs. ETOH	Ib-ETCl2	0.1N HCl	0.2N NaOH	Abs. ETOH	Ib-ETCl2	0.1N HCl	0.2N NaOH	Abs. ETOH	Ib-ETCl2
260	278	262	263	540	1439	534	534	25	19	25	24
260	278	262	263	388	1361	469	385	25	19	25	24
262	262	263	263	594	554	512	512	23	23	23	24
262	262	263	263	599	722	719	562	23	23	22	23
261	279	255	257	654	2037	716	462	24	19	26	24
257	279	263	263	430	1407	588	489	24	19	24	24
262	275	266	267	602	1607	682	707	19	16	19	18
262	272	265	267	756	1663	802	816	19	20	17	16
262	262	263	263	596	590	570	524	23	23	22	22
262	274	265	267	779	1731	973	790	19	18	19	19
256	271	256	257	415	1154	324	327	28	26	29	30
261	262	264	265	781	919	760	770	19	18	18	18
262	264	265	265	807	902	750	725	19	17	19	20
260	278	263	263	450	1530	534	505	25	19	24	22

primary and secondary amines. Identification of the compound was achieved through comparison of the retention time of the unesterified free compound with that of the esterified derivative(s). The peak shift technique was used quite effectively by Mule'[1] with extracts of tissues, urine, and blood. Figure 1 shows how effective the peak shift method was in forming esterified derivatives of morphine on the column by subjecting this drug to a homologous series of anhydrides. Retention data was obtained for the free drug, as well as the acetylated and propianated column derivative on a 2% SE-30 column at 215°C using an argon ionization detector. Unique differences were observed between 31 narcotic drugs representing 5 different chemical families.

Analytical use of gas-liquid chromatography was described by Wilkinson and Way,[85] whereby morphine was extracted from biological fluids and the trimethylsilyl ether derivatives prepared using Bis(trimethylsilyl) trifluoroacetamide as the silylating agent. A similar technique[86] involving charcoal adsorption and solvent extraction of morphine followed by GLC of the trimethylsilyl derivative was capable of detecting this drug for a period of 96 hours in urine.

Barbiturates

GLC has provided important advancements in the detection and identification of barbiturates as described in two excellent reviews.[87,88] Application of this technique to biological extracts was shown to be quite feasible.[82,83] Jain et al.[89] developed a method using fingertip blood, a simple extraction, and subsequent identification of the barbiturate on SE-30 using a flame ionization detector. Two gas chromatographic methods were described by Parker et al.[90] for the determination of barbiturates in blood and urine using an SE-30 and QF-1 mixed liquid phase column. The samples were extracted with an organic solvent containing an internal standard (tetraphenylethylene). Confirmation was achieved by the formation of a derivative on a solid injector and demonstrating a characteristic peak shift. The detectability of the methods ranged from 0.5 to 10 μg per 1 or 2 ml sample.

Street[91] demonstrated that a single injection of a mixture of *N,O*-bistrimethylsilylacetamide and barbiturate formed the trimethylsilyl derivatives of these drugs. The derivative peak shapes were then more symmetrical and the sensitivity greater than obtained with the parent drug. The application of

TABLE 4

Ultraviolet Absorption Spectra Data for Narcotic Analgesics Arranged According to Chemical Families[a]

Compound (free base)	Maximum wavelength, mμ		Absorptivity molar, Σ max		Minimum wavelength, mμ		Absorptivity molar, Σ min		Peak ratio, Σ max/Σ min		Δ mμ[b]	
	0.1N HCl	0.2N NaOH	0.1N HCl	0.2N NaOH	0.1N HCl	0.2N NaOH	0.1N HCl	0.2N NaOH	0.1N HCl	0.2N NaOH	0.1N HCl	0.2N NaOH
Iminoethanophenanthrenes												
1-3-Hydroxy-*N*-methyl-morphinan (levorphanol)	279	299	1621	2375	245	269	77	551	21.05	4.31	34	30
1-3-Hydroxymorphinan	279	298	1947	2927	245	269	102	652	19.09	4.49	34	29
1-3-Methoxy-*N*-methyl morphinan (levomethorphan)	278	279	1970	2092	245	249	108	214	18.24	9.77	33	30
1-3-Methoxymorphinan	278	279	2113	2265	245	249	139	226	15.20	10.02	33	30
1-3-Hydroxy-*N*-allylmorphinan (levallorphan)	279	299	2120	3157	245	269	130	740	16.30	4.27	34	30
Diarylalkoneamines[c]												
dl-Methadone	292		554		275		372		1.49		17	
l-Acetylmethadol	258		423		238		145		2.92		20	
d-Propoxyphene (Darvon®)	258		397		235		112		3.54		23	
Aryllpiperidines												
Pethidine (meperidine)	257	256	210	210	254	255	158	166	1.33	1.26	3	1
Norpethidine	257	257	198	198	254	254	150	157	1.32	1.26	3	3
Ketobemidone	280	299	2075	2941	250	271	336	1308	6.17	2.25	30	28
dl-Alphaprodine (nisentil)	257	257	195	201	254	254	137	147	1.42	1.37	3	3
Piminodine (Alvodine®)	257		357		250		328		1.09		7	
Benzomorphans												
dl-2′-Hydroxy-5,9-dimethyl-2-phenethyl-6,7-benzomorphan (phenozocine)	278	299	1944	2894	245	271	254	845	7.65	3.43	33	28
1-2′-Hydroxy-2,3,9-trimethyl-6,7-benzomorphan	278	299	1816	2684	245	270	211	726	8.60	3.70	33	29

TABLE 4 (continued)

2′-Hydroxy-5,9-dimethyl-2-(3,3-dimethylallyl)-6,7-benzomorphan	278	299	2071	3035	245	270	279	867	7.42	3.50	33	29
2′-Hydroxy-5,9-dimethyl-2-cyclopropylmethyl-6,7-benzomorphan (cyclazocine)	278	299	2061	3097	245	270	201	858	10.25	3.61	33	29

[a]From Mulé;[1] Courtesy of *Analytical Chemistry*.
[b]Difference between the maximum and minimum wavelength.
[c]Ultraviolet spectra data were not obtained for this group of 0.2N due to the apparent precipitation of the free base upon the addition of 19N NaOH to the 0.1N HCl sample. Data obtained in ethylene dichloride containing 25% isobutanol (v./v.) as follows:

	$m\mu_{max}$	$m\mu_{min}$	Σmax	Σmin
dl-Methadone	295	280	433	390
d-Propoxyphene	258	245	447	302
l-Acetylmethadol	259	256	550	494

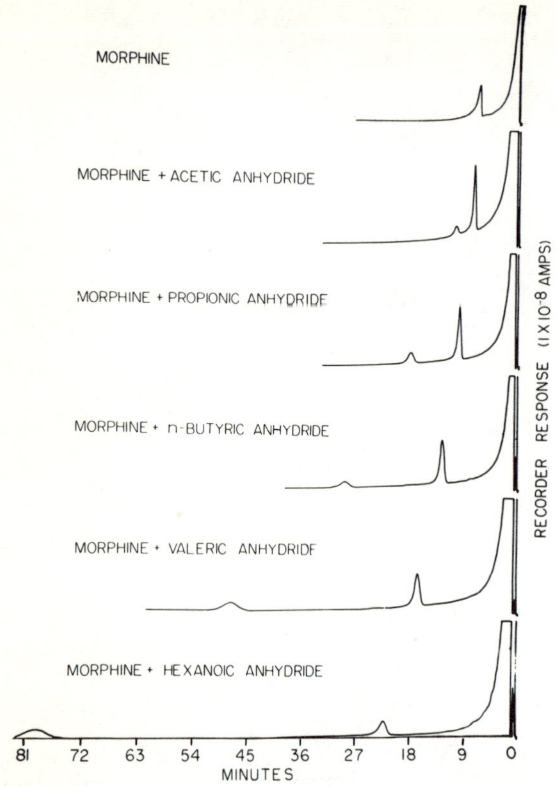

FIGURE 1. Gas-liquid chromatographic analysis of morphine. Five μg (5 μl) of morphine was injected into the GC followed by 5 μl of the anhydride. In ascending order of the homologous series of anhydrides, the retention times for the first and second peaks increased as follows: free, 6.94; acetic, 8.06, 11.34; propionic, 10.50, 18.37; *n*-butyric, 12.75, 29.06; valeric, 16.87, 48.19; and hexanoic 22.31, 79.50. Conditions: 2% SE-30 column; temperature of column and detector 215°C; inlet pressure 20 p.s.i.; outlet Atm; flow rate of argon carrier gas was 47 cc/min; ionization detector (radium-226) operated at 1000 V; relative gain 10^{-8} amperes.

derivative formation allows for ease of confirmation or identification of the drug in pure solution or from biological material. The *N-N'*-dimethyl derivatives of barbiturates[92] were also prepared by the addition of ethereal solution of diazomethane to a methanolic solution of the barbiturate. The application of this technique coupled with mass spectroscopy was extremely effective in the identification of barbiturates and their metabolites.

Sympathomimetic Amines

Fales and Pisano[93] described a GLC method using 4% SE-30 column and a GC equipped with an argon ionization detector that allowed the separation of β-phenethylamine, amphetamine, ephedrine, histamine, tyramine, tryptamine, dimethyltryptamine, and serotonin. The technique was especially applicable to the determination of amphetamine in urine.

Beckett and Rowland[94,95] have reported methods for the GLC determination of amphetamine in urine and blood. Essentially the biological material was extracted in diethyl ether, *N,N*-dimethylaniline added as an internal marker and the extract injected in the GC. The column consisted of 5% KOH and 10% carbowax 6000 and the GC was equipped with a hydrogen flame ionization detector. The method was effective in detecting 0.1 μg of amphetamine base/ml of urine. Similar methods were described[96] for the GLC detection of ephedrine and its congeners from urine. Acetone derivatives of the amines were used to further identify the compounds. A sensitive GLC method suitable for clinical and forensic purposes[97] was reported involving the precipitation of blood proteins, alkaline extraction with ether, and conversion of the phenethylamines to their corresponding acetamides. These authors reported retention data for over 50 compounds related to the phenethylamines. Bruce and Maynard[98] described a sensitive method for amphetamine and related amines which required the formation of heptafluorobutyl derivatives and the use of a GC equipped with an electron capture detector. Halogenated[99] derivatives, *N*-acetyl derivatives,[100] and trimethylsilyl derivatives of amines[101] were prepared from extracts of biological fluids which provided sensitivity, specificity, and rapid detection.

Psychosedatives

Methods for analyzing a wide variety of psychosedative drugs by GLC have been developed with direct applicability to biological materials. Proless and Lohman[102] described a simple solvent extraction at different pH values effecting a preliminary separation of the compounds into acid, neutral, and basic drugs from sera. The sedatives and tranquilizers including barbiturates, carbamates, glutarimides, succinimides, alcohols, hydantoins, phenothiazines, benzodiazepines, and dibenzepines were separated on XE-60 and OV-17 columns. The gas chromatographic determination of ethchlorvynol, paraldehyde, meprobamate, and carisoprodol in blood, urine, bile, and tissues was reported by Maes et al.[103] In all cases, the biological material was extracted and then separated on columns of Hi-Eff-3-BP for the drugs ethchlorvinyl, Hallcomid; M-18 for paraldehyde; SE-30 for meprobamate and carisoprodol. A gas chromatograph equipped with a flame ionization detector was used. In all cases, fatal as well as therapeutic levels of these drugs were easily detected.

The use of gas chromatography as a tool for rapid and detailed information concerning levels of psychosedative drugs in an unconscious patient was reported by Bloomer et al.[104] These investigators have identified in plasma using a one-step technique various sedatives, in particular the barbiturates, meprobamate, and glutethimide. The plasma was usually extracted at an alkaline and acid pH with subsequent separation on an SE-30 column with a gas chromatograph equipped with a radium source ionization detector. The method was reported to be sensitive to a level of 0.1 μg and was effective in detecting drug usage in 39 out of 41 unconscious patients.

Several methods with a degree of similarity were primarily designed for the detection of chlorpromazine,[105] thioridazine,[106] diazepam,[107,108] and glutethimide[109,110] from plasma by gas-liquid chromatography.

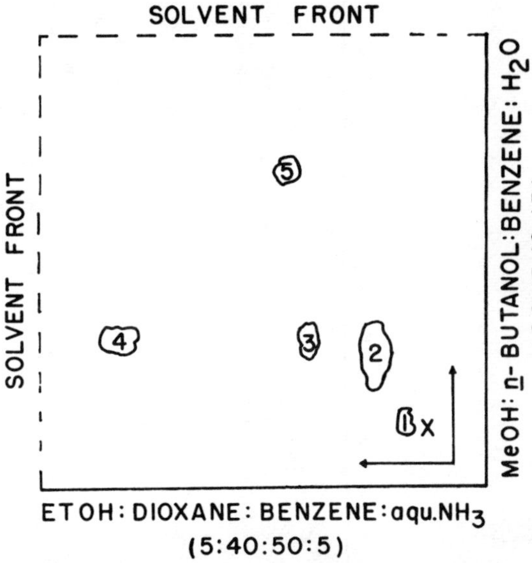

FIGURE 2. Two-dimensional thin layer chromatogram (silica gel G) of: (1) norcodeine; (2) morphine; (3) codeine; (4) dihydrohydroxycodeinone; (5) *N*-allylnormorphine extracted from human urine. The extract (about 10μg) was spotted and developed first in methanol:*n*-butanol: benzene: water (60:15:10:15, v/v), dried and then developed in ethanol: dioxane: benzene: ammonium hydroxide (5:40:50:5, v/v). The solvent fronts were allowed to rise 10 cm from the origin and the drugs were detected by spraying the TLC plate with the iodoplatinate reagent.

Thin-Layer Chromatography (TLC)

Narcotic Analgesics

Thin-layer chromatography has become the single most important tool for the detection, identification, and routine screening of urines and other biological materials for drugs of abuse. The method, essentially as described by Stahl,[111] has allowed for rapid, sensitive detection of chemical compounds and especially permits the use of reagents for detection (i.e. acids and alkalies) that normally destroy paper. Figure 2 shows that two dimensional thin-layer chromatography may be used to separate drugs that are quite similar and difficult to resolve by unidimensional chromatography.

Many methods[1-4,6,8,112-118] utilizing TLC were developed over the past few years for the detection of narcotic analgesics from biological materials. The author's laboratory has contributed significantly to this area of research and recently developed a column resin technique[31] which will be described in some detail.

Generally 25 ml of urine was applied to polypropylene columns containing about 1 g of the Amberlite XAD-2 resin. The flow rate was controlled and the resin eluted with 15 ml of chloroform:isopropanol (3:1, v/v). The organic solvents were shaken with 1 ml of saturated sodium bicarbonate and the separated organic phase evaporated to dryness in a water bath. The residue dissolved in methanol and applied equally to silica gel plates and sheets. The plates were developed in ethylacetate, methanol, water, NH_3 (85:10:3:1, v/v) and the sheets developed in chloroform, methanol, and NH_3 (90:10:1, v/v). The plates were sprayed with 0.3% ninhydrin acid, 5% H_2SO_4 iodoplatinate, and *p*-nitroaniline followed by NaOH. The polygram sheets were sprayed with 0.4% ninhydrin-acetone, $HgSO_4$, diphenylcarbazone, NaI, and iodoplatinate. These techniques were quite effective, unusually simple, rapid, inexpensive, and sensitive in detecting psychoactive drugs at concentrations ranging from 0.1 to 3 μg/ml of urine. Table 5 summarizes the results obtained with the various psychoactive drugs. In essence, the following comments were applicable: with the silica gel plates (system S_1), the iodoplatinate reagent was effective in detecting the narcotic analgesics and on polygram sheets (system S_2) both the NaI and iodoplatinate reagents were effective. Identification was made

TABLE 5

Thin-layer Chromatographic R_f x 100 Values Obtained With the Solvent System: Ethyl Acetate, Methanol, Water, Ammonia (85:10:3:1, v/v) (S_1) and Chloroform, Methanol, Ammonia (90:10:1, v/v) (S_2)

			Color reactions Silica gel plate – S_1 system							Color reactions Polygram silica gel sheets – S_2 system				
Drug	R_f	RR_f [a]	Ninhydrin acid + heating	5% H_2SO_4 + heating	Iodoplatinate	PNA + NaOH	Ultraviolet light longwave[b]	R_f	RR_f	Ninhydrin acetone UV + heating		H_gSO_4	Diphenylcarbazone	NaI + Iodoplatinate
Cocaine[c]	90	5.00	-----	-----	red-blue	-----	-----	94	4.95	----	d	----	-----	purple
Codeine	30	1.67	-----	------	blue	-----	-----	55	2.89	----	---	----	-----	purple-brown
Meperidine (Demerol®)	62	3.44	-----	-----	blue	-----	-----	85	4.47	----	d	----	-----	purple
Methadone[c] (Dolophine®)	80	4.44	-----	-----	red-blue	orange	-----	84	4.42	----	d	----	-----	brown
l-Methorphan	10	0.55	-----	-----	blue	-----	-----	69	3.63	----	green-blue	----	-----	purple
Morphine	18	1.00	-----	-----	blue	-----	-----	19	1.00	----	yellow	----	-----	blue
Pentazocine (Talwin®)	77	4.28	-----	-----	red-blue	-----	-----	56	2.95	----	blue	----	-----	purple
d-propoxyphene[c] (Darvon®)	94	5.22	-----	-----	red-blue	-----	-----	93	4.89	----	---	----	-----	purple
d-amphetamine (Dexedrine®)	42	2.33	-----	-----	e	orange-red	-----	50	2.63	purple	---	red	-----	e
Ephedrine	19	1.05	purple	-----	e	-----	-----	14	0.74	----	blue	red-purple	-----	e
Mescaline	22	1.22	light purple	-----	purple	orange-red	-----	37	1.95	purple	---	red-brown	-----	purple

TABLE 5 (continued)

Drug	R_f	RR_f[a]	Ninhydrin acid + heating	5% H_2SO_4 + heating	Idopolatinate	PNA + NaOH	Ultraviolet light longwave[b]	R_f	RR_f	Ninhydrin acetone UV + heating		H_gSO_4	Diphenylcarbazone	NaI + Iodoplatinate
Methamphetamine (Methedrine)	28	1.55	purple	-----	e	-----	-----	47	2.47	----	purple	red	-----	e
Methylphenidate (Ritalin®)	76	4.22	-----	-----	purple	-----	green	85	4.77	----	d	----	-----	purple
Phenylpropanolamine	31	1.72	purple	-----	e	orange-red	-----	16	0.84	light purple	---	red	-----	e
Phenmetrazine (Preludin®)	46	2.55	purple	-----	purple	-----	-----	69	3.63	----	d	----	-----	purple
Cyclohexylamine	20	1.11	light purple	-----	purple	orange-red	-----	23	1.21	purple	---	red	-----	green
Phenylethylamine	35	1.94	-----	-----	e	orange-red	-----	41	2.16	purple	---	red	-----	e
Nicotine[c]	56	3.11	-----	-----	blue	-----	-----	82	4.31	----	---	----		blue-gray
Quinine[f]	42	2.33	-----	-----	blue	-----	bright blue	43	2.26	----	---	f	-----	purple
Amitriptyline (Elavil®)	79	4.36	-----	-----	purple	-----	-----	89	4.68	----	light blue	----	-----	purple
Chlordiazepoxide (Librium®)	68	3.78	-----	-----	red-blue	-----	green-yellow	77	4.05	----	yellow	----	-----	purple
Chlorpheniramine (Chlortrimeton)	33	1.83	-----	-----	blue	-----	green	67	3.53	----	blue	----	-----	purple
Chlorpromazine (Thorazine®)	72	4.00	-----	reddish pink	purple-red	-----	blue	90	4.74	----	---	red-purple[g]	-----	purple
Diazepam (Valium®)	92	5.11	-----	-----	light red	-----	green-yellow	93	4.89	----	---	----	-----	purple[i]
Prochlorperazine (Compazine®)	52	2.89	-----	blue	purple	-----	blue	90	4.74	----	---	red-purple[g]	-----	blue
Promethazine (Phenergan)	70	3.89	-----	pink	purple	-----	-----	89	4.68	----	blue	brown[g]	-----	purple

TABLE 5 (continued)

Drug	R_f	RR_f[a]	Ninhydrin acid + heating	5% H_2SO_4 + heating	Iodoplatinate	PNA + NaOH	Ultraviolet light longwave[b]	R_f	RR_f	Ninhydrin acetone UV	+ heating	H_gSO_4	Diphenylcarbazone	NaI + Iodoplatinate
Thioridazine (Mellaril)	73	4.05	-----	blue	purple	-----	blue	88	4.63	----	green	yellow green[g]	-----	green-purple
Tripelennamine (Pyribenzamine)	60	3.33	-----	blue	blue	-----	blue	80	4.21	----	blue	----	-----	purple
Perphenazine (Trilafon®)	52	2.88	-----	light purple	purple	-----	blue	72	3.79	----	---	----	-----	purple
Allylisobutyl-barbital	36	2.00	-----	-----	-----	-----	-----	62	3.26	----	---	white [j]	white	i
Amobarbital (Amytal®)	86	4.78	-----	-----	-----	-----	-----	63	3.31	----	---	white [j]	purple	-----
Aprobarbital (Alurate®)	84	4.67	-----	-----	-----	-----	-----	58	3.05	----	---	white [j]	white	i
Barbital (Veronal®)	78	4.33	-----	-----	-----	-----	-----	50	2.63	----	---	white [j]	purple	-----
Diphenylhydantoin[c] (Dilantin®)	82	4.55	-----	-----	-----	-----	-----	54	2.84	----	d	white [j]	light purple	i
Glutethimide[c] (Doriden®)	92	5.11	-----	-----	-----	-----	-----	91	4.79	----	---	white [j]	purple	-----
Hexobarbital (Ortal®)	84	4.66	-----	-----	-----	-----	-----	86	4.53	----	---	white [j]	purple	-----
Meprobamate[h] (Equanil-Miltown®)	81	4.50	-----	-----	-----	-----	-----	34	1.79	----	---	white	-----	-----
Phenobarbital (Luminal®)	73	4.05	-----	-----	-----	-----	-----	46	2.42	----	---	white [j]	purple	-----
Pentobarbital (Nembutal®)	87	4.83	-----	-----	-----	-----	-----	59	3.10	----	---	white [j]	purple	-----
Secobarbital (Seconal®)	87	4.83	-----	-----	-----	-----	-----	70	3.68	----	---	white [j]	white	i

TABLE 5 (continued)

a. From Mulé,[31] Courtesy J. Chromatogr. $RR_f = R_f$ value relative to morphine.

b. The chromatograms were viewed under ultraviolet light prior to spraying with the sequence of chromogenic reagents and after spraying with 5% H_2SO_4 or H_gSO_4. All the drugs except meprobamate quench under the short wave ultraviolet light.

c. The metabolites of cocaine (ecgonine and benzoylecgonine) if extracted would provide R_f O in both systems. The metabolites of the following drugs were useful in the identification of the parent compound: methadone gave R_f values x 100 of 58 and 55 in S_1 and S_2 solvent system; nicotine gave R_f x 100 values of 36 and 22 in S_1 and 37 and 27 in S_2 solvent system; glutethimide gave R_f values x 100 of 88 in S_2 solvent system; diphenylhydantoin gave R_f values x 100 of 10 in S_2 solvent system; d-propoxyphene provided a streak from 56 down (up to 1" long) in S_1 solvent system.

d. Large concentrations of this drug may be partially decomposed and react.

e. May react when present in high concentration (50 ug or more) and provide a blue color.

f. The fluorescence of the spot intensifies after spraying with 5% H_2SO_4 or H_gSO_4 solution. The metabolic products of quinine with R_f values x 100 were: 30, 23, 07 in S_1 system and 33 in S_2 system.

g. Color observed after heating at 100° C for a few minutes.

h. Using a 25 ml sample of urine a gray spot was observed between 5 ug/ml and 25 ug/ml and a white spot above 25 ug/ml. This drug may be confirmed finally spraying the sheet (S_2) with 10% furfural-alcoholic solution followed by conc. HCl. A dark black spot appears after subjecting the sheet to heat (100°C)

i. After sodium iodide spray a yellow color reaction may be observed.

j. At low concentrations the white spot may fade into the gray background.

through the color changes induced as well as Rf values of the parent drug and/or metabolites.

Barbiturates

Thin-layer chromatography has been used widely for the detection of barbiturates, their metabolites, and other organic acids.[2,3,6,8,9,11,31,113,115-119] In almost all cases the biological material was extracted at an acidic pH ranging from 1 to 5, in an organic solvent, usually chloroform alone or in combination with an alcohol. Detection of these compounds on TLC plates most commonly was achieved through interaction with a mercury or silver salt followed by spraying with diphenylcarbazone.

The use of the XAD-2 resin column technique for the detection of barbiturates from urine was demonstrated quite nicely.[31] In comparison to other analytical extraction techniques,[3,4,6] the resin method was equal to or superior with respect to recovery of pentobarbital-^{14}C and phenobarbital-^{14}C (83 to 88%) from urine. Table 5 shows the Rf values, as well as the color reactions used to detect several barbiturates as well as glutethimide and diphenylhydantoin. The primary reagents used to detect these drugs were mercuric sulfate, followed by diphenylcarbazone. A few of the barbiturates (i.e. aprobarbital, secobarbital) provided a yellow color reaction with the NaI spray. Detection of these drugs was based upon the color reactions as well as the Rf values on the polygram silica gel sheets.

Sympathomimetic Amines

Thin-layer chromatography has become an important tool for the identification of amphetamine and related analogues from biological materials.[2,3,6,8,113-120] Quite commonly this group of drugs was extracted in organic solvents at alkaline pH 9 to 12 and detected with reagents like: ninhydrin; *p*-nitroaniline; *p*-dimethylaminobenzaldehyde; iodoplatinate; and NaI.

The sympathomimetic amines were extracted quite easily with the XAD-2 column resin method,[31] applied to silica gel thin-layer plates and sheets (see Table 5) developed in both the ethylacetate, methanol, water, and ammonia (85:10:3:1, v/v), and chloroform, methanol, and ammonia (90:10:1, v/v) solvent systems. On the silica gel plates a ninhydrin-acid spray followed by heating was effective in detecting methamphetamine (secondary amine) as well as some primary amines, i.e., mescaline, phenylpropanolamine. *P*-nitroaniline plus NaOH was used to identify as well as confirm the presence of primary amines (i.e., amphetamine). On the polygram silica gel sheets, ninhydrin-acetone followed by UV-irradiation allowed for the detection of primary amines, and heating the sheets provided reactions with secondary amines. Iodoplatinate reacted with the amines depending upon concentration of the drugs. The Rf values as well as the descriptive color reactions appear in Table 5. Sensitivity of detection ranged from 1 to 3 μg/ml of urine.

Psychosedatives

This group of drugs which includes the minor tranquilizers (benzodiazepines, carbamates), phenothiazines, amitriptyline, thioridazine, as well as some antihistamines, were easily detected by thin-layer chromatography.[2,3,4,6,8,113-121] Most of these drugs were extracted from biological materials at an alkaline pH with organic solvents and the extract applied to thin-layer plates and detected with general reagents such as iodine, iodoplatinate, and aqueous solutions of sulfuric acid.

The XAD-2 resin technique[31] was effective in adsorbing these drugs with subsequent elution (chloroform:isopropanol, 3:1, v/v) and application of the residue to silica gel thin-layer chromatograms. The results of these studies appear in Table 5. The Rf values as well as the color reactions with the various drugs on both the silica gel plates as well as the sheets were used to identify the individual psychosedative drugs.

Spectrophotofluorometry

Narcotic Analgesics

The feasibility and applicability of fluorometry to the analysis of drugs from biological material has been demonstrated.[122,123]

Brandt et al.[124] found that solutions of morphine in 0.1 N H_2SO_4 demonstrated fluorescence at 350 nm with the major peak at 285 nm. The intensity of emission decreased at pH 7 and at pH 10 to 12 was negligible. Codeine provided similar results, however, at pH 10 to 12, the intensity of the fluorescence of the codeine solution remained unchanged. The optimal range for the determination was 0.1 to 50 μg/ml.

A sensitive fluorometric method for the estimation of morphine in plasma and brain was developed by Kupferberg et al.[125] The method consisted of the ferri-ferrocyanide oxidation of morphine to pseudomorphine. The excitation wavelength was 250 nm with emission at 440 nm. As little as 0.1 μg of morphine was measurable in a tissue sample with relatively good precision and a high degree of specificity. Takemori[126] modified the fluorometric method of Kupferberg so that as little as 10 μg of morphine could be detected in plasma and cerebrospinal fluid.

Fulton[127] showed that a fluorescent product of morphine could be prepared by heating the drug in 0.5 cc of sulfuric acid, with subsequent dilution of the material in water and the addition of concentrated NH_4OH. Naudeau and Sobolewski[128] used essentially the same technique with a subsequent extraction into isobutanol. The compound was excited at 365 nm, with emission at 430 nm.

Utilizing the basic concept of acid, alkali treatment, a simple, sensitive and specific method for the fluorometric determination of morphine and quinine extracted from biological material was developed in the author's laboratory.[129] Peak excitation and emission spectra were 392 and 425 nm, respectively. Concentrations of 0.22 μg/ml of morphine and 0.10 μg/ml of quinine in urine were easily detected. The use of the automated turret spectrofluorometer (ATS) with this method has allowed the laboratory to easily screen thousands of urines daily for morphine and quinine.

A fluorometric method[130] was reported for the determination of meperidine in biological material following incubation of the material in a mixture of formaldehyde and concentrated sulfuric acid. Excitation and emission wavelengths were 275 and 440 nm, respectively. Sensitivity limits in plasma and urine were reported to be 300 μg/ml.

Barbiturates

The spectrofluorometric analysis of barbiturates has only recently gained some degree of interest. Udenfriend[131] reported the fluorescence characteristics of several barbiturates as well as general extraction procedures. The basic information was used to develop a method in blood[132] for pentobarbital. Using excitation maxima of 265 nm and emission maximum of 440 nm, these investigators found, following the administration of 200 mg of the drug, serum levels of 1.5 to 3 μg/ml at 2 hours, and about 1 μg/ml at 24 hours.

Swagzdis and Flanagan[133] developed a method for the fluorometric determination of amobarbital in plasma following extraction of the drug from plasma with butylether. The ether layer was reextracted with 1 N NaOH. Fluorescence was determined with excitation at 265 nm and emission at 410 nm. The concentration was proportional to fluorescence in the range of 0.3 to 3.0 μg/ml. In patients that received 65 mg of amobarbital, average plasma levels ranged from 1.0 to 1.3 μg/ml over a 3 to 7 hour time interval.

Sympathomimetic Amines

A spectrofluorometric procedure for the determination of amphetamine alone or in combination with other drugs was developed by Nix and Hume.[134] The determination was based upon the reaction of amphetamine with formaldehyde and acetylacetone to produce a fluorophore. The excitation and emission wavelengths of the lutidine derivative (fluorophore) of amphetamine were determined at 415 nm and 482 nm, respectively. The minimal detection limit was 0.26 μg/ml. Interference with this determination was observed with methamphetamine and phenethylamine.

An interesting fluorometric method for the analysis of amphetamines[135] was based upon the interaction between aliphatic and/or cyclic amines and 3-carboxy-7-hydroxy coumarin to yield fluorescent coumarin-amine salts. Excitation wavelength was 420 nm, emission wavelength at 450 nm. For amphetamine, a linear response was obtained from 7.4 to 118.4 μg/25 ml. The range of linearity for related analogues was from 4.4 to 118.4 μg/25 ml.

The fluorometric methods described for the sympathomimetic amines obviously were either for pure samples or mixtures of the drug in dosage form. The methods were not directly applicable to biological materials.

Psychosedatives

The native fluorescence of chlorpromazine and its sulfoxide metabolite was relatively weak, however, Mellinger and Keeler[136] found that on oxidation with potassium permanganate in 0.2 N H_2SO_4, most phenothiazines were converted to intensely fluorescent derivatives. All aspects of fluorescence associated with the phenothiazines including temperature, pH, concentration, oxidants, tissue, and serum extractions were thoroughly investigated.[137] Sensitivity for biological materials ranged between 2 to 5 μg/g of tissue for chlorpromazine.

Recently[138] a method was developed in which chlorpromazine and its metabolites reacted with dimethylaminonaphthyl sulfonyl chloride to provide fluorescent products. The method was applied to biological materials and apparently was effective in detecting nanogram quantities of the metabolites.

Methypyrlon (Noludar®)[139] and its metabolites were determined fluorometrically by treating the extract with alkali and the Folin-Ciocalten phenol reagent to produce a blue chromophore. Sensitivity of the assay was about 0.5 μg/ml and the linear range for fluorescence was observed to be 0.5 to 5.0 μg/ml.

Chlordiazepoxide (Librium®) was determined fluorometrically[140] along with its lactam metabolite in plasma. The sensitivity limit was 0.3 to 0.5 μg/ml of plasma.

SUMMARY

The primary purpose of this chapter was to review the most recent developments in the identification and detection of drugs that induce physical and/or psychic dependence.

The emphasis was upon detection in biological material which required extraction of the drugs and/or metabolites prior to analysis. Normally this was accomplished with an organic solvent at an alkaline pH for the organic bases and neutrals (narcotic analgesics, sympathomimetic amines, and certain psychosedatives) and an acid pH for the organic acids (barbiturates). The resin column technique was effective regardless of the chemical nature of the drug.

Qualitative and quantitative color tests were used to detect narcotic analgesics, barbiturates, sympathomimetic amines, and psychoactive drugs. All these tests have limited usefulness due to a lack of sensitivity and specificity associated with the color reaction.

Microcrystal tests were found useful in the identification of organic bases and in some cases, organic acids. The test was quite useful for materials in crystalline form, but normally required purification of extracts from biological material.

Ultraviolet spectrophotometry was used extensively for the analysis of narcotic analgesics and barbiturates, less so with the sympathomimetic amines and other psychoactive drugs. Although an extensive body of literature exists, the use of this technique is limited due to sensitivity and specificity associated with identification from biological materials. Purification was often required prior to analysis. However, ultraviolet spectrophotometry is still quite useful as a preliminary or adjunct test for identification when crystalline or powder forms of the drug are available.

Gas-liquid and thin-layer chromatography are essentially the methods of choice in identifying drugs subject to abuse extracted from biological material. All drugs may be detected at microgram or nanogram levels. The use of dual columns in gas chromatography and different solvent systems in thin-layer chromatography, coupled with sequential chromogenic spraying allows for positive identification of these drugs.

Spectrofluorometric detection of these drugs appears to offer a promising future, since sensitivity (nanograms), specificity (excitation, emission wavelengths), and rapidity of analysis are achieved. At the present time methods are available for the narcotic analgesics, but extensive research is required to develop more effective methods to make fluorometric analysis fully applicable to other drugs subject to abuse.

REFERENCES

1. Mulé, S.J., Determination of narcotic analgesics in human biological materials. Application of ultraviolet spectrophotometry, thin-layer and gas-liquid chromatography, *Anal. Chem.*, 36, 1907, 1964.

2. Mulé, S.J., Identification of narcotics, barbiturates, amphetamines, tranquilizers, and psychotomimetics in human urine, *J. Chromatogr.*, 39, 302, 1969.

3. Mulé, S.J., Routine identification of drugs of abuse in human urine. I. Application of fluorometry, thin-layer and gas-liquid chromatography, *J. Chromatogr.*, 55, 255, 1971.

4. Bastos, M.L., Kannanen, G.E., Young, R.M., Monforte, J.R., and Sunshine, I., Detection of basic organic drugs and their metabolites in urine, *Clin. Chem.*, 16, 931, 1970.

5. Taylor, J.F., Methods of chemical analysis, in *Narcotic Drugs: Biochemical Pharmacology,* Clouet, D.H., Ed., Plenum Press, New York, 1971, 17.

6. Davidow, B.D., Lipetri, N., and Quame, B., A thin-layer chromatographic screening procedure for detecting drug abuse, *Amer. J. Clin. Path.*, 50, 714, 1968.

7. Farmilo, C.G. and Genest, K., Alkaloids and related bases: identification, in *Toxicology Mechanisms and Analytical Methods*, Vol. II, Stewart, C.P. and Stolman, A., Eds., Academic Press, New York, 1961, 209.

8. Kaistha, K.K. and Jaffe, J.A., Extraction techniques for narcotics, barbiturates and central nervous system stimulants in a drug abuse screening program, *J. Chromatogr.*, 60, 83, 1971.

9. Sunshine, I., Maes, R., and Finkle, B., An evaluation of methods for the determination of barbiturates in biological materials, *Clin. Toxicol.,* 1, 281, 1968.

10. Curry, A.S., Barbiturates, in *Toxicology Mechanisms and Analytical Methods,* Vol. II, Stewart, C.P. and Stolman, A., Eds., Academic Press, New York, 1961, 153.

11. Cochin, J. and Daly, J.W., The use of thin-layer chromatography for the analysis of drugs. Isolation and identification of barbiturates and nonbarbiturate hypnotics from urine, blood and tissues, *J. Pharmacol. Exp. Ther.*, 139, 154, 1963.

12. Parker, K.D., Wright, J., Halpern, A.F., and Hine, C.H., The determination of barbiturates in blood and urine by gas-liquid chromatography with a peak shift for qualitative confirmation, *J. Forensic Sci.*, 8, 125, 1968.

13. Heyndrickx, A. and DeLeenheer, A., Toxicological analysis of weak amines (amphetamine, pervitin, preludin and ritalin) in pharmaceutical compounds and urine of persons suspected of doping, *J. De Pharmacie De Belgique,* 22, 59, 1967.

14. Beckett, A.H. and Rowland, M., Determination and identification of amphetamine in urine, *J. Pharm. Pharmacol.*, 17, 59, 1965.

15. Beckett, A.H., Tucker, G.T., and Moffat, A.C., Routine detection and identification in urine of stimulants and other drugs, some of which may be used to modify performance in sports, *J. Pharm. Pharmacol.*, 19, 273, 1967.

16. Lebish, P., Finkle, B.S., and Brackett, J.W., Determination of amphetamine, methamphetamine, and related amines in blood and urine by gas chromatography with hydrogen[1]-flame ionization detector, *Clin. Chem.*, 16, 195, 1970.

17. Haux, P. and Natelson, S., A practical method for the assay of phenothiazine in biologic fluids, *Amer. J. Clin. Path.*, 53, 77, 1970.

18. Cochin, J. and Daly, J.W., The use of thin-layer chromatography for the analysis of drugs. Identification and isolation of phenothiazine tranquilizers and of antihistamines in body fluids and tissues, *J. Pharmacol. Exp. Ther.*, 139, 160, 1963.

19. Sunshine, I., Use of thin-layer chromatography in the diagnosis of poisoning, *Amer. J. Clin. Pathol.*, 40, 576, 1963.

20. Tompsett, S.L., The detection and determination of phenothiazine drugs in urine, *Acta Pharmacol. Toxicol.*, 26, 303, 1968.

21. deSilva, A.J. and Paglisi, C.V., Determination of medazepam (Nobrian®), Diazepam (Valium®) and their major biotransformation products in blood and urine by electron capture gas-liquid chromatography, *Anal. Chem.*, 42, 1725, 1970.

22. deSilva, A. J., Schwartz, M. A., Stefanovic, B., Kaplan, J., and D'Arconte, L., Determination of Diazepam (Valium®) in blood by gas-liquid chromatography, *Anal. Chem.*, 36, 2099, 1964.

23. Tompsett, S.L., Nitrazepam (Mogadon®) in blood serum and urine and Librium® in urine, *J. Clin. Path.*, 21, 366, 1968.

24. Emmerson, J.L., Miya, T.S., and Yim, G.K.W., The distribution and metabolic state of carbon-14 meprobamate in the rat brain, *J. Pharmacol. Exp. Ther.*, 129, 89, 1960.

25. Sobolewski, G. and Nadeau, G., A scheme for the rapid identification in urine of commonly used sedatives, hypnotics and tranquilizers, *Clin. Chem.*, 6, 153, 1960.

26. Sunshine, I., Maes, R., and Faracie, R., Determination of glutethimide (Doriden®) and its metabolites in biologic specimens, *Clin. Chem.*, 14, 595, 1968.

27. Knowlton, M. and Goldbaum, L.R., An improved rapid method for the determination of glutethimide (Doriden®) in blood, *J. Forensic Sci.*, 14, 129, 1969.

28. Algeri, E.J., Katsas, G.G., and Luongo, M.A., Determination of ethchlorvynol in biologic mediums and report of two fatal cases, *Amer. J. Clin. Path.*, 38, 125, 1962.

29. Carr, D.J. and Crampton, R.F., Ethchlorvynol, *Brit. Med. J.*, 1, 262, 1963.

30. Cravey, R.H. and Baselt, R.C., Studies of the body distribution of ethchlorvynol, *J. Forensic Sci.*, 13, 532, 1968.

31. Mulé, S.J., Bastos, M.L., Jukofsky, D., and Saffer, E., Routine identification of drugs of abuse in human urine. II. Development and application of the XAD-2 resin column method, *J. Chromatogr.*, in press.

32. Ehrhich-Rogozinsky, S. and Cheronis, N.D., The identification and determination of morphine, *Microchem. J.*, 7, 336, 1963.

33. Bentley, K.W., *The Chemistry of the Morphine Alkaloids*, Oxford University Press (Clarendon), London, 1954.

34. Way, E.L. and Adler, T.K., The biological disposition of morphine and its surrogates, *Bull. W.H.O.*, 27, 359, 1962.

35. Brodie, B.B., Udenfriend, S., and Dill, W., The estimation of basic organic compounds in biological material. V. Estimation by salt formation with methyl orange, *J. Biol. Chem.*, 163, 335, 1947.

36. Woods, L.A., Cochin, J., Fornfeld, E.G., and Seevers, M.H., Estimation of morphine in biological materials, *J. Pharmacol. Exp. Ther.*, 111, 64, 1954.

37. Brodie, B.B., Udenfriend, S., and Taggart, J.V., The estimation of basic organic compounds in biological materials. IV. Estimation by coupling with diazanium salts, *J. Biol. Chem.*, 163, 327, 1947.

38. Turfitt, G.E., The identification of the clinically-important barbiturates, *Quart. J. Pharm. Pharmacol.*, 21, 1, 1948.

39. Koppanyi, T., Dille, S.M., Murphy, W.S., and Krop, S., Studies on barbiturates. II. Contributions to methods of barbital research, *J. Amer. Pharm. Ass.*, 23, 1074, 1934.

40. Riley, R.F., Krause, R.F., Steodman, L.T., Hunber, F.E., and Hodge, H.C., Cobalt color reactions of barbiturates, *Proc. Soc. Exp. Biol. Med.*, 46, 424, 1940.

41. Algeri, E.J. and Walker, J.T., Paper chromatography for identification of the common barbiturates, *Amer. J. Clin. Pathol.*, 22, 37, 1952.

42. Wickstrom, A. and Salvesen, B., The separation and identification of some barbiturates by paper partition chromatography, *J. Pharm. Pharmacol.*, 4, 98, 1952.

43. Curry, A.S., The detection of-bromallyl and barbiturates on paper chromatograms, *Acta Pharmacol. Toxicol.*, 13, 357, 1957.

44. Chatteu, L.G. and Levi, L., Identification and differentiation of sympathomimetic amines, *Anal. Chem.*, 31, 1581, 1959.

45. Pelka, J.R. and Metcalfe, L.D., Rapid colour test for detecting certain long chain diamines in the presence of monofunctional long-chain amines, *Anal. Chem.*, 38, 657, 1966.

46. Fontani, F. and Morandini, F., Colorimetric determination of amphetamine salts in dosage forms, *J. Pharm. Pharmacol.*, 27, 411, 1970.

47. Mellan, J.P. and Stiven, A.G., Detection of dexamphetamine sulfate in urine, *J. Med. Lab. Techn.*, 24, 285, 1967.

48. Dickens, G.J. and Ellis, A.C., The detection of amphetamine in urine by thin-layer chromatography, *J. Ass. Pub. Anal.*, 5, 103, 1967.

49. Forrest, F., Forrest, I., and Mason, A., Review of rapid urine tests for phenothiazine and related drugs, *Amer. J. Psych.*, 118, 300, 1961.

50. Haux, P. and Natelson, S., A practical method for the assay of phenothiazines in biologic fluids, *J. Clin. Path.*, 53, 77, 1970.

51. Frings, C.S. and Cohen, P.S., Rapid colorimetric method for the quantitative determination of Librium® (Chlordinzepoxide) in serum, *Amer. J. Clin. Path.*, 56, 216, 1971.

52. Madsen, O.D., Colorimetric determination of meprobamate in blood, *Clin. Chem. Acta,* 7, 481, 1962.

53. Harris, E.S. and Reik, J.J., Method for the determination of urinary meprobamate, *Clin. Chem.*, 4, 241, 1958.

54. Cravey, R.H. and Baselt, R.C., Studies of the body distribution of ethchlorvynol, *J. Forensic Sci.*, 13, 532, 1968.

55. Fulton, C.C., *Modern Microcrystal Tests for Drugs. The Identification of Organic Compounds by Microcrystalloscopic Chemistry*, Wiley-Interscience, New York, 1969.

56. Clarke, E.G.C., Microchemical differentiation between optical isomers of *N*-Methylmorphinan analgesics, *J. Pharm. Pharmacol.*, 10, 642, 1958.

57. Fulton, C.C., Qualitative tests for drugs, *J. Ass. Offic. Agri. Chem.*, 43, 262, 1960.

58. Clark, E.G.C., A note on the differentiation between *dextro* and *levo*-propoxyphene, *J. Pharm. Pharmacol.*, 15, 624, 1963.

59. Clarke, E.G.C. and Williams, M., Microchemical tests for the identification of alkaloids, *J. Pharm. Pharmacol.*, 7, 255, 1955..

60. Stephenson, C.H., *Some Microchemical Tests for Alkaloids,* Lippincot, Philadelphia, 1921.

61. Clarke, E.G.C., Microchemical identification of some modern analgesics, *Bull Narc.*, 11, 27, 1959.

62. Ono, M., Engelke, B.F., and Fulton, C., Procedures for assured identification of morphine, dihydromorphine, codeine, norcodeine, methadone, quinine, methamphetamine in human urine, *Bull Narc.,* 1, 31, 1969.

63. Peterson, H., *Methods for the Collection and Analysis of Horse Saliva and Urine for the Detection of Drugs,* 9th Revision, N.Y. State Racing Commission, New York, 1964.

64. Farmilo, C.G., Oestreicher, P.M., and Levi, L., Physical methods for the identification of narcotics. The ultraviolet spectrophotometric method, *Bull Narc. UN Dept. Soc. Affairs,* 6, 18, 1954.

65. Oestreicher, P.M., Farmilo, C.G., and Levi, L., Physical methods for the identification of narcotics. Ultraviolet spectral data for 90 narcotics and related compounds, *Bull Narc. UN Dept. Soc. Affairs,* 6, 42, 1954.

66. Bradford, L.W. and Brackett, J.W., Systematic procedure for the identification of dangerous drugs, poisons and narcotics by ultraviolet spectroscopy, *Microchem. Acta,* 3, 352, 1958.

67. Hilf, R., Castano, F.F., and Lichtbourn, G.H., Identification of alkaloids and related compounds by paper chromatography and ultraviolet spectrophotometry, *J. Lab. Clin. Med.*, 54, 634, 1959.

68. Kum–Tatt, L. and Farmilo, C.G., Preliminary report on the use of ammonium reineckate in the determination of opium alkaloids, *UN Secretariat Publ.*, 49, 31, 1957.

69. Levi, L. and Farmilo, C.G., Reineckate preparation of opium alkaloids, *Canad. J. Chem.*, 30, 783, 1952.

70. Gauties, J.A., Renault, J., and Rabiant, J., Ultraviolet spectrophotometric microdetermination of alkaloids as tetraphenylborides, *Amer. Pharm. Fran.*, 17, 4011, 1929.

71. Goldbaun, L.R., Determination of barbiturates, *Anal. Chem.*, 24, 1604, 1952.

72. Goldbaun, L.R., A ultraviolet spectrophotometric procedure for the determination of barbiturates, *J. Pharm. Exp. Ther.*, 94, 68, 1948.

73. Tompsett, S.C., Interference from the presence of other substances in detecting and determining barbiturates in biological material, *J. Clin. Path.*, 22, 291, 1969.

74. Wallace, J.E., Microdetermination of diphenylhydantoin in biological specimens by ultraviolet spectrophotometry, *Anal. Chem.*, 40, 978, 1968.

75. Rotondaro, R.A., Report on ultraviolet spectrophotometric methods for drugs: phenethylamines, *J. Ass. Off. Agric. Chem.*, 41, 509, 1958.

76. Keller, R.E. and Ellenbogen, W.C., The determination of *d*-amphetamine in body fluids, *J. Pharm. Exp. Ther.*, 106, 77, 1952.

77. Wallace, J.E., Biggs, J.D., and Ladd, S.I., Determination of amphetamine by ultraviolet spectrophotometry, *Anal. Chem.*, 40, 2207, 1968.

78. Wallace, J.E., Determination of ephedrine and certain related compounds by ultraviolet spectrophotometry, *Anal. Chem.*, 39, 531, 1967.

79. Knowlton, M. and Goldbaum, C.R., An improved method for the determination of gluthethimide (Doriden®) in blood, *J. Forensic Sci.*, 14, 129, 1969.

80. Lloyd, H.A., Fales, H.M., Highest, P.F., Vandenheuvel, W.J.A., and Wildman, W.C., Separation of alkaloids by gas chromatography, *Amer. Chem. Soc.*, 82, 3791, 1960.

81. Brochmann-Hanssen, E. and Furuys, T., Opium alkaloids – separation and identification by gas, thin-layer and paper chromatography, *J. Pharm. Sci.*, 53, 1549, 1964.

82. Kazyak, L. and Knoblock, E.C., Application of gas chromatography to analytical toxicology, *Anal. Chem.*, 35, 1448, 1963.

83. Parker, K.D., Fontan, C.R., and Kirk, P.L., Rapid gas chromatographic method for screening of toxicological extracts for alkaloids, barbiturates, sympathomimetic amines and tranquilizers, *Anal. Chem.*, 35, 356, 1963.

84. Anders, M.W. and Mannering, G.J., New peak-shift technique for gas-liquid chromatography, *Anal. Chem.*, 34, 730, 1962.

85. Wilkinson, G.R. and Way, E.L., Sub-microgram estimation of morphine in biological fluids by gas-liquid chromatography, *Biochem. Pharmacol.*, 18, 1435, 1969.

86. Ikekawa, N., Takayama, K., Hosoya, E., and Oka, T., Determination of morphine in urine by gas chromatography, *Anal. Biochem.*, 28, 156, 1969.

87. Anders, M.W. and Mannering, G.J., Application of gas chromatography to toxicology, in *Progress in Chemical Toxicology*, Vol. III, Stolman, A. Ed., Academic Press, New York, 1967, 121.

88. Brochmann-Hanssen, E., Gas chromatography and its application to pharmaceutical analysis, *J. Pharm. Sci.*, 51, 1017, 1962.

89. Jain, C.N., Fontan, C.R., and Kirk, P.L., Rapid extraction method for barbiturates from blood for gas-liquid chromatographic analysis, *Microchem. J.*, 8, 28, 1964.

90. Parker, K., Wright, J., Halpern, A., and Hine, C.H., The determination of barbiturates in blood and urine by gas-liquid chromatography with a peak shift for qualitative confirmation, *J. Forensic Sci.*, 8, 125, 1968.

91. Street, H.V., Gas-liquid chromatography of submicroamounts of drugs, *J. Chromatogr.*, 41, 358, 1969.

92. Gilbert, J.N.T., Millard, B.J., and Powell, J.W., Combined gas-liquid chromatography – mass spectrometry in the study of barbiturate metabolism, *J. Pharm. Pharmacol.*, 22, 897, 1970.

93. Fales, H.M. and Pisano, J.J., Gas chromatography of biologically important amines, *Anal. Chem.*, 3, 337, 1962.

94. Beckett, A.H. and Rowland, M., Determination and identification of amphetamine in urine, *J. Pharm. Pharmacol.*, 17, 59, 1965.

95. Rowland, M., Amphetamine, blood and urine levels in man, *J. Pharm. Sci.*, 58, 508, 1969.

96. Beckett, A.H. and Wilkinson, G.R., Identification and determination of ephedrine and its congeners in urine by gas chromatography, *J. Pharm. Pharmacol.*, 17, 104S, 1965.

97. Lehigh, P., Finkle, B.S., and Brackett, J.W., Determination of amphetamine, methamphetamine, and related amines in blood and urine by gas chromatography with hydrogen-flame ionization detector, *Clin. Chem.*, 16, 195, 1970.

98. Bruce, R.B., and Maynard, W.R., Determination of amphetamine and related amines in blood by gas chromatography, *Anal. Chem.*, 41, 977, 1969.

99. Noonan, J.S., Murdick, P.W., and Ray, R.S., A method for detecting amphetamine using gas chromatography of a halogenated derivative, *J. Pharmacol. Exp. Ther.*, 168, 205, 1969.

100. Toseland, P.A. and Scott, P.H., Determination of amphetamine as its *N*-acetyl derivative by gas-liquid chromatography, *Clin. Chem. Acta*, 25, 75, 1969.

101. Vanden Heuvel, W.J.A., Gas-liquid chromatography of the trimethylsilyl derivatives of several amines of biological interest, *J. Chromatogr.*, 36, 354, 1968.

102. Proless, H.F. and Lohman, H.J., Profile of sedatives and tranquilizers in serum as measured by gas-liquid chromatography, *Clin. Chem.*, 17, 222, 1971.

103. Maes, R., Hodnett, N., Landesman, H., Kananen, G., Finkle, B., and Sunshine, I., The gas chromatographic determination of selected sedatives (ethchlorvynol, paraldehyde, meprobamate and carisprodol) in biological material, *J. Forensic Sci.*, 14, 236, 1969.

104. Bloomer, H.A., Maddock, R.K., Sheehe, J.B., and Adams, E.J., Rapid diagnosis of sedative intoxication by gas chromatography, *Ann. Intern. Med.*, 72, 223, 1970.

105. Curry, S.H., Determination of nanogram quantities of chlorpromazine and some of its metabolites in plasma using gas-liquid chromatography with an electron capture detector, *Anal. Chem.*, 40, 1251, 1968.

106. Curry, S.H. and Mould, G.P., Gas chromatographic identification of thioridazine in plasma, and a method for the routine assay of the drug, *J. Pharm. Pharmacol.*, 21, 674, 1969.

107. Foster, L.B. and Frings, C.S., Determination of Diazepam (Valium®) concentrations in serum by gas-liquid chromatography, *Clin. Chem.*, 16, 177, 1970.

108. de Silva, J.A.F., Schwartz, M.A., Stefanovic, J.K., and D'Arcante, L., determination of Diazepam (Valium®) in blood by gas-liquid chromatography, *Anal. Chem.*, 36, 2099, 1964.

109. Grieveson, P. and Gordon, J.S., The assay of glutethimide in plasma, *J. Chromatogr.*, 44, 279, 1969.

110. Widdop, B., Rapid measurement of therapeutic levels of glutethimide in plasma, *J. Chromatogr.*, 47, 485, 1970.

111. Stahl, E., ed., *Thin-Layer Chromatography*, Springer-Verlag, New York, 1969.

112. Fujimoto, J.M. and Wang, R.I.H., A method of identifying narcotic analgesics in human urine after therapeutic doses, *Toxic. Appl. Pharmacol.*, 16, 186, 1970.

113. Coumbis, R.J., Fulton, C.C., Calise, J.P., and Rodriguez, C., The necessity of elution and identification of drugs indicated by thin-layer chromatography, *J. Chromatogr.*, 54, 245, 1971.

114. Cochin, J. and Daly, J.W., Rapid identification of analgesic drugs in urine with thin-layer chromatography, *Experientia*, 18, 294, 1962.

115. Heaton, A.M. and Blumberg, A.G., Thin-layer chromatographic detection of barbiturates, narcotics and amphetamines in urine of patients receiving psychotropic drugs, *J. Chromatogr.*, 41, 367, 1969.

116. Broich, J.R., Hoffman, D.B., Andryanskos, S., Galante, L., and Umberger, C.J., An improved method for rapid large-scale thin-layer chromatographic urine screening for drugs of abuse, *J. Chromatogr.*, 60, 95, 1971.

117. Vesell, E.S. and Passamanti, G.T., Utility of clinical chemical determinations of drug concentrations in biological fluids, *Clin. Chem.*, 17, 851, 1971.

118. Beny, D.J. and Grove, J., Improved chromatographic techniques and their interpretation for the screening of urine from drug-dependent subjects, *J. Chromatogr.*, 61, 111, 1971.

119. Schewda, P., Thin-layer chromatography of toxicologically significant substances on silica gel-coated glass plates and polyester sheets, *Anal. Chem.*, 39, 1019, 1967.

120. Dickes, G.J. and Ellis, A.C., The detection of amphetamine in urine by thin-layer chromatography, *J. Ass. Pub. Anal.*, 5, 103, 1967.

121. Cochin, J. and Daly, J.W., The use of thin-layer chromatography for the analysis of drugs. Identification and isolation of phenothiazine, tranquilizers and of anthihistamines in body fluids and tissues, *J. Pharmacol. Exp. Ther.*, 139, 160, 1963.

122. Udenfriend, S., *Fluorescence Assay in Biology and Medicine*, Vol. II, Academic Press, New York, 1969, 503.

123. deSilva, J.A.F., The use of spectrofluorometry in the analysis of drugs in biological materials, *J. Forensic Sci.*, 14, 184, 1969.

124. Brandt, R., Rogozinsky, S.R., and Cheronis, N.D., Spectrophotofluorometric method for the microdetection and estimation of morphine and codeine, *Microchem. J.*, 5, 215, 1961.

125. Kupferberg, H., Buckhalter, A., and Way, E.L., A sensitive fluorometric assay for morphine in plasma and brain, *J. Pharmacol. Exp. Ther.*, 145, 247, 1964.

126. Tabemori, A.E., An ultrasensitive method for the determination of morphine and its application in experiments *in vitro* and *in vitro*, *Biochem. Pharmacol.*, 17, 1627, 1968.

127. Fulton, C.C., Sulfomorphid and the purple fluorescence test, a new derivative test for morphine, *J. Amer. Pharm. Ass.*, 26, 726, 1937.

128. Naudeau, G. and Sobolewski, G., Fluorometric method for the analysis of morphine, *Canad. J. Biochem. Physiol.*, 36, 625, 1958.

129. Mulé, S.J. and Hushin, P.L., Semiautomated fluorometric assay for submicrogram quantities of morphine and quinine in human biological material, *Anal. Chem.*, 43, 708, 1971.

130. Dal Cortivo, L.A., DeMayo, M.M., and Weinberg, S.B., Fluorometric determination of microgram amounts of meperidine, *Anal. Chem.*, 42, 941, 1970.

131. Udenfriend, S., *Fluoresence Assay in Biology and Medicine*, Vol. I, Academic Press, New York, 1962.

132. Hollister, C.E., Kanter, S.L., and Clyde, D.J., Studies of prolonged action medication. III, *Clin. Pharmacol. Ther.*, 4, 612, 1963.

133. Swagzdis, J.E. and Flanagan, T.C., Spectrofluorometric determination of low concentrations of amobarbital in plasma, *Anal. Biochem.*, 7, 147, 1964.

134. Nix, C.R. and Hume, A.S., A spectrophotofluorometric method for the determination of amphetamine, *J. Forensic Sci.*, 15, 595, 1970.

135. Stewart, J.T. and Lotti, D.M., Fluorometric determination of amphetamines with 3-carboxy-7-hydroxycoumarin, *J. Pharmaceut. Sci.*, 60, 461, 1971.

136. Mellinger, T.J. and Keeler, C.E., Spectrofluorometric identification of phenothiazine drugs, *Anal. Chem.*, 35, 554, 1963.

137. Mellinger, T.J., Mellinger, E.M., and Smith, W.T., Urine analysis of phenothiazine drugs by spectrofluorometry, *Int. J. Neuropsychiat.*, 1, 466, 1965.

138. Kaul, P.N., Conway, M.W., Clark, M.L., and Huffine, J., Chloropromazine metabolism. I. Quantitative fluorometric method for 11 chlorpromazine metabolites, *J. Pharm. Sci.*, 59, 1745, 1970.

139. Randall, C.A., Iliev, V., and Brandman, O., Metabolism of methyprylon, *Arch. Int. Pharmacodyn.*, 106, 388, 1956.

140. Koechlin, B.A. and D'Arimte, L., The Determination of chlordiazepotide (Librium®) and of a metabolite of lactum character in plasma of humans, dogs and rats by a specific spectrofluorometric micro method, *Anal. Biochem.*, 5, 195, 1963.

PHYSIOLOGIC AND PHARMACOLOGIC ASPECTS OF DRUG DEPENDENCE

CHARACTERISTICS AND THEORIES RELATED TO ACUTE AND CHRONIC TOLERANCE DEVELOPMENT

C. C. Hug

TABLE OF CONTENTS

INTRODUCTION

Scope of the Chapter

Drug tolerance is a very broad subject involving a large number of substances from a variety of pharmacological classes. It is part of the even broader topic of adaptation to change in the environment.[65] In the case of drugs, the change is in the internal chemical environment of the organism.

The present chapter will be limited in scope to the phenomena of tolerance observed with the classes of psychoactive drugs most widely subject to dependence and abuse. These include a) narcotic analgesics, b) depressants such as ethyl alcohol, barbiturates, other sedative-hypnotic and minor tranquilizing agents, c) stimulants, d) hallucinogens, and e) cannabis preparations. The major effects of these five classes of psychoactive drugs are on the central nervous system, but important observations of tolerance have been made for a variety of tissues, and these will be included. The purposes of the chapter are to describe the characteristics of tolerance for each class of drugs and to review the mechanisms which conceivably could underlie the various phenomena of tolerance. Although many authors consider tolerance and physical dependence to be inextricably related phenomena, the latter is the subject of a separate chapter.

Because of the proliferation of review articles on the subject of tolerance, the reader will be referred to those discussions in which a specific topic is particularly well covered, and only a brief summary will be made herein. Hopefully, the burden of additional trips to the library will be adequately compensated by the choice of references and a minimum of redundancy.

Definitions

Drug refers to any chemical or substance used to produce an alteration or response (a pharmacologic effect) in a biological system (whole organism or an isolated component of the organism). *Drug tolerance* (or simply tolerance for the purposes of this chapter) is a state of decreased responsiveness of the system to a pharmacologic action of the drug, resulting from prior exposure of the system to that drug. It is defined in reference to the magnitude of response to the first dose of the drug, and it is expressed quantitatively as a reduction in the response to a subsequent dose of the same size, or, in some cases, as the increment of dosage required to produce a subsequent response equal in magnitude to the initial response. The definition declares that the state is acquired only by prior exposure to the drug (or a congener, see cross tolerance below), and thereby excludes a variety of other factors (genetic, environmental, developmental, pharmacologic, etc.) which may influence the responsiveness of the system to the drug. Obviously, it is essential to control experiments on tolerance for changes in responsiveness due to these other factors or arising spontaneously.

The characteristics of tolerance phenomena are multiple. Hence, it has become a common practice to qualify the term in a number of ways. When tolerance develops very rapidly following either a single dose or a few doses administered over a brief time, usually minutes to hours, it is designated *acute tolerance*[287] or *tachyphylaxis.* When tolerance develops after repeated administration of the drug over a longer period of time, usually days to months, it is termed *chronic tolerance.**

Cross tolerance may be defined as diminished responsiveness of the system to one drug, induced by the development of tolerance to another drug of a similar or dissimilar chemical structure or pharmacological action.[298] *Specific cross tolerance* denotes the fact that the test compound has the ability to evoke the same adaptive change (tolerance) as the original drug and that the two substances are mutually interchangeable in maintaining a state of tolerance. Generally, cross tolerance develops among drugs of the same pharmacological class.[74,151,295,370] Within each pharmalogical class, cross tolerance may develop more readily among compounds from the same chemical class,[295] although the latter is not always true. *Nonspecific cross tolerance*, in contrast, is usually a low-grade tolerance evident for compounds of different pharmacological classes (e.g., tolerance to general anesthetics in chronic alcoholics.[6,120,181])

General Characteristics of Tolerance

There are several quantitative characteristics of tolerance, which collectively provide a basis for: 1) accurately defining the specific phenomenon under consideration, 2) determining the factors which influence tolerance development, and 3) correlating physiological and biochemical alterations with changes in tolerance in the hope of identifying the mechanisms responsible for tolerance phenomena. In other words, in order to reduce confusion and controversy and to make significant progress in our understanding of tolerance, it is necessary that we be able to describe the phenomena quantitatively. The quantitative characteristics of tolerance include:

1. Relationship to dosage – Is a minimal dose required to induce tolerance? (As with any dose-effect relationship, it is difficult, often impossible, to determine accurately a threshold dose for tolerance development because of the variability inherent in the responses of biological systems, especially to weak stimuli.) Does tolerance develop progressively to each increment of dosage? Can tolerance be overcome and the effect elicited again by increasing the dose?

2. Time course – Is a minimal time of exposure to the drug required to induce tolerance? What is the rate of onset and the rate of disappearance of tolerance? (Disappearance of tolerance is particularly difficult to measure since each test dose has the potential to provoke renewed activity of the mechanisms responsible for tolerance.)

3. Degree of tolerance – How does the degree of tolerance relate to the dose of the drug? Is there a maximal degree of tolerance that can be developed? What is required to maintain a stable level of tolerance?

4. Extent of cross tolerance – To what drugs does cross tolerance develop and to what degree?

5. Residual effects – Are all the manifestations of tolerance completely reversible? Does it require the same drug administration procedure and time course to reintroduce tolerance in the system? Is the system qualitatively different after a cycle of tolerance than before?

It is readily apparent that tolerance does not necessarily develop to all of the effects of a given drug. Although it seems to be less well appreciated, it is clear that tolerance to different actions of a drug does not necessarily develop at the same rate and to the same extent.[172,298] Furthermore, there

*Many authors imply chronic-type tolerance when using the term tolerance alone; they specify acute tolerance or tachyphylaxis.

is considerable variation among species and among drugs, even from the same chemical or pharmacological class.[295] These points cannot be stressed too strongly, for they imply the necessity of avoiding unwarranted generalizations when discussing tolerance phenomena, and they lead to the suggestion that different mechanisms may underlie tolerance development to different effects of even the same drug in a single organism. In reality, it appears that highly specific types of compensation occur for individual types of drug action,[172,218] and in some cases, there may be more than one mechanism responsible for an apparently singular tolerance phenomenon.[172]

Relationship of Tolerance to Physical Dependence

Thus far, it appears that tolerance develops to some of the actions of all drugs which can induce physical dependence. However, there is no consistent qualitative or quantitative relationship between physical dependence and tolerance.[172,295] Certainly, tolerance develops to the effects of many drugs which do not induce physical dependence, and tolerance develops in non-nervous tissues which do not exhibit any signs of physical dependence when the drug is removed.[295] Thus, although the two phenomena may exhibit certain parallelisms, they are not necessarily related fundamentally. In fact, it has been suggested that tolerance relates to physical dependence largely as a means by which cells (specifically neurons) can be exposed to sufficiently high concentrations of drug so that significant degrees of physical dependence can be developed.[295] Without tolerance development the organism would succumb before sufficiently large concentrations could be achieved.

On the other hand, many authors have been struck by the fact that the same procedures used to induce physical dependence also serve to induce tolerance.[172] As a result, they have proposed that a common mechanism underlies both phenomena.

POTENTIAL MECHANISMS OF TOLERANCE

A brief, general discussion of the potential mechanisms of tolerance is useful in providing a framework for consideration of specific tolerance phenomena in subsequent sections of this chapter. Some of the potential mechanisms have limitations so they may be easily ruled out as significant factors in tolerance merely by observation or description of the particular tolerance phenomenon. On the other hand, the nature of some tolerance phenomena is such that it is conceivable that more than one mechanism may be responsible. Having a general knowledge of tolerance mechanisms, one will be less likely to accept a single mechanism and rule out other possibilities prematurely.

There are three major processes by which drug tolerance can occur.[108] First, the concentration of active drug molecules at the site of drug action could be reduced by a number of different mechanisms which can be classified under *altered biological disposition* of the drug. Second, the particular cells on which the drug acts directly could become less responsive in a number of ways which we will arbitrarily designate as *cellular mechanisms* of tolerance. Third, even though the drug continues to exert its effect at its site of action, the overall response (i.e., the response which is measured) could be diminished by various adjustments in other cells, *homeostatic mechanisms,* which tend to counteract the response. In the last category could be included both *physiologic* as well as *psychologic* ("learning") mechanisms of adjustment.

Since in many cases we are not yet able to distinguish between cellular and homeostatic mechanisms, it has been suggested that they be combined under the heading *functional tolerance.*[172] This suggestion has merit in emphasizing our lack of knowledge and possibly in reducing controversy based on semantics, but it also blurs certain distinctions which are useful in a theoretical formulation of mechanisms of tolerance.

Altered Biological Disposition

For the most part, alterations of absorption, metabolism, excretion and certain aspects of distribution would be expected to influence all drug actions equally. That is, the quantitative characteristics of all tolerance phenomena for a given drug in a given individual would be equivalent. Where differences in tolerance exist for different drug actions, it is unlikely that altered disposition of the drug could be the solely responsible mechanism.

Absorption

If tolerance were based on a diminished rate of absorption from a site of administration, then tolerance would not be manifest to doses of the drug administered by the intravenous route which by-passes the absorption mechanism. Except for the intestinal absorption of very few drugs,[200] none of which are considered to be drugs of dependence, specialized absorption processes have not been observed. Drug tolerance based on alterations of nonspecific absorption factors (e.g., diffusion, blood flow) would be manifest as cross tolerance to any other drug administered by the same route. Suffice it to state that absorption has not been implicated as a significant factor in any tolerance phenomena for the drugs under consideration here.

Metabolism

It is now widely recognized that a large number of drugs and other substances have the ability to stimulate the mechanisms responsible for their own metabolism in various tissues of the body, especially in the liver.[55,212] Where metabolism of the drug results in a product with less pharmacological activity than the original drug, stimulation of the metabolic process can serve as a mechanism of tolerance. Tolerance on this basis will likely be equivalent for all actions of the drug and will be manifest as a shortening of the duration of action and a lessening of the overall intensity of effect where the latter is measured as the area under the effect-duration curve. The maximum intensity of effect may also be lessened except when the test-dose of the drug is administered intravenously[108] or by any other route which permits a rate of absorption which is very rapid relative to the rate of metabolism. When tolerance is based on stimulation of metabolic inactivation of the drug, the intensity of response to the first dose of the drug should be reproduced merely by increasing the size of subsequent doses of the drug. And when the degree of drug effect is correlated with tissue concentrations of the drug, tolerance based on metabolism will not change the correlation (i.e., the same degree of effect will be evident at the same drug concentration in tolerant and naïve subjects). Any treatment preventing the increase in the rate of drug metabolism should also prevent tolerance development. However, the last point may be difficult to establish since many inhibitors of drug metabolism (e.g., SKF-525A) block both the increase as well as the base-line rate of metabolism,[212] thereby increasing the availability of active drug at its site of action in both tolerant and naïve subjects. Comparisons are difficult under these circumstances, and the increased concentration of drug at its site of action may tend to overcome functional types of tolerance. Finally, to the extent that a given drug stimulates the rate of metabolism of other drugs, cross tolerance will be manifest to these other drugs.

Excretion

Excretory processes which involve simple physical diffusion depend primarily on the concentration of the free (i.e., not protein bound) drug in plasma. Anything increasing plasma levels of the free drug will increase excretion, but at the same time, will tend to increase the level of active drug at its site of action. Hence, except for excretory processes involving specific transport mechanisms (e.g., organic acid and base secreting mechanisms of the proximal renal tubule[361]), significant degrees of tolerance are not likely to be based on augmentation of excretory processes. In the case of specialized renal excretory mechanisms, very few compounds are known to facilitate their own excretion (e.g., ammonium chloride,[275] penicillin[129]), and so far, the examples do not include any psychoactive drugs. For those drugs whose excretion is limited by pH-dependent non-ionic reabsorption,[249] a drug-induced change in urinary pH and body acid-base balance so as to increase the ionization of drug in the renal tubular fluid conceivably could promote more rapid excretion and thereby shorten the duration of action. However, no demonstration of such a mechanism of tolerance has been made.*

Distribution

Any drug-induced process for sequestering the drug at inactive sites (e.g., by increased binding to plasma proteins or to nonresponsive components of tissues, or by immunologic inactivation) could lower the drug concentration at its site of action (i.e., tolerance). Hypotheses of tolerance invoking immunologic phenomena[44] and inactivation of the drug by tissue components[343] have been put forth for the narcotics analgesics, but the evidence to support them is limited and contradictory.

*It is a theoretical possibility for the amphetamines and cocaine which are excreted more rapidly when the urine is acidic.[27,89] Long term use of high doses of these drugs is associated with markedly reduced food intake,[10,191] and this can lead to a metabolic acidosis with the production of a more acidic urine.

Cellular Mechanisms

Before our understanding of cellular mechanisms of tolerance is complete, we will necessarily have to understand the mechanism of drug action on the cells in question. At present, our understanding of both is lacking, almost completely so for most drugs acting in the central nervous system. Nevertheless, to the extent that we can postulate the nature of drug action on cells we can postulate cellular mechanisms of tolerance.

Most drugs interact with chemically specific sites or receptors located on the surface or within the cell, and the intensity of their effects is directly related to the number[13] (or possibly to the rate[270]) of drug-receptor interactions. Hence, anything that reduces the number (or rate) of such interactions will result in a diminished response of the system to the drug. All of the mechanisms of tolerance based on alterations of drug disposition reduce drug-receptor interactions by lowering the concentration of drug at the receptor site. It is conceivable that the concentration of free (active) drug could also be reduced by increased binding to inactive ("silent") receptors[49,50,52] in the immediate vicinity of the site of action or by diminished uptake of the drug at its site of action (e.g., altered membrane permeability).

On the other hand, the number of active receptors available for interaction with subsequent doses of the drug could be reduced through their continued occupation by previously administered drug molecules ("self-antagonism"). This assumes that the response of the system to the drug occurs only as a result of the initial drug-receptor interaction and disappears even though the drug-receptor complex persists.[14,355] Or, the combination of a drug and receptor could produce a conformational change in the receptor with a relatively long relaxation time. After dissociation of the drug-receptor complex, the altered receptor would have either a reduced affinity for the drug or a reduced ability to initiate the characteristic response.[273,274] Also, the receptors could become occupied with an inactive compound ("antagonist") synthesized from endogenous substances or from the drug itself. An antagonistic type of compound could also reduce the affinity of the receptor site for the drug without interacting directly with the receptor site (e.g., changing the conformation of the receptor by acting at an adjacent site: an allosteric effect).[12,108] Finally, the number of receptors could be diminished by decreased formation or increased catabolism of the receptors themselves.

Conversely, if the response to the drug is related to the proportion of the total number of receptors occupied by the drug, tolerance could arise from an increase in the total number of active receptors (increased synthesis, decreased destruction).[49,52] This concept has been formulated specifically for circumstances in which the receptor is an enzyme which is inhibited by the drug.[109,112,304] Inhibition of the enzyme results in diminished formation of the product (drug effect) which controls the rate of synthesis of the enzyme through a feedback mechanism. Lowered product formation initiates enzyme synthesis (i.e., increases the total number of receptors and increases the number which must be inhibited by the drug in order to produce its effect). Or along similar lines of thought, the drug interaction with the enzyme stabilizes the enzyme and thereby increases the amount of enzyme (receptors) to be inhibited by the drug.[109] Although the above hypotheses are plausible, they await identification and understanding of the intimate mechanisms of drug action for experimental verification.

For those drugs whose action is indirect and depends on their releasing a mediator substance, tolerance could be a manifestation of depletion of the mediator by the drug. This concept has been widely implicated in the tachyphylaxis developed in peripheral tissues (as opposed to the CNS) to a variety of drugs, and has been developed most elaborately and convincingly for peripheral autonomic nerves which release norepinephrine as a mediator.[22,60,108] Thus far, however, there is no direct or convincing evidence of drug tolerance arising from depletion of chemical mediators within the central nervous system, although such a mechanism is commonly suspected and has been the subject of much investigation.

Where the drug action is to prevent the release of a chemical mediator or to compete with the mediator for a receptor, tolerance to the drug's action could arise from increased synthesis or release of the endogenous substance. Alternatively, the blockade could be bypassed through use of an alternate mechanism or pathway. With some of these concepts, the distinctions between cellular and homeostatic mechanisms of tolerance become blurred.

For a stimulating discussion of metabolic adaptation in the brain, the reader is referred to the article by McIlwain.[233] Many of the concepts he reviews are theoretically applicable to the phenomena of drug tolerance. However, few of them have been studied seriously in relation to drug tolerance and there is little evidence to support or to refute them.

Homeostatic Mechanisms

Homeostasis or the constancy of the internal milieu is achieved by the function of feedback-sensitive control mechanisms (e.g., hormonal feedback on pituitary function) and the use of alternate physiologic mechanisms (e.g., blood pressure is maintained in the face of decreased cardiac output by an increase in total peripheral vascular resistance). Many examples of homeostatic mechanisms such as these are known for the intact organism. Obviously, such mechanisms serve to resist drug-induced alterations of bodily functions, and usually, the mechanisms are activated so rapidly that they limit the response to the first dose of the drug. In terms of drug tolerance, the question that arises is whether or not such homeostatic mechanisms can become progressively more effective ("hypertrophy"[128,218]) with each exposure to the drug so that the response to subsequent doses of the drug is smaller than that to the first dose.

An initial drug-induced response which requires a period of time to be completed and then is maintained could give the appearance of tolerance. For example, a drug acting on the thermoregulatory centers of the hypothalamus to lower body temperature of the dog will induce panting, which will persist until body temperature is lowered to the new set point. Additional doses of the drug can maintain the lowered body temperature by several alternate mechanisms but panting of the intensity seen after the first dose will not occur. Tolerance is apparent to the "panting response" but the initial hypothermic response is maintained.[218]

Behavioral (psychological or learned) tolerance could be considered to be a form of homeostasis in the sense that a subject whose performance is impaired by a drug could acquire new skills or functions to replace those which remain impaired and thereby regain the predrug level of performance. Tolerance development would represent relearning a task (originally learned in the drug-free state) under the influence of the drug. Cross tolerance between drugs would depend upon the resemblance (as perceived by the subject) of one drug state to the other.[172]

TOLERANCE TO NARCOTIC ANALGESICS

The narcotic analgesics, especially morphine and its chemical derivatives, have more often been the subject of investigations of drug tolerance than any other class of drugs. Numerous research reports have appeared and they have been reviewed periodically over the past 40 years.[43,73,74,145,280,293-296,298,331,363] These reviews are the source of much of the information presented herein. Unless indicated otherwise, the information relates primarily to morphine. It is generally true, however, that where observations have been made for other narcotic analgesics, they have been qualitatively similar to those for morphine.

Effects to which Tolerance Develops

Tolerance develops to many, but not all, of the effects of morphine (Table 1). It should be noted that the rates of appearance and disappearance and the degree of tolerance development may differ considerably for the different effects of morphine even within a single individual or species.[74,126,221,222,226,280] Moreover, there are notable examples of quantitative and qualitative differences in tolerance development between species of animals,[73,74,145,280] between individual narcotic analgesics,[76,126,145,295,301,373] and between experimental procedures used to demonstrate the phenomena.[4,46,87,126,329] These sources of variation have contributed confusion and controversy about tolerance to the narcotic analgesics, especially in relation to the mechanisms that may be involved.

Among the effects listed in Table 1, tolerance development has been studied widely for only a few: analgesia, narcosis, lethality, and alterations of behavior. Even for these effects, there are relatively few adequately controlled studies of a quantitative nature. Thus, the amount of information on which to base a discussion is limited, and in light of the above mentioned variability in tolerance characteristics between species, drug effects, etc., it is unwise to generalize. As an example of the hazard of generalization, consider

TABLE 1*

High-grade tolerance develops to:
- Analgesia
- Euphoria-dysphoria**
- Mental clouding
- Narcosis (sedation-sleep)
- Inhibition of REM sleep[184]
- Respiratory depression[184]
- Lethality due to respiratory depression[74,292]
- Hypotension and peripheral vasodilatation
- Hypothermia[117,208,225]
- Antidiuresis[142,143,213]
- Anorexia, nausea, and vomiting[221]
- Increased motor activity (mouse)[110,279,305]
- Alteration of spinal cord reflexes[222,365]
- Lenticular opacities (rodents)[314]

Moderate and variable degrees of tolerance develop to:
- Bradycardia

Minimal or no tolerance develops to:
- Miosis (man)
- Constipation and changes in gastrointestinal tone
- Convulsions
- Lethality due to convulsions[74,292]
- Antagonistic effects of nalorphine, cyclazocine, etc.[77]

*Individual references have not been given for effects where the tolerance development is well known and adequately described in many reviews.[73,74,150,280,295]

**Dysphoria is especially common for the narcotic antagonists and tolerance to this effect is observed with repeated administration.[77]

the often repeated statement that tolerance does not develop to the stimulant or excitatory* effects of morphine.[293,295,296] The statement is true when considering the convulsant action of morphine, but it is not true for another stimulant action of the drug, that of increased motor activity in the mouse.[110,279,305]

Characteristics of Tolerance

Acute vs. Chronic Tolerance

It has been a common practice to distinguish between acute and chronic tolerance to the various effects of morphine. A careful review of the literature suggests that, at least for some of the effects of morphine, the distinction is based more on the choice of dosage schedule to induce tolerance than on differences in the maximal rates at which various organ systems can develop tolerance. In fact, there is evidence to suggest that tolerance of a similar, if not identical, nature can be developed to certain effects of morphine by using either an acute or chronic dosage regimen.

Schmidt and Livingston first used the term "acute tolerance" to describe the rapid disappearance of the hypotensive responses in dogs given a series of large intravenous doses of morphine.[287] They later demonstrated that both the vasculature and the "vasomotor and respiratory centers" of the central nervous system participated in the development of acute tolerance.[288] Also, they reported that in the dog acute tolerance was evident to the narcotic (behavioral depressant) effects of the drug.[289]**

Martin and Eades[221] convincingly demonstrated that intravenous infusions of morphine (3 mg/kg/hour) over a 7½ to 8 hour period to dogs resulted in tolerance to the analgesic (withdrawal and skin twitch reflexes), narcotic (sedative), emetic and miotic effects of a test dose of morphine (10 mg/kg) administered 17 hours after termination of the infusion. They commented on the close similarity of tolerance phenomena induced by either acute or chronic treatment. On the other hand, Martin and Eades[222] could not demonstrate acute tolerance to the actions of intravenously infused morphine on spinal reflexes of the *chronic spinal dog* although high-grade tolerance to the spinal actions of morphine could be demonstrated in this preparation after it had received twice daily doses of morphine (10 mg/kg/dose) for a period of weeks.

Acute tolerance has been reported for the narcotic analgesic effects of analgesia,[58,175] hypotension,[85] and hypothermia[208] in rats, increased motor activity in mice,[110] and inhibition of electrically-induced contractions of the guinea pig ileum in vitro.[84,269,271]

Thus, it appears that distinctions between acute and chronic tolerance, at least for some of the effects of morphine, are based primarily on experimental design, specifically on the size of the dose and schedule of administration of the drug. In most cases there does not seem to be a fundamental difference between acute and chronic

*The words stimulation and excitation are used in the ordinary sense to describe the overt responses to drugs.

**While it is true that maximal tolerance to the hypotensive effect was observed within minutes to hours,[288] and that maximal tolerance phenomena to the narcotic effect were observed after one week,[289] this quantitative comparison is faulted because of the use of ether anesthesia in the studies of hypotension and because of the differences in the size and schedule of doses used to induce the two tolerance phenomena.

tolerance in terms of the tissues affected or the degree of tolerance that can be produced.

Dosage and the Onset of Tolerance

Even from reports such as those cited above, it is difficult to estimate the threshold dose or minimal exposure time required for the induction of tolerance to the narcotic analgesics. It is a commonly expressed clinical adage that tolerance to the analgesic and narcotic effects of morphine and related drugs in man is promoted by large, frequently administered doses and is minimized by giving small doses at widely spaced intervals.[74,156] One precise study of the development of tolerance to the activity increasing effects of levorphanol in mice[110] led to the same conclusion, that is, that the rate and degree of tolerance development are functions of the size of the dose and the frequency of administration. The latter study also demonstrated that while the rate of onset of tolerance to the activity increasing effects could be rapid, its development required a minimal period of time which may correspond to some rate limiting process with a half-time of approximately 16 hours in the mouse.

It has been suggested that even a single dose of morphine can induce tolerance to certain of its effects. In rats, one dose of morphine (10 or 20 mg/kg) appeared to reduce the analgesic response to a second dose given weeks to months later.[46,188] (Also see earlier references cited by Eddy.[74]) Martin and Eades[221] suggested that tolerance may play a role in recovery from the effects (analgesia, hypothermia, miosis) of a single dose of morphine on the basis of their finding that the recovery process followed a time course that was shorter than the time course estimated for disappearance of morphine from the brain of dogs.

It is clear that in order to maintain maximal degrees of tolerance to any of the effects of morphine studied thus far (analgesia, narcosis, behavioral alterations, lethality), the tolerant individual must be continuously exposed to the narcotic analgesic.[293,296] Hence, the minimal frequency of administration of a given size dose is determined by the rate of elimination of the specific drug. Any drug-free interval appears to result in a reduction of the degree of tolerance. This is the basis of the commonly reported experiences of addicts who become markedly intoxicated to a previously well tolerated dose of heroin after they have missed their usual injections for a few days.[204]

Degree of Tolerance

The extent of tolerance to morphine can be truly impressive, but the exact limits of tolerance vary for the individual effects. For example, tolerance to the emetic, antidiuretic, and hypotensive actions is essentially absolute in that once tolerance is established a dose of morphine no matter how large is unable to elicit a response, and there is no evidence of persistence of the initial response (i.e., urine flow and blood pressure recover to their predrug levels and are maintained there despite repeated administration of the drug).

On the other hand, tolerance to analgesia, euphoria, narcosis, respiratory depression, hypothermia, and, in man, lethality develops to each increment of dose.[220] But it is never absolute; that is, a sufficiently large dose of morphine can still elicit marked degrees of effect. The stepwise progression of tolerance to these effects can be dramatic in degree and seemingly could continue without end if it were not for the intervention of convulsions and death due to postconvulsive depression in all species with the apparent exception of man. Whereas a dose of 60 mg or less can cause respiratory arrest in nontolerant humans, addicts have received up to 2 g of morphine in 2½ hours and over 4 g per day without exhibiting clinically significant degrees of depression.[74]

In some cases tolerance may be more apparent than real. For example, in the case of respiratory depression to morphine in man, both the rate of respiration and the sensitivity of the respiratory center to carbon dioxide remain depressed throughout the period of chronic intoxication, although very large doses of morphine produce little additional depression of respiratory function.[224] Similarly, in dogs chronic morphine intoxication produces a persistent miosis and the change in pupil size after each stabilization dose of morphine is much reduced compared to that after the initial dose of morphine.[222] These effects of morphine persist at a near maximal level and little or no additional effect can be produced by larger doses of the drug (i.e., apparent tolerance).

Although very marked tolerance can be developed to morphine within a very short period of time (hours to days),[74] the most common pattern of development is by very gradual, "stair-case" increments of dosage.* Under these circumstances, tolerance first becomes evident as a shortening of the duration of drug action and then as a diminution of the peak effect as well.[295] It is possible for the addict to choose a dose that just balances his degree of tolerance so that he appears essentially normal and can carry out highly skilled technical operations. Although he experiences mild degrees of depression with each dose, it is short lived and only miosis, mild respiratory depression, and constipation persist.[74,150,220] Typically, however, addicts seek renewed euphoric and sedative effects by continuously increasing the frequency and size of the dose,[74,150,156] and thereby continuously elevate their tolerance to the effects of morphine-like drugs.

Disappearance of Tolerance

There are almost no precise studies of the disappearance of tolerance, possibly because of the difficulties inherent in doing such studies, especially in a single individual (i.e., each test dose has the potential for activating the tolerance mechanisms). Using groups of mice tolerant to the activity increasing effects of levorphanol, Goldstein and Sheehan[110] showed that the return to normal sensitivity to a test dose was evident within less than 24 hours and was complete 48 hours after the last dose (half-time approximately 20 hours). A puzzling finding in their study was that when the dosage interval for inducing tolerance was increased from 8 to 16 hours (without changing the size of the dose of levorphanol, 20 mg/kg/dose), the rate of recovery of sensitivity to the drug was slowed (half-time approximately 48 hours). No explanation for this observation is apparent.

All other experimental studies of tolerance report only rough estimates of the rate of its loss, but most of these indicate that marked reductions in tolerance are evident within a few days. The estimates are in line with the common clinical observation noted above, that addicts experience a marked diminution in their tolerance to the euphoric, depressant, and lethal effects of narcotic analgesics within a matter of days after their last dose.[204]

Seevers[293] suggested that the loss of tolerance parallels in a general way the detoxication and elimination of the drug from the body. He and his co-workers[295,296,298] also noted that there are apparent exceptions to this generalization. Some tissues (e.g., vascular smooth muscle) which gain tolerance rapidly appear to lose it rapidly, and tolerance to certain effects (e.g., emesis[272]) is quite persistent, even for months.

In regard to persistence of tolerance, the reports of Cochin and Kornetsky[46] and Kornetsky and Bain[188] are interesting and puzzling. These authors presented evidence that tolerance to the analgesic (hot-plate test) and behavioral depressant (swimming test) effects of morphine persisted from 6 to 12 or more months following either a single dose or termination of a period of daily administration of the drug. Others have reported that single doses of morphine have induced long-lasting tolerance to the analgesic[114] and hypothermic[208] effects in rats. Man retains some degree of tolerance to the hypothermic and emetic effects of morphine six months or more following termination of a cycle of addiction.[96] Although there are a few scattered statements to the effect that tolerance is more easily induced after an initial cycle of tolerance and dependence,[280] there are no definitive data to support the claim. Contrariwise, Goldstein and Sheehan[110] found no difference in the rate of tolerance development to a second or third cycle of tolerance to the activity increasing effects of levorphanol in mice.

Another long-lasting residuum of prolonged administration of morphine has been termed "post-tolerance sensitivity."[295,296,298] It is manifest in monkeys within a month or two after the last regular morphine injection as an increased sensitivity and exaggerated neurologic responses to a test dose of morphine (compared to the responses to a test dose before chronic administration of the drug). This increased susceptibility to morphine is said to persist for many months. Increased responsiveness to morphine has not been described in man in the postdependence period,[96] but long-lasting (4 to 6 months or more) alterations of physiologic functions, termed "protracted or secondary" abstinence,[225] have been described.[81,127,225]

Cross Tolerance

Eddy, the foremost authority on the relation-

*The addict usually has limited amounts of drug and money available to him. The physician wishes to maintain therapeutic effectiveness in his patients, and the experimenter wishes to minimize weight loss and debility among his subjects. For these reasons, gradual increments of dosage are employed.

ships between chemical structure and pharmacological activity of the narcotic analgesics, states[74] "that morphine-tolerant animals (including man) are generally tolerant to the narcotic effects of other morphine derivatives and of morphine-like analgesics, whatever their chemical type." Seevers and Deneau[295] state that "specific cross tolerance is developed to all narcotics with morphine-like properties... The term specific cross tolerance is used . . . to denote the fact that the test compound has the ability to evoke the same adaptive mechanisms as the original drug and that the two substances are mutually interchangeable in maintaining a state of tolerance following repeated administration." It should be noted that the last statement referring to mutual interchangeability was made with the implied qualifications that for equivalent interchangeability the dose and frequency of administration have to be chosen on the basis of relative narcotic analgesic potency and duration of action. These generalizations are based on the long-term experience of the authors. There are few systematic, quantitative studies of cross tolerance among the narcotic analgesics.

Continuing the work of Schmidt and Livingston[287,288] on acute vascular tolerance, Shideman and Johnson[301] observed only partial cross tolerance among morphine, meperidine, and methadone. Haggart (cited by Seevers and Deneau[295]) found cross tolerance between morphine and nalorphine, which in the presence of morphine antagonizes its effect, but when acting alone, produces hypotensive responses identical to those of morphine. Seevers and Deneau[295] indicated that cross tolerance to the peripheral vascular effects also exists among morphine, codeine, and thebaine although they do not give experimental evidence for the statement.

Isbell (quoted by Seevers and Woods[298]) reported that although there is cross tolerance to the narcotic and analgesic actions of morphine, methadone, meperidine, and their congeners, there are qualitative and quantitative differences. In the clinical setting it is generally recognized that signficant cross tolerance to analgesia exists among all narcotic analgesics when they are given in equivalent analgesic doses.[92,156,261] Although tolerance to methadone is reported to develop somewhat more slowly than to morphine,[145,150,295] it does reach a comparable level[145] and essentially complete cross tolerance to the euphoric and sedative effects is established to heroin and other morphine-like drugs. This cross tolerance is the fundamental principle underlying the use of methadone "blockade" in the treatment of narcotic addicts.[66,103]

Relatively small degrees of "nonspecific" cross tolerance are found between the narcotic analgesics and other classes of central nervous systems depressants.[295]

Tolerance to Opiate Antagonists

Tolerance develops to both the subjective and objective effects of cyclazocine and nalorphine including hallucinations, sedation, respiratory depression, and hypothermia, and there is cross tolerance between cyclazocine and nalorphine. However, tolerance does not develop to the antagonistic actions of these agents against morphine-like drugs.[77] The latter point is especially important in relation to the clinical use of cyclazocine to prevent the euphoric and other effects of heroin in the hope of deterring addicts from drug seeking behavior.[103,223]

Tolerance to Narcotic Analgesic Effects in vitro

Tolerance has been described for the growth-inhibiting action of morphine in cultured fibroblasts of heart and iris epithelium of the chick embryo,[73,74] and for cultured epithelial-like cells derived from a human cervical carcinoma.[56] But tolerance could not be demonstrated to the growth-suppressing effects of morphine in a human heteroploid epithelial-like cell line derived from a carcinoma of the cervix and maintained in continuous culture.[286] Whether or not these isolated tissues can serve as analogues for the nervous system in the development of tolerance remains an unsettled question,[309] but they may offer an opportunity to study cellular tolerance phenomena in systems somewhat less complicated than the intact organism.

Paton[269,271] and Fennessy et al.[84] reported that tolerance develops to the depressant action of morphine on the contractile activity of electrically-stimulated ileum from the guinea pig. However, the interpretation of the observations made by these authors as manifestations of tolerance has been questioned by others.[138,319]

Takemori[326-328] demonstrated that morphine added in vitro depresses the potassium-stimulated respiration of rat cerebral cortical slices, and that slices taken from rats given morphine, meperidine, or methadone on a chronic dosage schedule are tolerant to the respiratory depressant action of morphine added in vitro. The significance of Takemori's findings for the intact subject has not been determined.

Mulé[254-256] reported that morphine administered to guinea pigs or added in vitro stimulated the incorporation of radioactive phosphorus into phospholipids of cerebral cortical slices, and that chronic administration of morphine led to a reduction in the magnitude of this stimulation. The effect of morphine on the turnover of cerebral phospholipids has been related to the effects of morphine on calcium binding and transport by phospholipids.[256,257] The interactions of narcotic analgesics with calcium are complex[257] and beyond the scope of this discussion, but it is interesting to note that tolerance develops to the morphine-induced lowering of cerebral calcium concentrations in mice.[302] However, it is not certain that the effects observed are fundamental to the actions of narcotic analgesics or merely concomitant to the marked alterations of physiologic function induced by very large doses of morphine.

Mechanisms of Tolerance

Proposals of mechanisms of tolerance to the various effects of narcotic analgesics span the gamut of theoretical possibilities. In fact, some of them are strictly speculative with no experimental evidence to back them up. The order of discussion of the various hypotheses will follow approximately that found in the second section of this chapter.

It should be constantly kept in mind that more than one mechanism may be operating in tolerance to even a single effect of a drug. And in the case of the narcotic analgesics, the varied characteristics of tolerance to their different effects described above make it likely that more than a single mechanism underlies the overall tolerance to the actions of these drugs.

Altered Biological Disposition

Very early proposals of tolerance mechanisms related primarily to differences in the biological disposition of morphine in tolerant compared to nontolerant subjects. Where data were offered in support of a hypothesis, they were generally derived by methods which are unacceptable by current standards. Thus, many of the early hypotheses have either been disproven or simply ignored because they lack substantial support. These early hypotheses have been discussed elsewhere.[73,280] In addition, the reader is referred to the very complete summaries of the data on the biological disposition of narcotic analgesics by Way and Adler.[356,357]

Presently, it is generally held, on the basis of substantial negative evidence, that differences between tolerant and nontolerant subjects in terms of absorption, distribution,[137,163,238,258-260,282,346,371,374,380] metabolism,[45,162,193,238] and excretion[45,136,238,371] of narcotic analgesics are not sufficient to account in any major way for the differences in pharmacological responses observed in tolerant and nontolerant subjects. Although some of the studies have shown small quantitative differences between tolerant and nontolerant subjects, these differences are largely ignored in view of the dramatic degrees of tolerance that can be developed and because reports of differences for the most part have not been confirmed by other investigators. The observations that goldfish[159] and isolated tissues and cells maintained in a constant concentration of morphine developed tolerance to the effects of the drug even though they apparently do not metabolize it, further emphasize the necessity of looking beyond dispositional factors for explanations of tolerance to the narcotic analgesics.

One difference in the metabolism of drugs between tolerant and nontolerant male rats has been the subject of a large number of studies and discussions. Axelrod[19,20] observed a marked reduction in the ability of hepatic microsomes from tolerant (compared to nontolerant) male rats to *N*-demethylate several narcotic analgesics. Beckett et al.[28] proposed that morphine and other narcotic analgesics are adsorbed onto their receptor sites where they undergo *N*-demethylation to the nor-derivative which initiates the analgesic response. Axelrod[19] hypothesized that enzymes in the liver that *N*-demethylate narcotic drugs are closely related to the receptors for these drugs in the nervous system, and that continuous interaction of narcotic drugs with the receptors could inactivate the receptors (tolerance) just as continuous interaction of narcotic drugs with *N*-demethylating enzymes inactivated the enzymes. Both the hypothesis by Axelrod and that by Beckett et al. have received formidable challenges by Way and Adler, and the reader is referred to their extensive discussions[356,357] and to more recent publications for details.[5,37,42,162,177,178,379] The overall conclusion is that there are major, if not insurmountable, obstacles to be overcome before either or both hypotheses can be accepted as a basis of tolerance to the narcotic analgesics. Some of these obstacles are as follows: 1) *N*-dealkylation of narcotic analgesics can result in nor-derivatives which are more, equally or less potent than the parent compound depending on the specific drug and effect in question. 2) There is no consistent parallelism between the drug's analgesic potency and its ability to be *N*-demethylated in any species. 3) There is no apparent relationship between the times of onset and recovery of tolerance and inhibition of *N*-dealkylation. 4) The inhibition of *N*-dealkylation by chronic morphine administration has been observed only for male rats; it cannot be demonstrated either in vitro or in vivo for female rats or for either sex of any other species (mice, guinea pigs, rabbits, humans). Furthermore, the *N*-dealkylation reaction has not been detected in nervous tissue. 5) The inhibition of drug metabolism by chronic morphine administration is not limited to the *N*-dealkylation of narcotic analgesics. Inducers of drug metabolism such as phenobarbital induce *N*-dealkylation of narcotic analgesics but do not appear to alter the pharmacological actions of the latter compounds. As stated by Way and Adler,[356] "It may be concluded only that the role of *N*-demethylation in either promoting or limiting any of the pharmacological responses to morphine or its surrogates remains to be defined."

Inactivation of Narcotic Analgesics by Serum and Tissue Factors

Morphine-induced tolerance has been related to immunologic mechanisms by Cochin and Kornetsky.[46,47] Struck by their observations of long-persisting residual tolerance following a few doses or even a single dose of morphine and the time course of its development, they hypothesized that an antigen-antibody or similar mechanism develops to inactivate the drug in the tolerant individual. Attempts to transfer tolerance by transferring serum from tolerant to nontolerant subjects have produced inconsistent and conflicting results. Serum from morphine-tolerant rats and rabbits appeared to reduce the analgesic effectiveness of morphine when injected into mice.[47] Contrariwise, serum from tolerant dogs, monkeys, and humans was observed to *increase* the analgesic effectiveness of morphine in mice and the behavioral depressant effects (swimming) in rats.[185,189] Kiplinger and Clift[185] noted that the *potentiating factor* was not dialysable and suggested that it was a large molecular weight polypeptide or protein. The above observations have not been confirmed by independent investigators and, in fact, cannot be reproduced by the original authors.[44,47] Also, the work by Richter and Goldstein[282] on the concentrations of levorphanol in ultrafiltrates of brain tissue makes inactivation of the drug by binding to antibodies or large molecular weight substances unlikely. As far as the hypothesis of an immune-like mechanism of tolerance, we appear to be at the same point we were 30 years ago when Eddy[73] wrote (primarily in reference to tolerance to morphine-induced lethality), ". . . the evidence is conclusively against. . . production of a specific antibody as the mechanism of tolerance."

The reports describing transfer of tolerance by means of tissue preparations are equally confusing and inconclusive. Ungar and Cohen[343] first reported that brain tissue from morphine-tolerant dogs and rats contained a factor, thought to be a polypeptide, which when injected intraperitoneally in mice rendered them tolerant to the analgesic effects (tail pinch response) of morphine. Ungar and Galvan[344] later reported as did Tirri[334] that the tolerance factor was not detected in mice treated with morphine and that the potencies of extracts of brains from tolerant rats were quite variable in their ability to induce tolerance to the analgesic, hypothermic, and lethal effects of morphine in mice. More recently, Tulunay et al.[339] demonstrated that brain extracts from morphine-tolerant rats rendered naïve rats tolerant to morphine, an apparent confirmation of the work of Ungar et al. However, there are reports which conflict with those just cited. Two other groups[57,320] reportedly followed the procedure of Ungar and Cohen in preparing brain homogenates from morphine-tolerant rats, but were unable to detect tolerance to the analgesic effects of morphine in mice injected with the homogenate. On the other hand, Huidobro and Miranda[139] found that extracts of the whole bodies or of urine of mice tolerant to morphine (hot-plate test) contained a non-dialysable, water soluble factor (thought to be a polypeptide) which *increased* the analgesic and abstinence-suppressing effects of morphine in other mice. Thus, at the moment, the existence of morphine-induced tissue factors that can modify the responses to morphine when transferred to other subjects remains uncertain. And if present, one can only speculate on the role they may play in the development of tolerance to the narcotic analgesics.

The Role of Protein Synthesis

Because of reports of transferable tolerance factors of a polypeptide or protein nature, and because of the theoretical schemes relating tolerance to increased synthesis of enzymes[109,112] or receptors,[49,50,52] there has been an intense interest in the role of protein synthesis in the development of drug tolerance. Since no one has identified a specific protein involved in tolerance phenomena and since the nervous system and other tissues continuously synthesize and degrade a large number of proteins most of which are not likely to be directly related to tolerance phenomena, there has been little headway made by directly measuring the effects of narcotic analgesics on protein synthesis and nucleic acid metabolism.[41,59]

Rather, investigators have turned to examining the effects of inhibitors of nucleic acid function and protein synthesis on the development of tolerance to the narcotic analgesics. Thus far, the reports[48,58,59,206,316,322,358,376] are unanimous in concluding that such inhibitors prevent the development of tolerance to the effects of morphine and other narcotic analgesics. The inhibitors studied to date include actinomycin D,[48,58,59] 8-azaguanine,[322,376] cycloheximide,[206,358] 5-fluorouracil,[59] 6-mercaptopurine,[59] and puromycin.[316] In view of the generally marked toxicity associated with these inhibitors, there are serious reservations about the validity of conclusions based on their use. Most of the reports note that a large number of the animals given one of the inhibitors became sick or died. In one study,[206] the cumulative mortality in mice reached 60% after 13 days and 85% after 21 days of treatment with both morphine and cycloheximide. It is particularly noteworthy that the combination produced a much greater mortality than would be predicted by adding together the mortality figures for groups of mice given either one of the drugs alone (between 15 and 30% mortality for groups given either morphine or cycloheximide alone for 21 days). Obviously, any potential for toxicity due to the inhibitor or to its synergistic interactions with the narcotic analgesics makes interpretation of experiments employing such inhibitors difficult.

For example, the commonly used tests for analgesia are based on the ability of the animal to respond (withdrawal, vocalization, etc.) to a noxious stimulus. In naïve subjects, morphine depresses their response to noxious stimuli, and tolerance to morphine is manifest as recovery of responsiveness. Hence, prevention of tolerance development is indicated by depression of responsiveness. If the animal treated with morphine and one of the above inhibitors were unable to make the required response because of a toxic reaction, the latter could be mistaken for inhibition of tolerance development. While most of the experiments have included control animals given the inhibitor alone and showing normal responsiveness, such controls may not be adequate in view of the synergistic toxicity noted above for combinations of morphine and the inhibitor.

Cox et al.[56,58,59] have made a significant effort to reduce complications due to toxicity of the inhibitors by administering the inhibitor intracerebrally in small doses rather than systemically, and by studying acute tolerance produced over a three to seven hour period by infusion of morphine (thereby avoiding the delayed toxicity of the inhibitor). They have not yet completely ruled out toxic interactions as factors in their results. Nevertheless, their experiments are persuasive and lend considerable support to those hypotheses which depend on de novo synthesis of protein in the nervous system for the development of tolerance to the narcotic analgesics.

The Role of Receptors

The interaction of narcotic analgesics with their receptors is essential for the development of tolerance to their actions in responsive tissues. This statement is based primarily on the observations in rats, monkeys, and humans that simultaneous administration of one of the specific narcotic analgesic antagonists, nalorphine or levallorphan, along with morphine, antagonizes many of the actions of morphine and prevents the development of tolerance.[78,266,295,315] The question of immediate concern is whether or not the drug-receptor interaction per se can explain some of the phenomena of tolerance, perhaps by virtue of the drug continuing to occupy the receptor after the effect is over, thereby preventing access of other drug molecules to the receptor (self-antagonism) as is commonly assumed for membrane depolarizing agents such as nicotine, succinylcholine and decamethonium.[14,108,268] The reader is referred to a discussion of this concept of "receptor occupation" by Seevers.[294]

There are two groups of observations which support the concept of receptor occupation as a basis for tolerance to some of the actions of the narcotic analgesics. The first were those of Schmidt and Livingston[288,289] who noted that there was a progressive diminution and finally disappearance of the hypotensive responses to morphine with increasing dosage until a critical level was reached beyond which additional drug evoked no response. They concluded that tolerance was "conditioned simply upon the presence of a concentration of morphine that equals or exceeds a critical level, initiated as soon as that level is reached, and maintained only so long as the concentration of morphine remains at or above that level." There are no data to refute their hypothesis as it applies to *maximal* degrees of tolerance, and in fact, it is supported by requirements of dose-size and dose-interval to initiate and maintain high-grade tolerance. Of course, the persistence of low-grade tolerance long after administration of the drug has stopped is not easily explained by the receptor occupation concept.

Several authors[84,269,271] claim that tolerance develops in vitro to the depressant actions of morphine on electrically-stimulated segments of intestinal smooth muscle. Their claims are based on the observation of progressively smaller degrees of additional depression with successive additions of the same or larger concentrations of morphine to the bath. However, there are three points which must be recognized and emphasized. 1) The depression of the twitch by the initial small to moderate concentrations of morphine is maintained; it does not lessen even after hours of continued exposure.[319] The fact that larger and larger concentrations of morphine do not further depress the twitch may simply be a matter of maximal degree of effect (receptor saturation). 2) Very large doses of morphine may increase the twitch response which has been depressed by smaller doses.[84,269] This facilitation of the twitch response is probably the result of another action of morphine (e.g., to potentiate the actions of acetylcholine[138,269,271] and perhaps histamine[84]). 3) It does not seem possible to render the tissue tolerant by repeated additions of subliminal concentrations of morphine; that is, the additions of morphine accumulate and produce additive degrees of depression of the twitch.[138] 4) The return of the sensitivity of the electrically-stimulated smooth muscle to the depressant actions of morphine appears to parallel washout of morphine from the tissue, whether the morphine is added in vitro or injected into the animal prior to sacrifice.[138] Therefore, the saturation of receptors by morphine with *persistence of its effect* appears to be the basis of apparent "tolerance." By definition, tolerance involves a diminishing effect.

Axelrod's proposal for receptor inactivation by continued interaction with narcotic analgesic drugs has been discussed above.

Chemical Transmitters

There have been many attempts to link changes in tissue levels and turnover (metabolism, synthesis, and degradation) of chemical transmitters to the development of tolerance to various actions of the narcotic analgesics. Most of the putative transmitters, including acetylcholine,[362] catecholamines,[359] serotonin,[39,217,359] and histamine,[119,288] have been implicated at one time or another. So far, none of the changes in transmitter function can be assigned a fundamental role in the development of tolerance. Published reports frequently have been contradictory, and it is not certain in any case that the change observed is not merely coincidental or secondary to the fundamental mechanisms responsible for tolerance phenomena.

Of the recognized theoretical possibilities of mechanisms of tolerance based on alterations of neurochemical mediators (see section on cellular mechanisms), two have received particular emphasis in relation to the narcotic analgesics. The "transmitter surfeit" hypothesis of Paton[271] is based on the finding that morphine interferes with the release of acetylcholine from nervous elements in the gut and other organs including the central nervous system.[362] Paton proposes that as a result of this interference with release, acetylcholine accumulates in progressively larger concentrations in the nerve terminal until the proportion of stored acetylcholine released by an impulse is equal in absolute amount to that released before the addition of morphine and the degree of response is restored to its initial level (i.e., tolerance development). Thus far, there is no experimental evidence for a buildup of acetylcholine in nerve terminals, nor has there been a quantitative comparison of the amounts of the mediator released in the tolerant and nontolerant states.

A related hypothesis is that of Jaffe and Sharpless[158,300] and of Collier[51] who propose that as a result of "disuse" or decreased activity of certain neural pathways, there develops a supersensitivity in the tissues to one or more of the neurotransmitters that normally excite them. Supersensitivity develops in proportion to the degree of interruption in the flow of chemical impulses across the neuroeffector junctions. Tolerance arises as the diminution in transmitter release is offset by increasing sensitivity of the postsynaptic element. This hypothesis, though supported to some degree for certain drugs (e.g., pentobarbital) and neurotransmitters, has not been related by direct experimentation to the narcotic analgesics. It is mentioned here because of its potentially close relationship to Paton's hypothesis noted above and because of its contrast to the ideas of Martin discussed below.

Redundant or Alternate Pathways

On the basis of his observations of the effects of atropine and other non-narcotic drugs in the central nervous system, Martin[218,219] has proposed that there are functional systems which have parallel pathways consisting of elements which differ in their sensitivity to toxins (in the present case, to morphine and other narcotic analgesics). When one pathway is depressed by morphine, another parallel pathway which is insensitive to morphine increases its function ("hypertrophies") and becomes more effective in mediating the function (i.e., tolerance is manifest to the initial functional depression of the system by morphine). It should be noted, however, that the basic depressant action of morphine on the morphine-sensitive element of the system persists as long as morphine is present. (In fact, the hypothesis is offered to explain physical dependence as well as tolerance. Withdrawal of morphine allows the morphine-sensitive element to return to a normal level of activity which adds to that of the "hypertrophied" alternate element and leads to exaggerated function of the system and to manifestation of withdrawal phenomena.)

Again, direct experimental support for the redundancy hypothesis is lacking for the narcotic analgesics per se, but Martin et al.[219,224] offer evidence that certain depressant actions of morphine persist (e.g., decreased sensitivity of the respiratory center to carbon dioxide) even though the systems may exhibit functional tolerance to the drug (e.g., much larger doses of morphine produce little additional depression of the sensitivity of the respiratory center to carbon dioxide).

Homeostatic Mechanisms

In following his own admonition to consider tolerance to each of the actions of morphine separately rather than collectively, Martin[218] has convincingly demonstrated that tolerance to certain manifestations of morphine's actions is the result of normal coordination of physiologic function. For example, tolerance develops to panting induced by morphine in the dog. Panting is the usual mechanism by which body temperature can be lowered rapidly in the dog. Morphine apparently lowers the set point of the thermoregulatory centers and panting ensues. When body temperature declines to the new set point, panting ceases, but can be reinstituted by placing the dog in a hot environment. Thus, the degree of panting to subsequent doses of morphine will be determined by the amount of adjustment required to maintain body temperature at the lower level determined by the persistent action of morphine on the hypothalamic thermoregulatory centers.

Learning as a Factor in Tolerance

An interesting series of experiments by Mitchell and co-workers[4,86,179,180] demonstrated that rats given morphine and tested for analgesia (hot-plate method) on two separate occasions exhibited significantly less analgesia when tested after the second and subsequent doses of morphine (compared to the initial dose) regardless of the period of time (six hours or more) between the doses. The difference in the analgesic effectiveness of morphine was evident only in those groups of animals which were both given morphine and placed in the test situation (with the "hot"-plate set at either ambient or elevated temperatures) on the first occasion. Groups of rats given a first dose of morphine without testing or tested without first receiving morphine, could not be distinguished in their analgesic responses from naïve animals given morphine and tested both for the first time. The authors concluded that there is a drug-test interaction by which the animals acquire a significant degree of tolerance, which could be considered as an example of state-dependent learning.[172,239] It should be noted that in the experiments mentioned above, additional degrees of tolerance to the analgesic effects of morphine could be induced by chronic administration of the drug over a period of days. In other words, experience with the drug-test interaction is but one factor in the course of tolerance development to morphine.

Another example of the role of drug-test interactions in a diminishing sensitivity to morphine is found in an old report of Simon and Eddy.[308] These authors noted that the effect of a second dose of morphine was consistently less than that of the first dose on the maze performance of rats regardless of the time (up to four weeks) separating the two doses. Additional exposures to the maze or additional weekly doses of morphine between the initial dose-test and the second dose-test did not affect the degree of tolerance. Unfortunately, the experiment did not include control groups of animals which received neither morphine nor the maze test initially.

Learning has been related to tolerance in still another context, namely, that there are certain similarities between the development of tolerance and the acquisition of ability (learning). The similarities include time course for development, modification of the processes by similar factors (e.g., inhibitors of protein synthesis interfere with both), and reports of inter-animal transfer of memory and of tolerance by brain extracts.[342]

TOLERANCE TO GENERAL DEPRESSANTS OF THE CENTRAL NERVOUS SYSTEM

A major review of this subject by Kalant, LeBlanc, and Gibbins[172]* has just been published. There is no point in duplicating the effort and extensive discussions of these authors. Therefore, the following is a summary of the subject, which is based in part on their recent review. Additional references are cited where a particular point requires special emphasis or support from the literature.

The category of general depressants of the central nervous system comprises a large number and variety of chemical and pharmacological classes of drugs and poisons including alcohols, barbiturates, minor tranquilizers, gaseous and volatile anesthetics, organic solvents, etc. Over the years and still today, most of these substances have been used and abused for medical and nonmedical purposes, and in many instances, the results have included the development of tolerance.

When the pharmacology of the individual agents included in the category of general depressants is considered, one is impressed more with the similarities than with the differences found among the agents. And for the most part, the major differences are quantitative and related to differences in dispositional factors (tissue uptake, metabolism, etc.). The points of similarity include many of the features of tolerance to the effects of the depressants, and there is a widely held impression that cross tolerance is extensive among the general depressants. It seems appropriate then to consider tolerance phenomena for the general depressants as a single group.

In the discussion that follows, solvents and gases used as general anesthetics will be mostly ignored because 1) tolerance usually does not present a problem in their clinical use, 2) few studies have been made on tolerance development to these agents, and 3) the extent of tolerance development is probably not great in view of their rapid elimination from the body and the intermittent exposure which characterizes the use and abuse of these agents by most subjects.[54,192,209,265,309] On the other hand, there is no reason to believe that tolerance phenomena cannot develop when there is very frequent or continuous administration of volatile or gaseous depressants and there are anecdotal reports to that effect.[54,192,209] Also subjects tolerant to other general depressants demonstrate cross tolerance to general anesthetic agents.[6,120,156]

Tolerance to the Effects of Ethanol

Although all lower molecular weight alcohols can act as depressants, only ethanol has been subject to widespread social and medicinal use.

*The author wishes to thank Dr. Eugene Le Blanc for making available a preprint of the review which facilitated the preparation of this chapter.

Studies of tolerance development to the effects of alcohols are likewise confined almost entirely to ethanol. The principal pharmacologic effects of ethanol, including those on peripheral structures (e.g., gastrointestinal tract, cardiovascular system), can be attributed primarily, if not exclusively, to the actions of ethanol within the central nervous system.[167,168] Within the central nervous system, increasing concentrations of alcohol produce a progressive and simultaneous impairment of functions attributed to cortical and subcortical areas, with the preponderance of ethanol's actions being subcortical,[168] especially with small to moderate doses of the drug. At all levels of the central nervous system, the direct actions of ethanol are depressant; any apparent stimulation has been attributed to disinhibition produced by actions of ethanol on remote centers, particularly to its actions on the reticular cell core of the midbrain and brain stem. For example, increased excitability of the cerebral cortex, facilitation of spinal reflexes, and overt behavioral changes of an excitatory type have all been related to the suppression of inhibitory systems by ethanol (disinhibition or release phenomena).[167,168] Hence, the various effects characterizing mild to marked intoxication with alcohol lie on a spectrum of minimal to severe depression of neuronal activity. In the naïve, nontolerant individual, the effects include changes in behavioral, neurologic, autonomic, and endocrine functions, and in all cases the effects are manifestations of progressive depression of the respective systems in relation to increasing dosage in blood (and presumably in nervous tissue) concentrations of ethanol.[82,104,105,167,168,240,306] It should be noted, however, that there are considerable differences in the concentrations of ethanol required to produce different effects. Clearly detectable effects of ethyl alcohol are present at concentrations as low as 0.025 to 0.04% in blood (e.g., positional nystagmus, EEG arousal), whereas others become evident only at much higher levels (e.g., depression of spinal reflexes between 0.1 and 0.3% and cessation of respiration at 0.5% or higher depending on the species).[168] Failure to recognize these features of the pharmacology of ethanol has led to controversy and misunderstanding of tolerance phenomena. As for any other drug it is essential to specify the particular effect and dose range when considering tolerance to ethanol.

Although there are many reports concerning tolerance phenomena for ethanol, relatively few have been of quantitative nature. The techniques for measuring tolerance to the effects of alcohol and other depressant drugs have been reviewed.[172] Measures of tolerance to depressant drugs have included changes in 1) lethal dose, 2) EEG responses, 3) seizure threshold, 4) duration of loss of the righting reflex or sleep, (5) motor coordination (i. e., ability to maintain a position or perform a coordinated movement), and 6) various behavioral tests. In addition, attempts to measure tolerance to the effects of chronic ethanol intoxication on subjective feelings and mood[229] have been made. There is no *a priori* reason why any test based on measurement of a function which exhibits a dose-dependent change to a drug cannot be used to monitor the development and disappearance of tolerance to that particular drug effect. In choosing among possible tests, one should recognize 1) that tolerance does not necessarily develop at an equal rate to all the effects of a drug, 2) that it may be necessary to discriminate between the effects of relatively small increments of dosage where the degree of tolerance development is small, 3) phenomena which are objectively quantifiable and specific (i. e., based on a direct effect of the drug on a system rather than a nonspecific indication of the general state of the subject's well being) are generally more convincing and acceptable measures than those which are not objective and specific, and 4) that none of the tests of tolerance phenomena provide an indication of the mechanism(s) underlying the phenomena. The last point is particularly relevant to behavioral tests of tolerance where it may be impossible to measure separately changes in sensation, perception, reflex coordination, intellect, motivation, etc. The effects of alcohol on behavior and tolerance development to these effects have been reviewed by Goldberg[105,106] and Mello.[239]

Acute vs. Chronic Tolerance

Three types of observations lead to the suggestion that significant degrees of tolerance can develop acutely, even during a single exposure to ethanol. 1) Mellanby and many others[168,172] have reported that the degree of effect is greater during the rising (onset) phase of alcohol concentrations in venous blood than in the declining (recovery) phase. 2) The degree of intoxication at a given venous blood level is greater when that level is achieved rapidly than when it develops more slowly.[168] Both of these observations can be criticized on the basis that venous blood concentrations of ethanol may not have been representative of tissue concentrations at the times the measurements were made.[121,168,172] 3) However, this criticism cannot be raised for experiments in which relatively constant blood levels are maintained, and under such conditions, ataxia, nystagmus, ear drop, and diuresis induced by ethanol have diminished or disappeared.[172] As in the case of the narcotic analgesics, one wonders if differences in the rate of acquisition of tolerance to ethanol are based more on the choice of experimental conditions than on inherent limitations of the biological systems. Kalant[168] has stated that, "It is not unreasonable to speculate that the adaptation which occurs in the later portion of a single acute intoxication may involve essentially the same process as that which gives rise to the increased tolerance during repeated intoxication." Certainly the data do *not* support the often repeated statement that tolerance to the effects of alcohol develops only after years of repeated intoxication.[160]

Dosage and the Onset

Maximal degrees of tolerance to ethanol-induced impairment of motor function in rats can be developed within approximately 20 days of chronic administration of moderate doses.[8,197,351] Detectable degrees of tolerance are reported to develop within a few days to electroencephalographic and behavioral effects of ethanol in monkeys,[132] and to the depression of operant behavior in rats[199] And, as noted above, tolerance may be evident during a single exposure to the drug. Tolerance to a variety of effects in several species, including man, has been observed after two or three weeks of chronic administration,[172] but most of the studies have not attempted to detect the earliest possible evidence of tolerance.

The rate of tolerance development has been accelerated by increasing the daily dosage of ethanol. For example, maximal tolerance to the impairment of motor coordination in rats developed within 13 to 16 days at a daily dose of 6 g/kg[171] and in 19 to 22 days with a gradual increase from 3 to 9 g/kg/day.[197] A faster rate of tolerance development has been manifest by subjects given experience in the test situation under the influence of ethanol compared to those tested in the sober state and subsequently given the same quantities of alcohol.[38,171,172,239,253] The latter situations are comparable to the drug-test interactions described above for the development of tolerance to the analgesic actions of morphine. Kalant et al.[172] have suggested the term "behaviorally augmented tolerance" for situations in which the subjects appear to "learn" how to deal with the intoxicated state. It is interesting to note that tolerance based on experience in the intoxicated state is not necessarily limited to the specific test conditions but appears to generalize to other tests or conditions.[172,196]

Degree of Tolerance

Very few quantitative studies are available, but those few support the generally held impression that tolerance development is relatively low grade for most of the effects of ethanol, and that tolerance is easily overcome by simply increasing the dose.[172,295] LeBlanc et al.[197] have demonstrated that tolerance to ethanol-induced impairment of motor coordination in the rat involves an apparently parallel and progressive shift of the dose-response curve to the right. In other words, any degree of impairment produced by the initial dose of ethanol to a naïve subject can be produced after tolerance development by increasing the dose of alcohol. Newman and Lehman[262] also demonstrated an apparently parallel shift of the dose-response curve to the right as tolerance developed to the effects of alcohol on grossly observable behavior of dogs. The maximal degree of tolerance (estimated by the shift in the dose-response curve) was between 33%[197,262] and 50%.[171] Maynert and Klingman[231] determined the blood concentrations of alcohol at which dogs recovered from ataxia induced by intravenous doses of the drug. They observed a progressive increase in the concentrations at recovery up to a maximum of a 100% increase which was produced by a dose five times larger than that initially required to produce ataxia. Further increments of dosage did not lead to further increases in the plasma concentrations of ethanol at recovery. On the other hand, almost complete tolerance has been reported for the ethanol-induced elevation of electroshock seizure threshold in rats.[8]

It has been stated by many authors that tolerance does not develop to the lethal effects of ethanol, and there is no evidence to the contrary.[172,295] However, it has been suggested[172] that this may be the result of experimental limitations rather than a characteristic of biological systems, since it has not been possible to administer near lethal doses of ethanol on a regular basis without causing a marked deterioration in the physical well-being of the subject. An interesting observation which is of great importance in the interpretation of experiments on mechanisms of tolerance is that of Kalant et al.[171] who found that behaviorally-augmented tolerance developed more rapidly and reached the same magnitude as that developed by chronic administration of ethanol alone.

Disappearance of Tolerance and Residual Effects

The experiments of LeBlanc et al.[197] on tolerance to ethanol-induced impairment of motor coordination in rats demonstrated that there was a progressive shift of the dose-response curve to the left (i. e., recovery toward the control curve) after the chronic administration of ethanol was stopped. Detectable degrees of recovery were evident within the first week of abstinence and essentially complete recovery was observed within 12 days. In another series of experiments, these same authors[171] noted that although no residual tolerance could be detected 17 days after the last daily dose of ethanol, the rats reacquired the same maximal degree of tolerance in a shorter period of time than in the initial cycle of chronic administration of alcohol. In fact, there was a progressive reduction in the time required to reach maximal tolerance with each successive cycle (16 days on and 17 days off ethanol) of chronic administration of ethanol (i.e., the number of days to reach maximal tolerance in the first cycle was 13 to 16, in the second cycle was 7 to 13, and in the third cycle was 7, and in the fourth cycle was 4).

Tolerance to Effects of Ethanol in vitro

Apparently, contraction of the isolated frog heart is depressed by ethanol and despite the continued presence of ethanol in the perfusing solution, contractile activity gradually recovers.[172] Ethanol depresses the release of acetylcholine from cerebral cortical slices in vitro, and when the slices are prepared from animals tolerant to ethanol, the depressant effect of ethanol on acetylcholine release in vitro is no longer evident, even though the spontaneous rate of release is the same in tissues from nontolerant and ethanol-tolerant animals.[169]

Also, in brain slices, the rate of active transport of cations and the activity of Na, K-stimulated Mg-dependent adenosine triphosphatase (Na,K-ATPase) were both depressed by ethanol added in vitro.[154] When the spontaneous rate of transport and enzyme activity were measured in vitro in the absence of ethanol, they were higher in slices from ethanol-tolerant animals compared to nontolerant animals.[155] Perhaps the increase in the spontaneous activity was a manifestation of a tolerance mechanism; that is, a higher concentration of ethanol may be required to reduce the activities to the same absolute value in the alcohol-tolerant than in the control animals.

Dispositional Factors in Tolerance to Ethanol

There is considerable evidence[104,306] that in the naive subject the effects of ethanol correlate well with the doses administered, and correlate even better with the concentrations of alcohol in the blood. It is apparent that ethanol equilibrates rapidly between blood and the central nervous system[113,350] and that the rate of penetration from blood to brain is not altered by chronic administration of ethanol.[90,91,197,201] The importance of these facts to the analysis of tolerance mechanisms is obvious. Augmentation of the rate of elimination of alcohol from the blood as animals become tolerant is a potential tolerance mechanism which should be fairly easy to demonstrate. On the other hand, a reduction in the sensitivity of the tissue affected by ethanol can be detected by observing the recovery of function in the presence of blood alcohol levels which previously depressed the function. Both of these approaches to the problem of tolerance have been pursued widely in the case of ethyl alcohol.

Although a number of dispositional factors have been invoked at one time or another to explain tolerance phenomena for ethanol,[172,295] only an increased rate of metabolism of ethanol is seriously considered as a factor contributing to the development of tolerance.[172,241,242,244,285,295,348] Evidence for an increased rate of ethanol metabolism accompanying chronic administration of the drug has been conflicting.[172,244,295] However, it is now recognized that several factors (e.g., diet, schedule of alcohol administration, condition of the liver) determine the rate of ethanol metabolism, and where these have been adequately controlled, the experimental evidence is persuasive that chronic administration of ethanol is accompanied by an increased rate of ethanol metabolism.[125,147,183,246]

The biochemical basis of the augmentation of ethanol metabolism is not totally clear. First of all, there is uncertainty as to the rate limiting factor in ethanol metabolism; both limited alcohol dehydrogenase and a limited rate of reoxidation of reduced nicotinamide adenine dinucleotide phosphate[108,347] (formed during alcohol oxidation) have been suggested. Secondly, some authors have associated ethanol tolerance with increased activity of hepatic enzymes (alcohol dehydrogenase, catalase, microsomal oxidases) while others have denied a cause-effect relationship. (See reviews[210,244,347,348] for details and critical analyses.) Finally, it must be recognized that a number of factors influence the rate of ethanol metabolism in vivo and in vitro, and that in vitro experiments are subject to the introduction of artifacts and may not be representative of what is occurring in the intact organism.

It should be noted that the increased rate of ethanol metabolism was a function of the amount and duration of ethanol ingestion,[244,246] and that the increased rate diminished when alcohol administration was discontinued. There was no innate difference between alcoholics (in the abstinence phase) and nonalcoholics in their rate of metabolism of an acute dose of ethanol,[198] and both exhibited enhanced rates of metabolism to the same degree following chronic ingestion of alcohol.[242,244,245,285]

The magnitude of the increase in the rate of ethanol metabolism in vivo is relatively small, in the order of 60 to 100% over the control rate.[147,172,285] The significance of the small increase in the rate of elimination of ethanol has been discussed in detail by Kalant et al.[172] The essence of their conclusions is that while it is possible to attribute a shortening in the duration of the period of intoxication and a slight reduction of the peak intensity of intoxication to an enhanced rate of ethanol metabolism under certain conditions (low doses administered orally), there are other situations (large doses, parenteral administration) in which no significant changes in intensity would be evident because of the zero order kinetics of ethanol elimination. Furthermore, alterations in the rate of metabolism cannot account for the observations in alcohol-tolerant subjects of lesser degrees of functional impairment at blood levels equal to or greater than those clearly affecting nontolerant subjects.[90,91,161,172,197,202,231,239,262,295] Therefore, except for shortening the duration of action, enhancement of alcohol metabolism plays a relatively minor role in tolerance phenomena for ethanol. The primary basis of tolerance phenomena appears to involve unknown changes and mechanisms within the nervous system.

Tolerance to the Effects of Barbiturates

Most of the features of tolerance to barbiturates are analogous to those described for ethanol tolerance, and in fact, there is good evidence for the existence of cross tolerance between ethanol and the barbiturates. Differences that have been reported are largely quantitative and can be explained for the most part on the basis of dispositional factors.

It is important to recognize that individual barbiturates differ considerably among themselves in some of their physicochemical properties and in their distribution and fate in the body.[299] The most widely studied barbiturates in terms of tolerance phenomena include thiopental (rapid penetration of membranes and equilibration between plasma and tissues, very rapid onset and short duration of action, steep dose-response curve), pentobarbital (intermediate in rate of onset and duration of action, extensively metabolized in liver), phenobarbital and barbital (slow onset and long duration of action, shallow dose-response curve; barbital is excreted almost completely in the unmetabolized state). Such differences obviously must be kept in mind when one evaluates dosage intervals, metabolic fate, etc., as factors in tolerance phenomena.

Unfortunately, there is very limited information on the quantitative relationships of pharmacologic effects to plasma and nervous tissue concentrations of the barbiturates. In the case of thiopental,[216] and other barbiturates which equilibrate very rapidly between plasma and brain, one might expect to find close agreement between plasma and brain concentrations of the drug. Where there is a delay in reaching an equilibrium between plasma and nervous tissue (e. g., pentobarbital[216] and phenobarbital[36]) it would be expected that the intensity of effect would correlate more closely with brain than with plasma levels of the drugs, especially at early times after administration when the two are not yet in equilibrium. Thus far, two studies of pentobarbital in animals have demonstrated a relationship between brain levels of the drug and the duration (sleeping time[166]) or intensity (several behavioral tasks[211]) of its effects. On the other hand, there was practically no correlation between plasma levels of pentobarbital and the subjective reports of mood changes in man.[134]

In qualitative terms, the effects of the many barbiturates are almost identical to those of ethanol, and many of the same tests and types of experiments have been used in studies of tolerance phenomena. In general, there is a dose-related depression of nervous system functions. However, certain types of behavior are increased, while other behaviors are decreased when the subject is under the influence of barbiturates. As is claimed for ethanol, the primary action of barbiturates is a depressant one on all tissues including the central nervous system; overt signs of stimulation are generally attributed to depression of inhibitory systems, particularly those of the brain stem and midbrain reticular formation.[230] (On the other hand, there are data to support the view that certain barbiturates have the potential to stimulate neuronal cells directly.[68,303])

Acute Tolerance

Evidence of the development of acute tolerance to thiopental[31,70,231] and to pentobarbital[231] was found in the observations that as the size of a single dose was increased, the plasma concentrations at the time of disappearance of the effect (ataxia in dogs,[231] anesthesia in man[31,70]) also increased. In the case of the dogs, the increase in the plasma concentrations at recovery amounted approximately to a doubling when the dose producing ataxia was increased fivefold. It would appear that the nervous system can develop significant, if not maximal (see below), degrees of tolerance to the barbiturates (and other depressants[231]) very rapidly. Other evidence of acute tolerance to single doses has been presented for the thiopental-depression of cerebral oxygen consumption in dogs,[9] for pentobarbital-induced sleeping times in rats,[15,16] for amobarbital-induced sleeping time in mice,[264] for avoidance behavior in rats (including tolerance after single small doses given into the cerebral ventricles),[354] and for hexobarbital anesthesia in rabbits.[325] From these studies, it is not clear as to what latency existed for tolerance development since any drug remaining from the initial dose would have added to the second (test) dose and thereby obscured the detection of tolerance.[15,16,310,312,325,354] However, maximal degrees of tolerance were evident between 12 and 24 hours for pentobarbital sleeping time[15,16,312,354] and, if the intervals between the initial and test doses were 48 hours or longer, no tolerance to the test dose was detected.[15,16,312] A similar experiment with thiopental-induced sleeping time in rats indicated that maximal tolerance to a second dose occurred 21 hours after the initial dose.[310]

So far it is uncertain whether the degree of acute tolerance depends on the peak concentration of drug in the brain or on the intensity of the depression. It is claimed that the degree of acute tolerance does not depend in any major way on the duration of exposure to the drug,[231] but the data on which this claim is based are not convincing in view of the near impossibility of reducing the exposure time below the elimination time for a single dose. Maynert and Klingman have discussed the limited evidence which favors the conclusion that a common mechanism may underlie acute and chronic tolerance phenomena for general depressants.[231]

Onset and Degree of Tolerance

In light of the experiments just discussed, one must seriously entertain the notion that many of the published data concerning the onset of tolerance were determined more by a choice of a particular barbiturate and of the dosing and testing schedules than by any inherent limitations on the rate at which an organism can develop tolerance to the barbiturates and other general depressants. Kalant et al.[172] have summarized the past 30 years' literature related to the onset and degree of tolerance. It is evident that tolerance has been detected within a matter of days in mice, rats, rabbits, and dogs. In these same species, the degree of tolerance with few exceptions fell within the range of a 25 to 60% reduction in the effect. Jaffe and Sharpless[157] detected behavioral and neurological signs of tolerance, particularly evident as a shortening of the duration of action of intravenous pentobarbital in cats after five days of continuous intoxication. Fraser[95] has reviewed the development of tolerance in man and has noted that reaction time and motor coordination measures began to recover within four days and were essentially normal after seven days of administration of secobarbital or pentobarbital (0.4 g daily).

On the other hand, more than 70 days of regular administration passed before the number of hours of sleep per day decreased to the number found in the 30 days preceding daily administration of the drugs.

There are obvious difficulties in estimating the threshold dose for inducing tolerance to the barbiturates. In addition to the great variability in responding to minimally effective doses, it is necessary to take into account the differences in absorption from different routes of administration, the dosing schedule in relation to the rate of elimination, the particular effect under study (tolerance does not necessarily develop uniformly to all effects), and the fact that more than one mechanism probably underlies the development of tolerance.

Maximal degrees of tolerance, as measured by the decrease in the effect of a constant dose of drug or by estimating the increment of dose required to maintain a constant effect, fall within a relatively narrow and limited range (25 to 60% as noted above). The only attempts to study the change in dose-response relationships with the development of tolerance to the barbiturates have been those of Aston.[15,16] It appears from his studies that there is a parallel shift to the right (i. e., increasing doses are required to produce equivalent periods of loss of the righting reflex) as rats become tolerant to pentobarbital. The degree of shift was less for male (12%) than for female (40%) rats.[16]

It should be noted there can be marked variations in the degree of tolerance between individuals[95,145] and even within a single subject on different days.[145] The factors responsible for the variability are not known, but diet,[145] emotional excitement,[231] and drug interactions[285] can be suggested as possibilities. Despite the variability, there is a definite maximum dose of barbiturate which can be tolerated by each individual, and exceeding that dose by even a small amount (e. g., 0.1g added to a dose of 1 or 2 g) can produce a markedly increased degree of intoxication.[95]

Maynert and Klingman[231] have suggested that the degree of tolerance is less to greater degrees of neurologic impairment (e. g., ataxia vs. inability to walk at all). Moreover, it is commonly stated that there is little or no increase in the lethal dose after chronic administration of the barbiturates in doses sufficient to induce tolerance to the sedative and hypnotic effects.[116,145,295] The situation with the barbiturates is quite unlike that for the narcotic analgesics where subjects may acquire considerable tolerance to a dose of morphine which is 100 times the usual therapeutic dose,[95] and considerably above the lethal dose for nontolerant subjects.

Stevenson and Turnbull[324] have reported some interesting observations which lead to a note of caution on the interpretation of tolerance experiments, especially in relation to speculation about mechanism. They used the change in sleeping time (loss of the righting reflex) induced by chronic barbital administration as an index of tolerance and correlated this with the brain concentrations of barbital-^{14}C (test dose) and of total barbital (i.e., both the radioactive drug from the acute test dose and nonradioactive barbital from preceding maintenance doses). Although they observed no difference between control and barbital-treated (100 to 400 mg/kg/day for 32 days) rats in either the sleeping times or the concentrations of radioactive barbital in the brains following the test dose (see also 71, 381), they did find a progressive increase (up to 150% of control) in the *total* barbital concentrations in the brains of barbital-treated animals. Thus, tolerance was evident only as the increase in brain concentrations of total barbital upon awakening, and not by any change in the duration of sleeping time. Also of importance is that while measurements of the brain uptake of a single dose of radioactive barbital were not different in control and barbital-tolerant animals, the total content of the drug in brain was significantly higher in the tolerant rats. The latter observation demonstrates the validity of criticism directed at experiments in which tracer doses of a radioactive drug are used acutely to compare the distribution of drug in tolerant and nontolerant subjects. Finally, it is worth noting that chronic administration of barbital led to a marked shortening of the sleeping time to an acute dose of pentobarbital, and again, while the brain levels of radioactive pentobarbital at awakening were the same in control and barbital-treated animals, the concentration of total barbiturate (i.e., barbital plus pentobarbital) was seven times greater in the tolerant rats.

Disappearance of Tolerance and Residual Effects

In terms of acute tolerance to sleep induced by pentobarbital in rats, it appears that tolerance is lost sometime within 48 hours following a single dose, since little or no reduction in sleeping time was noted to subsequent doses given at intervals of 48 hours or longer.[15,16,312]

From the available studies, one can roughly estimate that a period of several days is required for the disappearance of tolerance following chronic administration of the barbiturates. Stevenson and Turnbull have noted that near maximal tolerance to the hypnotic effects of pentobarbital was evident two days after the last regular dose and that responding had returned to pretolerant levels after six days.[323,324] Similar time periods were noted for monkeys[377] and dogs,[231] and Isbell and Fraser have stated that tolerance was not evident following recovery from the withdrawal syndrome in barbiturate-dependent patients.[145]

Hypersensitivity or intolerance to the barbiturates has been described in scattered reports over the past 35 years.[15,145,352] Seevers and Tatum[297] observed that dogs first became tolerant and then abruptly became intolerant to daily doses of barbital that they had been receiving for a month or more. Whereas they had exhibited moderate degrees of depression during the course of chronic administration of large daily doses (60 to 100 mg/kg), they rather suddenly became severely intoxicated (stupor, prostration, anorexia). This was followed within a few days by the animal's death, and the investigators attributed the intolerance to pathologic changes observed in the nervous system at necropsy. Another possibility to be considered is cumulation of the barbital due to impairment of excretion.

More recently, Aston[15,18] reported a more subtle form of hypersensitivity to the hypnotic effect of pentobarbital. Rats exhibited a prolonged sleeping time to a third dose of pentobarbital approximately one month after receiving two successive daily doses of the drug. (Incidentally, it appeared that the first dose initiated tolerance since the sleeping time was less after the second than after the first dose.) The dose-response curve for the "post-tolerant" animal appeared to be shifted to the left in a parallel manner relative to that for the nontolerant rats. The mean increase in sensitivity was 14% in male rats[15] and 24% in female rats.[18] Also, it was noted that the anesthetic induction time was significantly shorter in the post-tolerant, hypersensitive rats. The explanation for this phenomenon is not yet clear. Certainly it does not represent a cumulative effect of the three doses of the drug, and it seems unlikely that the barbiturate hypersensitivity can be attributed to brain damage in this situation. It may reflect a decreased ability of the liver to metabolize pentobarbital; some investigators have reported that the drug metabolizing capability of the liver is reduced below normal following a period of increased metabolic capacity associated with the chronic administration of barbiturates.[323] This explanation is supported by the finding that post-tolerant hypersensitivity was evident to pentobarbital administered intraperitoneally but not to that injected into the cerebral ventricles.[324] It is not supported by Aston's report of no difference in the rate of disappearance of the drug from plasma of post-tolerant and nontolerant rats.[17]

Tolerance to the Effects of Barbiturates in vitro

The only report of tolerance development to a barbiturate in vitro is that of Goldstein[111] who observed that barbital suppressed the growth of *E. coli B* and inhibited the enzyme D-alanine oxidase. Cells grown in a barbital-containing medium accumulated greater than the usual amounts of alanine oxidase and racemase, which in turn overcame the inhibition of alanine metabolism by barbital.

Dispositional Factors in Tolerance to Barbiturates

Drug metabolism is the only dispositional factor to receive serious attention experimentally as a potential contributor to the development of tolerance to the barbiturates. Biotransformation of the barbiturates has been reviewed in detail[32,215,323,368] as has the well-known phenomenon of induction of drug metabolizing enzymes by barbiturates and other drugs.[55,212] Most of these reviews make note of the implications of an augmentation of drug metabolism for tolerance to the barbiturates. The subject has been discussed most recently by Remmer.[278] (Refer also to the chapter by Misra in this text.) From the extensive literature on these subjects, the following points seem clear. The chronic administration of any one of the many barbiturates to a variety of species is accompanied by a shortening of the duration of action (i.e., usually measured as the sleeping time or the period of loss of the righting reflex), which can be correlated with an increased rate of metabolism of the barbiturate by the liver (usually determined in vitro using hepatic microsomal preparations or in vivo by the rate of decline of plasma levels of the barbiturate). Although Remmer[277,278] has stated that a single anesthetic dose of hexobarbital in dogs was sufficient to stimulate drug metabolism and to increase the rate of decline of its concentration in plasma, it is not yet clear in quantitative terms what contribution biotransformation makes to the various phenomena of *acute* tolerance described above.[176]

Besides accounting for a shortened duration of action for those barbiturates which are metabolized rapidly and extensively in the liver, an increased rate of metabolism could contribute to a lessening of the peak intensity of the drug's effect in those cases where the drug does not equilibrate rapidly between plasma and nervous tissue, or where the drug is administered by routes (e.g., gastrointestinal, intraperitoneal) for which the venous blood flow is primarily through the liver by way of the portal circulation.

Because of the variety of drugs able to induce drug metabolism and because of the general nature of this induction (i.e., the increased biotransformation extends to a variety of drugs metabolized by a number of different reactions), changes in metabolism could potentially explain the development of cross tolerance as well as a number of drug interactions.

On the other hand, it is certain that drug metabolism alone is not the basis of all phenomena of tolerance to the barbiturates and other general depressants. It cannot explain tolerance phenomena related to recovery of function at plasma and brain concentrations of the drug which were associated with marked depression in the nontolerant subject. (See the extensive list of references cited by Kalant et al.[172]) It probably does not contribute significantly to tolerance development to barbital which is metabolized to a very limited extent in most species. And it probably does not explain tolerance developed to barbiturates administered into the cerebral ventricles.[354]

In summary, Remmer[278] has presented a scheme which arranges the barbiturates in a spectrum according to their duration of action and rate of metabolism. He concludes that augmentation of metabolism is the primary factor in tolerance to short-acting barbiturates (e.g., hexobarbital), while a change in sensitivity of the nervous system is the primary factor in tolerance to long-acting, slowly metabolized barbiturates (e.g., barbital and phenobarbital). For those barbiturates which are intermediate in their duration of action and rate of metabolism, both factors play a role with metabolism tending to be dominant. The apparent predominance of metabolism may be related to the facts that most studies of tolerance to the barbiturates have utilized measures of duration of action rather than intensity of effect, and the drug has been administered by the oral or intraperitoneal routes instead of intravenously.

Tolerance to the Effects of Other Sedative-Hypnotics and Minor Tranquilizers

Very few studies of tolerance to the effects of the drugs in these classes have been reported, and most of the published reports are not of a quantitative nature. It is usually presumed that tolerance to these drugs is essentially no different from that described for ethanol and the barbiturates because of the generally close similarity in the pharmacological actions of the depressant drugs. In general, it appears that the development of tolerance to the depressant drugs is comparable in degree to that observed for alcohol.[295]

Tolerance to the effects of meprobamate on the human electroencephalogram,[172] and on behavioral performance in rats[172] and cats[281,375] has been reported. Almost nothing is known about the nature of tolerance to meprobamate except that it is possible to augment the rate of metabolism of meprobamate by the hepatic microsomal system[172,212] and that, in addition, there is a diminished sensitivity of the nervous system in the tolerant state.[172]

Another chemical group of depressants which has received limited attention in studies of tolerance is the benzodiazepines. Tolerance is reported to develop to the following effects of chlordiazepoxide: depression of righting reflex in mice[107] and rats,[135] interference with ability of rats to maintain their position on an inclined plane[135] and of mice on a rotating rod,[107] reduction of spontaneous motor activity in mice,[107] elevation of the electroshock seizure threshold in mice,[107] and alterations of avoidance-escape behavior in mice.[107] In rats, the development of tolerance was accompanied by a doubling of the rate of disappearance of ^{14}C-

chlordiazepoxide from plasma and brain.[135] Tolerance to oxazepam[214] was selective on operant behavior in that it developed to the rate decreasing effect on the unpunished component but not to the rate increasing action on the punished component of a multiple schedule of reinforcement in rats. The authors felt that as tolerance developed to the depressant effect on the unpunished component that the stimulant effect on the punished behavior was unmasked. Lastly, acute tolerance has been observed to the depressant effects of diazepam on the linguomandibular reflex in cats, and has been attributed to metabolism of diazepam to *N*-desmethyl diazepam which antagonizes the depressant actions of diazepam.[25] The *N*-desmethyl compound is only weakly depressant itself and acute tolerance was not observed to its effects.[25] Diazepam-tolerant cats do not exhibit cross tolerance to other depressants of the linguomandibular reflex such as phenobarbital and methocarbomal.[26] On the other hand, one chronic alcoholic subject studied by de Silva et al. was able to tolerate daily doses of diazepam as high as 200 mg without major side effects, and the blood concentrations of diazepam and its major metabolite (*N*-demethylated diazepam, RO5-2180) were proportionally greater in this alcoholic subject that in nonalcoholic persons receiving lower doses and exhibiting mild intoxication.[25]

Maynert and Klingman[231] have reported the development of acute tolerance to ataxia induced in dogs by paraldehyde and trichloroëthanol, and they noted that tolerance was both qualitatively and quantitatively similar to that described above for ethanol and the barbiturates.

Cross Tolerance among Ethanol, Barbiturates, and Other Depressants

It is generally held that cross tolerance can exist between pharmacologically similar depressant drugs, even when they are from chemically distinct classes such as the alcohols, barbiturates, benzodiazepines, etc.[62,98,116,156,170,239,295,349,352] However, the experimental support for this concept is not unanimous.[170,172] There are several issues underlying the apparent contradictions concerning the subject of cross tolerance, especially as it relates to ethanol and the barbiturates.

The nature of depressant drug interactions is not adequately defined.[33,94,318] Although additive interactions are suggested by many authors, there is the distinct possibility that inhibitory or potentiative interactions may occur on the basis of augmentation or inhibition of drug metabolism in the liver.[172,212,285,337] Obviously, an understanding of the nature of the drug interactions is essential if we are to interpret experiments on cross tolerance.

The significance of induction of drug metabolizing enzymes in the liver for the phenomena of cross tolerance is not fully elucidated. While it seems clear that induction plays a prominent role in cross tolerance among nonalcoholic depressants,[21,170,212,278] the situation for cross tolerance between ethanol and other depressants is less certain.[170,182,242,248,285,311,313,332,335] However, in the reviewer's opinion, the best available evidence suggests strongly that the primary basis of cross tolerance between ethanol and the barbiturates is an alteration in the sensitivity of the nervous system, and that hepatic drug-metabolizing systems are probably involved minimally, if at all, in cross tolerance between ethanol and other depressant drugs in the intact animal.[124,170,182,248,276,335]

Just as tolerance to a single drug may be based on several different mechanisms, so too, cross tolerance may involve more than a single mechanism. Since, for the most part, we do not fully understand the tolerance mechanisms for any one drug, we are not in a position to do more than speculate about the possibilities for cross tolerance.

There are marked differences in the experimental procedures employed in studies published to date on cross tolerance, and few of the studies have included data on plasma and tissue levels of the drugs in question. The latter information is essential if we are to begin to identify and separate dispositional from functional mechanisms of cross tolerance.

Thus, while cross tolerance has been observed among the depressant drugs, little can be said in terms of the quantitative characteristics and mechanisms underlying the phenomena.

Mechanisms of Tolerance to Depressant Drugs

In this section only those mechanisms proposed specifically for tolerance to ethanol, the barbiturates and other general depressant drugs, will be considered. Theoretically, all of the mechanisms of tolerance enumerated in the second section could be entertained as possible explanations for tolerance to the effects of the depressant drugs. However, it seems clear from the data reviewed above, that alterations in the nervous system per se are significant, and quite possibly the predominant factors in tolerance phenomena for this class of drugs.

Jaffe and Sharpless[157,158,300] have attempted with only limited success to implicate their hypothesis of disuse supersensitivity in the development of tolerance to pentobarbital.

There are reports of experiments on the transfer of tissue factors from alcohol-tolerant rabbits[140] and barbital-dependent rats.[340] In the case of the rabbits, the intraperitoneal injection of a microsomal fraction of brain or liver from alcohol-tolerant rabbits lengthened the time of alcohol-induced anesthesia (measured as the absence of the corneal reflex) in naïve rabbits. The significance of this observation remains obscure, even in reference to the post-tolerance hypersensitivity to barbiturates described by Aston.[15,16] In the case of the rats, brain homogenates prepared from barbital-dependent rats decreased the sleeping time to hexobarbital in naïve rats injected intraperitoneally with the homogenate. It was noted, however, that the in vitro rate of hexobarbital metabolism by liver microsomes from rats receiving the brain homogenate was increased, and the authors attributed the apparent tolerance transfer to a stimulation of hexobarbital metabolism rather than to reduction in the sensitivity of the nervous system to the barbiturate.

There is a single report suggesting that increased brain levels of norepinephrine are responsible for x-radiation-induced tolerance to pentobarbital in rats.[250] The significance of this observation for drug-induced tolerance is not clear.

The role of state-dependent learning in the development of tolerance to ethanol has been discussed in detail elsewhere.[171,172,196,239] It should be emphasized that the only apparent difference between "learned" and "cellular" tolerance is one of rate of development. Kalant et al.[171] have shown that the *same maximal* degree of tolerance to ethanol is achieved more rapidly in rats tested repeatedly under the influence of alcohol compared to rats given repeated doses of alcohol before testing. The cellular effects of depressant drugs including ethanol have been reviewed elsewhere,[153,168,172] but they provide no clues as to mechanisms of tolerance.

Finally, Kalant et al.[172] have proposed an interesting mathematical or kinetic formulation in an attempt to interrelate the multiple factors which play a role in the development of tolerance (and physical dependence) to the nonopiate classes of psychoactive drugs. Their fundamental premise is that the stimulus to adaptation (i.e., tolerance and physical dependence) includes both the concentration of the drug in the body (actually the increment of concentration above the minimal threshold concentration) and the behavioral state of the animal (including the functional demands made upon the animal). The reader is referred to the discussion by Kalant et al.[172] The value of the kinetic model is that it offers a quantitative representation of a number of phenomena and thereby sets the stage for quantitative experimental analysis of tolerance phenomena and their component factors.

TOLERANCE TO STIMULANTS

A large number of drugs have the capacity to stimulate various portions of the central nervous system. Among the stimulants, cocaine and the amphetamines are the ones most subject to dependence and abuse. Cocaine and dextroamphetamine are considered to be prototypes of dependence in the stimulant class and will be emphasized in the discussion below.

Cocaine

Tolerance development to the effects of cocaine is questionable. Cocaine users have injected up to 10 g in a single day, but it has been noted that after a period of abstinence (presumably sufficient for loss of any tolerance that may have developed) these same large doses were tolerated equally well.[156,330] The latter observation coupled with the possibility of rapid elimination of cocaine from the body[89,367,372] suggests that the injection of even very large doses does not result in tolerance to cocaine. It has been stated categorically by several authors[75,150,190,220,295] that tolerance does not develop to the excitatory effects of cocaine. Rather, there appears to be an increased sensitivity to its stimulant effects when cocaine is administered repeatedly to animals including rats, rabbits, dogs, and monkeys.[69,330]

Amphetamines

Kramer et al.[191] described the patterns and effects of chronic amphetamine intoxication. Tremendous degrees of tolerance to certain effects of the amphetamines can be developed in human subjects. Whereas the usual therapeutic dose of dextroamphetamine taken orally is in the range of 10 to 20 mg daily,[141] oral doses as large as 250 to 1,000 mg daily are not unheard of where sufficient drug is available to dependent individuals.[115,141] Even more remarkable accounts of tolerance have been given for the use of amphetamines intravenously.[191,317] During the early phases of intravenous abuse, doses of 20 to 40 mg of dextroamphetamine or methamphetamine are injected three or four times daily. But with the development of tolerance, the dose and frequency of administration are increased to the point that 100 to 300 mg doses may be injected repeatedly throughout the day. Kramer et al.[191] cited the example of an individual who injected over 1,000 mg of methamphetamine every two hours up to a total of almost 15,000 mg in a single day apparently without serious morbidity. It is to be emphasized that such remarkable degrees of tolerance do not extend to all of the effects of the amphetamines. With repeated use, most individuals eventually exhibit toxic psychoses[10,156,295] and a variety of toxic physical effects.[79,174,191]

In man, marked tolerance develops to the euphoria[284] and apparently to the acutely lethal effects produced by amphetamines as described above.[10,115,190,191] Tolerance is also apparent to the actions of amphetamines on the cardiovascular system and pupils.[10,156] Little tolerance is evident to the awakening action of these drugs as judged from their continued effectiveness in the therapy of narcolepsy[141,190] and from the persistence of insomnia in the amphetamine abuser while he continues to take the drug (i.e., until exhaustion supervenes).[191] However, tolerance does appear to develop to the suppression of REM sleep by low doses of the various amphetamines.[267]

Tolerance to the anorexigenic actions of the amphetamines is difficult to evaluate. Rosenberg et al.[284] reported tolerance to appetite suppression in a carefully controlled study in human subjects. And from the therapeutic point of view in exogenous obesity, there is little question that the degree and duration of weight loss are limited.[10,79,141,174,190] There are, however, a number of factors that influence changes in body weight (e.g., physical activity, basal metabolic rate, water balance), and in some cases these factors may simply override the anorexigenic actions of amphetamine-like drugs and give the appearance of drug tolerance.[88,190,284] It is clear that the appetite remains suppressed and weight loss may be severe in the chronic amphetamine abuser while he continues to take the drug, even on a cyclic basis.[141,191]

Thus far, animal studies have failed to clarify the issue of tolerance to the anorexigenic actions of amphetamines. Dogs and rats appeared to demonstrate tolerance to the depression of food intake by amphetamines, but nevertheless maintained a significant reduction of body weight (compared to controls) throughout long-term experiments.[190,336] Tormey and Lasagna[336] suggested that since there was persistently increased motor activity in their amphetamine-treated rats, these animals would be expected to eat more than the control animals, and comparisons of food intake would tend to indicate the development of tolerance to the anorexia. On the other hand, indirect measurements of anorexia based on changes in body weight[341] may also be influenced by extraneous factors. For example, there is a transient decrease in water intake followed by a persistent polydipsia in rats treated chronically with amphetamines.[190,336] Such a sequence of changes in water balance would mimic those expected if a brief period of anorexia were to be followed by tolerance to the anorexigenic effects of the drug.

An equally complex situation exists with regard to the development of tolerance to the effects of amphetamines on spontaneous activity, excitability, and operant behavior in animals.[172,190] In terms of grossly observed reactions to amphetamines, it is reported that they become less intense with repeated administration of the drug to rats.[80,118] But when spontaneous motor activity is measured more accurately (e.g., by means of activity cages) it is consistently found that tolerance does *not* develop to the hyperactivity produced by dextroamphetamine in rodents.[80,190,291,336,341] If anything, the animals may exhibit even greater degrees of stimulation to a constant dose of amphetamine.[190] Somewhat surprising are the reports[190,345] that tolerance *does* develop to the augmentation of spontaneous activity of mice, rats, and cats injected with methamphetamine; hypoactivity replaces the initial hyperactivity. No explanation can be offered for this discrepancy between dextroamphetamine and methamphetamine which are usually considered to be essentially identical in terms of their actions on the central nervous system.[27,141,234]

It seems clear from the initial studies of Schuster et al.[290,291] that tolerance does not develop uniformly to the effects of amphetamines on operant behavior. *d*-Amphetamine initially reduced the number of food rewards obtained by rats during two different types of food-reinforced schedules; as daily administration of the drug continued, tolerance became evident over a period of 30 days. In contrast, repeated administration of dextroamphetamine increased the rate of responding in a shock avoidance situation for as long as the drug was administered. On the basis of their observations, Schuster et al.[290] hypothesized: "Behavioral tolerance will develop in those aspects of the organism's repertoire where the action of the drug is such that it disrupts the organism's behavior meeting the enviornmental requirement for reinforcements. Conversely, where the actions of the drug enhance, or do not affect the organism's behavior in meeting reinforcement requirements we do not expect the development of behavioral tolerance." This interesting hypothesis is compatible with a recent report by Uehling,[341] but additional studies are required to reconcile it with earlier reports and to rule out other possible interpretations of the data.[190] In the meantime, it should serve to direct greater attention to the important possibilities of studying tolerance to the amphetamines as it relates to behavioral phenomena. Other effects of amphetamines in animals to which tolerance has been reported include lethality,[80] hyperthermia,[122] piloerection,[118] cardiovascular stimulation,[72] and sympathomimetic effects on smooth muscle.[396]

Almost nothing can be specified about the quantitative characteristics of tolerance to the amphetamines. Tachyphylaxis has been demonstrated for the peripheral sympathomimetic actions,[72,369] but a careful study has not been made for the other effects of the amphetamines. From anecdotal and clinical case reports one gains the impression that tremendous degrees of tolerance can be developed to certain effects of the amphetamines, while little or no tolerance may be evident to other actions of the drug. But here again, no attempt has been made to quantitate the changes.

Essentially nothing is known about the time course of tolerance. It has been detected in rats as early as the second or third day for the hyperthermic response to daily doses of amphetamine[122] and for the stimulation of spontaneous activity by methamphetamine.[190] In contrast, tolerance developed only very gradually to the effects of d-amphetamine on operant behavior in rats.[390] There is a single report of persistence of tolerance beyond a few days after cessation of chronic administration of dextroamphetamine.[290]

Finally, there are clinical impressions of cross tolerance among the amphetamines,[156] but cross tolerance has not been reported between the amphetamines and cocaine or other stimulant drugs. Cross tolerance has been shown not to develop between dextroamphetamine and LSD.[11,284]

As one would expect, there is a great deficiency in our understanding of the mechanisms underlying tolerance to the amphetamines. One recent study[83] of the disposition of the d-^{3}H-amphetamine in tolerant and nontolerant cats did not reveal any differences between the two groups. However, it is still not clear as to whether or not amphetamines can induce their own metabolism and thereby contribute to the development of tolerance to their effects.[172]

In fact, the only tolerance phenomenon to receive serious study with regard to mechanism is that of the action of amphetamines on the cardiovascular system. It is generally accepted that the amphetamines are indirectly acting sympathomimetics which produce stimulation of cardiac and vascular muscle by releasing norepinephrine from the endings of the nerves innervating the muscle.[108,141] Experiments based on this hypothesis have led Axelrod and others[21,22] to conclude that tachyphylaxis occurs as a result of amphetamine-induced depletion of the stores of norepinephrine in peripheral nerve endings. Brodie et al.[30] have shown that dextroamphetamine is metabolized to *p*-hydroxynorephedrine in various tissues and have suggested that the latter compound may be responsible for persistent depletion of norepinephrine from peripheral nerve endings. In turn, the metabolite may act as an ineffective, false transmitter released from adrenergic nerve endings in amphetamine-tolerant tissues.

Many attempts have been made to apply hypotheses developed for drug action on the peripheral autonomic nervous system to drug actions within the central nervous system. In the case of the amphetamines, there is limited evidence to support the concept that their actions within the central nervous system are related to the release of catecholamines,[251] and that the development of tolerance is accompanied by a persistent depletion of norepinephrine[118,203] and the accumulation of *p*-hydroxynorephedrine which may act as a false transmitter.[203]

Other Stimulants

Kosman and Unna[190] have summarized the few scattered reports of tolerance to other stimulants of the amphetamine-class. It appears that as far as they have been studied, tolerance phenomena for pipradrol, methylphenidate, and phenmetrazine do not differ essentially from those described above for dextroamphetamine and methamphetamine.

Caffeine

Tolerance to caffeine has been discussed by Colton et al.[53] The effects to which tolerance regularly develops in coffee drinkers include diuresis, salivation, bradycardia, and disturbances of sleep patterns (primarily a delay in onset of sleep). In all cases, tolerance is of a low grade and can be overcome by increasing the dose of caffeine. Although the data are limited, Colton et al.[53] have suggested that the basis of tolerance is a reduced sensitivity of the nervous system rather than an alteration in the biotransformation of caffeine. They also note that the reduction in caffeine-induced bradycardia may result in part from the direct stimulant actions of caffeine on the myocardium.

Nicotine

There is an extensive old literature on the subject of tolerance to nicotine that has been summarized along with the sparse reports of recent years by Larson, Haag, and Silvette.[194,195] There is little consistency to be found among the various reports which include studies of a variety of species, a large range of doses and dosage schedules, and a spectrum of effects induced by various tobacco preparations and by nicotine per se. The most common deficiency of these studies is the failure to regulate dosage size and frequency in relation to the duration of action of nicotine. As will be noted from most of the tolerance phenomena mentioned in this chapter, it is necessary to maintain a fairly constant state of intoxication in order to produce a stable level of tolerance. One cannot be certain that this condition was met for nicotine in most of the studies cited by Larson et al., especially in view of the very brief duration of action observed after parenteral administration of nicotine.

The impression gained from Larson et al. is that tolerance to nicotine is low-grade, rapidly lost after the last dose, different in degree for the different effects of nicotine, and quite variable in quantitative characteristics even among individuals of the same species. Regular smoking of tobacco products by man is associated with a reduction in (i.e., tolerance to) the nausea, light-headedness, and other discomforting symptoms described by the naive smoker. In some cases, these effects may reappear in the experienced smoker after a period of abstinence. There seems to be only minimal tolerance, if any, to the mild central nervous system stimulation and electrocardiographic changes produced by the regular use of tobacco. Human subjects do not consistently increase their daily dosage of nicotine (i.e., in terms of the number of cigarettes) in order to continue to enjoy the effects of smoking.

Tachyphylaxis to nervous system stimulation and to changes in heart rate and vascular resistance appears to be a consistent observation when successive doses are repeated within a fraction of an hour. Under such circumstances, even the lethal dose for animals has been elevated to a significant degree (Hug, unpublished data). One explanation for this type of acute tolerance relates to the well-known actions of nicotine to first stimulate and then to depress autonomic ganglia. This biphasic action on ganglia, including the adrenal medulla, could explain changes in the hemodynamic responses to nicotine given in rapidly repeated doses. In turn, the changes in hemodynamic responses could result in an altered distribution of nicotine to various body tissues, including the central nervous system. Evidence for the last point is found in the observation that there was a markedly reduced uptake of radioactive nicotine and of antipyrine (an agent which distributes freely to total body water) by the brain when these were administered after an initial dose of nicotine or any one of several other ganglionic blocking agents compared to the uptake found in the brains of animals given an initial injection of saline. The reduction in nicotine concentrations in the brain correlated inversely with an elevation of the convulsive-$dose_{50}$ (Hug, unpublished results). Other examples of tachyphylaxis are reported for isolated skeletal and smooth muscle preparations. (See Larson et al. for details.)

TOLERANCE TO HALLUCINOGENS (PSYCHOTOMIMETICS)

Although there are a variety of chemical and biological products capable of inducing hallucinations and other features of psychosis, only three principal hallucinogens, D-lysergic acid diethylamide (LSD-25), mescaline, and psilocybin, will be considered herein. In spite of the wide recognition of rather dramatic degrees of tolerance to certain of the effects of these drugs, relatively little attention has been paid to the subject in review articles[99,130,131] and in the experimental laboratory. Most of the literature on tolerance to the hallucinogens is descriptive in nature; almost nothing is known about the quantitative characteristics and mechanisms of tolerance to these drugs. Perhaps these deficiencies in our knowledge relate to the limitations of using animals for the study of drugs which primarily affect psychological processes (i.e., mood, thought patterns, etc.).

In man, the principal hallucinogens mentioned above produce changes in autonomic functions (including tachycardia, systolic hypertension, hyperthermia, mydriasis), in somatic reflexes (lowered threshold and increased amplitude of the kneejerk), and in mental status (alterations of mood, thinking, sensory perception, hallucinations) which can be measured by clinical observation and subjective questionnaires. Abramson et al.,[1] Isbell et al.,[144,146,149,151,152,370] and others[23] have convincingly demonstrated that direct tolerance develops within a few days to the above mentioned effects when a subject receives small daily doses of LSD, mescaline or psilocybin. However, it is to be noted that the magnitude of tolerance did not appear to be equivalent for the various effects.

In rats, tolerance has been described for certain of the effects of LSD and mescaline on behavior (bar pressing,[11,102,333] conditioned avoidance,[228,321] rope climbing,[100] and apparent confusion[101]) and on autonomic functions (mydriasis[102] and piloerection[101]). On the other hand, tolerance was *not* demonstrated for LSD-induced bradycardia,[101] respiratory arrest,[102] or alterations of running to escape shock.[102]

In other species, tolerance was evident to the effects of LSD on ambulation in goats,[187] on escape-running in cats,[228] and on behavior and electroencephalographic activity in rabbits.[24] Behavioral and postural changes induced by mescaline in the awake dog became progressively less with repeated doses, but there was no diminution in the mydriasis or respiratory depression caused by repeated doses of mescaline. Tolerance was not apparent to the behavioral and autonomic effects produced by very large daily doses (1 mg/kg) of LSD in the rhesus monkey.[164] From the above, the impression is gained that the choice of drug, size of dose, and species are important determinants in tolerance development to the hallucinogens. Unfortunately, the variation in experimental conditions among the various studies precludes any definitive conclusions on these points.

Observations related to dosage schedules and the time course of tolerance development are interesting though somewhat confusing. For example, Freedman et al.[100] reported that acute tolerance to impairment of rope climbing ability in rats developed when a period of 6 hours or less separated successive doses of LSD, that chronic tolerance required a dosage interval of approximately 24 hours, and that no tolerance developed if doses were separated by 8 to 22 hours or by more than 72 hours. A satisfactory explanation for this series of observations has not been offered.

Tachyphylaxis or acute tolerance has been reported for hypotensive responses to mescaline in the pentobarbital-anesthetized dog,[123] but not to behavioral, somatic and autonomic effects in man given a second dose six hours after the first.[23]

Tolerance to the LSD experience in man was evident to a second dose given at 24 hours and was virtually complete after three to four daily doses.[130,146] In rats, tolerance to the effects of daily doses of LSD on bar pressing behavior was apparent on the second day and complete within seven to eight days,[11,102] while that to depression of the rate of rope climbing was evident on the second day and complete as early as three or four days.[100,101] Tolerance to psilocybin interference with operant behavior paralleled that seen with LSD.[11] Interestingly, tolerance developed in rats more slowly (requiring up to ten days) and erratically to the effects of mescaline on rope climbing than to its effects on bar pressing for a food reinforcement (complete within two to three days).[101]

An interesting but unexplained observation is that the degree of tolerance to LSD in goats given daily microgram doses oscillated with time; that is, maximal degrees of tolerance were evident every five to six days despite a constant daily dosage schedule continued over a period of weeks.[187]

In terms of dose size, tolerance appears to develop less readily to larger doses of LSD[102] and psilocybin[11] in rats. And, as noted above, very large dâily doses of LSD failed to induce tolerance in monkeys.[164] Also, the route of administration may be important since it has been claimed that rats tolerant to mescaline injected into the cerebral ventricles were not tolerant to equivalent doses (in terms of behavioral disruption) given intraperitoneally.[333]

Man loses his tolerance to LSD by abstaining from its use for a period of three to five days.[35,146] The only reference to loss of tolerance in animals relates to mescaline-induced alterations of conditioned avoidance in rats; tolerance was evident up to eight weeks after the last 25 mg/kg dose of the drug.[321]

Cross tolerance has been demonstrated in man for LSD and mescaline,[23,370] for LSD and psilocybin,[2,151] for LSD and *N, N*-dimethyltryptamine,[283] and for LSD and several of its chemical analogues.[2,3,149] Similar examples of cross tolerance have been demonstrated in the rat.[11] There appears to be no cross tolerance between LSD and *d*-amphetamine in either man[152,284] or rats,[11,186] but amphetamine derivatives which possess greater potency as hallucinogens do induce cross tolerance to LSD in rats.[186] The generally accepted conclusion is that cross tolerance is primarily based on similarity of pharmacological actions rather than on resemblance of chemical structures.[151,370] There is a fairly close correlation between psychotomimetic potencies and the ability to induce cross tolerance to LSD.[149] However, there appears to be no cross tolerance between LSD and cannabis products.[148,307]

Very little is known about the mechanisms of tolerance to the hallucinogens. Studies of biological disposition of these agents in the body have not yet been extended to the tolerant state. Little is known about the biochemical mechanisms of action for the hallucinogens. Several authors have attempted to relate the effects of LSD to its interactions with serotonin[7,64,130,228] and other putative neurotransmitters.[130,131] However, a number of experimental observations cannot be reconciled by any one of the hypotheses put forth thus far. And none of the hypotheses provide an adequate explanation of the dramatic degrees of tolerance developed to LSD and the other hallucinogens.

Finally, it should be noted that while repeated experiences with LSD-like drugs may lessen one's anxiety about using the drug and possibly alter the intensity of its effects through one's learning to cope with the situation, it is clear that these factors alone cannot explain the remarkable tolerance developed by man and animals to some of the effects of psychotomimetics.[11,101,102]

TOLERANCE TO CANNABIS AND RELATED DRUGS

There are few answers to questions about the development of tolerance to the effects of *cannabis sativa*, its constituent chemicals and their semisynthetic derivatives. The studies up to 1938, reviewed by Walton[353] and many others reported up to recent times, suffer from inadequate experimental design (at least by current standards) and from lack of a standardized drug preparation with a known quantity and purity of chemical ingredients. The latter problem is accentuated by the instability of some cannabinols under ordinary storage conditions. While these deficiencies have been remedied in certain recent investigations, there remains a paucity of information about the quantitative and qualitative characteristics of tolerance to cannabis. Very few studies involving long-term administration of cannabis products have been reported, almost none for man. The availability of tetrahydrocannabinols (THC) and their chemical analogues in pure form offers the opportunity to obtain the needed experimental data. Additionally, application of the newly-developed analytical methods for THC and its derivatives should permit identification and quantitation of the pyrolysis products inhaled while smoking cannabis preparations.

From the data presently available, there appear to be two types of change in the sensitivity of an individual to cannabis used repeatedly, tolerance and sensitization.

Tolerance has been reported for the following effects of cannabis, cannabis extracts, or Δ^9-THC in animals: a) alterations of psychomotor activity including bar pressing operant behavior,[99] rope climbing,[99] maze performance,[130] open field behavior[227] in rats, and operant key pecking in pigeons;[29,235] b) altered locomotor activity in mice,[252] rats,[252] and dogs;[63] and c) hypothermia in rats.[207] Conversely, tolerance did not develop to the attenuation of the electroencephalogram or to the grossly observable behavioral changes induced in rabbits by daily doses of Δ^9-THC (3 mg/kg/day for six days).[205]

In man, the situation regarding tolerance to cannabis is not at all clear, primarily because there has been only one formal study of the effects of chronic cannabis intoxication. Williams et al.[366] reported that human subjects became tolerant to the effects of "pyrahexyl compound" and smoking marijuana on the electroencephalogram, autonomic functions and psychomotor activity. The principal changes in response over the course of the 26 to 31-day periods of ad libitum administration were a reduction in the drug-induced tachycardia and hyperthermia, a return of depressed alpha EEG activity to predrug levels, a loss of the euphoria, and the appearance of lassitude and indolence in place of the increased psychomotor activity. These changes occured even though the daily dose of pyrahexyl compound increased from 60 mg to as much as 2,400 mg. It appeared that tolerance developed to each increment of dosage. By comparison, there was a much less impressive increase in the number of marijuana cigarettes smoked daily, although the changes in response were similar to those observed with pyrahexyl compound.

Most studies involving human subjects have compared experienced cannabis users with naive individuals. Here the results are somewhat confusing and in great need of clarification. Although there is little tendency for most regular users to increase the dose,[54,75] it is apparent that certain effects of cannabis become modified after repeated experiences with the drug. Several authors have noted that regular users appear to control some of the psychological and behavioral effects while subjectively "high" and to perform certain functions better than nonusers given the same dose.[54,247,360] Such observations suggest the presence of a form of tolerance in the experienced user.

On the other hand, it is commonly stated that the naïve individual fails to experience many of the effects of marijuana during his initial trials with it. After several trials using the same dosage he may begin to detect the rather subtle effects of this drug. Still later in his experiences with the drug, it may be noted that he achieves his customary "high" with lower doses of marijuana. The latter phenomenon has been referred to as sensitization or "reverse tolerance."[360]

Confusion about the changes in one's sensitivity to marijuana with repeated use can probably be attributed to the fact that it is difficult to detect and to measure the subtle effects of a weak form of the drug. In such cases, variability is likely to be great, and the effects will be dependent on a variety of factors in addition to the drug itself. Most studies in animals have employed unquestionably effective doses of the drug to induce tolerance. Perhaps in man, tolerance will be clearly and consistently demonstrable when sufficiently large doses of cannabis products are used.

Cross tolerance has been observed for the behavioral suppression produced in pigeons by various tetrahydrocannabinol derivatives including Δ^9-THC, Δ^8-THC, synhexyl, and DHMP (the dimethylheptyl derivative of synhexyl).[29,236] Cross tolerance could not be demonstrated between Δ^9-THC and lysergic acid diethylamide (LSD-25) in man,[148] nor between Δ^9-THC and mescaline or LSD-25 in rats.[307] There are some indications that cross tolerance develops between ethyl alcohol and cannabis in man[165] and in rats.[263] Cannabis is known to possess sedative-hypnotic-anesthetic properties in addition to its hallucinogenic actions.[67,133,148,364] The mechanisms of tolerance to cannabis and its psychoactive constituents are unknown. There is a single report to the effect that SKF-525A, an inhibitor of many drug metabolism reactions in the liver, reversed the tolerance to Δ^9-THC in animals.[63]

One can only speculate about the mechanisms of sensitization or reverse tolerance to cannabis and its products. Speculation includes the following: 1) induction of enzymes converting THC to a pharmacologically more potent metabolite, 2) cumulation of THC or an active metabolite, 3) learned response, 4) increased sensitivity of tissues to THC. The first two points are supported by the observations that: 1) THC is converted to 11-hydroxy-THC in the body[93] and this metabolite is equally or more active than THC;[40] 2) the pharmacological effects of THC were greater when it was administered intraperitoneally than when it was injected subcutaneously[237] (i.e., the venous outflow from the peritoneum is primarily through the liver by way of the portal circulation); 3) the rate of disappearance of THC (presumably by biotransformation in the liver) is more rapid in human chronic marijuana smokers compared to human subjects who have not previously used cannabis products;[198] and 4) the metabolites of THC persist for one week or longer in human volunteers.[198]

The speculation that sensitization to marijuana is a learned response is logical in view of the fact that marijuana is a weak form of cannabis. Hence, its effects are probably influenced strongly by a number of factors other than the drug itself, especially those related to expectations for the drug experience and to the anxiety and excitement centered about the use of an illegal drug. In addition, as a person gains experience, his technique of smoking may improve in terms of efficiency so that he delivers greater quantities of the active ingredients to his lungs and circulation. Finally, the variability in the potency of marijuana supplies cannot be ignored as a coincidental factor in the sensitization phenomena. There are no reports of a change in the sensitivity of tissues to cannabis products when they are administered repeatedly.

REFERENCES

1. Abramson, H. A., Jarvik, M. E., Gorin, M. H., and Hirsch, W. M., Lysergic acid diethylamide (LSD-25): XVII. Tolerance development and its relationship to a theory of psychosis, *J. Psychol.*, 41, 81, 1956.

2. Abramson, H. A. and Rolo, A., Lysergic acid diethylamide (LSD-25). 38. Comparison with action of methylsergide and psilocybin on test subjects, *J. Asthma Res.*, 3, 81, 1965.

3. Abramson, H. A., Sklarofsky, B., Baron, M. O., and Fremont-Smith, N., Lysergic acid diethylamide (LSD-25) antagonists. II. Development of tolerance in man to LSD-25 by prior administration of MLD-41 (1-methyl-d-lysergic acid diethylamide), *A. M. A. Arch. Neurol. Psychiat.*, 79, 201, 1958.

4. Adams, W. J., Yeh, S. Y., Woods, L. A., and Mitchell, C. L., Drug-test interaction as a factor in the development of tolerance to the analgesic effect of morphine, *J. Pharmacol. Exp. Ther.*, 168, 251, 1969.

5. Adler, T. K., Studies on morphine tolerance in mice. I. *In vivo* N-demethylation of morphine and N- and O-demethylation of codeine, *J. Pharmacol. Exp. Ther.*, 156, 585, 1967.

6. Adriani, J. and Morton, R. C., Drug dependence: Important considerations from the anesthesiologists' viewpoint, *Anesth. Analg. Cur. Res.*, 47, 472, 1968.

7. Aghajanian, G. K., Sheard, M. H., and Foote, W. E., LSD and mescaline: Comparison of effects on single units in the midbrain raphé, *Psychotomimetic Drugs*, Efron, D. H., Ed., Raven Press, New York, 1970, 165.

8. Allan, F. D. and Swinyard, C. A., Evaluation of tissue tolerance to ethyl alcohol by alterations in electroshock seizure threshold in rats, *Anat. Rec.*, 103, 419, 1949.

9. Altenberg, B. M., Michenfelder, J. D., and Theye, R. A., Acute tolerance to thiopental in canine cerebral oxygen consumption studies, *Anesthesiology,* 31, 443, 1969.

10. A. M. A. Committee on Alcoholism and Addiction, Dependence on amphetamines and other stimulant drugs, *J.A.M.A.*, 197, 1023, 1966.

11. Appel, J. B. and Freedman, D. X., Tolerance and cross-tolerance among psychotomimetic drugs, *Psychopharmacologia,* 13, 267, 1968.

12. Ariens, E. J., Receptor theory and structure-action relationships, *Advances Drug Res.*, 3, 235, 1966.

13. Ariens, E. J., Simonis, A. M., and van Rossum, J. M., Drug receptor interaction: Interaction of one or more drugs with one receptor system, in *Molecular Pharmacology,* Vol. I, Ariens, E. J., Ed., Academic Press, New York, 1964, 119.

14. Ariens, E. J., Simonis, A. M., and van Rossum, J. M., The relation between stimulus and effect, in *Molecular Pharmacology,* Vol. I, Ariens, E. J., Ed., Academic Press, New York, 1964, 395.

15. Aston, R., Quantitative aspects of tolerance and posttolerance hypersensitivity to pentobarbital in the rat, *J. Pharmacol. Exp. Ther.*, 150, 253, 1965.

16. Aston, R., Acute tolerance indices for pentobarbital in male and female rats, *J. Pharmacol. Exp. Ther.*, 152, 350, 1966.

17. Aston, R., Latent hypersensitivity to pentobarbital in the rat, *Proc. Soc. Exp. Biol. Med.*, 121, 623, 1966.

18. Aston, R. and Hibbeln, P., Induced hypersensitivity to barbital in the female rat, *Science,* 157, 1463, 1967.

19. Axelrod, J., Possible mechanisms of tolerance to narcotic drugs, *Science,* 125, 263, 1956.

20. Axelrod, J., The enzymatic N-demethylation of narcotic drugs, *J. Pharmacol. Exp. Ther.*, 117, 322, 1956.

21. Axelrod, J., Cellular adaptation in the development of tolerance to drugs, in *The Addictive States,* Wikler A., Ed., Res. Publ. Ass. Nerv. Ment. Dis., Vol. 46, Williams & Wilkins, Baltimore, 1968, 247.

22. Axelrod, J., Gordon, E., Hertting, G., Kopin, I. J., and Potter, L. T., On the mechanism of tachyphylaxis to tyramine in the isolated rat heart, *Brit. J. Pharmacol.*, 19, 56, 1962.

23. Balestrieri, A. and Fontonari, D., Acquired and crossed tolerance to mescaline, LSD-25 and BOL-148, *A.M.A. Arch. Gen. Psychiat.*, 1, 279, 1959.

24. Baran, L. and Longo, V. G., Instrumental reward discrimination in rabbits, EEG and behavioral effects of a series of lysergic acid derivatives, *Acta Physiol. Lat. Amer.*, 14, 125, 1964.

25. Barnett, A. and Fiore, J. W., Acute tolerance to diazepam in cats and its possible relationship to diazepam metabolism, *Europ. J. Pharmacol.*, 13, 239, 1971.

26. Barnett, A. and Fiore, J. W., Acute tolerance to diazepam in cats; lack of cross-tolerance to phenobarbital and methocarbamol, *Europ. J. Pharmacol.*, 14, 301, 1971.

27. Beckett, A. H. and Brookes, L. G., The effects of chain and ring substitution on the metabolism, distribution and biological action of amphetamines, in *Amphetamines and Related Compounds,* Costa, E. and Garattini, S., Eds., Raven Press, New York, 1970, 109.

28. Beckett, A. H., Casy, A. F., and Harper, N. J., Analgesics and their antagonists: Some steric and chemical considerations. Part III. The influence of the basic group on the biological response, *J. Pharm. Pharmacol.*, 8, 874, 1956.

29. Black, M. B., Woods, J. H., and Domino, E. F., Some effects of (-)-trans-tetrahydrocannabinol and cannabis derivatives on schedule-controlled behavior, *Pharmacologist,* 12, 258, 1970.

30. Brodie, B. B., Cho, A. K., and Gessa, G. L., Possible role of p-hydroxynorephedrine in the depletion of norepinephrine induced by d-amphetamine and in tolerance to this drug, in *Amphetamines and Related Compounds*, Costa, E. and Garattini, S., Eds., Raven Press, New York, 1970, 217.

31. Brodie, B. B., Mark, L. C., Lief, P. A., Bernstein, E., and Papper, E. M., Acute tolerance to thiopental, *J. Pharmacol. Exp. Ther.*, 102, 215, 1951.

32. Bush, M. T. and Sanders, E., Metabolic fate of drugs: Barbiturates and closely related compounds, *Ann. Rev. Pharmacol.*, 7, 57, 1967.

33. Coldwell, B. B., Wiberg, G. S., and Trenholm, H. L., Some effects of ethanol on the toxicity and distribution of barbiturates in rats, *Canad. J. Physiol. Pharmacol.*, 48, 254, 1970.

34. Carlini, E. A., Tolerance to chronic administration of *Cannabis sativa* (marihuana) in rats, *Pharmacology*, 1, 135, 1968.

35. Carlini, E. A., Hamaoui, A., Bieniek, D., and Korte, F., Effects of (-) Δ^9-trans-tetrahydrocannabinol and a synthetic derivative on maze performance of rats, *Pharmacology*, 4, 359, 1970.

36. Cassano, G. B., Ghetti, B., Gliozzi, E., and Hansson, E., Autoradiographic distribution study of "short acting" and "long acting" barbiturates: ^{35}S-thiopentone and ^{14}C-phenobarbitone, *Brit. J. Anesth.*, 39, 11, 1967.

37. Castro, J. A. and Gillette, J. R., Species and sex differences in the kinetic constants for the N-demethylation of ethyl-morphine by liver microsomes, *Biochem. Biophys. Res. Commun.*, 28, 426, 1967.

38. Chen, C. S., A study of the alcohol-tolerance effect and an introduction of a new behavioral technique, *Psychopharmacologia* (Berlin), 12, 433, 1968.

39. Cheney, D. L., Goldstein, A., Algeri, S., and Costa, E., Narcotic tolerance and dependence: Lack of relationship with serotonin turnover in the brain, *Science*, 171, 1169, 1971.

40. Christensen, H. D., Freudenthal, R. I., Gidley, J. T., Rosenfeld, R., Boegli, G., Testino, L., Brine, D. R., Pitt, C. G., and Wall, M. E., Activity of Δ^8- and Δ^9-tetrahydrocannabinol and related compounds in the mouse, *Science*, 172, 165, 1971.

41. Clouet, D. H., Protein and nucleic acid metabolism, in *Narcotic Drugs, Biochemical Pharmacology*, Clouet, D. H., Ed., Plenum Press, New York, 1971, 216.

42. Clouet, D. H. and Ratner, M., The effect of altering liver microsomal N-demethylase activity on the development of tolerance to morphine in rats, *J. Pharmacol. Exp. Ther.*, 144, 362, 1964.

43. Cochin, J., Possible mechanisms in development of tolerance, *Fed. Proc.*, 29, 19, 1970.

44. Cochin, J., Role of possible immune mechanisms in the development of tolerance, in *Narcotic Drugs, Biochemical Pharmacology*, Clouet, D. H., Ed., Plenum Press, New York, 1971, 432.

45. Cochin, J., Haggart, J., Woods, L. A., and Seevers, M. H., Plasma levels, urinary and fecal excretion of morphine in non-tolerant and tolerant dogs, *J. Pharmacol. Exp. Ther.*, 111, 74, 1954.

46. Cochin, J. and Kornetsky, C., Development and loss of tolerance to morphine in the rat after single and multiple injections, *J. Pharmacol. Exp. Ther.*, 145, 1, 1964.

47. Cochin, J. and Kornetsky, C., Factors in blood of morphine-tolerant animals that attenuate or enhance effects of morphine in non-tolerant animals, in *The Addictive States*, Wikler, A., Ed., Res. Publ. Ass. Nerv. Ment. Dis., Vol. 46, Williams & Wilkins, Baltimore, 1968, 268.

48. Cohen, M., Keats, A. S., Krivoy, W., and Ungar, G., Effect of actinomycin D on morphine tolerance, *Proc. Soc. Exp. Biol. Med.*, 119, 381, 1965.

49. Collier, H. O. J., A general theory of the genesis of drug dependence by induction of receptors, *Nature*, 205, 181, 1965.

50. Collier, H. O. J., Tolerance, physical dependence and receptors, *Advances Drug Res.*, 3, 171, 1966.

51. Collier, H. O. J., Supersensitivity and dependence, *Nature,* 220, 228, 1968.

52. Collier, H. O. J., Humoral transmitters, supersensitivity, receptors and dependence, in *Scientific Basis of Drug Dependence,* Steinberg, H., Ed., Grune and Stratton, New York, 1969, 49.

53. Colton, T., Gosselin, R. E., and Smith, R. P., The tolerance of coffee drinkers to caffeine, *Clin. Pharmacol. Ther.*, 9, 31, 1968.

54. Commission of Inquiry into the Non-Medical use of Drugs: Interim Report, LeDain, G., chairman, Queen's Printer for Canada, Ottowa, Canada, 1970, 82 and 108.

55. Conney, A. H., Pharmacological implications of microsomal enzyme induction, *Pharmacol. Rev.,* 19, 317, 1967.

56. Corssen, G. and Skora, I. A., "Addiction" reactions in cultured human cells, *J.A.M.A.,* 187, 328, 1964.

57. Cox, B. M. and Ginsburg, M., Is there a relationship between protein synthesis and tolerance to analgesic drugs?, in *Scientific Basis of Drug Dependence,* Steinberg, H., Ed., Grune and Stratton, New York, 1969, 77.

58. Cox, B. M., Ginsburg, M., and Osman, O. H., Acute tolerance to narcotic analgesic drugs in rats, *Brit. J. Pharmacol.*, 33, 245, 1968.

59. Cox, B. M. and Osman, O. H., Inhibition of the development of tolerance to morphine in rats by drugs which inhibit ribonucleic acid or protein synthesis, *Brit. J. Pharmacol.*, 38, 157, 1970.

60. Crout, J. R., Muskus, A. J., and Tredelenburg, U., Effect of tyramine on isolated guinea-pig atria in relation to their noradrenaline stores, *Brit. J. Pharmacol.*, 18, 600, 1962.

61. de Silva, J. A. F., Koechlin, B. A., and Bader, G., Blood level distribution patterns of diazepam and its major metabolite in man, *J. Pharm. Sci.*, 55, 692, 1966.

62. Devenyi, P. and Wilson, M., Barbiturate abuse and addiction and their relationship to alcohol and alcoholism, *Canad. Med. Ass. J.*, 104, 215, 1971.

63. Dewey, W. L., Harris, L. S., Howes, J. F., and Kenedy, J. S., Pharmacological effects of some active constituents of marihuana, *Pharmacologist*, 11, 278, 1969.

64. Diaz, J- L.. and Huttunen, M. O., Persistent increase in brain serotonin turnover after chronic administration of LSD in the rat, *Science,* 174, 62, 1971.

65. Dill, D. B., Adolph, E. F., and Wilber, C. G., Eds., *Handbook of Physiology,* Section 4: Adaptation to the Environment, American Physiological Society, Washington, D. C., 1964.

66. Dole, V. P. and Nyswander, M. E., A medical treatment for diacetylmorphine (heroin) addiction, *J.A.M.A.*, 193, 646, 1965 and *J.A.M.A.*, 195, 972, 1966.

67. Domino, E. F., Clinical pharmacology of marihuana and its derivatives, *Univ. Mich. Med. Cent. J.*, 37, 1, 1971.

68. Downes, H., Perry, R. S., Ostlund, R. E., and Karler, R., A study of the excitatory effects of barbiturates, *J. Pharmacol. Exp. Ther.*, 175, 692, 1970.

69. Downs, A. W. and Eddy, N. B., The effect of repeated doses of cocaine in the rat, *J. Pharmacol. Exp. Ther.*, 46, 199, 1932.

70. Dundee, J. W., Price, H. L., and Dripps, R. D., Acute tolerance to thiopentone in man, *Brit. J. Anesth.*, 28, 344, 1956.

71. Ebert, A. G., Yim, G. K. W., and Miya, T. S., Distribution and metabolism of barbital-^{14}C in tolerant and nontolerant rats, *Biochem. Pharmacol.*, 13, 1267, 1964.

72. Eble, J. N. and Rudzik, A. D., Interaction between amphetamine and sympathomimetic agents on the cardiovascular system, in *Amphetamines and Related Compounds,* Costa, E. and Garattini, S., Eds., Raven Press, New York, 1970, 513.

73. Eddy, N. B., Tolerance and addiction, in *The Pharmacology of the Opium Alkaloids,* Part I, Pub. Health Rep. Suppl., 165, Kreuger, H., Eddy, N. B. and Sumwalt, M., Eds., 1941, 687.

74. Eddy, N. B., The phenomena of tolerance, in *Origins of Resistance to Toxic Agents,* Sevag, M. G., Reid, R. D., and Reynolds, O. E., Eds., Academic Press, New York, 1955, 223.

75. Eddy, N. B., Halbach, H., Isbell, H., and Seevers, M. H., Drug dependence: Its significance and characteristics, *Bull. W.H.O.,* 32, 721, 1965.

76. Eddy, N. B., Lee, L. E., and Harris, C. A., The rate of development of physical dependence and tolerance to analgesic drugs in patients with chronic pain. Comparison of morphine, oxymorphone and anileridine, *Bull. Narc.,* 11 (1), 3, 1959.

77. Eddy, N. B. and Martin, W. R., Drug dependence of specific opiate antagonist type, *Fortschritte in Theorie, Klinik und Praxis,* 3, 73, 1970.

78. Eddy, N. B., Piller, M., Pirk, L. A., Schrappe, O., and Wende, S., The effect of the addition of a narcotic antagonist on the rate of development of tolerance and physical dependence to morphine, *Bull. Narc.,* 12 (4), 1, 1960.

79. Edison, G. R., Amphetamines: A dangerous illusion, *Ann. Intern. Med.,* 74, 605, 1971.

80. Ehrich, W. E. and Krumbhaar, E. B., The effects of large doses of Benzedrine Sulfate on the albino rat: Functional and tissue changes, *Ann. Intern. Med.,* 10, 1874, 1937.

81. Eisenman, A. J., Sloan, J. W., Martin, W. R., Jasinski, D. R., and Brooks, J. W., Catecholamine and 17-hydroxycorticosteroid excretion during a cycle of morphine dependence in man, *J. Psychiat. Res.,* 7, 19, 1969.

82. Ekman, G., Frankenhaeuser, M., Goldberg, L., Hagdahl, R., and Myrsten, A. L., Subjective and objective effects of alcohol as functions of dosage and time, *Psychopharmacologia,* 6, 399, 1964.

83. Ellison, T., Okun, R., Silverman, A., and Siegel, M., Metabolic fate of amphetamine in the cat during development of tolerance, *Arch. Int. Pharmacodyn.,* 190, 135, 1971.

84. Fennessy, M. R., Heimans, R. L. H., and Rand, M. J., Comparison of effect of morphine-like analgesics on transmurally stimulated guinea-pig ileum, *Brit. J. Pharmacol.,* 37, 436, 1969.

85. Fennessy, M. R. and Rattray, J. F., Cardiovascular effects of intravenous morphine in the anesthetized rat, *Europ. J. Pharmacol.,* 14, 1, 1971.

86. Ferguson, R. K., Adams, W. J., and Mitchell, C. L., Studies of tolerance development to morphine analgesia in rats tested on the hot plate, *Europ. J. Pharmacol.,* 8, 83, 1969.

87. Ferguson, R. K. and Mitchell, C. L., Pain as a factor in the development of tolerance to morphine analgesia in man, *Clin. Pharmacol. Ther.,* 10, 372, 1969.

88. Fineberg, S. K., Anorexigenic drugs in perspective, *J. Amer. Geriat. Soc.,* 15, 51, 1967.

89. Fish, F. and Wilson, W. D. C., Excretion of cocaine and its metabolites in man, *J. Pharm. Pharmacol.,* 21, 135S, 1969.

90. Fleming, R. and Stotz, E., Experimental studies in alcoholism. I. The alcohol content of blood and cerebrospinal fluid following oral administration in chronic alcoholism and the psychoses, *A.M.A. Arch. Neurol. Psychiat.,* 33, 492, 1935.

91. Fleming, R. and Stotz, E., Experimental studies in alcoholism. II. The alcohol content of the blood and cerebrospinal fluid following intravenous administration of alcohol in chronic alcoholism and the psychoses, *A.M.A. Arch. Neurol. Psychiat.,* 35, 117, 1936.

92. Foldes, F. F., Swerdlow, M., and Siker, E. S., *Narcotics and Narcotic Antagonists,* Charles C Thomas, Springfield, Ill., 1964, 84.

93. Foltz, R. L., Fentiman, A. F., Jr., Leighty, E. G., Walter, J. L., Drewes, H. R., Schwartz, W. E., Page, T. F., Jr., and Truitt, E. B., Jr., Metabolite of (-)-trans Δ^8-tetrahydrocannabinol: Identification and synthesis, *Science,* 168, 844, 1970.

94. Forney, R. B. and Hughes, F. W., Interaction between alcohol and psycho-pharmacological drugs, in *Int. Encyclopedia Pharmacol. Ther.*, Sect. 20, Vol. II, *Alcohols and Derivatives*, Tremolieres, J., Ed., Pergamon Press, New York, 1970, 445.

95. Fraser, H. F., Tolerance to and physical dependence on opiates, barbiturates, and alcohol, *Ann. Rev. Med.*, 8, 427, 1957.

96. Fraser, H. F. and Isbell, H., Comparative effects of 20 mgm of morphine sulfate on non-addicts and former morphine addicts, *J. Pharmacol. Exp. Ther.*, 105, 498, 1952.

97. Fraser, H. F., Isbell, H., Wikler, A., Belleville, R. E., Essig, C. F., and Hill, H. E., Minimum dose of barbiturates required to produce physical dependence, *Fed. Proc.*, 15, 423, 1956.

98. Fraser, H. F., Wikler, A., Isbell, H., and Johnson, N. K., Partial equivalence of chronic alcohol and barbiturate intoxications, *Quart. J. Stud. Alcohol*, 18, 541, 1957.

99. Freedman, D. X., The psychopharmacology of hallucinogenic agents, *Ann. Rev. Med.*, 20, 409, 1969.

100. Freedman, D. X. and Aghajanian, G. K., Time parameters in acute tolerance, cross tolerance, and antagonism to psychotogens, *Fed. Proc.*, 18, 390, 1959.

101. Freedman, D. X., Aghajanian, G. K., Ornitz, E. M., and Rosner, B. S., Patterns of tolerance to lysergic acid diethylamide and mescaline in rats, *Science*, 127, 1173, 1958.

102. Freedman, D. X., Appel, J. B., Hartman, F. R., and Molliver, M. E., Tolerance to behavioral effects of LSD-25 in rat, *J. Pharmacol. Exp. Ther.*, 143, 309, 1964.

103. Freedman, A. M., Zaks, A., Resnick, R., and Fink, M., Blockade with methadone, cyclazocine, and naloxone, *Int. J. Addict.*, 5, 507, 1970.

104. Gibbins, R. J., Kalant, H., and LeBlanc, A. E., A technique for accurate measurement of moderate degrees of alcohol intoxication in small animals, *J. Pharmacol. Exp. Ther.*, 159, 236, 1968.

105. Goldberg, L., Quantitative studies on alcohol tolerance in man. The influence of ethyl alcohol on sensory, motor, and psychological functions referred to blood alcohol in normal and habituated individual, *Acta Physiol. Scand.*, 5, Suppl. 16, 5, 1943.

106. Goldberg, L., Behavioral and physiological effects of alcohol in man, *Psychosomat. Med.*, 28, 570, 1966.

107. Goldberg, M. E., Manian, A. A., and Efron, D. H., A comparative study of certain pharmacologic responses following acute and chronic administration of chlordiazepoxide, *Life Sci.*, 6, 481, 1967.

108. Goldstein, A., Aronow, L., and Kalaman, S. M., *Principles of Drug Action*, Harper and Row, New York, 1968, 284.

109. Goldstein, A. and Goldstein, D. B., Enzyme expansion theory of drug tolerance and physical dependence, in *The Addictive States*, Wikler, A., Ed., Res. Publ. Ass. Res. Nerv. Ment. Dis., Vol. 46, Williams & Wilkins, Baltimore, 1968, 265.

110. Goldstein, A. and Sheehan, P., Tolerance to opioid narcotics. I. Tolerance to the "running fit" caused by levorphanol in the mouse, *J. Pharmacol. Exp. Ther.*, 169, 175, 1969.

111. Goldstein, D. B., Effects of barbital on amino acid metabolism in *Escherichia coli*, *Molec. Pharmacol.*, 1, 31, 1965.

112. Goldstein, D. B. and Goldstein, A., Possible role of enzyme inhibition and repression in drug tolerance and addiction, *Biochem. Pharmacol.*, 8, 48, 1961.

113. Gostomzyk, V. J. G., Dilger, D., and Dilger, K., Arteriovenose Konzentrationdifferenzen in Niersen-und Hirngefassen bei intravenoser Infusin, *Z. Klin. Chem. Klin. Biochem.*, 8, 17, 1970.

114. Green, A. F. and Young, P. A., A comparison of heat and pressure analgesiometric methods in rats, *Brit. J. Pharmacol.*, 6, 572, 1951.

115. Griffith, J., A study of illicit amphetamine drug traffic in Oklahoma City, *Amer. J. Psychiat.*, 123, 560, 1966.

116. Gruber, C. M. and Keyser, G. F., A study of the development of tolerance and cross tolerance to barbiturates in experimental animals, *J. Pharmacol. Exp. Ther.*, 86, 186, 1946.

117. Gunne, L. M., The temperature response in rats during acute and chronic morphine administration: A study of morphine tolerance, *Arch. Int. Pharmacodyn.*, 129, 416, 1960.

118. Gunne, L. M. and Lewander, T., Brain catecholamines during chronic amphetamine intoxication, in *The Addictive States*, Wikler, A., Ed., *Res. Publ. Ass. Nerv. Ment. Dis.*, Vol. 46, Williams & Wilkins, Baltimore, 1968, 106.

119. Haggart, J., On the mechanism of the vascular action of morphine, Doctoral Dissertation, University of Michigan, 1955, *Dissertation Abstracts*, 15, 1631, 1955.

120. Han, Y. H., Why do chronic alcoholics require more anesthesia?, *Anesthesiology*, 30, 341, 1969.

121. Harger, R. N. and Forney, R. B., The aliphatic alcohols, in *Progress in Chemical Toxicology*, Vol. 1, Stolman, A., Ed., Academic Press, New York, 1963, 53.

122. Harrisson, J. W. E., Ambrus, C. M., and Ambrus, J. L., Tolerance of rats toward amphetamine and methamphetamine, *J. Amer. Pharm. Ass.*, 41, 539, 1952.

123. Hasko, M. J., Jr. and Tislow, R., Acute tolerance to mescaline in the dog, *Fed. Proc.*, 15, 440, 1956.

124. Hatfield, G. K., Modification of drug action by repeated ethanol treatment in the rat, *Quart. J. Stud. Alcohol*, 29, 190, 1968.

125. Hawkins, R. D., Kalant, H., and Khanna, J. M., Effects of chronic intake of ethanol on rate of ethanol metabolism, *Canad. J. Physiol. Pharmacol.*, 44, 241, 1966.

126. Heifetz, S. A. and McMillan, D. E., Development of behavioral tolerance to morphine and methadone using the schedule-controlled behavior of the pigeon, *Psychopharmacologia*, 19, 40, 1971.

127. Himmelsbach, C. K., Studies on the relation of drug addiction to the autonomic nervous system: Results of cold pressor tests, *J. Pharmacol. Exp. Ther.*, 73, 91, 1941.

128. Himmelsbach, C. K., With reference to physical dependence, *Fed. Proc.*, 2, 201, 1943.

129. Hirsch, G. H. and Hook, J. B., Stimulation of renal organic acid transport and protein synthesis by penicillin, *J. Pharmacol. Exp. Ther.*, 174, 152, 1970.

130. Hoffer, A., D-Lysergic acid diethylamide (LSD): A review of its present status, *Clin. Pharmacol. Ther.*, 6, 183, 1965.

131. Hoffer, A. and Osmond, H., *The Hallucinogens*, Academic Press, New York, 1967.

132. Hogans, A. F., Moreno, O. M., and Brodie, D. A., Effects of ethyl alcohol on EEG and avoidance behavior of chronic electrode monkeys, *Amer. J. Physiol.*, 201, 434, 1961.

133. Hollister, L. E., Marihuana in man: Three years later, *Science*, 172, 21, 1971.

134. Hollister, L. E. and Clyde, D. J., Blood levels of pentobarbital sodium, meprobamate, and tybamate in relation to clinical effects, *Clin. Pharmacol. Ther.*, 9, 204, 1968.

135. Hoogland, D. R., Miya, T. S., and Bousquet, W. F., Metabolism and tolerance studies with chlordiazepoxide-2-^{14}C in the rat, *Toxic. Appl. Pharmacol.*, 9, 116, 1966.

136. Hug, C. C., Jr., Mellett, L. B., and Cafruny, E. J., Stop-flow analysis of the renal excretion of tritium-labeled dihydromorphine, *J. Pharmacol. Exp. Ther.*, 150, 259, 1965.

137. Hug, C. C., Jr. and Oka, T., Uptake of dihydromorphine-^{3}H by synaptosomes, *Life Sci.*, 10, 201, 1971.

138. Hug, C. C., Jr. and Villarreal, J. E., unpublished observations.

139. Huidobro, F. and Miranda, H., The presence in mice chronically treated with morphine of a substance(s) that modifies morphine responses, *Biochem. Pharmacol.*, 17, 1099, 1968.

140. Iida, S., Kanno, M., and Nakamura, K., An increased sensitivity to alcohol in rabbits treated with a certain factor contained in a microsomal subfraction of the brain, *Jap. J. Pharmacol.*, 19, 409, 1969.

141. Innes, J. R. and Nickerson, M., Drugs acting on postganglionic adrenergic nerve endings and structures innervated by them (sympathomimetic drugs), in *The Pharmacological Basis of Therapeutics*, 4th ed., Goodman, L. S. and Gilman, A., Eds., Macmillan, New York, 1970, 478.

142. Inturrisi, C. E. and Fujimoto, J. M., Studies on the antidiuretic action of morphine in the rat, *Europ. J. Pharmacol.*, 2, 301, 1968.

143. Inturrisi, C. E. and Fujimoto, J. M., The development of tolerance to the antidiuretic effect of morphine in the mouse, *Toxic. Appl. Pharmacol.*, 13, 258, 1968.

144. Isbell, H., Belleville, R. E., Fraser, H. F., Wikler, A., and Logan, C. R., Studies on lysergic acid diethylamide (LSD-25). I. Effects in former morphine addicts and development of tolerance during chronic intoxication, *A. M. A. Arch. Neurol. Psychiat.*, 76, 468, 1956.

145. Isbell, H. and Fraser, H. F., Addiction to analgesics and barbiturates, *Pharmacol. Rev.*, 2, 355, 1950.

146. Isbell, H., Fraser, H. F., Wikler, A., and Belleville, R. E., Tolerance to diethylamide of lysergic acid, *Fed. Proc.*, 14, 354, 1955.

147. Isbell, H., Fraser, H. F., Wikler, A., Belleville, R. E., and Eisenman, A. J., An experimental study of the etiology of "rum fits" and delirium tremens, *Quart. J. Stud. Alcohol*, 16, 1, 1955.

148. Isbell, H. and Jasinski, D. R., A comparison of LSD-25 with (-)-Δ^9- trans-tetrahydrocannabinol (THC) and attempted cross-tolerance between LSD and THC, *Psychopharmacologia*, 14, 115, 1969.

149. Isbell, H., Miner, E. J., and Logan, C. R., Cross tolerance between d-2-brom-lysergic acid diethylamide (BOL-148) and d-diethylamide of lysergic acid (LSD-25), *Psychopharmacologia*, 1, 109, 1959.

150. Isbell, H. and White, W. M., Clinical characteristics of addiction, *Amer. J. Med.*, 14, 558, 1953.

151. Isbell, H., Wolbach, A. B., Wikler, A., and Miner, E. J., Cross tolerance between LSD and psilocybin, *Psychopharmacologia*, 2, 147, 1961.

152. Isbell, H., Wolbach, A., and Rosenberg, D., Observations on direct and cross tolerance with LSD and dextroamphetamine in man, *Fed. Proc.*, 21, 416, 1962.

153. Israel, Y., Cellular effects of alcohol. A review, *Quart. J. Stud. Alcohol*, 31A, 293, 1970.

154. Israel, Y., Kalant, H., and LeBlanc, A. E., Effects of lower alcohols on potassium transport and microsomal adenosine triphosphatase activity of rat cerebral cortex, *Biochem. J.*, 100, 27, 1966.

155. Israel, Y., Kalant, H., LeBlanc, E., Bernstein, J. C., and Salazar, I., Changes in cation transport and (Na,K)-activated adenosine triphosphatase produced by chronic administration of ethanol, *J. Pharmacol. Exp. Ther.*, 174, 330, 1970.

156. Jaffe, J. H., Drug addiction and abuse, in *The Pharmacological Basis of Therapeutics*, 4th ed., Goodman, L. S. and Gilman, A., Eds., Macmillan, New York, 1970, 276.

157. Jaffe, J. H. and Sharpless, S. K., The rapid development of physical dependence on barbiturates, *J. Pharmacol. Exp. Ther.*, 150, 140, 1965.

158. Jaffe, J. and Sharpless, S. K., Pharmacological denervation supersensitivity in the central nervous system: A theroy of physical dependence, in *The Addictive States*, Wikler, A., Ed., *Res. Publ. Ass. Nerv. Ment. Dis.*, Vol. 46, Williams & Wilkins, Baltimore, 1968, 226.

159. Jansen, G. A. and Greene, N. M., Morphine metabolism and morphine tolerance in goldfish, *Anesthesiology,* 32, 231, 1970.

160. Jellinek, E. M., *The Disease Concept of Alcoholism,* Hillhouse Press, Highland Park, N. J., 1960.

161. Jetter, W. W., Studies in alcohol. II. Experimental feeding of alcohol to non-alcoholic individuals, *Amer. J. Med. Sci.,* 196, 487, 1938.

162. Johannesson, T., Rogers, L. A., Fouts, J. R., and Woods, L. A., Tolerance to morphine and codeine analgesia and hepatic enzyme microsomal drug metabolism in the rat, *Acta Pharmacol. Toxicol.,* 22, 255, 1965.

163. Johannesson, T. and Woods, L. A., Analgesic action and brain and plasma levels of morphine and codeine in morphine tolerant, codeine tolerant and non-tolerant rats, *Acta Pharmacol. Toxicol.,* 21, 381, 1964.

164. Jonas, S. and Downer, J. deC., Gross behavioral changes in monkeys following administration of LSD-25, and development of tolerance to LSD-25, *Psychopharmacologia,* 6, 303, 1964.

165. Jonas, R. T. and Stone, G. C., Psychological studies of marijuana and alcohol in man, *Psychopharmacologia,* 18, 108, 1970.

166. Jori, A., Blanchetti, A., and Prestini, P. E., Relations between barbiturate brain levels and sleeping time in various experimental conditions, *Biochem. Pharmacol.*, 19, 2687, 1970.

167. Kalant, H., The pharmacology of alcohol intoxication, *Quart. J. Stud. Alcohol,* 22 Suppl. 1, 1, 1961.

168. Kalant, H., Effects of ethanol on the nervous system, *Int. Encyclopedia Pharmacol. Ther.,* Sect. 20, Vol. 1, *Alcohols and Derivatives,* Tremolieres, J., Ed., Pergamon Press, New York, 1970, 189.

169. Kalant, H. and Grose, W., Effects of ethanol and pentobarbital on release of acetylcholine from cerebral cortex slices, *J. Pharmacol. Exp. Ther.*, 158, 386, 1967.

170. Kalant, H., Khanna, J. M., and Marshman, J., Effect of chronic intake of ethanol on pentobarbital metabolism, *J. Pharmacol. Exp. Ther.,* 175, 318, 1970.

171. Kalant, H., LeBlanc, A. E., and Gibbins, R. J., Pharmacological and behavioral variables in the development of alcohol tolerance, reported to the Committee on Problems of Drug Dependence, Feb. 16-17, 1971, Toronto, Ontario, Vol. II, 1283.

172. Kalant, H., LeBlanc, A. E., and Gibbins, R. J., Tolerance to, and dependence on, some non-opiate psychotropic drugs, *Pharmacol. Rev.,* 23, 135, 1971.

173. Kalant, O. J., *The Amphetamines: Toxicity and Addiction,* University of Toronto Press, Toronto, 1966.

174. Kales, A., Heuser, G., Kales, J. D., Rickles, W. H., Jr., Rubin, R. T.,Scharf, M. B., Ungerleider, J. T., and Winters, W. D., Drug dependency: Investigations of stimulants and depressants, *Ann. Intern. Med.*, 70, 591, 1969.

175. Kaneto, H., Shimomura, K., Kamei, C., et al., Acute tolerance to continuous subcutaneous infusion of morphine, *Folia Pharmacol. Jap.,* 66, 487, 1970.

176. Kato, R., Analysis and differentiation of the mechanism in the development of drug tolerance, *Jap. J. Pharmacol.*, 17, 499, 1967.

177. Kato, R. and Onoda, K., Effect of morphine administration on the activities of microsomal drug-metabolizing enzyme systems in liver of different species, *Jap. J. Pharmacol.*, 16, 217, 1966.

178. Kato, R. and Takanaka, A., Lack of chronic morphine effects on the induction of drug-metabolizing enzymes of liver microsomes by phenobarbital in female rats, *Chem. Pharm. Bull.*, 15, 1419, 1967.

179. Kayan, S. and Mitchell, C. L., Further studies on the development of tolerance to the analgesic effect of morphine, *Arch. Int. Pharmacodyn. Ther.*, 182, 287, 1969.

180. Kayan, S., Woods, L. A., and Mitchell, C. L., Experience as a factor in the development of tolerance to the analgesic effect of morphine, *Europ. J. Pharmacol.*, 6, 333, 1969.

181. Keilty, S. R., Anesthesia for the alcoholic patient, *Anesth. Anal. Cur. Res.*, 48, 659, 1969.

182. Khanna, J. M. and Kalant, H., Effect of inhibitors and inducers of drug metabolism on ethanol metabolism *in vivo*, *Biochem. Pharmacol.*, 19, 2033, 1970.

183. Khanna, J. M., Kalant, H., and Bustos, G., Effects of chronic intake of ethanol on rate of ethanol metabolism. II. Influence of sex and of schedule of ethanol administration, *Canad. J. Physiol. Pharmacol.*, 45, 777, 1967.

184. Khazan, N., Weeks, J. R., and Schroeder, L. A., Electroencephalographic, electromyographic and behavioral correlates during a cycle of self-maintained morphine addiction in the rat, *J. Pharmacol. Exp. Ther.*, 155, 521, 1967.

185. Kiplinger, G. F. and Clift, J. W., Pharmacological properties of morphine-potentiating serum obtained from morphine-tolerant dogs and men, *J. Pharmacol. Exp. Ther.*, 146, 139, 1964.

186. Knoll, J. and Vizi, E. S., Cross-tolerance between para-bromomethamphetamine (V-111) and LSD-25, *Pharmacology*, 4, 278, 1970.

187. Koella, W. P., Beaulieu, R. F., and Bergen, J. R., Stereotyped behavior and cyclic changes in response produced by LSD in goats, *Int. J. Neuropharmacol.*, 3, 397, 1964.

188. Kornetsky, C. and Bain, G., Morphine: Single dose tolerance, *Science*, 162, 1011, 1968.

189. Kornetsky, C. and Kiplinger, G. F., Potentiation of an effect of morphine in the rat by sera from morphine-tolerant and abstinent dogs and monkeys, *Psychopharmacologia* (Berlin), 4, 66, 1963.

190. Kosman, M. E. and Unna, K. R., Effects of chronic administration of the amphetamines and other stimulants on behavior, *Clin. Pharmacol. Ther.*, 9, 240, 1968.

191. Kramer, J. C., Fischman, V. S., and Littlefield, D. C., Amphetamine abuse, *J.A.M.A.*, 201, 305, 1967.

192. Krug, D. C., Sokol, J., and Nylander, L., Inhalation of commercial solvents: A form of defiance among adolescents, in *Drug Addiction in Youth*, Harms, E., Ed., Pergamon Press, New York, 1965, 36.

193. Kuhn, H. F. and Friebul, H., Die Ausscheidung von Codein und Codeinmetaboliten im Harn codeingewohnter Ratten und Meerschweinchen, *Med. Exp.*, 7, 225, 1962.

194. Larson, P. S., Haag, H. B., and Silvette, H., *Tobacco: Experimental and Clinical Studies*, Williams & Wilkins, Baltimore, 1961, 517.

195. Larson, P. S., Haag, H. B., and Silvette, H., *Tobacco: Experimental and Clinical Studies*, Supplement I, Williams & Wilkins, Baltimore, 1968, 257.

196. LeBlanc, A. E., Gibbins, R. J., and Kalant, H., Training under the influence of ethanol as a factor in the development of tolerance and physical dependence in the rat, reported to the Committee on Problems of Drug Dependence, February 16-18, 1970, Washington, D. C., 6627.

197. LeBlanc, A. E., Kalant, H., Gibbins, R. J., and Berman, N. D., Acquisition and loss of tolerance to ethanol by the rat, *J. Pharmacol. Exp. Ther.*, 168, 244, 1969.

198. Lemberger, L., Tamarkin, N. R., Axelrod, J., and Kopin, I. J., Delta-9-tetrahydrocannabinol: Metabolism and disposition in long-term marijuana smokers, *Science*, 173, 72, 1971.

199. Lester, D., Self-maintenance of intoxication in the rat, *Quart. J. Stud. Alcohol*, 22, 223, 1961.

200. Levine, R. R. and Pelikan, E. W., Mechanisms of drug absorption and excretion: Passage of drugs out of and into the gastrointestinal tract, *Ann. Rev. Pharmacol.*, 4, 69, 1964.

201. Levy, J., Contribution a l'etude de l'accoutumance experimentale aux poisons. I. Alcoolisme experimental, *Bull. Soc. Chim. Biol.*, 17, 13, 1935.

202. Levy, J., Contribution a l'etude de l'accoutumance experimentale aux poisons. III. Alcoolisme experimental. L'accoutumance a l'alcool peut-elle être considérée comme une consequence de l'hyposensibilite cellulair?, *Bull. Soc. Chim. Biol.*, 17, 47, 1935.

203. Lewander, T., Catecholamine turn-over studies in chronic amphetamine intoxication, in *Amphetamines and Related Compounds,* Costa, E. and Garattini, S., Eds., Raven Press, New York, 1970, 317.

204. Light, A. B., Physiologic aspects of opium addiction, *J.A.M.A.*, 96, 823, 1931.

205. Lipparini, F., DeCarolis, A. S., and Longo, V. G., Aeuropharmacological investigation of some trans-tetrahydro-cannabinol derivatives, *Physiol. Behav.*, 4, 527, 1969.

206. Loh, H. H., Shen, F-H., and Way, E. L., Inhibition of morphine tolerance and physical dependence development and brain serotonin synthesis by cycloheximide, *Biochem. Pharmacol.*, 18, 2711, 1969.

207. Lomax, P., Acute tolerance to the hypothermic effect of marijuana in the rat, *Res. Commun. Chem. Path. Pharmacol.*, 2, 159, 1971.

208. Lotti, V. J., Lomax, P., and George, R., Acute tolerance to morphine following systemic and intracerebral injection in the rat, *Int. J. Neuropharmacol.*, 5, 35, 1966.

209. Louria, D. B., *The Drug Scene*, McGraw-Hill, New York, 1968, 46.

210. Lundquist, F., Enzymatic pathways of ethanol metabolism, in *Int. Encyclopedia Pharmacol. Ther.*, Sect. 20, Vol. I, *Alcohols and Derivatives,* Tremolieres, J., Ed., Pergamon Press, New York, 1970, 95.

211. Maickel, R. P., Cox, R. H., Jr., Miller, F. P., Segal, D. S., and Russell, R. W., Correlation of brain levels of drugs with behavioral effects, *J. Pharmacol. Exp. Ther.*, 165, 216, 1969.

212. Mannering, G. J., Significance of stimulation and inhibition of drug metabolism in pharmacological testing, in *Selected Pharmacological Testing Methods*, Vol. 3, Berger, A., Ed., Marcel-Dekker, New York, 1968, 51.

213. Marchand, C. and Denis, G., Diuretic effect of chronic morphine treatment in rats, *J. Pharmacol. Exp. Ther.*, 162, 331, 1968.

214. Margules, D. L. and Stein, L., Increase of "antianxiety" activity and tolerance of behavioral depression during chronic administration of oxazepam, *Psychopharmacologia*, 13, 74, 1968.

215. Mark, L. C., Metabolsim of barbiturates in man, *Clin. Pharmacol. Ther.*, 4, 504, 1963.

216. Mark, L. C., Burns, J. J., Brand, L., Campomanes, C. I., Trousof, N., Papper, E. M., and Brodie, B. B., The passage of thiobarbiturates and their oxygen analogs into brain, *J. Pharmacol. Exp. Ther.*, 123, 70, 1958.

217. Marshall, I. and Grahame-Smith, D. G., Unchanged rate of brain serotonin synthesis during chronic morphine treatment and failure of parachlorophenylalanine to attenuate withdrawal syndrome in mice, *Nature,* 228, 1206, 1970.

218. Martin, W. R., A homeostatic and redundancy theory of tolerance to and dependence on narcotic analgesics, in *The Addictive States*, Wikler, A., Ed., Res. Publ. Ass. Nerv. Ment. Dis., Vol. 46, Williams & Wilkins, Baltimore, 1968, 206.

219. Martin, W. R., Pharmacological redundancy as an adaptive mechanism in the central nervous system, *Fed. Proc.*, 29, 13, 1970.

220. Martin, W. R., Drug Dependence, in *Drill's Pharmacology in Medicine*, 4th ed., DiPalma, J. R., Ed., McGraw-Hill, New York, 1971, 362.

221. Martin, W. R. and Eades, C. G., Demonstration of tolerance and physical dependence in the dog following short term infusion of morphine, *J. Pharmacol. Exp. Ther.*, 133, 262, 1961.

222. Martin, W. R. and Eades, C. G., A comparison between acute and chronic physical dependence in the chronic spinal dog, *J. Pharmacol. Exp. Ther.*, 146, 385, 1964.

223. Martin, W. R., Gorodetsky, C. W., and McClane, T. K., An experimental study in the treatment of narcotic addicts with cyclazocine, *Clin. Pharmacol. Ther.*, 7, 455, 1966.

224. Martin, W. R., Jasinski, D. R., Sapira, J. D., Flanary, H. G., Kelly, O. A., Thompson, A. K., and Logan, C. R., The respiratory effects of morphine during a cycle of dependence, *J. Pharmacol. Exp. Ther.*, 162, 182, 1968.

225. Martin, W. R. and Jasinski, D. R., Physiologic parameters of morphine dependence in man: Tolerance, early abstinence, protracted abstinence, *J. Psychiat. Res.*, 7, 9, 1969.

226. Martin, W. R., Wikler, A., Eades, C. G., and Pescor, F. T., Tolerance to the physical dependence on morphine in rats, *Psychopharmacologia*, 4, 247, 1963.

227. Masur, J., Martz, R. M. W., and Carlini, E. A., Effects of acute and chronic administration of *cannabis sativa* and (-) Δ^9 -trans-tetrahydrocannabinol on the behavior of rats in an open-field arena, *Psychopharmacologia*, 19, 388, 1971.

228. Matthies, H., Schmidt, J., and Pohle, W., Toleranzerscheinungen bei der Beeinflussung bedingter Reaktionen durch Noradrenalin, Serotonin und Lysergsäurediäthylamid, *Acta Biol. Med. German*, 11, 849, 1963.

229. Mayfield, D. G., Psychopharmacology of alcohol, *J. Nerv. Ment. Dis.*, 146 (I), 314 and (II), 322, 1968.

230. Maynert, E. W., Sedatives and hypnotics. II. Barbiturates, in *Drill's Pharmacology in Medicine*, 4th ed., DiPalma, J. R., Ed., McGraw-Hill, New York, 1971, 250.

231. Maynert, E. W. and Klingman, G. I., Acute tolerance to intravenous anesthetics in dogs, *J. Pharmacol. Exp. Ther.*, 128, 192, 1960.

232. Maynert, E. W. and van Dyke, H. B., The metabolism of barbiturates, *Pharmacol. Rev.*, 1, 217, 1949.

233. McIlwain, H., Metabolic adaptation in the brain, *Nature*, 226, 803, 1970.

234. McLean, R. A., Adrenergic drugs, in *Medicinal Chemistry*, 2nd ed., Burger, A., Ed., Interscience, New York, 1960, 592.

235. McMillan, D. E., Harris, L. S., Frankenheim, J. M., and Kennedy, J. S., 1-Δ^9-trans-tetrahydrocannabinol in pigeons: Tolerance to the behavioral effects, *Science*, 169, 501, 1970.

236. McMillan, D. E., Harris, L. S., Turk, R. F., and Kennedy, J. S., Development of marked behavioral tolerance to 1-Δ^9-tetrahydrocannabinol (Δ^9-THC) and cross tolerance to 1-Δ^8-tetrahydrocannabinol (Δ^8-THC) in the pigeon, *Pharmacologist*, 12, 258, 1970.

237. Mechoulam, R., Marihuana chemistry, *Science*, 168, 1159, 1970.

238. Mellett, L. B. and Woods, L. A., The distribution and fate of morphine in the non-tolerant and tolerant monkey. *J. Pharmacol. Exp. Ther.*, 116, 77, 1956.

239. Mello, N. K., Some aspects of the behavioral pharmacology of ethanol, in *Psychopharmacology, A Review of Progress, 1957-1967*, Efron, D. H., Cole, J. O., Levine, J., and Wittenborn, J. R., Eds., PHS Publ. No. 1836, U.S. Govt. Printing Office, Washington, D.C., 1968, 787.

240. Mello, N. K. and Mendelson, J. H., Alterations in states of consciousness associated with chronic ingestion of alcohol, in *Neurobiological Aspects of Psychopathology*, Zubin, J. et. al., Eds., Grune and Stratton, New York, 1969, 183.

241. Mello, N. K. and Mendelson, J. H., Experimentally induced intoxication in alcoholics: A comparison between programmed and spontaneous drinking, *J. Pharmacol. Exp. Ther.*, 173, 101, 1970.

242. Mendelson, J. H., Biochemical pharmacology of alcohol, in *Psychopharmacology, A Review of Progress, 1957-1967*, Efron, D. H., Cole, J. O., Levine, J., and Wittenborn, J. R., Eds., PHS Publ. No. 1836, U.S. Govt. Printing Office, Washington, D.C., 1968, 769.

243. Mendelson, J. H., Ethanol-1-C^{14} metabolism in alcoholics and nonalcoholics, *Science*, 159, 319, 1968.

244. Mendelson, J. H., Biological concomitants of alcoholism, *New Eng. J. Med.*, 283, 24, 1970.

245. Mendelson, J. H., Stein, S., and McGuire, M. T., Comparative psychophysiological studies of alcoholic and non-alcoholic subjects undergoing experimentally induced ethanol intoxication, *Psychosom. Med.*, 28, 1, 1966.

246. Mendelson, J. H., Stein, S., and Mello, N. K., Effects of experimentally induced intoxication on metabolism of ethanol-1-C^{14} in alcoholic subjects, *Metabolism*, 14, 1255, 1965.

247. Meyer, R. E. et al., Administration of marijuana to heavy and casual users, Amer. Psychiat. Ass. Meeting, Wash. D. C., May 1971.

248. Mezey, E., Effect of phenobarbital administration on ethanol oxidizing enzymes and on rates of ethanol degradation, *Biochem. Pharmacol.*, 20, 508, 1971.

249. Milne, M. D., Scribner, B. H., and Crawford, M. A., Non-ionic diffusion and excretion of weak acids and bases, *Amer. J. Med.*, 24, 709, 1958.

250. Miletich, D. J., Bradley, S. L., and Strike, T. A., The effect of sympathomimetic amines on radiation-induced tolerance to pentobarbital in the rat, *Proc. Soc. Exp. Biol. Med.*, 134, 403, 1970.

251. Moore, K. E., Carr, L. A., and Dominic, J. A., Functional significance of amphetamine-induced release of brain catecholamines, in *Amphetamine and Related Compounds*, Costa, E. and Garattini, S., Eds., Raven Press, New York, 1970, 371.

252. Moreton, J. E. and Davis, W. M., Effects of Δ-9-tetrahydrocannabinol on locomotor activity and phases of sleep, *Pharmacologist*, 12, 258, 1970.

253. Moskowitz, H. and Wapner, M., Studies on the acquisition of behavioral tolerance to alcohol, *Quart. J. Stud. Alcohol*, 25, 619, 1964.

254. Mulé, S. J., Effect of morphine and nalorphine on the metabolism of phospholipids in guinea pig cerebral cortex slices, *J. Pharmacol. Exp. Ther.*, 154, 370, 1966.

255. Mulé, S. J., Morphine and the incorporation of P_i^{32} into brain phosholipids of nontolerant, tolerant and abstinent guinea pigs. *J. Pharmacol. Exp. Ther.*, 156, 92, 1967.

256. Mulé, S. J., Effect of morphine and nalorphine on brain phospholipid metabolism, in *The Addictive States*, Wikler, A., Ed., Res. Publ. Ass. Nerv. Ment. Dis., Vol. 46, Williams & Wilkins, Baltimore, 1968, 32.

257. Mulé, S. J., Inhibition of phospholipid-facilitated calcium transport by central nervous system-acting drugs, *Biochem. Pharmacol.*, 18, 339, 1969.

258. Mulé, S. J. and Gorodetzky, C. W., Physiologic disposition of H^3-cyclazocine in non-tolerant, tolerant and abstinent dogs, *J. Pharmacol. Exp. Ther.*, 154, 632, 1966.

259. Mulé, S. J., Redman, C. M., and Flesher, J. W., Intracellular disposition of H^3-morphine in the brain and liver of nontolerant and tolerant guinea pigs, *J. Pharmacol. Exp. Ther.*, 157, 459, 1967.

260. Mulé, S. J. and Woods, L. A., Distribution of N-C^{14}-Methyl labeled morphine: I. In central nervous system of nontolerant and tolerant dogs, *J. Pharmacol. Exp. Ther.*, 136, 232, 1962.

261. Murphree, H. B., Clinical pharmacology of potent analgesics, *Clin. Pharmacol. Ther.*, 3, 473, 1962.

262. Newman, H. W. and Lehman, A. J., Nature of acquired tolerance to alcohol, *J. Pharmacol. Exp. Ther.*, 62, 301, 1938.

263. Newman, L. M., Lutz, M. P., Gould, M. H., and Domino, E. F., Δ^9-Tetrahydrocannabinol and ethyl alcohol: Evidence for cross-tolerance in the rat, *Science*, 175, 1022, 1972.

264. Nurmand, L. B., On the acute tolerance to barbamil, *Farmakol. Toksik.*, 32, 41, 1969.

265. Nylander, I., "Thinner" addiction in Sweden, in *Drug Addiction in Youth*, Harms, E., Ed., Pergamon Press, New York, 1965, 49.

266. Orahovats, P. D., Winter, C. A., and Lehman, E. G., The effect of N-allynormorphine upon the development of tolerance to morphine in the albino rat, *J. Pharmacol. Exp. Ther.*, 109, 413, 1953.

267. Oswald, I., Effects on sleep of amphetamine and its derivatives, in *Amphetamines and Related Compounds*, Costa, E. and Garrattini, S., Eds., Raven Press, New York, 1970, 865.

268. Paton, W. D. M., Transmission and block in autonomic ganglia, *Pharmacol. Rev.*, 6, 59, 1954.

269. Paton, W. D. M., The action of morphine and related substances on contraction and on acetylcholine output of coaxially stimulated guinea-pig ileum, *Brit. J. Pharmacol. Chemother.*, 12, 119, 1957.

270. Paton, W. D. M., A theory of drug action based on the rate of drug receptor combination, *Proc. Roy. Soc. B.*, 154, 21, 1961.

271. Paton, W. D. M., A pharmacological approach to drug dependence and drug tolerance, in *Scientific Basis of Drug Dependence*, Steinberg, H., Ed., Grune and Stratton, New York, 1969, 31.

272. Plant, O. H. and Pierce, I. H., Studies of chronic morphine poisoning in dogs. I. General symptoms and behavior during addiction and withdrawal, *J. Pharmacol. Exp. Ther.*, 33, 329, 1928.

273. Rang, H. P. and Ritter, J. M., A new kind of drug antagonism: Evidence that agonists cause a molecular change in acetylcholine receptors, *Molec. Pharmacol.*, 5, 394, 1969.

274. Rang, H. P. and Ritter, J. M., On the mechanism of desensitization at cholinergic receptors, *Molec. Pharmacol.*, 6, 357, 1970.

275. Rector, F. C., Jr., Seldin, D. W., and Copenhaver, J. H., The mechanism of ammonia excretion during ammonium chloride acidosis, *J. Clin. Invest.*, 34, 20, 1955.

276. Reinhard, J. F. and Spector, E., Effects of phenobarbital, phenylbutazone, 3,4-benzpyrene, or 3-methylcholanthrene on ethanol metabolism in the rat, *Toxic. Appl. Pharmacol.*, 17, 12, 1970.

277. Remmer, H., Gewohnung au Hexobarbital durch beschleunigten Abbau, *Arch. Int. Pharmacodyn.*, 152, 346, 1964.

278. Remmer, H., Tolerance to barbiturates by increased breakdown, in *Scientific Basis of Drug Dependence*, Steinberg, H., Ed., Grune and Stratton, New York, 1969, 111.

279. Rethy, C. R., Smith, C. B., and Villarreal, J. E., Effects of narcotic analgesics upon locomotor activity and brain catecholamine content of the mouse, *J. Pharmacol. Exp. Ther.*, 176, 472, 1971.

280. Reynolds, A. K. and Randall, L. O., *Morphine and Allied Drugs*, University of Toronto Press, Toronto, 1957.

281. Richelle, M., A note on behavioral tolerance to meprobamate, *J. Exp. Anal. Behav.*, 8, 45, 1965.

282. Richter, J. A. and Goldstein, A., Tolerance to opioid narcotics. II. Cellular tolerance to levorphanol in mouse brain, *Proc. Nat. Acad. Sci. U.S.A.*, 66, 944, 1970.

283. Rosenberg, D. E., Isbell, H., Miner, E. J., and Sogan, C. R., The effect of N, N-dimethyltryptamine in human subjects tolerant to lysergic acid diethylamide, *Psychopharmacologia*, 5, 217, 1964.

284. Rosenberg, D. E., Wolbach, A. B., Jr., Miner, E. J., and Isbell, H., Observations on direct and cross-tolerance with LSD and d-amphetamine, *Psychopharmacologia*, 5, 1, 1963.

285. Rubin, E. and Lieber, C. S., Alcoholism, alcohol, and drugs, *Science*, 172, 1, 1971.

286. Ruffin, N. E., Reed. B. L., and Finnin, B. C., Effects of morphine withdrawal on cells in continuous culture, *Life Sci.*, 8, 671, 1969.

287. Schmidt, C. F. and Livingston, A. E., Reactions of the circulation to morphine, *J. Pharmacol. Exp. Ther.*, 33, 284, 1928.

288. Schmidt, C. F. and Livingston, A. E., The action of morphine on the mammalian circulation, *J. Pharmacol. Exp. Ther.*, 47, 411, 1933.

289. Schmidt, C. F. and Livingston, A. E., The relation of dosage to the development of tolerance to morphine in dogs, *J. Pharmacol. Exp. Ther.*, 47, 443, 1933.

290. Schuster, C. R., Dockens, W. S., and Woods, J. H., Behavioral variables affecting the development of amphetamine tolerance, *Psychopharmacologia*, 9, 170, 1966.

291. Schuster, C. R. and Zimmerman, J., Timing behavior during prolonged treatment with *dl*-amphetamine, *J. Exp. Anal. Behav.*, 4, 327, 1961.

292. Seevers, M. H., Animal experimentation in studying addiction to newer synthetic analgesics, *Ann. N.Y. Acad. Sci.*, 51, 98, 1948.

293. Seevers, M. H., Adaptation to narcotics, *Fed. Proc.*, 13, 672, 1954.

294. Seevers, M. H., Termination of drug action by tolerance development, *Fed. Proc.*, 17, 1175, 1958.

295. Seevers, M. H. and Deneau, G. A., Physiological aspects of tolerance and physical dependence, in *Physiological Pharmacology*, Vol. 1, Root, W. S. and Hofmann, F. G., Eds., Academic Press, New York, 1963, 565.

296. Seevers, M. H. and Deneau, G. A., Animals in toxic environments: mammals and narcotic analgesics, in *Handbook of Physiology*, Section 4, *Adaptation to the Environment*, American Physiological Society, Washington, D.C., 1965, 809.

297. Seevers, M. H. and Tatum, A. L., Chronic experimental barbital poisoning, *J. Pharmacol. Exp. Ther.*, 42, 217, 1931.

298. Seevers, M. H. and Woods, L. A., The phenomena of tolerance, *Amer. J. Med.*, 14, 546, 1953.

299. Sharpless, S. and Jaffe, J., Hypnotics and sedatives. I. The barbiturates, in *The Pharmacological Basis of Therapeutics*, 4th ed., Goodman, L. S. and Gilman, A., Eds., Macmillan, New York, 1970, 98.

300. Sharpless, S. and Jaffe, J., Withdrawal phenomena as manifestations of disuse supersensitivity, in *Scientific Basis of Drug Dependence*, Steinberg, H., Ed., Grune and Stratton, New York, 1969, 67.

301. Shideman, F. E. and Johnson, H. T., Acute vascular tolerance to morphine, isonipecaine (Demerol), and methadon (Amidone) in the dog, *J. Pharmacol. Exp. Ther.*, 92, 414, 1948.

302. Shikimi, T., Kaneto, H., and Hano, K., Changes of brain calcium content in normal and morphinized mice after the administration of morphine, *Jap. J. Pharmacol.*, 17, 135, 1967.

303. Shulman, A., The pharmacology of barbiturates, *Med. J. Aust.*, 1, 1199, 1970.

304. Shuster, L., Repression and de-repression of enzyme synthesis as a possible explanation of some aspects of drug action, *Nature*, 189, 314, 1961.

305. Shuster, L., Hannam, R. V., and Boyle, W. E., Jr., A simple method for producing tolerance to dihydromorphone in mice, *J. Pharmacol. Exp. Ther.*, 140, 149, 1963.

306. Sidell, F. R. and Pless, J. E., Ethyl alcohol: Blood levels and performance decrements after oral administration to man, *Psychopharmacologia* (Berlin), 19, 246, 1971.

307. Silva, M. T. A., Carlini, E. A., Claussen, U., and Korte, F., Lack of cross-tolerance in rats among (-) Δ^9-trans-tetrahydrocannabinol (Δ^9-THC), cannabis extract, mescaline and lysergic acid diethylamide (LSD-25), *Psychopharmacologia*, 13, 332, 1968.

308. Simon, A. K. and Eddy, N. B., Studies of morphine, codeine, and their derivatives. V. The use of maze-trained rats to study the effect on the central nervous system of morphine and related substances, *Amer. J. Psychol.*, 47, 597, 1935.

309. Simon, E. J., Single cells, in *Narcotic Drugs, Biochemical Pharmacology*, Clouet, D. H., Ed., Plenum Press, New York, 1971, 310.

310. Singh, J. M., Clinical signs and development of tolerance to thiopental, *Arch. Int. Pharmacodyn. Ther.*, 187, 199, 1970.

311. Singh, J. M., Comparison between acute and chronic administration of ethyl alcohol on the development of tolerance to pentobarbital, *Arch. Int. Pharmacodyn. Ther.*, 189, 123, 1971.

312. Singh, J. M., Fiegenschue, B., and Schexnaydre, C., Development of tolerance to pentobarbital, *J. Pharm. Sci.*, 59, 1020, 1970.

313. Singh, J. M., Trahan, P., and Liljeberg, J. A., The reversal of developed tolerance to pentobarbital by ethyl alcohol, *Arch. Int. Pharmacodyn. Ther.*, 184, 334, 1970.

314. Smith, A. A., Adrenergic regulation of the lenticular response to opioids in mice, in *The Addictive States*, Wikler, A., Ed., Res. Publ. Ass. Nerv. Ment. Dis., Vol. 46, Williams & Wilkins, Baltimore, 1968, 74.

315. Smith, A. A., Inhibitors of tolerance development, in *Narcotic Drugs, Biochemical Pharmacology*, Clouet, D. H., Ed., Plenum Press, New York, 1971, 424.

316. Smith, A., Karmin, M., and Gavitt, J., Blocking effects of puromycin, ethanol, and chloroform on the development of tolerance to an opiate, *Biochem. Pharmacol.*, 15, 1877, 1966.

317. Smith, D. E., Physical vs. psychological dependence and tolerance in high-dose methamphetamine abuse, *Clin. Toxicol.*, 2, 99, 1969.

318. Smith, S. E. and Herxheimer, A., Toxicity of ethanol-barbiturate mixtures, *J. Pharm. Pharmacol.*, 21, 869, 1969.

319. Smith, T. C., Failure to show tolerance to opioid in guinea pig ileum, *Fed. Proc.*, 30, 277, Abs., 1971.

320. Smith, S. E. and Takemori, A. E., Lack of transfer of morphine tolerance by administration of rat cerebral homogenates, *Proc. Soc. Exp. Biol. Med.*, 127, 1167, 1968.

321. Smythies, J. R. and Sykes, E. A., The effect of mescaline upon the conditioned avoidance response in the rat, *Psychopharmacologia*, 6, 163, 1964.

322. Spoerlein, M. T. and Scrafani, J., Effects of time and 8-azaguanine on the development of morphine tolerance, *Life Sci.*, 6, 1549, 1967.

323. Stevenson, I. H. and Turnbull, M. J., Hepatic drug-metabolizing enzyme activity and duration of hexobarbitone anesthesia in barbitone-dependent and withdrawn rats, *Biochem. Pharmacol.*, 17, 2297, 1968.

324. Stevenson, I. H. and Turnbull, M. J., The sensitivity of the brain to barbiturate during chronic administration and withdrawal of barbitone sodium in the rat, *Brit. J. Pharmacol.*, 39, 525, 1970.

325. Stumpf, C. and Chiari, I., Echte Gewohnung un Hexobarbital, *Naunyn Schmiedeberg Arch. Exp. Path. Pharmacol.*, 251, 275, 1965.

326. Takemori, A. E., Studies on cellular adaptation to morphine and its reversal by nalorphine in cerebral cortical slices of rats, *J. Pharmacol. Exp. Ther.*, 135, 89, 1962.

327. Takemori, A. E., Cross-cellular adaptation to methadone and meperidine in cerebral cortical slices from morphinized rats, *J. Pharmacol. Exp. Ther.*, 135, 252, 1962.

328. Takemori, A. E., The effects of morphine, other opioids and their derivatives on the metabolism of the cerebral cortex, in *The Addictive States*, Wikler, A., Ed., Res. Publ. Ass. Nerv. Ment. Dis., Vol. 46, Williams & Wilkins, Baltimore, 1968, 53.

329. Tamayo, L. and Contreras, E., Effect of training on the analgesic action of morphine, *Europ. J. Pharmacol.*, 11, 96, 1970.

330. Tatum, A. L. and Seevers, M. H., Experimental cocaine addiction, *J. Pharmacol. Exp. Ther.*, 36, 401, 1929.

331. Tatum, A. L. and Seevers, M. H., Theories of drug addiction, *Physiol. Rev.*, 11, 107, 1931.

332. Tephly, T. R., Tinelli, F., and Watkins, W. D., Alcohol metabolism: Role of microsomal oxidation *in vivo*, *Science*, 166, 627, 1969.

333. Tilson, H. A. and Sparber, S. B., Differences in tolerance to mescaline produced by peripheral and direct central administration, *Psychopharmacologia*, 19, 313, 1971.

334. Tirri, R., Transfer of induced tolerance to morphine and promazine by brain homogenate, *Experientia*, 23, 278, 1967.

335. Tobon, F. and Mezey, E., Effect of ethanol administration on hepatic and drug-metabolizing enzymes and on rates of ethanol degradation, *J. Lab. Clin. Med.*, 77, 110, 1971.

336. Tormey, J. and Lasagna, L., Relation of thyroid function to acute and chronic effects of amphetamine in the rat, *J. Pharmacol. Exp. Ther.*, 128, 201, 1960.

337. Trenholm, H. L., Maxwell, W. B., Paul, C. J., Wiberg, G. S., and Coldwell, B. B., Biochemical aspects of the interaction of ethanol with barbiturates, *Canad. J. Biochem.*, 48, 706, 1970.

338. Truitt, E. B., Pharmacological activity in a metabolite of 1-trans-Δ^8-tetrahydrocannabinol, *Fed. Proc.*, 29, 619, 1970.

339. Tulunay, F. C., Kiran, B. K., and Kaymakcalan, S., Transfer of morphine tolerance in rats by brain extracts, *J. Pharm. Pharmacol.*, 22, 871, 1970.

340. Turnbull, M. J. and Stevenson, I. H., Tolerance experiments with barbitone-dependent rats, *J. Pharm. Pharmacol.*, 20, 884, 1968.

341. Uehling, B. S., Effects of chronic d-amphetamine sulfate administration during development in rats, *Int. J. Neuropharmacol.*, 8, 43, 1969.

342. Ungar, G., Ed., *Molecular Mechanisms in Memory and Learning*, Plenum Press, New York, 1970.

343. Ungar, G. and Cohen, M., Induction of morphine tolerance by material extracted from brain of tolerant animals, *Int. J. Neuropharmacol.*, 5, 183, 1966.

344. Ungar, G. and Galvan, L., Conditions of transfer of morphine tolerance by brain extracts, *Proc. Soc. Exp. Biol. Med.*, 130, 287, 1969.

345. Utena, H., Behavioral abberations in methamphetamine-intoxicated animals and chemical correlates in the brain, *Prog. Brain Res.*, 21, 192, 1966.

346. Van Praag, D. and Simon, E. J., Studies on the intracellular distribution and tissue binding of dihydromorphine-7, 8-H^3 in the rat, *Proc. Soc. Exp. Biol. Med.*, 122, 6, 1966.

347. Videla, L. and Israel, Y., Factors that modify the metabolism of ethanol in the rat liver and adaptive changes produced by its chronic administration, *Biochem. J.*, 118, 275, 1970.

348. von Wartburg, J. P. and Papenberg, J., Biochemical and enzymatic changes induced by chronic ethanol intake, in *Int. Encyclopedia Pharmacol. Ther.*, Sect. 20, Vol. II, *Alcohols and Derivatives*, Tremolieres, J., Ed., Pergamon Press, New York, 1970, 301.

349. Wahlström, G. and Widerlöv, E., Interaction and acute cross tolerance between ethanol and hexobarbitone in the rat, *J. Pharm. Pharmacol.*, 23, 58, 1971.

350. Wallgren, H., Absorption, diffusion, distribution and elimination of ethanol. Effect on biological membranes, in *Int. Encyclopedia Pharmacol. Ther.*, Sect. 20, Vol. 1, *Alcohols and Derivatives*, Tremolieres, J., Ed., Pergamon Press, New York, 1970, 161.

351. Wallgren, H. and Lindbohm, R., Adaptation to ethanol in rats with special reference to brain tissue respiration, *Biochem. Pharmacol.*, 8, 423, 1961.

352. Wahlström, G., Changes in hexobarbital anesthesia threshold in rats induced by repeated long-term treatment with barbital or ethanol, *Psychopharmacologia*, 19, 366, 1971.

353. Walton, R. P., *Marihuana: America's New Drug Problem*, J. B. Lippincott, Co., Philadelphia, 1938, 128.

354. Warburton, D. M., Modified sensitivity to pentobarbital in a continuous avoidance situation, *Psychopharmacologia* (Berlin), 13, 387, 1968.

355. Waud, D. R., Pharmacological Receptors, *Pharmacol. Rev.*, 20, 49, 1968.

356. Way, E. L. and Adler, T. K., The pharmacologic implications of the fate of morphine and its surrogates, *Pharmacol. Rev.*, 12, 383, 1960.

357. Way, E. L. and Adler, T. K., The biological disposition of morphine and its surrogates, *Bull W.H.O.*, 25, 227, 1961; 26, 51, 1962; 26, 261, 1962; 27, 359, 1962.

358. Way, E. L., Loh, H. H., and Shen, F-H., Morphine tolerance, physical dependence, and synthesis of brain 5-hydroxytryptamine, *Science*, 162, 1290, 1968.

359. Way, E. L. and Shen, F-H., Catecholamines and 5-hydroxytryptamine, in *Narcotic Drugs, Biochemical Pharmacology*, Clouet, D. H., Ed., Plenum Press, New York, 1971, 229.

360. Weil, A. T., Zinberg, N. E., and Nelsen, J. M., Clinical and psychological effects of marijuana in man, *Science*, 162, 1234, 1968.

361. Weiner, I. M., Mechanisms of drug absorption and excretion: The renal excretion of drugs and related compounds, *Ann. Rev. Pharmacol.*, 7, 39, 1967.

362. Weinstock, M., Acetylcholine and cholinesterase, in *Narcotic Drugs, Biochemical Pharmacology*, Clouet, D. H., Ed., Plenum Press, New York, 1971, 254.

363. Wikler, A., Sites and mechanisms of action of morphine and related drugs in the central nervous system, *Pharmacol. Rev.*, 2, 435, 1950.

364. Wikler, A., Clinical and social aspects of marijuana intoxication, *Arch. Gen. Psychiat.*, 23, 320, 1970.

365. Wikler, A. and Frank, K., Hindlimb reflexes of chronic spinal dogs during cycles of addiction to morphine and methadone, *J. Pharmacol. Exper. Ther.*, 94, 382, 1948.

366. Williams, E. G., Himmelsbach, C. K., Wikler, A., Ruble, D. C., and Lloyd, B. N., Studies on marijuana and pyrahexyl compound, *Public Health Rep.*, 61, 1059, 1946.

367. Williams, R. T., *Detoxication mechanisms*, John Wiley & Sons, New York, 1959.

368. Williams, R. T. and Parke, D. V., The metabolic fate of drugs, *Ann. Rev. Pharmacol.*, 4, 85, 1964.

369. Winder, C. V., Anderson, M. M., and Parke, H. C., Comparative properties of six phenethylamines, with observations on the nature of tachyphylaxis, *J. Pharmacol. Exp. Ther.*, 93, 63, 1948.

370. Wolbach, A. B., Jr., Isbell, H., and Miner, E. J., Cross tolerance between mescaline and LSD-25 with a comparison of the mescaline and LSD reactions, *Psychopharmacologia*, 3, 1, 1962.

371. Woods, L. A., Distribution and fate of morphine in non-tolerant and tolerant dogs and rats, *J. Pharmacol. Exp. Ther.*, 112, 158, 1954.

372. Woods, L. A., McMahon, F. G., and Seevers, M. H., Distribution and metabolism of cocaine in the dog and rabbit, *J. Pharmacol. Exp. Ther.*, 101, 200, 1951.

373. Woods, L. A., Wyngaarden, J. B., and Seevers, M. H., Addiction potentialities of 1,1-diphenyl-1-(3-dimethylaminopropyl)-butanone-2 hydrochloride (Amidone) in the monkey, *Proc. Soc. Exp. Biol. and Med.*, 65, 113, 1947.

374. Wuepper, K. D. and Woods, L. A., The distribution of free N-C^{14}-methyl labeled levorphanol in the CNS of non-tolerant dogs, non-tolerant and tolerant monkeys, *Fed. Proc.*, 19, 272, 1960.

375. Xhenseval, B. and Richelle, M., Behavioral effects of long-term treatment with meprobamate in cats, *Int. J. Neuropharmacol.*, 4, 1, 1965.

376. Yamamoto, I., Inoki, R., Tamari, Y., and Iwatsubo, K., Inhibitory effect of 8-azaguanine on the development of tolerance in the analgesic action of morphine, *Jap. J. Pharmacol.*, 17, 140, 1967.

377. Yanagita, T. and Takahashi, S., Development of tolerance to and physical dependence on barbiturates in rhesus monkeys, *J. Pharmacol. Exp. Ther.*, 172, 163, 1970.

378. Yanagita, T., Takahashi, S., Ishida, K., and Funamoto, H., Voluntary inhalation of volatile anesthetics and organic solvents by monkeys, *Jap. J. Clin. Pharmacol.*, 1, 13, 1970.

379. Yeh, S. Y. and Woods, L. A., The effect of tolerance and withdrawal on the *in vivo* metabolism of N-C^{14}-methyl-dihydromorphine in the rat, *J. Pharmacol. Exp. Ther.*, 169, 168, 1969.

380. Yeh, S. Y. and Woods, L. A., Maternal and fetal distribution of H^3-dihydromorphine in the tolerant and nontolerant rat, *J. Pharmacol. Exp. Ther.*, 174, 9, 1970.

381. Yoshikawa, H., Mechanism of development of tolerance to pentobarbital, *Folia Pharmacol. Jap.*, 66, 214, 1970.

THEORIES RELATED TO PHYSICAL DEPENDENCE

A. Wikler

TABLE OF CONTENTS

INTRODUCTION

Except for the "dual action" theory of physical dependence on morphine proposed by Tatum, Seevers, and Collins in 1929,[1] (the original form of which has been discarded by Seevers and Deneau[2]) theories related to physical dependence not only on opioids, but also on barbiturates, certain nonbarbiturate sedatives, "minor tranquilizers," and on ethanol, generally postulate one or another sort of "counter-adaptation" to the agonistic actions of these drugs, which results in the development of "latent hyperexcitability" of the central nervous system that becomes manifest as an abstinence syndrome when the drug in question is withdrawn abruptly. At least in the case of dependence on morphine or other opioids, such a hypothesis is strongly suggested by the fact that in general, the direction of change in directly observable physiological variables during the "primary" (or "early" or "acute") abstinence syndrome is opposite to that produced by the drug in the nontolerant state. Thus, in nontolerant human subjects, morphine constricts the pupil and depresses respiratory rate; while little, if any tolerance develops to the miotic effect of morphine during chronic administration of the drug, partial tolerance to the respiratory-depressant effect does supervene. However, in the "primary" abstinence syndrome, miosis gives way to mydriasis, and bradypnea to tachypnea. To account for such, and other autonomic changes during cycles of morphine addiction, Himmelsbach[3] proposed a "homeostatic" counter-adaptive theory of morphine tolerance and physical dependence. According to this theory, through its actions on hypothalamic centers, morphine disturbs homeostasis in the nontolerant subject. In response to this "stress," autonomic adjustments take place which partially restore homeostasis. With repeated administration of morphine, such adjustments gain strength "disproportionately," so that continued presence of the drug is required to maintain a new level of homeostasis. When the drug is withdrawn abruptly, the "equilibrium" which had been achieved is lost, and the unchecked, counter-adaptive changes in autonomic function become manifest as the abstinence syndrome. That such counter-adaptive changes are associated with "latent hyperexcitability" of the autonomic nervous system is indicated by Himmelsbach's[4] observation that vasopressor responses to a standard cold stimulus were greater, and recovery after removal of the stimulus was slower in morphine-tolerant subjects than in normal subjects.

During the primary morphine-abstinence syndrome, the reversal of agonistic effects of morphine on the somatic nervous system is more difficult to recognize in the intact human or animal subject, but the phenomenon is striking in the chronic spinal dog[5] or man.[6] Thus, in the nontolerant chronic spinal dog, single doses of morphine depress the flexor and crossed extensor reflexes, while enhancing the ipsilateral extensor thrust and exerting little effect in either direction on the knee jerk. During regular administration of morphine, four times daily, tolerance develops to the depressant effects of morphine on the flexor and crossed extensor reflexes[5] and, as was shown later by Martin,[7] to the excitant effects on the ipsilateral extensor thrust. About 17 hours after abrupt withdrawal of morphine, the flexor and crossed extensor reflexes become hyperactive, while the ipsilateral extensor thrust becomes difficult to elicit. At about 41 hours of morphine-abstinence, the paralyzed lower limbs exhibit spontaneous "running" movements which may persist for as long as 96 hours.[5] To account for these findings, Wikler[8] suggested that during the development of tolerance, "cellular adaptation" to the depressant effects of morphine takes place in the spinal cord and that these "counter-adaptations" are "released" when morphine is withdrawn abruptly. The same sequence of changes in reflexes can be "precipitated" by a single dose of nalorphine in morphine-tolerant chronic spinal dogs[9] or in chronic spinal man.[6] One possible interpretation of this phenomenon is that, by antagonizing the agonistic actions of morphine, the "cellular counter-adaptations," previously held in check by morphine, are suddenly "unmasked." However, Wikler and Carter[9] noted that in the chronic spinal dog, the sequence of changes in reflexes could be "precipitated" by nalorphine even before there was any evidence of tolerance to morphine. Moreover, when "running" movements were "precipitated" by nalorphine in the morphine-tolerant preparation, administration of morphine increased the amplitude of these "running" movements in contrast to their disappearance when morphine administration was reinstituted after "running" movements had appeared following abrupt withdrawal of morphine. In view of these observations, Wikler and Carter[9] suggested that ". . .the processes responsible for physical dependence begin very early during morphine addiction, possibly after a single dose, that they are distinct from those which subserve tolerance, and that they are 'masked' by the narcotic actions of morphine. *N*-allylnormorphine appears to antagonize the narcotic effects of morphine, thereby 'unmasking' such physical dependence as had developed." Also, Wikler[8] pointed out that the observations on the nalorphine-precipitated hindlimb morphine-abstinence syndrome just cited are compatible with the "dual action" theory of physical dependence. As revised by Seevers and Deneau,[2] the "excitant" actions of morphine postulated in the "dual action" theory play only a minor role in the very early phases of the morphine-withdrawal syndrome, but a more significant one in the nalorphine-precipitated abstinence syndrome in both acutely and chronically morphine-tolerant subjects. In such individuals, nalorphine not only "unmasks" the adaptive responses to the depressant actions of morphine, but also intensifies the abstinence syndrome as a whole by "unmasking" the direct excitant actions of morphine.

Newer theories of physical dependence may be viewed essentially as attempts to explain the mechanisms involved in the development of "counter-adaptation" and "latent hyper-excitability" during continued exposure of the central nervous system to drugs that produce physical dependence. Although the data on which some of these theories are based were acquired with drugs other than opioids, they are "aimed" at offering an explanation of tolerance to and physical dependence on morphine. Implicit in all of them is the morphine model of "reversal" described above, although what is held to be "reversed" depends on the specific pattern of agonistic actions of the drug, or the class of drugs under consideration. Though differing considerably in the degrees of "reduction" attempted by them (formulations in terms of "brain tissue," "neuronal circuits," "receptors," or "enzymes"), these theories are not mutually exclusive. Indeed, with relatively minor modifications, any one of them can be restated in such a way as to fit the data presently adduced in support of any of the others. However, each theory has heuristic value in its own right and hopefully, successive reformulations of them in the light of new data acquired by research at all levels of "reduction" will, eventually, lead to a "unified" theory of physical dependence.

In the sections that follow, the general outlines of a selected number of newer theories of physical dependence will be presented first and later, some special factors pertaining to the opioid, barbiturate-sedative, and ethanol abstinence syndromes individually, will be reviewed.

GENERAL THEORIES OF PHYSICAL DEPENDENCE

"Disuse Supersensitivity" ("Pharmacological Denervation Supersensitivity")

Jaffe and Sharpless[10] have proposed that, in a manner analogous to the development of "pharmacological denervation supersensitivity" in peripheral tissues,[11-13] "latent hyperexcitability" of postsynaptic elements in the central nervous system can develop as a consequence of prolonged "disuse" of the synapses in question either through continuous local pharmacological blockade, or through continuous reduction of neural activities converging on such synapses as a result of the agonistic effects of a given drug elsewhere in the brain. In support of this hypothesis are data indicating that the time-courses of development of "latent hyperexcitability" during continued drug administration, and of subsidence of "hyperexcitability" after withdrawal of the drug, are consistent with the known time-courses of the development of physical dependence and of abstinence phenomena, respectively. Thus, by testing pentylenetetrazol-induced seizure thresholds 22 to 24 hours after the last dose of pentobarbital, Jaffe and Sharpless[14] were able to show that in the cat, such thresholds were significantly lower than control values even after only 26 hours of chronic pentobarbital intoxication (in anesthetic doses) and continued to fall as chronic intoxication on pentobarbital was maintained. Maximal "supersensitivity" to pentylenetetrazol was achieved in 2 to 3 weeks; after abrupt withdrawal of pentobarbital, such seizure thresholds rose gradually toward control values over time-courses that were the more prolonged (three to over six days), the longer the period of chronic pentobarbital intoxication had been. Similarly, Friedman and Jaffe[15] and Friedman, Jaffe, and Sharpless[16] demonstrated that in the mouse, the muscarinic cholinergic agent, pilocarpine, produces a dose-dependent fall in rectal temperature, presumably through a central action, inasmuch as this hypothermic response is blocked by the antimuscarinic agent, scopolamine (a tertiary compound), but not by its quaternary analog, methscopolamine. Testing hypothermic responses to pilocarpine (i.p.) 24 hours after withdrawal of scopolamine (p.o., in drinking water), they found that the pilocarpine dose-hypothermic response curve was shifted to the left after continuous ingestion of scopolamine for five days to four weeks, and that the hyperresponsiveness to pilocarpine lasted longer after four weeks of scopolamine treatment than after five days. Evidence for tolerance to scopolamine (decreased effectiveness in blocking pilocarpine-induced hypothermia) and for a scopolamine-abstinence syndrome (spontaneous fall in rectal temperature on withdrawal of scopolamine) was also obtained.

Though proposing "disuse hypersensitivity" (or "disuse adaptation") as a possible mechanism in the development of physical dependence, Jaffe and Sharpless[10] note that intracellular changes in neurons constantly exposed to the presence of a foreign agent may also play a role ("direct, pharmacogenic or chemogenic adaptation").

"Pharmacological Redundancy"

In a series of publications, Martin and his associates[7,17-19] have developed a theory of *chronic* tolerance and physical dependence. The main features of this are (1) that for the mediation of a given brain function, there are not only "primary" neural pathways that normally serve this purpose, but also "redundant" pathways that are normally less, or not at all activated in the mediation of that function; (2) that the "primary" and "redundant" pathways are differentially sensitive to chemical agents (neurohumors, drugs); (3) that the activities of both the "primary" and "redundant" pathways are subject to tonic inhibition "upstream" from the effector tissues expressing that function by negative feedback loops from those effector tissues; (4) that if the "primary" pathway is selectively blocked *for prolonged periods of time* by a chemical agent at a site "downstream" from the site of negative feedback inhibition in the "primary" pathway, and *if such blockade results in decreased activation of the effector tissues,* then the consequent diminution of tonic negative feedback inhibition of the "redundant" pathways will result in increased activation and eventually, "hypertrophy" of them (chronic tolerance); and (5) when the selective blockade of the "primary" pathway is removed (e.g., by drug withdrawal, or administration of a drug-anatagonist), the effector tissues are activated by neural impulses arriving not only through the now restored "primary" pathway, but also through the hypertrophied "redundant" pathways, resulting in an abstinence syndrome, the time-course of which corresponds to that required for reestablishment of negative feedback inhibition of both the "primary" and "redundant" pathways, and eventual recession of "hypertrophy" in the latter.

It should be noted that, according to this theory, mere "occupation" by a drug of a receptor site in the "primary" pathway is not sufficient to unleash the chain of events that leads to hypertrophy of the "redundant" pathways; for this to happen, the drug must exert agonistic effects. Thus, naloxone, the specific opioid-antagonist that presumably occupies the same receptor site as morphine, but has virtually no agonistic actions, does not produce physical dependence.[20] Also, in the case of agonists that do produce physical dependence, their blocking effects in the "primary" pathway persist despite the development of tolerance and physical dependence. Thus, in studies on the effects of morphine upon the responsiveness of the respiratory center to carbon dioxide inhalation in man, Martin et al.[18] found that in nontolerant subjects, the slope of the respiratory minute volume (l./min) – carbon dioxide partial pressure (mm Hg) curve was 1.5, with a threshold ("intercept," for respiratory minute volume of 10 l./min) of 51.7 pCO_2; after administration of morphine, 15 mg/70 kg, the corresponding values were 1.2 and 60.1, and after 30 mg/70 kg, 1.1 and 62.8 (differences between effects of 15 and 30 mg/70 kg not significant). In subjects receiving 60 mg/70 kg 4 times daily for periods up to 8 months, "pre-drug" values (4 to 5 hours after the last previous dose) ranged from 1.8 to 1.9 (slope) and 61.0 to 62.1 (threshold). Though these values did not differ significantly from pre-drug control values, these investigators concluded that, all data considered, respiratory sensitivity to CO_2 was less during dependence than in the control period. Similarly, Martin and Jasinski[21] noted that in morphine-tolerant subjects, "pre-drug" respiratory rate remained significantly depressed, compared to control values in the nontolerant state. The studies on responsivity of the respiratory center to carbon dioxide[18] also yielded evidence that despite the continued agonistic effects of morphine, partial tolerance does develop to its respiratory-depressant effects, and that this can be explained on the assumption of "redundancy." Thus, in subjects "stabilized" on morphine, 60 mg/70 kg 4 times daily, single doses of 60 or 120 mg/70 kg of morphine produced much smaller changes (in slopes and thresholds of the respiratory minute volume-carbon dioxide partial pressure curves) than did 15 or 30 mg/70 kg of morphine in the nontolerant state. Inasmuch as there is no evidence of increased destruction or inactivation of morphine in the tolerant state and, as noted above, morphine continues to exert its agonistic actions on respiration during tolerance, the data can be explained by assuming that in the tolerant subjects, the "primary" respiratory pathway was already blocked maximally by morphine, and that respiration was maintained by morphine-insensitive, hypertrophied "redundant" circuits. The data obtained during morphine withdrawal are also consistent with this view. Thus, 20 hours after the last dose of morphine, the slope was increased from 1.5 in the control, nontolerant state to 3.1 (difference significant).[18] In keeping with this observation is the characteristic hyperpnea during the primary morphine abstinence syndrome.[21] It may be remarked, however, that the data are also consistent with the "disuse supersensitization" theory. Thus, if it is assumed that the site of morphine blockade lies "distal" to the CO_2-sensitive neurons, but "proximal" to internuncials innervating the ventral horn ganglion cells of the diaphragm and thoracic musculature, and that neural outflow to the ganglion cells, though diminished, is not halted completely even by maximally effective doses of morphine, then in consequence of "less use" over time, the ganglion cells would become supersensitive to the neurohumor (acetylcholine) released by those impulses evoked by carbon dioxide that do "get through" the morphine blockade, with all the consequences for tolerance and physical dependence predicated in the "pharmacological redundancy" theory. However, support for the "pharmacological redundancy" theory (as opposed to the "disuse supersensitization" theory) would be afforded if it could be shown that in the morphine-tolerant (as compared with the nontolerant) state there is an increased respiratory response, not to acetylcholine (presumed to be the neurohumor activating the ventral horn ganglion cells) or to cholinomimetic agents, but to some other neurohumor (or precursor, or mimicker thereof) postulated to mediate transmission in hypertrophied, redundant pathways.

Strong evidence for the existence of "redundant" pathways has been acquired by Martin and Eades[17] and Martin[19] using the flexor reflex in the chronic spinal dog as a simplified model of the central nervous system. In this preparation, neither phenoxybenzamine (alpha-adrenergic antagonist) nor chlorpromazine (alpha-adrenergic and tryptaminergic antagonist) affects the flexor reflex; atropine (muscarinic cholinergic antagonist) does have a small but significant effect.[19] Nevertheless, facilitation of the flexor reflex and production of stepping ("running") movements by the adrenergic agonists, methoxamine and amphetamine, are antagonized by phenoxybenzamine and chlorpromazine; the same effects of tryptaminergic drugs (tryptamine, LSD, psilocin, mescaline, DOM) are antagonized by chlorpromazine and cyproheptadine (also a tryptaminergic antagonist), but not by phenoxybenzamine; and the likewise similar effects of cholinergic agonists (physostigmine and oxotremorine) are antagonized by atropine, but not phenoxybenzamine. One model of "pharmacological redundancy" that can be constructed to explain these results postulates that the segmental reflex arc for the flexor reflex is neither adrenergic, nor tryptaminergic, nor cholinergic (except possibly at the ventral horn ganglion cell synapse), but that there are suprasegmental adrenergic, tryptaminergic, and cholinergic facilitatory pathways ("redundant") to the segmental internuncial cells subserving the flexor reflex arc which can be activated by appropriate agonists. This, and other models of "pharmacological redundancy" are described by Martin.[19]

As noted earlier, augmentation of the flexor reflex and spontaneous "running" movements are characteristic of the morphine-abstinence syndrome in the chronic spinal dog, and this preparation has the capacity for development of a high level of chronic tolerance.[5,7] It would be expected then, that hypertrophy of adrenergic, tryptaminergic, and/or cholinergic "redundant" spinal pathways would play a role in these phenomena. Atropine, but not phenoxybenzamine, has been found to depress the flexor reflex in the morphine-abstinent chronic spinal dog, suggesting that cholinergic neurons (which may or may not be "redundant") do play such a role.[17] Data on cyproheptadine have not come to the attention of this reviewer.

The implications of the "pharmacological redundancy" theory for *acute* tolerance and physical dependence and for "protracted abstinence" will be mentioned only briefly here. While recruitment of "redundant" pathways may play some role in the development of acute tolerance to morphine, the more important mechanism in this situation appears to be partial restoration of autonomic functioning through responses of homeostatic regulatory systems to the abnormal conditions (hypothermia, hypocapnia) created by the actions of morphine on "homeostats" (lowering or raising their regulatory "set points"). If, after the new state of homeostatic equilibrium has been established, a morphine-antagonist is administered, the "set points" of the homeostats are immediately restored to normal levels and the homeostatic regulatory systems now respond vigorously to the still-persisting abnormal environmental conditions ("acute precipitated abstinence syndrome"), until these are dissipated.[7,22] On the other hand, slow regression of hypertrophied, pharmacologically redundant pathways may account for "protracted abstinence";[21] thus, Sloan and Eisenman[23] have shown that changes in brain and adrenal catecholamine levels are detectable five months after withdrawal of morphine in dependent rats.

"New Receptors"

Modeling his hypothesis on Ehrlich's "side-chain theory," Sakel[24] proposed that in the "vegetative nervous system," sympathetic neurons are normally activated by a combination of their "side-chains" (receptors) with a circulating hormone (tentatively identified as "adrenaline"). Morphine also combines with these "side-chains," but this combination does not excite the neuron. Inasmuch as there are now fewer "side-chains" that can combine with the excitant hormone, the neuron assumes a state of subthreshold quiescence ("unterschwellige Ruhe"), which is experienced subjectively as "euphoria." Inactivation of some "side-chains" by morphine constitutes a biological stimulus for the formation of new hormone-receptive "side-chains" in a more abundant fashion ("in reichlicherer Weise") than before. As more "side-chains" are available for combination with excitant hormone, the initial effect of morphine is reversed – the neuron is overexcited ("überregt"), and larger doses of morphine are required to inactivate the excess number of "side-chains" and to reduce their number to the level required for "euphoria" (tolerance). In consequence, still more "side-chains" are formed and the cycle is repeated. In a saturated ("gesättigter") morphinist, the neuron is covered with an excessively large number of "side-chains;" however, all but those required for maintenance of a "normal" level of activation (by combination with circulating hormone) are inactivated by combination with morphine. However, when morphine is suddenly withdrawn, all of the "side-chains" become free to combine with circulating hormone, the neuron is intensely overexcited and consequently an abstinence syndrome appears as a supernormal excitation of the "vegetative nervous system," which continues over a time-course corresponding to that of the falling away ("abfallen") of the excess "side-chains" (which are not regenerated since the morphine-stimulus is lacking).

A more elaborate theory of "new receptors" to explain tolerance and physical dependence has recently been proposed by Collier.[25,26] According to this theory, receptors may be "silent" (receptor-drug combination produces no observable effect) or "pharmacological" ("active," in that the receptor-drug combination does produce an effect). The number of "silent" or "pharmacological" receptors may be increased ("induction") or decreased ("reduction") in adaptation of the cell to distortion of its functioning by an excess or deficiency of a chemical substance. Induction of "silent" receptors or reduction of "pharmacological receptors" could account for tolerance to drugs without physical dependence – e.g., certain drugs induce "silent receptors" for themselves, while others reduce the number of pharmacological receptors that are available for combination with them. To explain tolerance with physical dependence, interactions between pharmacological receptors, neurohumoral transmitter substances, and drugs are postulated. Thus, one type of interaction described is very similar to that proposed by Sakel (see above): by occupation of receptors for an endogenous excitatory transmitter, the drug induces new pharmacological receptors for the transmitter (tolerance), and after drug withdrawal, removal of the surplus receptors lags behind the disappearance of the drug molecules from the cell (abstinence syndrome). Another type of interaction is compatible with the "disuse supersensitivity" and "pharmacological redundancy" theories previously described: by whatever mechanism, the drug reduces the supply of an excitatory transmitter, thereby inducing new pharmacological receptors for that transmitter (tolerance); on withdrawal of the drug, the supply of transmitter is restored to normal before the surplus pharmacological receptors are removed (abstinence syndrome). A third type of interaction hypothesized is not predicated on the "disuse supersensitization" and "pharmacological redundancy" theories: the supply of an endogenous inhibitory transmitter is increased, in consequence of which the number of pharmacological receptors is decreased (tolerance); on drug withdrawal, the supply of transmitter falls to normal levels more rapidly than the normal number of pharmacological receptors are restored (abstinence syndrome due to deficiency of inhibitory pharmacological receptors). Collier[26] also discusses the possible roles played by the transmitter substances, acetylcholine and norepinephrine, in connection with morphine tolerance and physical dependence.

"Enzyme Expansion"

A number of sedative drugs stimulate their own metabolism by nonspecific liver microsomal enzyme induction. Among these are phenobarbital, pentobarbital, hexobarbital, meprobamate, glutethimide, and chlopromazine, but not morphine or meperidine.[27] Also, ethanol induces a liver microsomal ethanol-oxidizing enzyme which is distinct from liver alcohol dehydrogenase.[28] Increase in liver alcohol dehydrogenase activity during ethanol consumption has been reported by some investigators,[29,30] but denied by others.[28] Such enzyme inductions could result in lowering of blood levels and decrease in the effects of the drugs involved during chronic administration (tolerance), but not in the development of physical dependence. In the case of ethanol, this type of tolerance has been termed "metabolic tolerance," in contradistinction to "tissue tolerance" which is accompanied by physical dependence.[31] However, the term, "tissue tolerance" does not imply that metabolic alterations in "tissues" (as distinct from increased catabolism of the drug itself) are not involved in the development of tolerance with physical dependence.

In 1961, Shuster[32] and Goldstein and Goldstein[33] proposed metabolic theories of tolerance with physical dependence that are quite similar to each other. In Shuster's theory, morphine acts at two sites: (1) by inhibiting the action or synthesis of a neurohumoral transmitter, thereby causing analgesia, sedation, and other characteristic morphine effects; and (2) by either "de-repressing" the synthesis of the enzyme concerned with synthesis of the neurohumoral transmitter, or by "repressing" the synthesis of an enzyme which destroys the neurohumoral transmitter. In consequence of the second action, the concentration (activity) of the neurohumoral transmitter-synthesizing enzyme steadily increases with continued administration of morphine, thereby reducing the effects of the first action (tolerance). When morphine is withdrawn, both actions of the drug cease and, because of the greatly increased levels of neurohumoral transmitter-synthesizing enzyme still present, an excess of the transmitter supervenes, with reversal of the agonistic effects of morphine (abstinence syndrome), the time-course of which corresponds to that required for decline of the transmitter-synthesizing enzyme to normal levels. The same train of events can be precipitated by nalorphine in the tolerant state through antagonizing the inhibitory actions of morphine at the first site. In Goldstein and Goldstein's theory, further elaborated in 1968,[34] only one site of action of the inhibitory drug is postulated – namely, at the receptor of the transmitter-synthesizing enzyme. "Expansion" of this enzyme could result from either of two mechanisms: (1) "de-repression" consequent to decrease in the level of the natural "repressor" of that enzyme, namely, the product of its catalytic action, the transmitter substance; or (2) "stabilization" of the transmitter-synthesizing enzyme against its own catabolism. The consequence of these mechanisms for tolerance and physical dependence would be the same as those postulated in Shuster's theory.

Expressed in terms of transmitter-synthesizing "enzyme expansion," these theories would seem to differ from the "receptor expansion" ("new receptor") theory in that the former is "presynaptic" and predicates an increased level of transmitter-synthesizing enzyme during dependence, while the latter is "post-synaptic" and predicates an increase in number of "pharmacological receptors" during dependence. However, the "enzyme expansion" theory could be applied as well to explain a postulated increase in "pharmacological receptors" during dependence by merely substituting "cellular receptor protein-synthesis" for the site of drug-inhibitory action, the receptor in question being that which combines with a neurohumoral transmitter. In effect, then, one problem for "unification" of the general theories of physical dependence reviewed resolves itself into ascertaining whether it is the level of transmitter-synthesizing enzyme protein, or cellular receptor-synthesizing enzyme protein, that is increased in the "tissue-tolerant" state.

SPECIAL FACTORS RELATED TO PHYSICAL DEPENDENCE

Opioids

Oxidative metabolism – In vitro, the increase in oxygen consumption of cortical slices produced by electrical stimulation is inhibited by meperidine,[35] and that produced by K^+ ion is inhibited by morphine, methadone, or meperidine.[36-39] Furthermore, the same concentration of morphine (1×10^{-3}M) in vitro failed to inhibit K^+ ion-stimulated respiration in cortical slices from rats made tolerant to morphine in vivo, and "cross-adaptation" was shown for methadone, and to a lesser extent for meperidine.[38] Such "adaptation" was not found in cortical slices from morphine-tolerant rats given nalorphine 30 minutes before sacrifice.[38] The specificity of such cross-adaptation for opioids is indicated by the absence of cross-adaptation of morphine-adapted cortical slices to the depressant effects of pentobarbital or ethanol.[40] Though the in vitro concentrations of opioids needed to show these effects were inordinately high, the findings do suggest as Takemori[39] points out, that brain mitochondrial respiratory enzyme systems may be one of the "receptor sites" for opioid action. Whether or not "adaptation" to the effects of opioids at this site is merely an example of tolerance, or a cause of tolerance to other effects of these drugs in the intact organism, is not clear.

***N*-demethylating enzymes** – Axelrod[41,42] reported that *N*-demethylation of morphine and other opioids by rat liver in vitro decreased progressively as the animals acquired tolerance to morphine in vivo and that chronic administration of nalorphine with morphine in vivo reduced both the rates of the development of tolerance and the decrease in liver *N*-demethylating enzyme activity. These data were interpreted as an indication that *N*-demethylating enzyme receptor sites are inactivated by continuous interaction with opioids and become "unavailable" for such drugs. Alternatively, the data could be explained in terms of induction of "silent" receptors (tolerance without physical dependence).[25,26]

Catecholamines – Changes in levels of brain norepinephrine (NE), adrenal NE and epinephrine (E), and of both catecholamines in the urine after single doses of morphine during tolerance and in abstinence (by withdrawal of morphine or precipitation by nalorphine) have been studied in the rat, dog, and/or rabbit by Gunne,[43-46] Sloan,[23,47] Maynert,[48,49] and their associates. Though there are some differences in details, the findings on which there is general agreement may be summarized as follows. Single doses of morphine produce a decrease in brain NE only when the effects of the drug are grossly "excitant" (best seen in the cat); however, adrenal E decreases with or without "excitement" (cat, dog, rabbit, rat).[49] In the morphine-tolerant state, brain NE concentrations remain unchanged in dogs,[46] but in the rat, brain NE and adrenal E increase as tolerance to the depressant effects of morphine develop, and excitant effects of the drug (with hyperthermia) become predominant.[46-49] During the early abstinence period (morphine-withdrawal or nalorphine-precipitation) no change is noted in brain NE[46,49] or adrenal E[49] of rats (which exhibit hypothermia), but brain NE (and dopamine) falls markedly in dogs (which exhibit marked excitement and hyperthermia). In the urine, the output of NE and E is greatly increased both in the dog[46] and the rat;[23] that of E peaking somewhat earlier than NE, both returning to normal in two weeks, but NE falling to subnormal levels for several months thereafter in the rat.[23]

It is very difficult to judge whether the changes in brain catecholamines are causes or consequences of tolerance and physical dependence. The fact that brain NE levels are not increased in morphine-tolerant dogs would suggest that the increased levels found in the brains of morphine-tolerant rats are due to increased synthesis of NE in response to increased utilization of this neurohumor in a species in which "excitatory" effects of morphine (increased activity and oxygen consumption, hyperthermia) predominate after tolerance to its depressant effects has been established. Similarly, the greatly increased urinary excretion of NE (and E) in the early morphine-abstinence period in both dog and rat, may reflect even greater utilization of these neurohumors in consequence of enhanced activation of the "ergotrophic" (predominantly sympathetic) system not only in the dog, which is obviously "excited," but also in the rat (increased frequency of "wet dog" shakes, hyperalgesia), despite its deceptive "sedated" appearance when not handled.

On the other hand, at least in the rat, the data could be interpreted as indicative of a causal role of changes in brain NE in the development of tolerance to and physical dependence on morphine. However, in the formulation of such a concept, it is not necessary to assume that the actions of NE in the brain are "excitatory." The analgesic actions of morphine are antagonized by reserpine,[50-52] suggesting that this "depressant" effect of morphine may be mediated by NE, though mediation by serotonin cannot be ruled out. Assuming that NE exerts inhibitory actions in the central nervous system, Collier[26] suggested that the increased brain concentration of NE in the morphine-tolerant rat may "inactivate" NE receptors (tolerance) and when brain levels of NE fall after withdrawal of morphine ("best seen in the dog"), central inhibition is reduced because less than the normal number of NE receptors are available ("excitatory" abstinence phenomena). In this connection, it is interesting to note that during the early morphine abstinence period in the chronic spinal dog, phenoxybenzamine did not merely fail to suppress the hyperactivity of the flexor reflex, but actually increased its amplitude.[17] Such a result would be expected from Collier's hypothesis, since phenoxybenzamine would reduce still further the number of receptors available for the "inhibitory" transmitter, NE. However, this interpretation is clouded by the data on the effects of amphetamine which augments the flexor reflex in the "normal" chronic spinal dog, presumably through release of NE because this action of amphetamine is antagonized by reserpine treatment and by phenoxybenzamine.[17] Complicating the interpretation of the mode of action of amphetamine is Martin's[53] observation that reserpine did not antagonize the behavioral effects of amphetamine *above* the level of transection in the "normal" chronic spinal dog (whether or not reserpine actually enhanced such effects of amphetamine is not stated). Perhaps these apparently conflicting data could be reconciled by assuming that amphetamine releases NE and that NE is "inhibitory," but whether "depression" or "excitation" results, depends on what is "inhibited" – a response ("depression") or a response-inhibiting mechanism ("excitation"). Both above and below the level of transaction, the "normal" and morphine-tolerant, physically dependent chronic spinal dog may differ in regard to response-inhibitory mechanisms.

Serotonin (5-hydroxytryptamine, 5-HT) – That continued protein synthesis is involved in the development of tolerance to morphine is suggested by observations that concomitant administration of actinomycin D[54] or cycloheximide[55] with morphine retards the development of tolerance to the analgesic effects of morphine in mice. Way et al.[55] also reported that concomitant administration of cycloheximide with morphine retards the development of physical dependence in mice ("jumping" response to naloxone). That the protein in question may be that concerned with the synthesis of 5-HT is suggested by evidence reported by Way et al:[55] (a) brain levels of 5-HT are greatly increased after administration of a monoamine oxidase inhibitor (pargyline) in mice made tolerant to morphine by morphine injections or by morphine-pellet implantation, but not in nontolerant controls, two weeks after pellet-removal; and (b), single or a few doses of *p*-chlorophenylalanine (which inhibits the hydroxylation of tryptophan and reduces brain levels of 5-HT in the mouse) reduced the analgesic effect of single doses of morphine (thermal tail-flick threshold method), and the incidence of "jumping" responses to naloxone (morphine-abstinence phenomenon) after six days of administration of morphine subcutaneously at eight hour intervals.

The hypothesis that increased synthesis of 5-HT is responsible for the development of morphine-tolerance and physical dependence implies that 5-HT mediates pain and other central events that are depressed or inhibited by morphine. If so, then *p*-chlorophenylalanine (which reduced brain 5-HT levels) should have analgetic actions, but there is no evidence. Also, as morphine-tolerant mice (with increased 5-HT levels) are not "hyperalgesic," it would be necessary to postulate that, in addition to "inducing" brain 5-HT synthesis, morphine blocks receptors for 5-HT on cells of the central nervous system, as in peripheral tissues.[56] It should be noted also that brain 5-HT levels are not increased in morphine-tolerant dogs or rats.[46,57]*

Acetylcholine – Paton[58] found that in the

*The role of altered serotonin metabolism in the development of tolerance to and physical dependence on opioids has been called into question by the results of further investigations. Shen et al.[107] were able to confirm the findings of Way et al.[55] that in mice made tolerant to morphine by subcutaneous implantation of a morphine (75mg) pellet for 3 or 4 days, brain levels of serotonin increased significantly (to twice their control values) during the first 30 minutes after administration of the monoamine oxidase inhibitor, pargyline (75mg/kg i.p.). Furthermore, Shen et al.[107] found that in such morphine-tolerant mice, brain levels of 5-hydroxyindole acetic acid (5-HIAA) increased significantly after administration of probenecid (100 mg/kg i.p.) which blocks transport of 5-HIAA from the central nervous system to the blood. These findings would seem to be in accord with the conclusion drawn by Way et al.[55] that morphine-tolerance is associated with increased turnover of brain serotonin. Supporting this conclusion also are the findings of Shen et al.[107] that concomitant administration of naloxone with morphine injections prevented not only the development of tolerance and physical dependence, but also the initial (0 to 30 minutes) increase in brain serotonin levels after administration of pargyline. However, these investigators also reported some findings that are not easily reconciled with this conclusion. Thus, administration of *p*-chlorophenylalanine (PCPA), 320 mg/kg i.p., one day prior to morphine-pellet implantation guinea pig ileum suspended in Krebs solution and stimulated electrically through coaxial electrodes, twitch responses were depressed by morphine added to the bath, but tolerance to this effect developed quickly either on prolonged exposure to the same concentration of the drug or to increasing concentrations. On washing morphine out, the twitch response decreased again, but could be *restored* by adding morphine to the bath ("dependence"). As in the morphine-tolerant state, the preparation was fully responsive to acetylcholine, it was concluded that morphine does not act as a cholinergic blocking agent, nor does it depress the contractility of the intestine itself, and therefore, must act by blocking the release of acetylcholine from postganglionic nerve endings in the intestine. This was confirmed by direct assay of acetylcholine in the bath after electrical stimulation of the esernized guinea pig ileum in the absence and in the presence of morphine in the bath.

These data indicate that, at least in the intestine, morphine can act through blocking the release of acetylcholine. As Paton[58] points out, morphine has no such action on autonomic ganglia or skeletal nerve-muscle junctions, nor does it affect neural transmission at these loci. It is possible, therefore, that morphine may act in the central nervous system by blocking the release of acetylcholine at some of the synapses where it does block neural transmission.

The type of morphine-"dependence" described by Paton is more difficult to relate to physical dependence in organisms with a central nervous system. In general, it is reminiscent of the detoxification-inhibition and detoxification-excitation ("Entgiftungshemmung" and "Entgiftungserregung") phenomena observed by

Footnote continued from page 367.
inhibited the development of tolerance to the analgesic effect of morphine (tail-flick method) by about 50%, but did not inhibit the development of physical dependence, as measured by the "jumping" response to naloxone, 8 mg/kg. Nor was the "jumping" response to naloxone, 8 mg/kg reduced in mice pretreated with PCPA and tested after 5 and 10 injections of morphine, 40 mg/kg. s.c. (given 3 times daily); inhibition of the development of physical dependence was observed when morphine injections were continued (total of 15 or 19 injections), but only when the test-dose of naloxone was reduced from 8 to 4 mg/kg in one strain of mice, whereas in another strain, the "jumping" response to 8 mg/kg of naloxone was observed in only 1 of 7 PCPA-pretreated, compared with 9 of 11 nonpretreated mice that had received 15 or 19 injections of morphine. Complicating interpretation of changes in brain serotonin further, is the statement of Shen et al.[107] that preliminary findings indicate that depletion of brain stores of serotonin and catecholamines with reserpine appears to further decrease markedly the analgesic response to morphine in morphine-tolerant mice. These investigators conclude that tolerance to and physical dependence on morphine is associated with changes in serotonin turnover, but a casual relationship has not been established.

Similarly, Maruyama et al.[108] doubt that there is a causal relationship between opioid tolerance and physical dependence on the one hand, and changes in brain serotonin metabolism on the other. Like Way et al.,[55] these investigators found that brain serotonin turnover (pargyline method) is increased three days after morphine-pellet implantation, but they noted that the extent of this increase depends on the strain of mice. Furthermore, they also found that administration of PCPA or reserpine before morphine-pellet implantation did not decrease the incidence of "jumping" to either naloxone or naloxone plus pargyline, and that there were no significant differences in brain serotonin turnover between mice that "jumped" and in mice that did not "jump". On the other hand, they found that administration of PCPA prior to commencement of morphine injections did reduce the development of tolerance to the analgesic effects of morphine (writhing test) and cross-tolerance to other opioids, though such pretreatment failed to alter the incidence of "jumping" to naloxone.

That the "pargyline method" may not be a valid one for measurement of brain serotonin turnover is indicated by the failure of Cheney et al.[109] to find any differences in the "conversion index" (tryptophan to serotonin in brain) at any time up to 160 minutes after intravenous injection of radioactive (^{3}H-) tryptophan of mice which had had implantations of morphine (75 mg)-pellets for 3.7 days and of "sham-implanted" mice, and in the fractional rate constants (K_S) for turnover of brain serotonin in the two groups. Cheney and his associates[110,111] were also unable to demonstrate that PCPA, in doses sufficient to reduce brain levels of serotonin to approximately one third of its control value, had any effect on the development of tolerance to levorphanol-induced "running" activity in mice with prior 3.7-day morphine-pellet implantations or on the rate of development of such tolerance in mice receiving injections of levorphanol, 20 mg/kg twice daily (with PCPA, 320 mg/kg once daily), or on the degree of tolerance to levorphanol-analgesia (hot plate method) in mice that had received PCPA, 320 mg/kg daily beginning 3 days prior to twice-daily levorphanol injections, 20 mg/kg, for 3 or 7 days; nor did daily PCPA (320 mg/kg) injections, started 3 days before morphine (75 mg)-pellet implantation, elevate the ED_{50} for naloxone-induced "jumping" 3 days after such implantation, compared with mice similarly implanted but not treated with PCPA. Interestingly, these investigators[111] found that although PCPA did not alter the rate of development of tolerance to levorphanol-induced "running," the values for the latter (light beam crossings) were consistently higher in mice receiving injections of both PCPA and levorphanol than in mice receiving levorphanol alone. Such "potentiation" was antagonized by administration of 5-hydroxytryptophan concomitantly with PCPA and levorphanol, suggesting that inhibitory serotonergic neurons impinge on the neuronal pathway for the opioid-induced "running fit" in mice, and that opioids may either block serotonin release or serotonin receptors; however, they point out that this model does not apply to analgesia.

Kuyer and Wijsenbeek[59] in studies on isolated smooth muscle preparations. They found that when a number of nonopioid substances (including physostigmine, pilocarpine, and muscarine) were added to the bath, the characteristic effects of each of these agents subsided after some time, but when the drug was washed out, the effects on the preparation exerted initially by the drug reappeared. Paton's guinea pig ileum type of morphine-"dependence" is not without parallel in "higher" organisms. Thus, "prostrated" patients and chronic decorticated dogs[60] in severe morphine-abstinence are dramatically restored to a "normal" level of activity by a "pick-up" dose of morphine. On the other hand, physostigmine can mimic the morphine-abstinence syndrome in "normal" chronic spinal dogs.[5,17]

Barbiturates

In contrast to the profusion of data and, even more so, of theories about the biochemical-physiological basis of tolerance to and physical dependence on opioids, corresponding information for barbiturates, nonbarbiturate sedatives, and "minor tranquilizers" is remarkable for its paucity. Data on changes in pentylenetetrazol-seizure thresholds during chronic pentobarbital intoxication have been reviewed in connection with the "disuse supersensitivity" theory (second section of this chapter). Other data have recently been reviewed by Wikler and Essig.[61] Among these are the results of a number of investigations by Essig, which may be summarized as follows. Ablation of the cerebellum does not alter the pattern or frequency of generalized seizures in dogs abruptly withdrawn from sodium barbital after a period of chronic intoxication.[62] In contrast, after prior bilateral decortication, the daily dose level of barbital required for the occurrence of withdrawal seizures is elevated, and such seizures are altered in pattern, consisting of tonic extension of the extremities and generalized trembling, preceded by "sham rage."[63] Focal cortical lesions produced by injection of aluminum hydroxide into the cerebral cortex of dogs chronically intoxicated with barbital resulted in the occurrence of both generalized and focal, contralateral seizures (usually at different times) after abrupt withdrawal of the drug, suggesting that the focal and most of the generalized seizures developed in two separate functional systems.[64] Neither diphenylhydantoin[65] nor chlorpromazine[66] proved to be effective in reducing the frequency of barbital-withdrawal seizures in intact dogs. Nor did reserpine, iproniozid, hydrazine, scopolamine, alpha-methyl-DOPA, or a number of aminoacids exert any protective effects. However, amino-oxyacetic acid (AOAA), which inhibits GABA alpha-ketoglutaric acid transaminase and elevates GABA levels in the brain,[67,68] significantly reduced the predictable number of barbital-withdrawal seizures as long as the substitution of AOAA was maintained. However, several of the animals died while receiving AOAA and the remaining dogs had seizures when administration of AOAA was discontinued.[69] It appears to be doubtful, therefore, that barbiturate-withdrawal seizures are due to a "GABA deficiency" state; rather, the "protection" afforded by AOAA could have been related to its anticonvulsant properties[67] in a nonspecific sense. The older literature on the effects of barbiturates upon cerebral oxidative metabolism, including "uncoupling" of oxidation from phosphorylation, was reviewed *in extenso* by Wikler,[70] but at the present time, there seems to be little basis for relating such metabolic changes to physical dependence.

Ethanol

In most respects, the phenomena associated with chronic intoxication and withdrawal of barbiturates and ethanol are, at least qualitatively, very similar. Behaviorally, acute and chronic intoxication with either barbiturates or alcohol are characterized by varying degrees of clouding of the sensorium, drowsiness, ataxia, impaired performance on psychomotor tasks, and emotional lability. Below critical dose levels for each type of drug, a substantial degree of tolerance to these effects can develop within two weeks of chronic drug administration.[71,72] In the case of ethanol, such tolerance is accompanied by a progressive decline in blood ethanol levels[72] and in electroencephalographic changes,[73] as well as by acceleration of the rate of metabolism of ethanol[74] (which is of the same order of magnitude in alcoholic and nonalcoholic subjects[75]). In the case of barbiturates, tolerance to the effects of chronic administration of "moderate" doses of barbiturates has also been reported,[76] but data on blood barbiturate levels during such tolerance are not available. However, when the daily dosage of either barbiturates or ethanol exceeds the critical level, signs of intoxication[72,77] and the characteristic electroencephalographic changes[73,78] reappear, and only a mild degree of tolerance subsequently develops. During this stage of chronic intoxication, blood ethanol levels remain markedly elevated[72,73] (barbiturate levels have not been studied).

With continued intoxication on either barbiturates or ethanol, a state of physical dependence develops, the degree of which is related positively to the daily dose level and duration of drug intake.[79-81] On abrupt withdrawal of barbiturates or ethanol, abstinence syndromes ensue which, except for certain details, are remarkably similar both in character and in the sequence of events.[72,77,80,82] In their complete forms, three successive stages can be distinguished: (1) within 12 to 24 hours after withdrawal of barbiturates, and as early as 6 to 8 hours after withdrawal of ethanol, tremulousness, restlessness, nausea, insomnia, anorexia, anxiety, diaphoresis, and, in the case of ethanol withdrawal, visual hallucinations; (2) generalized seizures, more commonly 24 to 48 hours after barbiturate withdrawal and 7 to 48 hours (over 90% of cases) after ethanol withdrawal; and[83] (3) confusion, disorientation, agitation, severe autonomic disturbances, gross tremors, insomnia, anorexia, visual, and sometimes auditory hallucinations, delusions ("delirium tremens"). Also common to the barbiturate and ethanol abstinence syndromes is markedly increased susceptibility to evocation of myoclonic jerks of the face and neck, spreading to the extremities, by intermittant photic stimulation; if stimulation is prolonged, generalized seizures with loss of consciousness may follow. Susceptibility to photomyoclonus peaks 4 to 7 days and usually disappears by 14 days after withdrawal of barbiturates;[84] in the case of the ethanol abstinence syndrome, the corresponding times are 33 to 45 hours (or earlier) and 111 hours after the last drink.[83,85]

However, there are some differences. In the case of ethanol, morning tremulousness, uneasiness, and nausea often occur, allegedly "while drinking." That these phenomena are actually "prodromal" signs of abstinence is indicated by their disappearance after resumption of drinking. Such phenomena, and even "major" ethanol withdrawal phenomena (convulsions and delirium) may be associated with substantial blood alcohol levels which, however, had fallen from still higher levels at which no abstinence signs occurred; evidently, the occurrence of abstinence phenomena is related to the *rate of decline* in blood (and tissue) ethanol concentration, not to its absolute level.[72,80] The most striking differences are found in the electroencephalograms during chronic intoxication, and especially after drug withdrawal, from daily doses of either drug sufficient to produce abstinence phenomena of comparable severity. Mixtures of increased fast and abnormally slow activity characterize the electroencephalograms of subjects chronically intoxicated with "short-acting" barbiturates (amobarbital, pentobarbital, secobarbital),[78] while generalized slowing typifies the electroencephalograms during chronic ethanol intoxication.[73,86] On withdrawal of "short-acting" barbiturates, a variety of abnormalities, including paroxysmal, high amplitude 4 c.p.s. spike-and-wave discharges appear during the second or third day of abstinence, and may persist up to 8 days, even in subjects who do not exhibit overt seizures of any kind.[78] In contrast, the electroencephalogram after withdrawal of ethanol is remarkably free from such gross abnormalities;[73] in one study, transient, inconspicuous 4-5, 6, and 9 c.p.s. bifrontal discharges could be detected, but only between the 15th and 19th hours of abstinence.[73] Interestingly, this time period corresponds to the time period of peak incidence for spontaneous ethanol withdrawal seizures (13 to 24 hours).[83]

In regard to physiological mechanisms that underlie the barbiturate and ethanol abstinence syndromes, evidence of "latent hyperexcitability" of the central nervous system is common to both. Thus, progressive lowering of thresholds for experimentally induced seizures has been demonstrated in the cat after chronic intoxication with pentobarbital[14] and in the mouse with ethanol.[87] Recently, Wolfe, Victor, and their associates[88-90] have demonstrated a close temporal relationship between respiratory alkalosis and hypomagesemia on the one hand, and the "minor" features of the ethanol abstinence syndrome on the other (in their terminology, "minor" symptoms include not only tremulousness, anxiety, and visual hallucinations but also convulsions). Thus, the time course for increase in arterial pH, decrease in arterial pCO_2 and fall in serum magnesium levels corresponds closely with that of the onset and development of the "minor" ethanol withdrawal phenomena and with increased photomyoclonic susceptibility. Also, all of these changes are directly related to the amount and duration of ethanol consumption prior to withdrawal and to the severity of the abstinence syndrome. Furthermore, during the period of increased photomyoclonic susceptibility, the myoclonic responses are stopped promptly by intravenous injection of magnesium sulfate, 3.0 g. Suggestive, but not conclusive data were obtained, indicating that carbon dioxide inhalation may reduce the intensity of the "minor" ethanol abstinence phenomena. These investigators[80] point out that in nonalcoholic patients with respiratory obstructive disease, excessive mechanical ventilation may increase blood pH and produce disorientation, hallucinations, tremor, hyperreflexia, general muscular irritability, seizures, and hyperpyrexia. Tentatively, they propose the following sequence of events in the genesis of the ethanol abstinence syndrome: the respiratory center is chronically depressed by ethanol; on withdrawal, "rebound" hyperexcitability of the respiratory center occurs, leading to hyperventilation, lowering of blood pCO_2 with consequent reduction of cerebral blood flow, and elevation of blood pH with consequent shift of magnesium ion from blood to bone and other intracellular sites (urinary output of magnesium ion is decreased during the early abstinence period). Reduction of cerebral blood flow and hypomagnesemia would then produce the "minor" ethanol withdrawal phenomena, including convulsions. Presumably, such mechanisms would not be sufficient to account for the "major" ethanol abstinence phenomena (delirium tremens) because, although hypomagnesemia is generally found in this stage,[90] the serum magnesium levels may be much higher than on admission in some patients.[80,88] Likewise, elevation of blood pH and lowering of blood pCO_2 levels are declining by the time of onset of delirium tremens, although a "secondary" fall in blood pCO_2 occurs as the delirium continues.[80,90] Comparable data for the barbiturate and opioid abstinence syndromes are not available. It may be pointed out, however, that hyperventilation[21] and "supersensitivity" of the respiratory center to CO_2[18] are characteristic of the human morphine withdrawal syndrome, but convulsions and delirium are not. However, in very severe morphine-abstinence syndromes precipitated by nalorphine, delirium has been observed in man[91] and convulsions in the dog.[49] Certainly, therefore, the studies on blood pH, pCO_2 and magnesium levels should be extended to the barbiturate and opioid abstinence syndromes as well. In the absence of such information, judgment on whether derangement of these variables plays a role in the genesis of all three types of drug-abstinence syndromes must be suspended.

Data on the inhibitory effects of ethanol on the active transport of sodium and potassium ions in nerve cells, on the effects of ethanol on energy metabolism, and neurotransmitter function, as well as aminoacid metabolism and transport have been reviewed by Israel,[92] but there appears to be little information on changes in these variables during the ethanol abstinence syndrome. Perhaps this is due to the difficulties in developing an animal model of this syndrome that obtained in the past. In recent years, however, such models have been developed in the dog,[93;94] in the mouse[95,96] and in the monkey,[97] so progress in the elucidation of the mechanisms underlying the ethanol abstinence syndrome should be accelerated.

PHYSICAL DEPENDENCE – BEHAVIOR – RELAPSE

This survey of "theories related to physical dependence" should include at least brief mention of the possible role of physical dependence in the perpetuation of drug-seeking behavior and in relapse. This problem has been investigated mainly with reference to opioid-dependence. At least some aspects of the morphine-abstinence syndrome can be classically conditioned[98-100] and stimuli frequently associated with suppression of the morphine-abstinence syndrome can acquire secondary (conditioned) operant-reinforcing properties, the potency of which long outlasts the "primary," and probably also the "secondary" ("protracted") morphine-abstinence syndrome.[101] Both of these types of conditioning processes may play a powerful role in "motivating" the formerly morphine-dependent individual to relapse, given the necessary stimulus conditions (e.g., environments and/or people previously associated with morphine-abstinence and morphine-acquisition).[102-104] For optimal success in treatment, therefore, experimental extinction of such conditioned responses after drug withdrawal should be carried out. In the case of opioid dependence, post-withdrawal "stabilization" on a narcotic antagonist for a limited period of time, as proposed by Martin et al.,[105] together with self-administration of opioids (nonreinforcing under conditions of narcotic antagonist-blockade) should accomplish this end. Theoretically, there would seem to be no reason why similar conditioning processes should not operate in the cases of barbiturate and ethanol dependence as well, but specific antagonists for these drugs are not available (disulfiram is not an ethanol-antagonist in the same sense as cyclazocine or naloxone is a narcotic antagonist, and "Antabuse Therapy" is a form of "aversion" treatment, not extinction through nonreinforcement).[106]

REFERENCES

1. Tatum, A. L., Seevers, M. H., and Collins, K. H., Morphine addiction and its physiological interpretation based on experimental evidence, *J. Pharmacol. Exp. Ther.*, 36, 447, 1929.

2. Seevers, M. H. and Deneau, G. A., A critique of the "dual action" hypothesis of morphine physical dependence, *Arch. Int. Pharmacodyn.*, 140, 514, 1961.

3. Himmelsbach, C. K., With reference to physical dependence, *Fed. Proc.*, 2 201, 1943.

4. Himmelsbach, C. K., Studies on the relation of drug addiction to the autonomic nervous system: results of cold pressor tests, *J. Pharmacol. Exp. Ther.*, 73, 91, 1941.

5. Wikler, A. and Frank, K., Hindlimb reflexes of chronic spinal dogs during addiction to morphine and methadone, *J. Pharmacol. Exp. Ther.*, 94, 382, 1948.

6. Wikler, A. and Rayport, M., Lower limb reflexes of a chronic "spinal" man in cycles of morphine and methadone addiction, *Arch. Neurol. Psychiat.*, (Chicago), 71, 160, 1954.

7. Martin, W. R., A homeostatic and redundancy theory of tolerance to and dependence on narcotic analgesics, in *The Addictive States*, Wikler, A., Ed., Res. Publ. Ass. Nerv. Ment. Dis., Vol. 46, Williams & Wilkins, Baltimore, 1968, 206.

8. Wikler, A., *Opiate Addiction. Psychological and Neurophysiological Aspects in Relation to Clinical Problems*, Charles C Thomas, Springfield, Ill., 1953.

9. Wikler, A. and Carter, R. L., Effects of single doses of *N*-allylnormorphine on hindlimb reflexes of chronic spinal dogs during cycles of morphine addiction, *J. Pharmacol. Exp. Ther.*, 109, 92, 1953.

10. Jaffe, J. H. and Sharpless, S. K., Pharmacological denervation supersensitivity in the central nervous system: a theory of physical dependence, in *The Addictive States*, Wikler, A., Ed., Res. Publ. Ass. Nerv. Ment. Dis., Vol. 46, Williams & Wilkins, Baltimore, 1968, 226.

11. Emmelin, N. and Murén, A., The sensitivity of submaxillary glands to chemical agents studied in cats under various conditions over long periods, *Acta Physiol. Scand.*, 26, 221 1952.

12. Fleming, W. W. and Trendelenburg, V., The development of supersensitivity to norepinephrine after pretreatment with reserpine, *J. Pharmacol. Exp. Ther.*, 133, 41, 1961.

13. Emmelin, N., Supersensitivity following "pharmacological denervation," *Pharmacol. Rev.*, 13, 16, 1961.

14. Jaffe, J. H. and Sharpless, S. K., The rapid development of physical dependence on barbiturates, *J. Pharmacol. Exp. Ther.*, 150, 140, 1965.

15. Friedman, M. J. and Jaffe, J. H., A central hypothermic response to pilocarpine in the mouse, *J. Pharmacol. Exp. Ther.*, 167, 34, 1969.

16. Friedman, M. J., Jaffe, J. H., and Sharpless, S. K., Central nervous system supersensitivity to pilocarpine after withdrawal of chronically administered scopolamine, *J. Pharmacol. Exp. Ther.*, 167, 45, 1969.

17. Martin, W. R. and Eades, C. G., Pharmacological studies of spinal cord adrenergic and cholinergic mechanisms and their relation to physical dependence on morphine, *Psychopharmacologia,* (Berlin), 11, 195, 1967.

18. Martin, W. R., Jasinski, D. R., Sapira, J. D., Flanary, H. G., Kelly, O. A., Thompson, A. K., and Logan, C. R., The respiratory effects of morphine during a cycle of dependence, *J. Pharmacol. Exp. Ther.*, 162, 182, 1968.

19. Martin, W. R., Pharmacological redundancy as an adaptive mechanism in the central nervous system, *Fed. Proc.*, 29, 13, 1970.

20. Jasinski, D. R., Martin, W. R., and Haertzen, C. A., The human pharmacology and abuse potential of *N*-allylnoroxymorphone (naloxone), *J. Pharmacol. Exper. Ther.*, 157, 420, 1967.

21. Martin, W. R. and Jasinski, D. R., Physiological parameters of morphine dependence in man – tolerance, early abstinence, protracted abstinence, *J. Psychiat. Res.*, 7, 9, 1969.

22. Martin, W. R. and Eades, C. G., A comparison between acute and chronic physical dependence in the chronic spinal dog, *J. Pharmacol. Exp. Ther.*, 146, 385, 1964.

23. Sloan, J. W. and Eisenman, A. J., Long persisting changes in catecholamine metabolism following addiction to and withdrawal from morphine, in *The Addictive States,* Wilker, A., Ed., Res. Publ. Ass. Nerv. Ment. Dis., Vol. 46, Williams & Wilkins, Baltimore, 1968, 96.

24. Sakel, M., Theorie der Sucht, *Z. Ges. Neurol. Psychiat.*, 129, 639, 1930.

25. Collier, H. O. J., A general theory of drug dependence by induction of receptors, *Nature*, (London), 205, 181, 1965.

26. Collier, H. O. J., Tolerance, physical dependence and receptors, in *Advances in Drug Research,* Vol. 3, Harper, N. J. and Simmonds, A. B., Eds., Academic Press, New York, 1966, 171.

27. Conney, A. H., Pharmacological implications of microsomal enzyme induction, *Pharmacol. Rev.*, 19, 317, 1967.

28. Lieber, C. S. and de Carli, L. M., Ethanol oxidation by hepatic microsomes: adaptive increase after ethanol feeding, *Science*, 162, 917, 1968.

29. Schlesinger, K., Bennet, E. L., Hebert, M., and McClearn, G. E., Effects of alcohol consumption on the activity of liver enzymes in C57BL (Crg) mice, *Nature,* (London), 209, 488, 1966.

30. Khanna, J. M., Kalant, H., and Bustos, G., Effects of chronic intake of ethanol on rate of ethanol metabolism, *Canad. J. Physiol. Pharmacol.*, 45, 777, 1967.

31. Wikler, A., Electroencephalographic changes associated with chronic alcoholic intoxication and the alcohol abstinence syndrome, *Amer. J. Psychiat.*, 113, 106, 1956.

32. Shuster, L., Repression and de-repression of enzyme synthesis as a possible explanation of some aspects of drug action, *Nature,* (London), 189, 314, 1961.

33. Goldstein, D. B. and Goldstein, A., Possible role of enzyme inhibition and repression in drug tolerance and addiction, *Biochem. Pharmacol.*, 8, 48, 1961.

34. Goldstein, A. and Goldstein, D. B., Enzyme expansion theory of drug tolerance and physical dependence, in *The Addictive States,* Wikler, A., Ed., Res. Publ. Ass. Nerv. Ment. Dis., Vol. 46, Williams & Wilkins, Baltimore, 1968, 265.

35. McIlwain, H., Actions of haloperidol, meperidine and related compounds on the excitability and ion content of isolated cerebral tissue, *Biochem. Pharmacol.*, 13, 523, 1964.

36. Takemori, A. E., Cellular adaptation to morphine in rats, *Science,* 133, 1018, 1961.

37. Takemori, A. E., Studies on cellular adaptation to morphine and its reversal by nalorphine in cerebral cortical slices of rats, *J. Pharmacol. Exp. Ther.*, 135, 89, 1962a.

38. Takemori, A. E., Cellular adaptation to methadone and meperidine in cerebral slices from morphinized rats, *J. Pharmacol. Exp. Ther.*, 135, 252, 1962b.

39. Takemori, A. E., The effects of morphine, other opioids and their derivatives on the metabolism of the cerebral cortex, in *The Addictive States,* Wilker, A., Ed., Res. Publ. Ass. Nerv. Ment. Dis., Vol. 46, Williams & Wilkins, Baltimore, 1968, 53.

40. Takemori, A. E., Studies on morphine-adapted cerebral cortical slices of rats, *Fed. Proc.*, 21, 177, 1962.

41. Axelrod, J., The enzymatic *N*-demethylation of narcotic drugs, *J. Pharmacol. Exp. Ther.*, 117, 332, 1956.

42. Axelrod, J., Possible mechanism of tolerance to narcotic drugs, *Science,* 124, 263, 1956.

43. Gunne, L.-M., The excretion of noradrenaline and adrenaline in the urine of rats during chronic morphine administration and drug abstinence, *Psychopharmacologia,* (Berlin), 2, 214, 1961.

44. Gunne, L.-M., Catecholamine metabolism and morphine abstinence, *Ann. N. Y. Acad. Sci.*, 96, 205, 1962.

45. Gunne, L.-M., Catecholamines and 5-hydroxytryptamine in morphine tolerance and withdrawal, *Acta Physiol. Scand.*, 58, (Supplementum 204), 1, 1963.

46. Gunne, L.-M., and Lewander, T., Long-term effects of some dependence-producing drugs on the brain monoamines, in *Molecular Basis of Some Aspects of Mental Activity,* Vol. 2, Walaas, O., Ed., Academic Press, New York, 1967, 75.

47. Sloan, J. W., Brooks, J. W., Eisenman, A. J., and Martin, W. R., The effect of addiction to and abstinence from morphine on rat tissue catecholamine and serotonin levels, *Psychopharmacologia,* (Berlin), 4, 261, 1963.

48. Maynert, E. W. and Klingman, G. I., Tolerance to morphine, I, Effects on catecholamines in the brain and adrenal glands, *J. Pharmacol. Exp. Ther.*, 135, 285, 1962.

49. Maynert, E. W., Catecholamines metabolism in the brain and adrenal medulla during addiction to morphine and in the early abstinence period, in *The Addictive States,* Wikler, A., Ed., Res. Publ. Ass. Nerv. Ment. Dis., Vol. 46, Williams & Wilkins, Baltimore, 1968, 89.

50. Schneider, J. A., Reserpine antagonism of morphine analgesia in mice, *Proc. Soc. Exp. Biol. Med.*, (New York), 87, 614, 1954.

51. Sigg, E. B., Caprio, B., and Schneider, J. A., Synergism of amines and antagonism of reserpine to morphine analgesia, *Proc. Soc. Exp. Biol. Med.*, (New York), 97, 97, 1958.

52. Schaumann, W., Beeinflussung der analgetischen Wirkung des Morphins durch Reserpin, *Naunyn Schmiedeberg Arch Pharm. Exp. Path.*, 235, 1, 1958.

53. Martin, W. R., Discussion, in *The Addictive States,* Wikler, A., Ed., Res. Publ. Ass. Nerv. Ment. Dis., Vol. 46, Williams & Wilkins, Baltimore, 1968, 116.

54. Cohen, M., Keats, A. S., Krivoy, W., and Ungar, G., Effect of actinomycin D on morphine tolerance, *Proc. Soc. Exp. Biol. Med.*, (New York), 119, 381, 1965.

55. Way, E. L., Loh, H. H., and Shen, F.-H., Morphine tolerance, physical dependence and synthesis of 5-hydroxytryptamine, *Science,* 162, 1290, 1968.

56. Gaddum, J. H. and Picarelli, Z. P., Two kinds of tryptamine receptors, *Brit. J. Pharmacol.*, 12, 323, 1957.

57. Maynert, E. W., Klingman, G. L., and Kaji, H. K., Tolerance to morphine. II. Lack of effect on brain 5-hydroxytryptamine and γ-aminobutyric acid, *J. Pharmacol. Exp. Ther.*, 135, 296, 1962.

58. Paton, W. D. M., The action of morphine and related substances on contraction and on acetylcholine output of coaxially stimulated guinea pig ileum, *Brit. J. Pharmacol.*, 12, 119, 1957.

59. Kuyer, A. and Wijsenbeek, I. A., Über Entgiftungserregung und Entgiftungshemmung, *Arch. Ges. Physiol.*, 154, 16, 1913.

60. Wikler, A., Reactions of dogs without neocortex during cycles of addiction to morphine and methadone, *Arch. Neurol. Psychiat.*, (Chicago), 67, 672, 1952.

61. Wikler, A. and Essig, C. F., Withdrawal seizures following chronic intoxication with barbiturates and other sedative drugs, in *Epilepsy*, Vol. 4, Modern Problems of Pharmacopsychiatry, Neidermeyer, E., Ed., Karger, Basel/New York, 1970, 170.

62. Essig, C. F., Barbiturate withdrawal convulsions in decerebellate dogs, *Int. J. Neuropharmacol.*, 3, 453, 1964.

63. Essig, C. F., Convulsive and sham rage behaviors in decorticate dogs during barbiturate withdrawal, *Arch. Neurol.*, (Chicago), 7, 471, 1962.

64. Essig, C. F., Focal convulsions during barbiturate abstinence in dogs with cerebrocortical lesions, *Psychopharmacologia* (Berlin), 3, 432, 1962.

65. Essig, C. F. and Carter, W. W., Failure of diphenylhydantoin to prevent barbiturate withdrawal convulsions in dogs, *Neurology*, (Minneapolis), 12, 481, 1962.

66. Essig, C. F. and Fraser, H. F., Failure of chlorpromazine to prevent barbiturate withdrawal convulsions, *Clin. Pharmacol. Ther.*, 7, 466, 1966.

67. Eidelberg, E., Baxter, C. F., Roberts, E., Saldias, C. A., and French, J. D., Anticonvulsant properties of hydroxylamine and elevation of cerebral gamma-aminobutyric acid in cats, *Proc. Soc. Exper. Biol. Med.*, (New York), 101, 815, 1959.

68. Wallach, D. P., Studies on the GABA pathway, I, The inhibition of gamma-aminobutyric acid alpha-ketoglutaric acid transaminase *in vitro* and *in vivo* by U-7524 (amino-oxyacetic acid), *Biochem. Pharmacol.*, 5, 323, 1961.

69. Essig, C. F., Anticonvulsant effect of amino-oxyacetic acid during barbiturate withdrawal in the dog, *Int. J. Neuropharmacol.*, 2, 199, 1963.

70. Wikler, A., *The Relation of Psychiatry to Pharmacology*, Williams & Wilkins, Baltimore, 1968.

71. Belleville, R. E. and Fraser, H. F., Tolerance to some effects of barbiturates, *J. Pharmacol. Exper. Therap.*, 120, 469, 1957.

72. Isbell, H., Fraser, H. F., Wikler, A., Belleville, R. E., and Eisenman, A. J., An experimental study of the etiology of "rum fits" and delirium tremens, *Quart. J. Stud. Alcohol*, 16, 1, 1955.

73. Wikler, A., Pescor, F. T., Fraser, H. F., and Isbell, H., Electroencephalographic changes associated with chronic alcoholic intoxication and the alcohol abstinence syndrome, *Amer. J. Psychiat.*, 113, 106, 1956.

74. Mendelson, J. H., Stein, S., and Mello, N. K., Effects of experimentally induced intoxication on metabolism of ethanol 1-C^{14} in alcoholic subjects, *Metabolism*, 14, 1255, 1965.

75. Mendelson, J. H., Ethanol-1-C^{14} metabolism in alcoholics and non-alcoholics, *Science*, 159, 319, 1968.

76. Essig, C. F. and Fraser, H. F., Electroencephalographic changes in man during use and withdrawal of barbiturates in moderate dosage, *Electroenceph. Clin. Neurophysiol.*, 10, 649, 1958.

77. Isbell, H., Altschul, S., Kornetsky, C. H., Eisenman, A. J., Flanary, H. G., and Fraser, H. F., Chronic barbiturate intoxication. An experimental study, *Arch. Neurol. Psychiat.*, (Chicago), 64, 1, 1950.

78. Wikler, A., Fraser, H. F., Isbell, H., and Pescor, F. T., Electroencephalograms during cycles of addiction to barbiturates in man, *Electroenceph. Clin. Neurophysiol.*, 7, 1, 1955.

79. Fraser, H. F., Wikler, A., Essig, C. F., and Isbell, H., Degree of physical dependence induced by secobarbital or pentobarbital, *J.A.M.A.*, 166, 126, 1958.

80. Victor, M. and Wolfe, S. M., The causation and treatment of the alcohol withdrawal syndrome, in *Alcoholism: Progress in Research and Treatment,* Bourne, P. and Fox, R., Eds., Academic Press, New York, 1971, in press.

81. Mendelson, J. H. and La Dou, J., Experimentally induced chronic intoxication and withdrawal in alcoholics. Pt. 2. Psychophysiological findings, *Quart. J. Stud. Alcohol,* Suppl. 2, 14, 1964.

82. Victor, M. and Adams, R. D., The effect of alcohol on the nervous system, in *Metabolic and Toxic Diseases of the Nervous System,* Res. Publ. Ass. Nerv. Ment. Dis., Vol. 32, 526, 1953.

83. Victor, M. and Brausch, C., The role of abstinence in the genesis of alcoholic epilepsy, *Epilepsia,* 8, 1, 1967.

84. Wulff, M. H., The barbiturate withdrawal syndrome. A clinical and electroencephalographic study, *Electroenceph. Clin. Neurophysiol.,* Suppl. 14, 173, 1959.

85. Victor, M., The pathophysiology of alcoholic epilepsy, in *The Addictive States,* Wikler, A., Ed., Res. Publ. Ass. Nerv. Ment. Dis., Vol. 46, Williams & Wilkins, Baltimore, 1968, 431.

86. Weiss, A. D., Victor, M., Mendelson, J. H., and La Dou, J., Experimentally induced chronic intoxication and withdrawal in alcoholics. Pt. 7, electroencephalographic findings, *Quart. J. Stud. Alcohol,* Suppl. 2, 96, 1964.

87. McQuarrie, D. G. and Fingl, E., Effect of single doses and chronic administration of ethanol on experimental seizures in mice, *J. Pharmacol. Exp. Ther.,* 124, 264, 1958.

88. Wolfe, S. M. and Victor, M., The relationship of hypomagnesemia and alkalosis to alcohol withdrawal symptoms, *Ann. N. Y. Acad. Sci.,* 162, 973, 1969.

89. Wolfe, S. M., Mendelson, J., Ogata, M., Victor, M., and Mello, N. K., Respiratory alkalosis and alcohol withdrawal, *Trans. Ass. Amer. Physicians,* 82, 344, 1969.

90. Wolfe, S. M. and Victor, M., The physiological basis of the alcohol withdrawal syndrome, in *Recent Advances in Studies of Alcoholism,* Mello, N. K. and Mendelson, J. H., Eds., U.S. Govt. Printing Office, Washington, D. C., in press.

91. Wikler, A., Fraser, H. F., and Isbell, H., *N*-allylnormorphine: effects of single doses and precipitation of acute "abstinence syndromes" during addiction to morphine, methadone or heroin in man (post-addicts), *J. Pharmacol. Exp. Ther.*, 109, 8, 1953.

92. Israel, Y., Cellular effects of alcohol, *Quart. J. Stud. Alcohol,* 31, 293, 1970.

93. Essig, C. F. and Lam, R. C., Convulsions and hallucinatory behavior following alcohol withdrawal in the dog, *Arch. Neurol.,* (Chicago), 18, 626, 1968.

94. Essig, C. F., Jones, B. E., and Lam, R. C., The effect of pentobarbital on alcohol withdrawal in dogs, *Arch. Neurol.,* (Chicago), 20, 554, 1969.

95. Freund, G., Alcohol withdrawal syndrome in mice, *Arch. Neurol.,* (Chicago), 21, 315, 1969.

96. Goldstein, D. B. and Pal, N., Alcohol dependence produced in mice by inhalation of ethanol: grading of the withdrawal reaction, *Science,* 172, 288, 1971.

97. Ellis, F. W. and Pick, J. R., Dose - and time- dependent relationships in ethanol-induced withdrawal reactions, *Fed. Proc.,* 30, 568, 1971 (abs.).

98. Wikler, A., Conditioning factors in opiate addiction and relapse, in *Narcotics,* Wilner, D. M. and Kassebaum, G. G., Eds., McGraw-Hill, New York, 1965, 85.

99. Wikler, A. and Pescor, F. T., Classical conditioning of a morphine-abstinence phenomenon, reinforcement of opiod-drinking behavior and "relapse" in morphine-addicted rats, *Psychopharmacologia,* (Berlin), 10, 255, 1967.

100. Goldberg, S. R. and Schuster, C. R., Conditioned nalorphine-induced abstinence changes: persistence in post morphine-dependent monkeys, *J. Exp. Anal. Behav.*, 14, 33, 1970.

101. Wikler, A., Pescor, F. T., Miller, D., and Norrell, H., Persistent potency of a secondary (conditioned) reinforcer following withdrawal of morphine from physically dependent rats, *Psychopharmacologia,* (Berlin), 20, 103, 1971.

102. Wikler, A., Recent progress in research on the neurophysiological basis of morphine addiction, *Amer. J. Psychiat.*, 105, 329, 1948.

103. Wikler, A., On the nature of addiction and habituation, *Brit. J. Addict.*, 57, 73, 1961.

104. Thompson, T. and Ostlund, W., Susceptibility to readdiction as a function of the addiction and withdrawal environments, *J. Comp. Physiol. Psychol.*, 60, 388, 1965.

105. Martin, W. R., Gorodetzdy, C. W., and McClane, T. K., An experimental study in the treatment of narcotic addicts with cvclazocine, *Clin. Pharmacol. Ther.*, 4, 455, 1966.

106. Wikler, A., Some implications of conditioning theory for problems of drug abuse, *Behav. Sci.*, 16, 92, 1971.

107. Shen, F. S., Loh, H. H., and Way, E. L., Brain serotonin turnover in morphine tolerant and dependent mice, *J. Pharmacol. Exp. Ther.*, 175, 427, 1970.

108. Maruyama, Y., Hayashi, G., and Takemori, A. E., Relation between 5-hydroxytryptamine (5-HT) and tolerance and physical dependence in mice, *The Pharmacologist*, 12, 231, 1970.

109. Cheney, D. L., Goldstein, A., Algeri, S., and Costa, E., Narcotic tolerance and dependence: lack of relationship with serotonin turnover in brain, *Science,* 171, 1169, 1971.

110. Cheney, D. L., Goldstein, A., and Sheehan, P., Rate of development of brain tolerance and physical dependence in mice treated with opiates, *Fed. Proc.*, 29, 685, 1970.

111. Cheney, D. L. and Goldstein, A., The effect of *p*-chlorophenylalanine on opiate-induced running, analgesia, tolerance and physical dependence in mice, *J. Pharmacol. Exp. Ther.*, 177, 309, 1971.

ELECTROPHYSIOLOGY OF DRUGS OF DEPENDENCE

M. Fink

TABLE OF CONTENTS

INTRODUCTION

The W.H.O. Expert Committee on Drug Dependence lists more than 100 compounds under international narcotics control, presumably as drugs with high dependence liability in man.[1] To this list, which includes opiate derivatives, cocaine, and cannabis, we must add the 107 sympathomimetic hallucinogens (as lysergide, psilocybin), amphetamines, barbiturates, and benzodiazepines (as diazepam, chlordiazepoxide) named by an earlier W.H.O. Expert Committee.[2] Despite their length, these lists omit such widely used substances of dependence as ethyl alcohol, the xanthines (caffeine, theophylline, theobromine) in coffee, tea, cocoa, and maté, and nicotine in tobacco. In its 1969 report, the W.H.O. Expert Committee[3] adopted the following definitions:

"*Drug.* Any substance that, when taken in the living organism, may modify one or more of its functions."

"*Drug abuse.* Persistent or sporadic excessive use inconsistent or unrelated to acceptable medical practice."

"*Drug dependence.* A state, psychic and sometimes also physical, resulting from the interaction between a living organism and a drug, characterized by behavioral and other responses that always include a compulsion to take the drug on a continuous or periodic basis in order to experience its psychic effects, and sometimes to avoid the discomfort of its absence. Tolerance may or may not be present. A person may be dependent on more than one drug."

The definitions of dependence are based on social and behavioral criteria, not on any characteristic biologic, biochemical, or neurophysiologic aspects of their use.

Modern electrophysiological techniques have increased in sophistication and complexity since the string galvanometer used by the early pioneers less than a century ago. Progress has been particularly marked in the measurement of the changes in the human cerebral electroencephalogram (EEG) since the first descriptions by Berger in 1929. Psychoactive drugs useful in clinical practice exhibit characteristic changes in the EEG of man. These changes are drug specific; they are related to the dose, route, and rate of administration, and are directly related to the behavioral effects of the drugs.[4,5] An early systematic view of the relation of EEG changes to behavior was described in a study of morphine and nalorphine. Increased synchronization of EEG rhythms and an increase in slow wave activity were accompanied by subjective reports of euphoria, relaxation, and drowsiness; while desynchronization of frequencies was accompanied by anxiety, hallucinations, fantasies, illusions, or tremors.[6] This hypothesis has been verified and extended to encompass a greater range of EEG changes in frequencies, amplitude, variability, and pattern, sufficient to provide criteria for nine classes of compounds.[4,5]

These observations have encouraged the development of a theory of a direct association between changes in electrophysiological events and alertness, mood, thought processes, and perception.[5,7] Many of the compounds studied by these methods are defined as drugs of dependence, and it is the purpose of this report to summarize these data, to classify the EEG events in man, and to attempt a justification of 'dependence' in EEG terms.

GENERAL

Chronic Drug Administration

For drugs of dependence, particularly those with high abuse potential, the central effects following their injection, ingestion, or inhalation are rapid in onset and usually short in duration. The more rapid the onset, the more likely are the central effects to have a bimodal character, as we have described for pentothal[8] and heroin (diacetylmorphine).[9-11] The development of tolerance in behavioral indices is accompanied by sequential changes in the EEG, such that successive doses of equal strength excite fewer and fewer central effects – a manifestation of tolerance in the central nervous system.[10] While not studied in detail, cross tolerance may also be observed in EEG indices, as in the blockade of heroin by methadone.[9,10,12]

Withdrawal from many substances is accompanied by behavioral sequellae of insomnia, irritability, mood depression, and seizures, and these are also associated with specific EEG events, as for barbiturates,[13] alcohol,[14] and fenfluramine and imipramine.[15]

Among the nine EEG classes,[4,5] drugs of dependence are of three classes: drugs which stimulate fast frequencies with increased synchronization and amplitudes, as the barbiturates; drugs which stimulate fast frequencies with desynchronization of frequencies and decreased amplitudes, as the amphetamines and lysergide; and drugs which enhance the abundance of alpha activity, and increase the synchronization of frequencies, as the opiates and alcohol.

Acute Drug Administration

It is characteristic of the use of dependence-producing drugs that the most rapid introduction is preferred – inhalation and intravenous administration being preferred to oral, intramuscular, or subcutaneous routes.

On acute administration at high dosage additional short-term EEG effects may be seen with accompanying changes in behavior. The short-term effects are most critical for the definition of abuse potential, and may be separated into two classes: drugs which yield high voltage slow waves, including seizure-like patterns, and drugs that yield a rapid and prolonged period of EEG desynchronization. The first pattern is characteristic for alcohol,[14] opiates,[10,11] and barbiturates,[16,17] and the second is found with amphetamines,[17] lysergide, and cocaine.[4,5]

Accompanying EEG seizure activity are sensations of floating, dissociation from the immediate external environment, intensified bodily sensations, and a separation from pain, anxiety, and immediate concerns. Accompanying acute desynchronization of EEG frequencies, subjects also report changes in perception, dissociation from the immediate environment, heightened internal bodily sensations, and a "distance" from thoughts and feelings of pain, anxiety, and immediate preoccupations. Accompanying both EEG patterns, there is a 'turning inward' of thought processes, a decrease in ability to discriminate percepts, and an inability to focus on the future or the past – a preoccupation with the immediate present.

It is this dissociation from the ongoing events of conscious life and preoccupation with internal sensations that has been invested by mystics and poets with symbols of a 'higher' brain function, allowing novel interpretations to thought processes. Such alterations in brain functions can be achieved by nondrug means as well. Altered consciousness with decreased perception, discrimination, and dissociation from the present occurs in the dream state (accompanied by EEG desynchronization and concurrent rapid eye movements); the zen, hypnotic, or meditation states (accompanied by hypersynchronous alpha activity and decreased beta activity); and in delirium (accompanied by increases in delta and beta activities, increased voltages, burst-like activity, without response to eye opening).[18]

Tolerance

The short-term, rapid events in the central nervous system are characteristic for the pleasurable states described by those dependent on drugs. Unfortunately, the more rapidly a compound affects the central nervous system, the more rapidly are defensive biochemical processes stimulated. An accompaniment of the use of these drugs is the development of tolerance – increasing dosages are necessary to achieve the same or greater degrees of central effect. One concept of prevention of opiate dependence is based on a concept that blockade of the central effects, either directly (as with such specific narcotic antagonists as naloxone and cyclazocine) or by cross tolerance (as with synthetic opiates of long duration, as methadone and acetylmethadol) will prevent the gratification of self-administered drugs and reinforcement of dependence.[19] In subjects receiving cyclazocine, naloxone, or methadone, the administration of heroin in the usual doses fails to excite either a central effect or the usual behavioral effects. However, as our subjects rapidly discover, it is possible to overcome this "relative" blockade by large doses of heroin or morphine. With large doses, the central effects, including EEG seizure-like activity, synchronization, and slow wave activity can be observed.[9,11]

Thus, the characteristic central changes of drugs of dependence lie, in part, in the specific changes in the EEG they excite (the EEG pattern has relevance, as may be seen in the difference in abuse potential of opiates and cocaine compared to imipramine and pentelenetetrazol), and in part, in the rate at which these changes are stimulated. The common basis for drugs with abuse potential is their solubility and ready availability to the central nervous system and the rapid discharge of these effects, so that the subject can be ready for another stimulation in a short period of time. Oswald et al. have recently emphasized that drugs of dependence need not be drugs of abuse, suggesting that those of abuse are those that are rapidly detoxified, which may indeed be relevant.[15]

SPECIFIC EEG PATTERNS

Opiates and Antagonists

Diacetylmorphine and methadone – The effects of heroin and methadone have been reviewed recently in reports from this laboratory.[9-11] Volavka et al.[11] summarized the EEG effects on acute administration of heroin (20 to 25 mg/2 cc/2 minutes) as occurring in two phases. An early response occurs within the first 4 minutes of injection, and is characterized by an increase in alpha amplitudes, decrease in alpha frequency, and an increase in alpha spindling. The late response develops from 5 to 30 minutes after the start of injection, with a decrease in alpha abundance, an increase in theta and delta activities, and frequent paroxysmal activity. In that study, two clinical grand mal seizures were observed, and these were in addition to those reported earlier from the same laboratory.[9] Though more detailed, these EEG patterns are similar to earlier reports of the acute administration of morphine and methadone.[10]

We have not observed the effect of chronic administration of heroin in the laboratory, but have studied the changes with methadone. The subjects received methadone in gradually increasing increments until a daily dosage of 100 mg/day was established (usually requiring 40 days). Weekly EEG records demonstrated a progressive decrease in the mean alpha frequency, an increase in the percent time alpha activity, a decrease in beta activity, and increased theta activity, both random and in bursts. Voltages increased, and the variability of the frequencies decreased. When a maintenance dose was established, these changes gradually diminished, and the pre-methadone patterns again emerged, except that fast frequencies remained less and the mean alpha frequency remained lower. We interpreted the return of the records to pre-methadone levels as indicative of the development of tolerance.[10]

To patients receiving 100 mg methadone daily, we have given varying doses of heroin (25, 50, 75 mg) at different periods (4 to 72 hours) after a daily dose of methadone to assess the duration of blockade.[12] Using both behavioral and EEG criteria, we observed the duration of blockade to be approximately 60 hours for 25 mg, 48 hours for 50 mg, and 36 hours for 75 mg heroin. The heroin-induced decrease in mean alpha frequency and the increase in theta activity did not occur in these subjects when the behavioral effects were blocked, but were apparent when the dose exceeded the extent of the blockade.

Narcotic antagonists – In these experiments we also studied the EEG effects of the narcotic antagonists, cyclazocine and naloxone. On acute and chronic administration of 1 to 5 mg daily, cyclazocine elicited EEG changes characterized by increased theta and beta activity, increased variability of frequencies and amplitudes, and decreased mean amplitudes – a pattern classified as similar to imipramine, a clinical antidepressant.[20] Naloxone, however, failed to stimulate any EEG effects when given by itself to post-addicts and normal male volunteers.[10,11]

In post-addicts who were given single daily oral doses of cyclazocine (4 to 5.5 mg/day), the administration of heroin (25mg) elicited neither EEG nor behavioral effects for periods up to 26 hours after a single dose, averaging 20 hours.[20] Similarly with naloxone, the administration of heroin had neither behavioral nor central effects up to 24 hours after single oral doses of 2.4 to 3.0 g.[21]

In another series of experiments, we administered 0.7 mg naloxone intravenously immediately after heroin, at the time when the EEG and behavioral effects were most prominent, and noted an immediate cessation of the EEG and the behavioral effects.[21] In subjects first given naloxone, intravenous heroin had no EEG effect. In three subjects, in whom heroin stimulated a clinical grand mal seizure, and in numerous others in whom EEG hypersynchrony was prominent, the intravenous administration of naloxone (0.7 to 1.0 mg) produced an immediate (30 to 90 seconds) reversal of seizure activity and restitution of the pre-heroin EEG patterns, occasionally with increases in alpha percent time and in mean alpha frequency.[9,11]

Barbiturates and Benzodiazepines

These sedative drugs stimulate a characteristic spindling of beta (18 to 26 Hz) frequencies, accompanied by an increased synchronization of frequencies, increased amplitudes, and decreased variability measures. The EEG response is dose and rate specific, and is dependent on the mental state of the subject. The barbiturate spindling response to amobarbital and pentothal is so characteristic, it was the basis for many studies classifying subpopulations of the mentally ill[22] and for servo-control studies of anesthesia.[23]

In dose-response studies, we observed that the amount of beta activity and the amount of induced theta/delta activities were intimately dependent on dose and rate of administration. The beta activity is prominent when dosages of amobarbital approximate 0.5 mg/kg/40 seconds and for pentothal at 4 mg/kg/2 minutes. Increasing the dose of barbiturate or shortening the time of intravenous administration stimulates an increase in delta activity.[16] The EEG response to pentothal is so rate and dose dependent that Schwartz et al.[8] were able to characterize the response in mathematical terms.

In another study, we measured the EEG changes to two doses of oral amobarbital (50 mg, 100 mg) and distinguished these from dextroamphetamine (10 mg). Also, in this study the profile of a sedative anorexigenic, fenfluramine (40 mg), was found to be similar to amobarbital and distinguishable from dextroamphetamine.[17]

The benzodiazepines elicit similar EEG responses. We examined the EEG activity of intravenous diazepam in doses of 0.14 mg/kg/2 minutes in normal male volunteers and observed increased beta activity, decreased alpha activity, and some increase in theta activity.[24] In chronic studies of a short-acting benzodiazepine, tybamate, given to opiate-dependent subjects in an effort to develop narcotic blockade, we observed similar EEG changes, which persisted during the chronic administration of high doses.[25]

Many EEG studies of benzodiazepines and barbiturates focus on the effect of single doses used as soporifics, usually given shortly before bedtime. The effects on the duration of various sleep stages, including REM, are measured. REM time is usually reduced during the first nights of administration, gradually returning to baseline levels, with a significant increase in REM time on the first post-withdrawal night ("REM rebound").[26] The gradual return of REM activity, even when drug administration continues, and REM rebound are evidence of the development of tolerance. Withdrawal effects are also prominent, often with the development of seizure activity in the EEG, and clinically, in subjects who have taken high doses of barbiturates for extended periods.[13]

Drugs which elicit beta spindling in the 18 to 26 Hz bands have some clinical effects in common. Their use is associated with a reduction of anxiety; tolerence develops and dosages must be increased to maintain efficacy; withdrawal, if rapid, is associated with EEG and clinical seizures, tremulousness, and irritability; the compounds effectively suppress grand mal seizures; and drugs of this class exhibit synergism and cross tolerance among the members and with ethyl alcohol. The similarity of the EEG and accompanying behavioral effects suggests that these compounds have common biochemical effects on the central nervous system, highly specific for the elicitation of spindling activity.

Ethyl Alcohol

We have not examined alcohol in systematic studies. The literature indicates that the acute administration of alcohol bears dose-specific relations to the accompanying EEG changes.[14] These are characterized by a slowing of the dominant frequency, increased theta and delta activity, and an initial reduction in amplitudes. With continued administration, tolerance to the central effects develops, and increasing dosages are necessary to stimulate both the EEG and the behavioral effects. In subjects who have used high doses of alcohol for extended periods, delirium may occur, accompanied by characteristic EEG patterns of this syndrome – increased theta and delta activity, decreased alpha activity, and an increase in low voltage, mixed fast frequencies. In alcoholic patients in acute withdrawal, high voltage hypersynchrony and clinical seizures may occur. From its EEG profiles, we would anticipate that the effects of alcoholic delirium may be antagonized by THA (tetrahydroaminacrin), and reduced to a stupor by the administration of a phenothiazine, following our studies of drug interactions in delirium.[18]

Sympathomimetic Hallucinogens

Lysergide, mescaline, amphetamine, methamphetamine, and cocaine are hallucinogens with similar central and behavioral effects. Their central activity is ascribed usually to similar effects on sympathomimetic amines. Their EEG effects are characterized by an increase in the mean frequency, a reduction in slow and alpha activities, and a decrease in mean amplitudes. Beta activity, when prominent, is variable in frequency and low in voltage.[4,27] These drugs exhibit similar EEG effects, their differences depending on dosage, duration of administration, the rate of onset of central effects, and the characteristics of the population studied. With lysergide, for example, administration in therapy-resistant schizophrenics is associated with little EEG or behavioral effects, even at high dosages (to 10 gamma/kg). In severe epileptics with continuous hypersynchrony and delta/theta bursts, lysergide elicits an increase in alpha activity, a manifestation of the shift of frequencies to a higher dominant frequency.

Lysergide is a drug of slow onset, even on intravenous administration, and is thus distinguishable from other drugs of dependence. However, cocaine, dextroamphetamine, and methamphetamine are rapid in onset and I would anticipate the development of a diphasic EEG response on their intravenous administration.

Tolerance to lysergide develops rapidly, and cross tolerance to mescaline has been studied. These compounds are antagonized by phenothiazines, given either before or after the onset of the central effects.[27] The blockade of amphetamines by phenothiazines has led to the study of fluphenazine enanthate as an antagonist in the therapy of amphetamine dependence.[28]

On chronic administration, tolerance to the EEG changes is readily observed, as these changes parallel the behavioral effects. As a consequence, various observers have failed to find a 'characteristic' EEG profile for chronic amphetamine users.

Cannabis

There are few published studies of the central effects of cannabis and its derivatives. Research has been inhibited by the poor quality of the material and governmental proscription. However, during the past four years, standardized materials have been made available, the constituents have been identified and some synthesized, and the governmental agencies have relaxed their restrictions on research. Research is now actively in progress and these observations are preliminary.

Cannabis is rapidly effective on inhalation. Its central effects have an onset during smoking, and the changes are dose related. In male volunteers, dosages rated under 8 mg THC-delta-9 yielded little central or peripheral (heart rate) effects. At 20 mg THC rated material, the EEG changes occurred within 4 minutes during smoking and were characterized by an increase in alpha activity with a reduction in beta and theta activities.[29] These changes were accompanied by increases in heart rate and deficits in memory tasks.[30] In subjects allowed to smoke early in the evening, spontaneous drowsiness and stage-1 sleep patterns were reduced by the high dose cannabis.

Some reports associate chronic cannabis use with psychosis and abnormal EEG.[31] Ongoing studies of chronic cannabis users in Jamaica and in Greece have not found a characteristic 'abnormal' EEG pattern. In laboratory studies in New York, five college enrolled, middle-class volunteer males smoked the equivalent of 14 mg THC-delta-9 THC cannabis for each of 21 consecutive days, without untoward behavioral effects and without persistent EEG effects.[32]

The phenomenon of tolerance has been reported in behavioral tasks in animal trials using high doses of THC-delta-9, but an EEG demonstration of this phenomenon has not yet been made. The interaction of cannabis with other drugs and the effects of acute withdrawal are also problems under study.

DISCUSSION

Drugs of dependence are of diverse structure and origin, with few behavioral effects in common. Their EEG patterns, also, are varied. If all the drugs of dependence listed in the introduction were examined, the variety of central effects would be greater. Drugs of dependence are defined according to their behavioral effects and to the extent that the behavioral and EEG effects of psychoactive compounds have a direct relationship, we would anticipate that drugs of dependence would also show these intimate relationships, and they do, on acute and chronic administration and during withdrawal. The drugs examined in this summary are characterized by rapid onset and short duration of central action, rapid development of tolerance, and withdrawal symptoms when dosage is suddenly terminated. For each of these clinical effects there are parallel, recordable, and measurable changes in CNS measures, particularly if the more recently developed methods of quantification of the alert EEG are examined. These observations are consistent with the EEG behavioral association theory of psychoactive drugs[4,5] and also provide a basis for a systematic reexamination and reclassification of drugs of dependence.

Using EEG measures, Oswald et al.[15] recently suggested that some drugs of dependence were not drugs of abuse because they induced dysphoric effects either early in their use or during withdrawal and because their withdrawal period was prolonged, i.e., they cleared the metabolic pathways of the body slowly, in a matter of days. This distinction provides another interesting basis for study.

Among the constructs used by the W.H.O. Expert Committee, that of "psychic dependence" seems a weak interpretation of the available data. It is as likely that detailed studies of the central effects of psychoactive compounds will establish persistent central patterns which would justify a single hypothesis or definition of dependence, based on physical tissue responses. Such a foundation for a classification would do much to relieve the endless arguments and sophistry, as to drugs to be proscribed and those to be allowed medical use and study, so characteristic of governmental and intergovernmental committees today. The paradigm of self-stimulation studies in animals provides a useful model in support of a biological or physical view of dependence. The EEG studies summarized here provide another.

After many years of limited study, the resurgence of interest in the opiates, their antagonists, cocaine, alcohol, and cannabis, with governmental support instead of proscription, provides the basis for optimism that the phenomenon of tolerance may yield to systematic study, provide a basis for a more rational view of dependence, and a more rational governmental and societal attitudes to drugs to be proscribed and drugs to be legalized for public use.

SUMMARY

The extensive list of compounds classified by expert committees as drugs of dependence is reviewed and the EEG patterns of opiates (and their antagonists), alcohol, barbiturates and benzodiazepines, sympathomimetic hallucinogens, and cannabis are examined. The compounds are characterized by acute central nervous system effects, rapid in onset, and short in duration. They exhibit diverse EEG patterns, directly related to the diversity of their behavioral effects – observations that are consistent with the theory of association of EEG and behavior with psychoactive drugs in man.

EEG methods may be useful in the study of the central effects of dependence, tolerance, cross tolerance, and to clarify the inadequate definition of physical and 'psychic' dependence.

REFERENCES

1. WHO Expert Committee on Drug Dependence, *Wld. Hlth. Org. Tech. Rep. Ser.*, 460, 41, 1970.
2. WHO Expert Committee on Drug Dependence, *Wld. Hlth. Org. Tech. Rep. Ser.*, 437, 13, 1970.
3. WHO Expert Committee on Drug Dependence, *Wld. Hlth. Org. Tech. Rep. Ser.*, 407, 6, 1969.
4. Fink, M., EEG classification of psychoactive compounds in man: Review and theory of behavioral association, in *Psychopharmacology – A Review of Progress, 1957-1967*, Efron, D. and Cole, J., Eds., U.S. Govt. Printing Office, Washington, D.C., 1969, 497.
5. Fink, M., EEG and human psychopharmacology, *Annu. Rev. Pharmacol.*, 9, 241, 1969.
6. Wikler, A., Clinical and electroencephalographic studies on the effects of mescaline, *n*-allylnormorphine and morphine in man, *J. Nerv. Ment. Dis.*, 120, 157, 1954.

7. Fink, M., Quantitative EEG classification of psychoactive drugs in man, in *The Nature of Sleep,* Jovanovic, U. J., Ed., Wurzburg, in press.

8. Schwartz, J., Feldstein, S., Fink, M., Shapiro, D. M., and Itil, T., Evidence for a characteristic EEG frequency response to thiopental, *Electroencephalogr. Clin. Neurophysiol.,* 31, 149, 1971.

9. Zaks, A., Bruner, A., Fink, M., and Freedman, A. M., Intravenous diacetylmorphine (heroin) in studies of opiate dependence, *Dis. Nerv. Syst. (Suppl.)*, 30, 89, 1969.

10. Fink, M., Zaks, A., Volavka, J., and Roubicek, J., Electrophysiological studies of opiates and antagonists in man, *Narcotic Drugs, Biochemical Pharmacology,* Clouet, D., Ed., Plenum Press, New York, 1971, 452.

11. Volavka, J., Zaks, A., Roubicek, J., and Fink, M., Electrographic effects of diacetylmorphine (heroin) and naloxone in man, *Neuropharmacology,* 9, 587, 1970.

12. Zaks, A., Fink, M., and Freedman, A., Duration of methadone induced cross-tolerance to heroin, *Br. J. Addict.*, 66, 226, 1971.

13. Essig, C. and Fraser, H., Electroencephalographic changes in man during use and withdrawal of barbiturates in moderate dosage, *Electroencephalogr. Clin. Neurophysiol.,* 10, 649, 1958.

14. Wallgren, H. and Barry, H., *Actions of Alcohol,* Elsevier, Amsterdam, 1970.

15. Oswald, I., Lewis, S. A., Dunleavy, D. L. F., Brezinova, V., and Briggs, M., Drugs of dependence though not of abuse: Fenfluramine and imipramine, *Br. Med. J.*, 3, 70, 1971.

16. Itil, T., Elektroencephalographische Studien Bei Psychosen Und Psychotropen Medikamenten, Monograph, Ahmet Sait Matbaasi, Istanbul, 1964.

17. Fink, M., Shapiro, D. M., and Itil, T., EEG profiles of fenfluramine, amobarbital and dextroamphetamine in normal volunteers, *Psychopharmacologia,* 22, 369, 1971.

18. Itil, T. and Fink, M., Anticholinergic drug induced delirium (experimental modification, quantitative EEG and behavioral correlations), *J. Nerv. Ment. Dis.,* 143, 492, 1966.

19. Fink, M., A rational therapy of opiate dependence: Narcotic antagonists, Zarofenetis, C., Ed., International Conference on Drug Abuse, University of Michigan Press, Ann Arbor, in press.

20. Fink, M., Itil, T. M., Zaks, A., and Freedman, A. M., EEG patterns of cyclazocine, a narcotic antagonist, in *Neurophysiological and Behavioral Aspects of Psychotropic Drugs*, Karczmar, A. G. and Koella, W. P., Eds., Charles C Thomas, Springfield, Ill., 1969, 62.

21. Fink, M., Zaks, A., Sharoff, R., Mora, A., Bruner, A., Levit., S., and Freedman, A. M., Naloxone in heroin dependence, *Clin. Pharmacol. Ther.*, 9, 568, 1968.

22. Fink, M., Neurophysiological response strategies in the classification of mental illness, in *The Role and Methodology of Classification in Psychiatry and Psychopathology,* U.S. Govt. Printing Office, Washington, D.C., 1968, 535.

23. Mayo, C. W., Bickford, R., and Faulconer, A., Electroencephalographically controlled anesthesia in abdominal surgery, *J.A.M.A.,* 144, 1081, 1950.

24. Simeon, J., Spero, M., and Fink, M., Clinical and EEG studies of doxepin: interim report, *Psychosomatics,* 10, 14, 1969.

25. Veress, F., Major, V., Fink, M., and Freedman, A. M., High-dose tybamate therapy of heroin dependence, *J. Clin. Pharmacol.,* 9, 232, 1969.

26. Kales, A., *Sleep Physiology and Pathology,* J. B. Lippincott, Philadelphia, 1969.

27. Itil, T. M., Electroencephalography and pharmacopsychiatry, *Mod. Prob. Pharmacopsychiat.,* 1, 163, 1968.

28. Jaffe, J., Psychopharmacology and opiate dependence, in *Psychopharmacology – A Review of Progress, 1957-1967,* Efron, D., Cole, J., Levine, J., and Wittenborn, J., Eds., Washington, D. C., U. S. Govt. Printing Office, 1969, 853.

29. Volavka, J., Dornbush, R., Feldstein, S., Clare, G., Zaks, A., Fink, M., and Freedman, A., Marijuana, EEG and behavior, *Proc. N. Y. Acad. Sci.,* 191, 206, 1971.

30. Dornbush, R., Fink, M., and Freedman, A., Marijuana, memory and perception, *Am. J. Psychiat.,* 128, 194, 1971.

31. Freedman, A. and Fink, M., Cannabis psychosis, in: Biochemical and Pharmacologic Aspects of Drug Dependence, van Praag, H. M., Ed., E. F., Bohn, Amsterdam, 1972, 85.

32. Dornbush, R., Volavka, J., Clare, G., Zaks, A., and Fink, M., 21-Day Administration of Cannabis in Male Volunteers, in preparation.

NEUROPATHOLOGY OF DRUGS OF DEPENDENCE

L. Roizin, M. Halpern, M. M. Baden, M. Kaufman, S. Hashimoto, J. C. Liu, and B. Eisenberg

TABLE OF CONTENTS

INTRODUCTION

Although the behavioral aspects of psychotropic agents are well known since the time of "Corpus Hippocraticum" (4th century B.C.),[1-3] the tissue reactions and especially those of the CNS are still in the early phases of exploration.[4]

Because of space limitation we will limit our review to the most salient neuropathologic, histochemical, and ultracellular reactions associated with the current most commonly abused addictive drugs in man and experimental conditions.

OPIATES AND NARCOTICS

Morphine

Tissue reactions to drugs are related principally to their pharmacodynamic properties which they exercise through direct or indirect mechanisms. Neuropathologic lesions (cellular and architectural) may be minimal, nonspecific, or absent in rapid-acting toxicity or/and deaths occurring within a short time after drug intake. The survival period must be long enough to permit development of lesions.

Acute morphine toxicity is associated with engorgement of larger veins (with dark blood) or severe congestion of blood vessels with diapedesis of erythrocytes, perivascular hemorrhages, and cerebral edema. In some cases, the white matter of the brain appears studded with hemorrhagic petchiae.[5]

In chronic morphine addicts moderate atrophy of the frontal lobe was noted. Histologically, fibrous thickening of the leptomeninges, degenerative changes of the cortical nerve cells (particularly pyramidal) with patchy loss of neurons, nonspecific lipid degeneration of the Ganglion cells, microglia and endothelial cells of the blood vessels were noted. Fibral thickening of the walls of small vessels were also encountered.[5,6]

In experimental animals (rabbits, guinea pigs, and cats) surviving up to 20 days, various histopathologic alterations such as pyknosis of small and medium pyramidal cells, loss of tigroid material, swelling, homogenization or vesicle formation in the cytoplasm of neurons, clumping of nuclear chromatin, bead-like swellings of dendrites, and focal hemorrhages in various parts of the CNS[7] were detected. In more chronic conditions (after 20 days survival) morphologic alterations with fatty degeneration were prominent, particularly in the cerebral cortex, corpus striatum, and Ammon's horn.

Heroin

According to several investigators,[8-12] the most common pathologic findings in heroin addicts are represented by hepatitis (viral), particularly periportal variant from 29 to 70% according to various authors, hepatotoxic degeneration, pulmonary complications (embolic) pneumonia or lung abscesses or both, upper respiratory tract pneumonia, bronchopneumonia, acute pulmonary congestion, pulmonary edema, pulmonary fibrosis or granulomas or both, cardiovascular complications; endocarditis (subacute bacterial, including Staphylococci, enterococci, Escherichia coli, Candida klebsiella, Aerobacter, Pseudomonas aeruginosa); brain abscess (phycomycotic);[13] thrombophlebitis and septicemia; skin lesions (cellulitis or necrotic subcutaneous nonpurulent lesions); and nonspecific encephalopathy[14] which will be discussed in more detail in the chapter on methadone.

Fatalities in Miscellaneous Chronic Opiate Addiction

The most prominent neuropathological findings consist of proliferation of the fibrous elements of the leptomeninges, edema of the brain, and changes of the cortical neurons, including mild chromatolysis of Purkinje's cells, lipid infiltration, pyknosis, satellitosis, and progressive degeneration leading to patchy neuronal loss.

Symmetrical softening of the globus pallidus and early softening of the cerebral cortex, including laminar necrosis of Ammon's horn similar to cerebral anoxia, were observed in cases who survived large doses of an opiate (patopon).[7] It is not certain whether such changes are the intercurrent effects (depression) on the respiratory and cardiac centers with the resulting anoxic effects or whether they may be related to histotoxic anoxia (secondary vasomotor reactions).[15]

In relation to the mode of action of these toxic agents, it is important to remember that solutions with molecular weight below 500 pass through the placenta and that its permeability increases in the latter months of pregnancy.[16] Having passed the placental barrier, most substances accumulate in the fetal blood in concentrations up to twice as high as those in the maternal blood. The blood-brain barrier is more permeable in the newborn than in the adult. Furthermore, the fetal vulnerability to noxious agents and anoxia is particularly more prominent in the first trimester of gestation. Also, children are generally more vulnerable than adults to morphine and their derivatives while elderly people, undernourished and infirm as well as under stress, have decreased tolerance to toxicity.[17-19]

Recent biochemical and histochemical studies have been concerned with distribution and metabolism of morphine,[20,21] effects of morphine on acetylcholine metabolism,[22-24] and effects of morphine on the catecholamines in the nerve cells[25] and their excretion.[26] These studies seem to suggest that they may be the possible target sites as well as interaction loci between the structural and chemical processes or their intermediary metabolism. In relation with the latter, we would like to recall the significance of the drug effects upon the ultracellular organelles, their respective units and subunits.

Methadone

The recently-developed methadone treatment for the withdrawal of narcotic drug dependence has renewed and stimulated the interest in its pharmacological properties. Table 1 summarizes the most common adverse and toxicologic methadone reactions in tolerant (heroin addicts enrolled, "drop-outs", or discharged from methadone maintenance program) and nontolerant (adults and children) cases following the use of methadone for maintenance of heroin withdrawal or detoxification abuse and accidental or suicidal overdosages.

The percentages of methadone fatalities reported by various investigators differ in relation to a variety of individual chemicopharmacodynamic, medical, psychiatric (including behavioral disorders), biological, and environmental (including socio-economical and ecological) conditions, which will be reviewed in more detail in the last section of this chapter on neuropathology. Although several methadone fatalities have been reported in the medical literature,[12, 27-41] no microscopic or neuropathologic findings have been described.

Our neuropathologic studies disclosed a variety of questionable to moderate nonspecific neuronal degenerative changes in various anatomotopographic regions of the central nervous system and liver. The latter were visualized as being more prominent in lipid-staining techniques. In the liver, the hepatic cells showed frequently moderate to prominent sudanophilia (Figures 1 and 2) and in three cases mild to pronounced hepatitis (Figures 3 and 4).

TABLE 1

Tabulation of the Most Significant Clinico-pathologic Findings in 14 Methadone Fatalities of Heroin-Dependent Patients

Methadone (Human Cases)

Case #	Age and Sex	Drug and Dosage*	Duration of treatment	Clinical findings (drug habits)	Toxicologic findings and General Comments
4821 (B.R.)	52; M	Methadone (180 mg before death)	Meth. progr.	alcohol; codeine; barbiturates (addiction to all; cardiac disorders)	Urine: Morphine: + – Methadone: + Quinine: + Codeine: – Barbiturates: –
4825 (D.H.)	19; M	Methadone	unknown →	Heroin addict Methadone	No Urine
4830 (W.D.)	24; M	Methadone 140 mg per day	2 mos. →	Heroin addict for 4 years; Heroin and Methadone	Urine: Methadone: very strongly + Morphine: – Quinine: –

TABLE 1 (continued)

Case #	Age and Sex	Drug and Dosage*	Duration of treatment	Clinical findings (drug habits)	Toxicologic findings and General Comments
4831 (P.P.)	19; F	Methadone 90 mg per day	Meth. progr.	Heroin addict; asthma Methadone	Urine: Methadone: + very faint reaction, traces
4838 (P.C.)	22; M	Methadone (20 mg BID) thorazine: (75 mg tid) Methadone overdosage	Meth. progr.	Heroin addict; Methadone Thorazine Clorox	Urine: Morphine: – Quinine: – Methadone: + Barbiturates: – Unknown Others: +
4856 (J.J.)	30; M	Methadone overdosage	Meth. progr.	Heroin and Methadone	Urine: Morphine: + – Quinine: – Methadone: –
4882 (R.J.)	32; M	Methadone overdosage	unknown →	Heroin addict and Methadone	found in street No urine
4928 (J.J.)	65; M	Methadone 80 mg; Heroin ?	1 mo. Meth. progr. Narcotics 40 yrs.	Heroin and Meth.; Quinine; Naline; Digitalis; Darvan; cardiac disorders	Urine and serum: +
4939 (B.M.)	18; F	Methadone 100 mg before death	unknown		collapsed at a party; flat ECG. pneumothorax. Insufficient amount of urine.
4957	20; M	Heroin overdosage ?	Methadone program	Heroin and Methadone	Urine: Morphine: + Quinine: – Methadone: – Barbiturates: –
4972	58; M	Methadone overdosage	Methadone program	Narcotics: 10 yrs. +	Urine: Methadone: +
4986	18; M	Methadone overdosage	not on Methadone program	Heroin addict	Urine: Morphine: + Quinine: + Methadone: + Unknown Others +
4989 (J.F.)	31; M	Methadone (80 mg)	unknown	Alcohol (severe)	Urine: Morphine: – Quinine: – Methadone: +
4997	23; M	Methadone overdosage	unknown		Urine: Morphine: – Quinine: – Methadone: +

*prior to demise

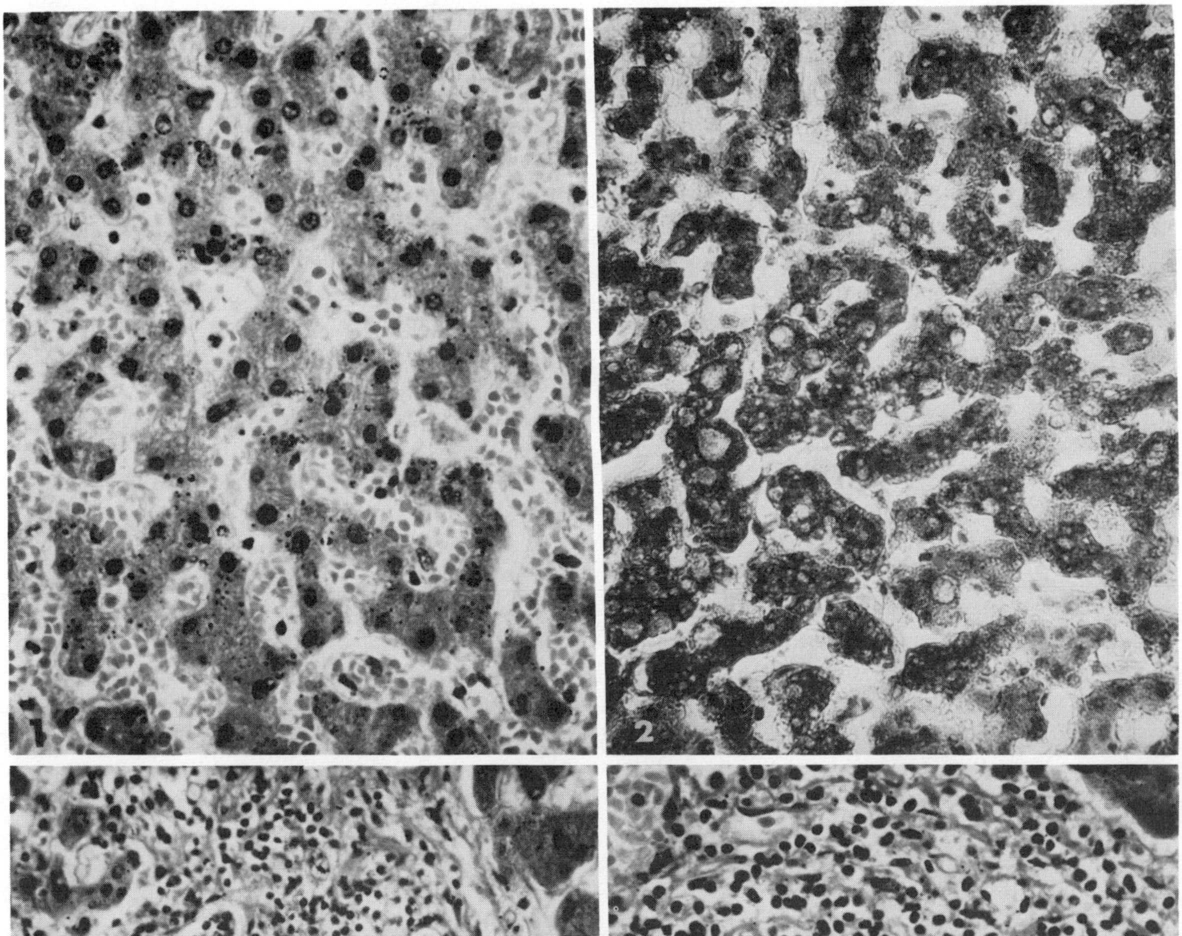

FIGURES 1 - 4. Liver showing various degrees of degenerative changes affecting, in particular, the hepatic cells and deposits of variable amounts of lipid stainable material in the structural alterations of the liver. (1) Hematoxylin and Eosin stain, magnification: 640x; (2) Sudan III method, magnification: 400x. (3) and (4): Hepatitis, inflammatory exudate consisting predominantly of mononuclear cells. Hematoxylin and Eosin stain; magnification: (3) 480x and (4) 640x.

Additional clinicopathologic and histopathologic findings were similar to those observed in heroin addicts. These consisted of cardiovascular disorders (subacute bacterial and, at times, fungus endocarditis, left or right side, in some instances with rapid destruction of the valve, cardiac perforation, and sudden death); phlebitis and thrombophlebitis, local and diffuse abscess formation with sequelae as described in heroin cases; liver diseases (hepatitis, postnecrotic cirrhosis); lung diseases (pulmonary edema, recurrent pulmonary emboli of septic character); and skin lesions as previously described. The causes of death in patients in methadone maintenance programs were attributed to alcoholism (see discussion on drug interactions), barbiturate and amphetamine abuse, trauma, liver disease, heroin abuse, coronary arteriosclerosis or cerebral hemorrhage, and bacterial meningitis.[12]

Among the histochemical studies of particular interest are the cytoarchitectural and anatomotopographic distribution of the G-6-P (glucose-6-phosphatase), Ac.P. (acid phosphatase), and TPP (thiamine pyrophosphatase) enzyme reaction products. Distinctive reactions have been noted in relation to the duration of the incubation and according to cytomorphologic patterns of the cerebral cortex, striatum, thalamus, hypothalamus, mesencephalon, pons, medulla, cerebellum, and spinal cord. Various degrees of neuronal morphologic changes, distribution, and concentration of the enzyme reaction patterns were noted in various anatomo-topographic regions of the central nervous system. Glial reactions (particularly astrocytes) appeared more prominent along or in the vicinity of blood vessels and with the increase of the incubation time became more prominent as compared with the neurons. Vascular and perivascular reactions appeared particularly more prominent in TPP preparations (Figure 5). Also of particular interest were the presence of some senile plaques in two cases.

It is also of particular significance to note that, in various animals, some vascular lesions were noted. These were principally characterized by unusual perivascular glia hyperplasia and hypertrophy. Since there was no tissue necrosis or degeneration, it was assumed that these latter reactions were caused probably by increased vascular permeability (Figures 6 and 7).

The electron microscope studies of human material present the well-known difficulties caused by postmortem changes. However, certain findings, in the light of the experimental observation, are considered of significance; for instance, in the CNS, changes of the ultrastructure and distribution of the RER (rough endoplasmic reticulum) and SER (or Golgi system, Figures 8 and 9) ribosomes, polymorpho-metabolosomes or PMS (matrix and membranes), synaptosomes, and their subunits (including contents of the presynaptic terminals, vesicles, and pre- and postsynaptic membranes, as well as the synaptic cleft). Degenerative changes within the vascular walls and in the perivascular region were noted in several cases. Degenerative processes associated with osmiophilic products and structures of variable density, composition, and configuration were noticed in basal ganglia and cerebellum (Figure 10). Of particular significance, is the presence of axonal dystrophies as well as some senile plaque-like formations (Figure 11). The most salient ultrastructural changes of the liver were expressed by alterations, and, at times, disorganization of the fine membranes of the endoplasmic reticulum, related subunits, PMS, as well as MVB (multivesicular body) in addition to abnormal presence of lipid products, glycogen granules, and necrobiotic material undergoing various degrees of metabolization or digestion (Figure 12).

STIMULANTS OF THE CNS

Amphetamines

Toxic reactions[42-46] and "amphetamine psychosis" (chronic course and dementia) with reversible and irreversible organic changes of the brain are well known.[47,48] Lesions of vascular character expressed by congestion and subdural and subarachnoid petechiae have been reported in some amphetamine fatalities.[49] Biochemical studies[50,51] detected a decrease of aerobic lactic acid formation in the brains of patients and experimental animals with chronic amphetamine intoxication. More recent biochemical and metabolic investigations[52] support the view that the central stimulatory action of the amphetamine and its peripheral sympathomimetic effects are mediated through the release of catecholamines. It has been suggested that the adrenergic receptor could be a component of the adenyl cyclase system.[53] As far as the brain tissue is concerned, subcellular distribution studies of adenyl cyclase are compatible with synaptic localization[54] and extrapolation

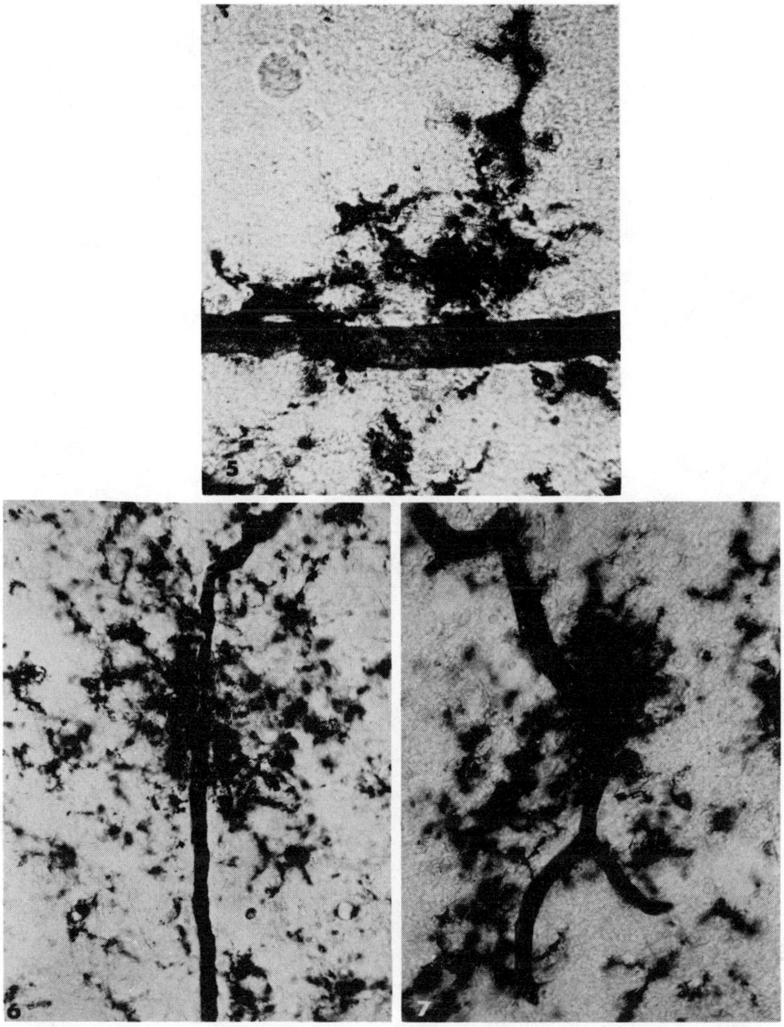

FIGURES 5 - 7. Various degrees of perivascular glial reactions associated with increased vascular permeability (as described in the text). TPP method; (5) frontal lobe cortex, magnification: 1000x; (b) frontal lobe cortex, magnification: 360x; and (c) cerebellum, magnification: 540x.

from studies with pineal gland homogenates suggests a postsynaptic localization.[55] Furthermore, electron microscope examinations of CNS affected by experimental chronic methamphetamine intoxication[56] disclosed coalescence of membranes between axons at the nerve endings and between axons and dendrites and an increased number with hypertrophy and increase of endoplasmic reticulum within the cytoplasm of neurons. Some of these ultrastructural findings may be indicative of possible disturbances of neural conduction and transmission mechanisms in the CNS.

Cocaine and Its Derivatives

Acute toxic fatalities due to respiratory failure have been observed not only after overdoses but also following therapeutic doses.[57] In these instances, edema and congestion of the meninges and nervous tissues, early chromatolysis, and pyknosis of neurons were also prominent.[5,57] In chronic conditions, fatty changes in the blood vessels, the "cortical and ganglionic" neurons and microglia, in addition to chromatolysis (particularly in the Ammon's horn),[57,58] vacuole formation and condensation of the nuclear chromatin in nerve cells were widespread through-

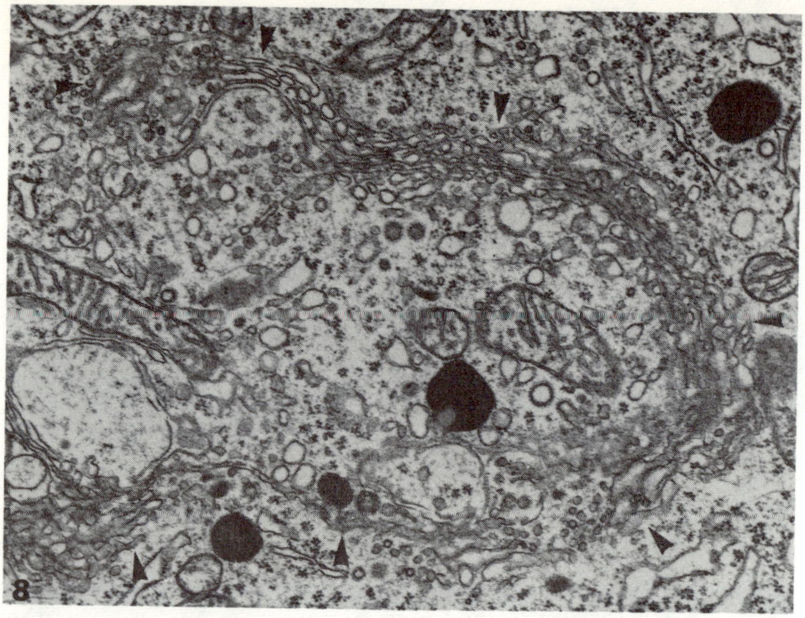

FIGURE 8.

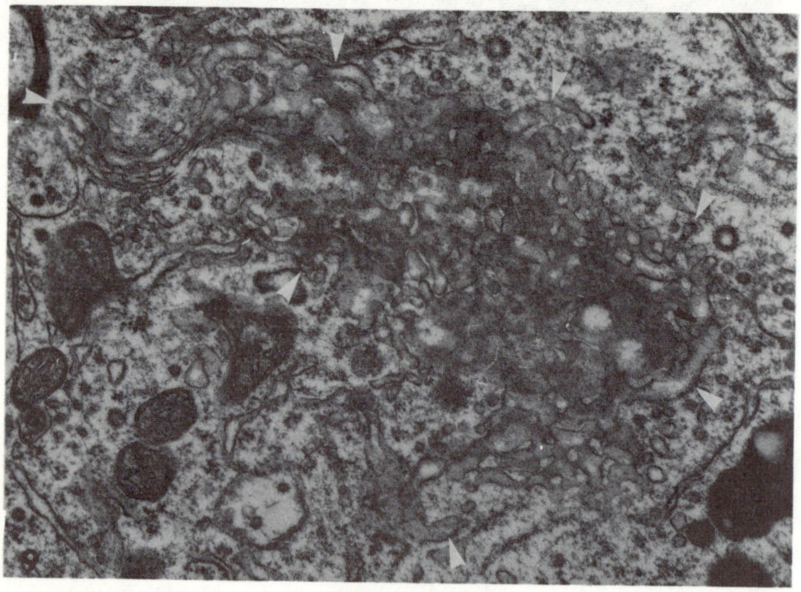

FIGURE 9.

FIGURES 8 and 9. Various degrees of ultrastructural alterations (8) and disorganization (9) of the endoplasmic reticulum, particularly of the Golgi complex (see arrows). Uranyl acetate and lead citrate counterstains. RCA-EMU-3G. Magnifications: (8): 26,000x; (9): 33,800x.

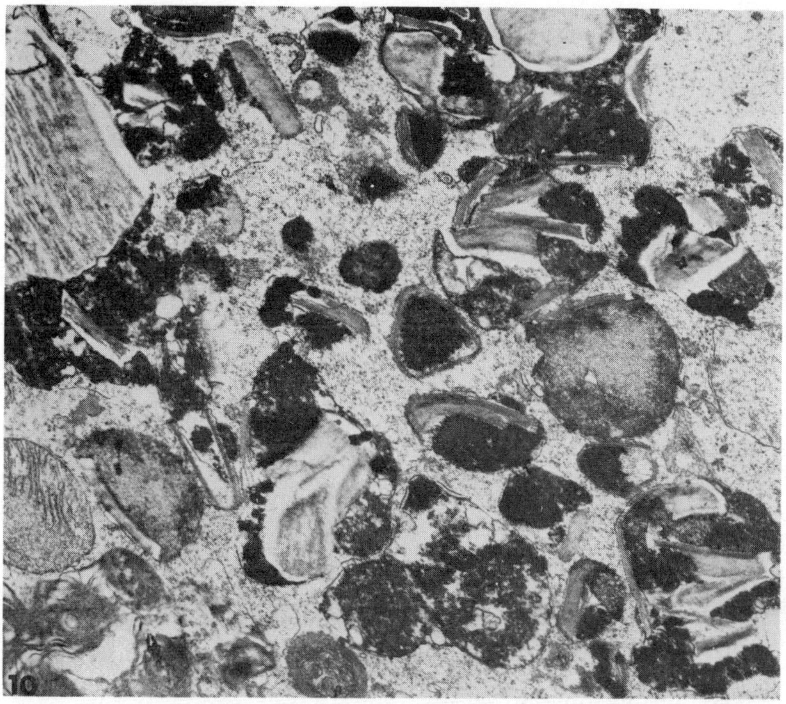

FIGURE 10. Cerebellum (dentate nucleus). Degenerative processes associated with osmiophilic products and ultrastructures of variable composition and configurations. Uranyl acetate and lead citrate counterstains. RCA,EMU-3G. Magnification: 26,000x.

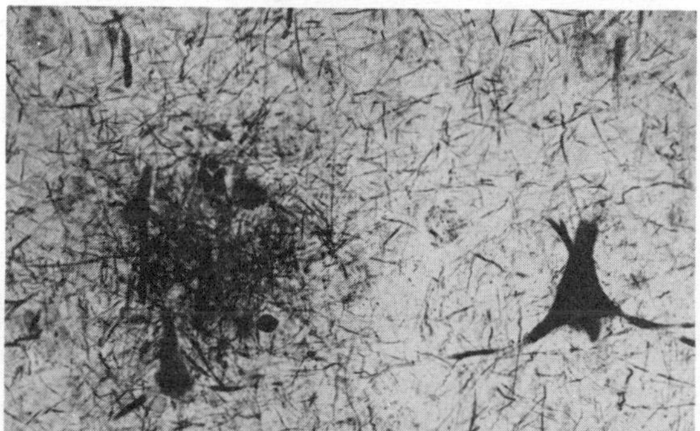

FIGURE 11. Frontal cortex. Senile plaque formation in the middle layer of the cerebral cortex. Acid phosphatase method. Magnification: 1,280x.

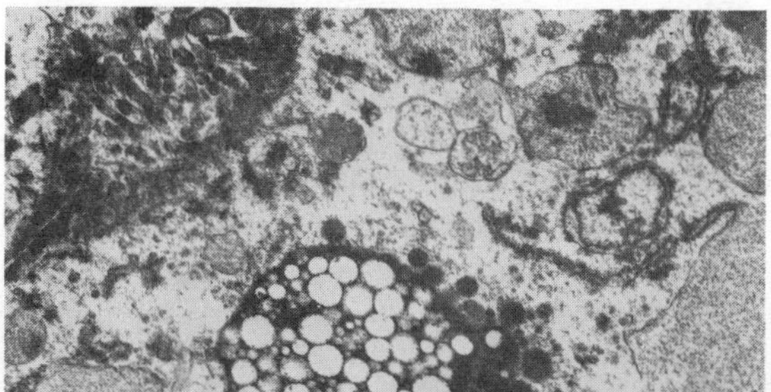

FIGURE 12. Liver. Degenerative changes involving the ultrastructural organization of the hepatic parenchyma. Uranyl acetate and lead citrate. RCA,EMU-3G; magnification: 26,000x.

out the CNS. Thrombosis of the small blood vessels of the brain was additionally evident in experimental animals.[59]

CENTRAL NERVOUS SYSTEM DEPRESSANTS

Barbiturates

Most cases of barbiturate toxicity either recover or demise during the acute phase.[60,61] In fatal intoxication nonspecific alterations with chromatolysis of the cortical neurons, acute disease of Nissl (widespread swelling), particularly nuclear, marked meningeal reaction (aseptic), medullary hemorrhage and mild brain edema[62] were described. The most prominent neuropathologic findings in prolonged survival (in a vegetative state), the cerebral cortex, and basal ganglia (especially globus pallidus) show all degrees of laminar necrosis from cell degeneration to "scar formation."[5,63,64] The lesions seem to be due to anoxia and display the same distribution as cases of anoxia due to other agents, although sparing Sommer's sector and Purkinje cells.[61] The character of the lesions seems to be related to the length of survival, the patient's habituation to the drug, and the actual dose ingested. The anoxia is produced by the depression or paralysis of the medullary respiratory center, inhibition of the respiratory enzymes at the cellular level,[65] and possibly by vasomotor spasms, thus resembling other hypoxic poisons. In the chronic barbiturism, mild intellectual deterioration and lessening of will power become associated with cortical atrophy of the brain.[66] This encephalopathy results from the progressive degeneration of the cortical neurons with their final disappearance. There is no responsive gliosis to the loss of neurons. In a case of combined barbiturate dependence and opiate intoxication, the CNS pathology consisted of bilateral necrosis of the basal ganglia, small necrotic foci throughout the cerebral hemispheres and cerebellum, small areas of demyelination in the white matter of the encephalon, considerable degeneration of the neurons of the inferior olives of the cerebellar folia, progressive reaction of the astroglia, metamorphosis of microglia into compound granular corpuscles and degeneration of the spinal tracts in the spinal cord. Liver, spleen, kidney, and lungs showed no significant changes.[67]

The synergistic effect between ethyl alcohol and phenobarbital was demonstrated in a series of rats.[68] The maximum sublethal dose of one drug and half of the other caused a high percentage of fatalities in animals. Three medicolegal cases occurring in a usual community indicated similar fatal synergism, i.e., the combination of phenobarbital and ethyl alcohol.

HALLUCINOGENIC DRUG REACTIONS

Δ^9 Tetrahydrocannabinol

(THC) is the principal component of cannabis sativa (hemp plant). Hashish is derived from the flowering top of the female plant and the marijuana consists of chopped plant material. To some extent, these drugs resemble alcohol as well as LSD.[69,70]

Marijuana (or Marihuana)

Some people assert that this drug improves artistic or creative endeavors, whereas others believe that its abuse does not result in physical dependence. However, psychosomatic (hypermotility, congestion of cilliary vessels and oropharyngitis, chronic bronchitis and asthma, hypoglycemia, and bulimia) and toxic reactions demonstrate that it has real similarities with other drugs of dependence in the sense that marihuana is basically a multi-causal problem.[71] For instance, we will begin with supplementing the previously mentioned disturbances with the following adverse effects: a reduced fertility among women who regularly smoke marihuana, change in the user's sex drive, possible early abortion and liver damage,[72] severe body tremors and tachycardia, nausea, vomiting, and diarrhea, diffuse aching pains, hypotension, non-oliguric renal failure, thrombocytopenia and leukopenia after i.v. injection,[73] arteritis,[74] transverse myelitis,[75] encephalopathy and paraplegia,[14] hepatotoxicity,[76] cerebral atrophy,[77] neuronophagia, vacuolization of the cytoplasm and nuclei of the cortical neurons,[5] and teratogenic activity.[78,79]

Hashish

The chemistry and pharmacology of hashish[80-82] as well as marihuana are discussed respectively in separate chapters of this book. However, in relation with our topic of discussion, it is significant to emphasize that hashish is five to ten times more potent than marihuana.

Since the focus of attention regarding the smoking of the various products of *Cannabis sativa* has been directed toward the behavioral or psychological aspects, in this review we will emphasize in particular the adverse and toxicologic effects. American soldiers who smoked large quantities of hashish for several months[83] experienced respiratory dysfunctions and diseases (dyspnea, inspiratory rales, expiratory wheezes, increased bronchopulmonary markings, bronchitis, cough, and asthma), opacification of sinuses, increased nasal secretions and irritations, rhinopharyngeal symptoms, oropharyngitis and uvular edema, recurrent urticaria, acne, abdominal cramps, and diarrhea. In view of the fact that asthma and rhinopharyngitis may be the results of allergies, the possibility that hashish may be an allergen was investigated.[83] These studies were not contributory, indicating that hashish was not a primary allergen. However, by virtue of irritating capacity upon the mucosa of the oropharyngo-laryngeal and respiratory system, hashish may have potentiating allergic tendencies. It is also important to note the occurrence of a general collapse after intravenous injection of hashish,[84] and that by the fluorescent method some investigators[85] revealed the effect of hashish smoke sublimate on hypothalamic noradrenaline. The influence of hashish on human EEG has been studied in 27 hashish-addicted soldiers, ages 20 to 25 years who have been hashish smokers from 1 to 9 years.[86] While confusion was generally accompanied by increased stabilization of alpha rhythm in these cases, hallucinations, delusions, dizziness, and headaches were associated with "disorganization of the tracing or tendency to it."

In regard to the neural tissue reactions and histochemical effects of hashish in the CNS, it is interesting to note that in a brain of a dog who died about three months after consuming a large amount of hashish,* microscopic examinations revealed marked variations in concentration and distribution of the reaction products of acid phosphatases, thiamine-pyrophosphatase, and glucose-6-phosphatase in the neurons and some glial elements in various anatomotopographic regions of the CNS. It is also of interest to note that various phases of senile plaque formations were detected in the hippocampal gyrus, though the estimated age of the dog was about two years.

LSD, Mescaline, and DOM (2, 5-dimetoxy-4-methyl-amphetamine hydrochloride)

As a result of the interest in hallucinogens by most diversified professions such as the medical, biological, social, religious, legislative, and creative and performing arts, and, due to sensational publicity of the mass media communication systems, frequent misunderstandings or misconceptions have confused the evaluation of objective facts which are diluted in an exuberant and kaleidoscopic literature. Fortunately, several excellent scientific symposia, as well as critical reviews of the medical, biological, and psychiatric literature have been published.[87-92] Since many narcotic drug-dependent patients intermittently or occasionally experiment for "kicks" with some of the hallucinogens that also induce adverse or toxic effects[93-111] and interact with other drugs, we will mention briefly only some of the most significant toxicologic and neuropathologic findings. In experimental investigations with variable doses of LSD, we[112] noticed nuclear vacuolization associated with disappearance of nuclear chromatin and intranuclear Nissl staining granules, cytoplasmic fragmentation, as well as depletion of Nissl substance and neuronal degeneration in cerebral cortex nerve cells of rats. Some hepatic cells also displayed nuclear vacuolization resembling those in the cerebrum. Dogs subjected to acute and chronic intoxication with lysergic acid diethylamide[113] have shown "high frequent waves" of low amplitude, similar to those observed with mescaline and in the first stage of barbiturate intoxication. Acid and alkaline phosphatases in the CNS of the LSD-affected animals revealed some qualitative changes as compared with the control including some significant alterations in the liver and kidneys. Reversible changes and decrease of Nissl substance with concomitant alterations of the nucleus and nucleolus, contraction of oligodendroglia and, at times, increased number of glia were observed also in adult mammalian brain cultures after administration of LSD-25.[114]

In view of the fact that the teratogenic effects of psychotropic agents, including hallucinogens, will be described in a separate chapter of this book, we will limit our discussion to electron microscope examinations based on some personal

*This study was carried out in cooperation with Drs. G. Gold and J. Silverman.

studies.[115] Concentrated doses of LSD-25, DOM, and mescaline administered to various strains of pregnant mice during the early phases of gestation (first week) induced teratogenic effects such as resorptions, miscarriages, stillborn, early and late embryonal or fetal deaths, stunted and small offspring, defective development of one extremity or tail, and occasionally exencephalia. In the latter, the most significant ultracellular changes affected the fine structural organization of the nucleolar-nuclear correlates, the nuclear membranes, the endoplasmic reticulum, the distribution of RNA, and variations in distribution of mitochondria or polymorphometabolosomes (PMS), lysosomes, and multivesicular bodies. In adult animals, it was particularly prominent: modifications of the rough and smooth components of the endoplasmic reticulum and irregular distribution of RNA which was frequently associated with qualitative and quantitative alterations of PMS and lysosomes. Variations of the presynaptic terminal content and modification of the osmiophilic density and extension at the level of the synaptic cleft and subsynaptic webb were noted. These findings seem to indicate possible ultrastructural modifications at the interneuronal communication level.

MISCELLANEOUS NEUROPSYCHOTROPIC DRUG INTERACTIONS

Among neuropsychotropic drug interactions, a large percentage of drug-dependent patients indulge more commonly in the combined use of tranquilizers and/or antidepressive agents. Since the adverse reactions, histo- and neuropathologic, histochemical, and ultracellular (in vivo and in vitro) in human and experimental conditions have been recently reviewed in detail, and because of space limitation, the interested reader is referred to other general references.[9,116-124]

DISCUSSION

Our studies on the morbidity and mortality of narcotic drug dependence reveal that the pathogenic mechanisms that drug-induced diseases process (Toxo-Synpathies) may be also caused by the accumulative effects of participating drugs or combination of reciprocally potentiating, aggravating, and precipitating cofactors.[125] The simultaneous occurrence of multiple chemicodynamics and the living organization interactions intensify the toxopathogenesis of the independent drug's vulnerability. These are represented by multiple factors such as:

Anatomo-Functional Cofactors

The structural organization of the CNS is characterized by the differential embryological metamorphosis and evolution of its morphological and histochemical constituents, functional and metabolic plurality, and the diversified or selective pathological tissue reaction patterns. At a closer examination the neuron or the anatomo-functional unit of the CNS is endowed and capable, within normal conditions, to perceive, assimilate, store, and elaborate metabolic and biophysical (action potentials) energy. These intracellular activities are patterned through nuclear-nucleolar, PMS, endoplasmic reticulum, lysosomes, multivesicular bodies (including their accessory units and subunits), microsomes, neurofilaments, and neurotubules. Since the neurons are in constant contact with neighboring and distant neuronal organizations, in order to carry the aforementioned functions the neuron must be prepared, upon perception of appropriate stimuli, to convey (deliver) its "quantum" energy to its anatomo-physiological and metabolic correlates. This interneuronal assignment is accomplished through the very fine communicating mechanisms represented by the elaborate network of the neuronal processes and innumerable synaptosomes. Current electron microscope studies indicate that (1) the membrane systems enclose the cell and its organelles, compartmentalize their interior, delineate systems for the direction or channeling of the intermediary metabolites or metabolic processes, and (2) the physicochemical properties of the membranes are expressed by particular configuration of molecules. These are arranged in multiple species of repeating units (within a membrane system) and serve as a miniaturized base for characteristic spectra of enzyme systems or assemblies.* Within this framework, the membranes also control or direct the traffic of electrolytes and colloidal systems. Thus, the membrane-enzyme associated

*Each membrane-bound enzyme serves in a dual capacity: (a) as one of a group of catalysts in a sequential biochemical process and (b) as an integral constituent of the membrane.

systems represent the molecular basis of the metabolic and physiological mechanisms in neural tissue, i.e., their synergistic functions mediate the cybernetics of the specialized activities and regulate the flow of the living cellular energy. These biological cycles involve fixation, release, transport (translocation) and transformation or use of energy for mechanical, synthesis, digestive, secretory, and bioelectrical (action potentials), activities. Recent observations have also disclosed that various biophysical, biochemical, and morbigenous agents can act as stabilizers or disorganizers of the membrane-bound enzyme systems. This condensed summary of the complex structural and histochemical organization of the CNS is aiming not only to recall its diversified anatomo-physiological characteristic of the CNS but, in particular, to focus attention on the many areas where biochemical and biophysical phenomena or drugs and disease processes may influence or alter the functions of the cells and their mechanisms of communication up to the molecular framework.

In this light, the qualitative and quantitative variations of the oxidoreduction and hydrolytic enzyme systems may be attributed to some of the following conditions: (1) morphologic characteristics of the correlated anatomo-topographic regions of the CNS (from the cellular to the molecular level of organization), (2) heterogeneous metabolism (structurally dependent), and (3) correlated physiological activities. However, for clearer understanding and better evaluation of the mode of action of drugs and their potential pathogenicity, the role of the following cofactors should be also considered.

Biochemical Cofactors

The wide range effects of the pharmacodynamic properties of the chemical agents on the rate of enzyme activity, transfer or conduction mechanisms, stimulation or inhibition of synthetic processes suggest that each drug may have several sites of actions which may or may not coincide with other drugs or factors. Thus, two or more drugs, as encountered in chemotherapy, frequently induce unexpected reactions because of synergistic or antagonistic effects on key tissue processes, i.e., ATP synthesis, oxidoreduction mechanisms, biogenic amine metabolism (inhibition of storage or liberation and depletion) causing variations in the concentration of neurochemical mediators at receptor sites or along the neuronal transmission pathways (at the pre- or postsynaptic levels), protein synthesis, lipid membrane integrity, neural barrier permeability, etc. In relation to our topic under discussion, of particular interest, is the tendency of the "current polypharmacology" or the multiple drug intake and the toxicity due to the interaction between drugs ("toxic cocktail"). Tranquilizers and hypnotics potentiate the cerebral depressant effect of each other and alcohol potentiates the reactions of both of them. The combination may cause fatal toxicity in cases where both the amount of alcohol and the dosage of each of these drugs were moderate. In patients treated with MAO inhibitors, a fatal hypertensive crisis may be induced by sympathomimetic agents, such as adrenaline, ephedrine, and amphetamine; phenothiazines and imipramine may cause excitement, hyperthermia, and coma. When the patient has previously used hypotensives, dangerous shock may develop in anesthesia as a result of exhaustion of catecholamines. The concomitant administration of salicylates, phenylbutazone derivatives, broad-spectrum antibiotics, clofibrate, or alcohol may increase and prolong the effect of anticoagulants to such a degree as to cause severe hemorrhages because of reduced prothrombin. Conversely, a drug may reduce the pharmacological activity of another by stimulating its metabolic inactivation. Barbiturates stimulate the metabolism of anticoagulants, thereby lowering the anticoagulant activity. When the administration of the barbiturate is stopped, severe bleeding may occur. Severe and protracted hypoglycemia occur in diabetics treated with sulfonylurea agents (tolbuamide, tolasamide) and especially after chlorpropamide (half-life of 33 hrs). This potentiation may occur in elderly patients and in patients with impaired renal function. The interaction may occur not only with long-acting sulfonamides, but also when short-acting sulfonamides are administered. Moreover, for the proper evaluation of the reversible and irreversible pathologic processes, the following accessory biological cofactors should be considered.

Biological Cofactors

Environmental or metereopatic variants – Death records during the "London fog" (December 5-9, 1952) show that about 4,000 more deaths occurred than would have been expected on the basis of the data from previous years.[125] During another similar episode, many patients presented symptoms of acute bronchiolitis without the evidence of infection.[126] Respiratory insufficiency due to hypoxaemia associated with hypercapnia (as in cases of bronchial asthma hyphoscoliosis and severe anemia) may cause alarming dangerous or comatose states when narcotics or sedatives, in otherwise normal doses, are administered.[127]

Nutritional variants – These are related to both insufficient quantity, and deficient quality of food (poor in proteins and vitamins, rich in carbohydrates). Many drug addicts have poor appetites, erratic eating habits, and suffer from digestive disorders as well as malabsorption. It has also been demonstrated that laboratory animals subjected to partial starvation and nutritional stress are more susceptible to toxic adverse reactions as compared with controls.

Geographical differences – Recently it has been reported that nephrotoxicity has been increased in Switzerland following the use of analgesics with phenacitin.[128]

Individual and Stressor Cofactors

Many investigators[94,129,130] have compared the initial symptoms of adverse reactions to the peak of an "iceberg," i.e., the most extensive and most damaging part is beneath the surface. The stressor effects of a physical and chemical character upon the CNS, neurohormonal, and psychogenic mechanisms are well known[131-133] and for this reason they are not reviewed here, except to mention that they are also acting as potentiating mechanisms through neurogenic and neurohumoral (including the electrolytes) homeokinetic mechanisms. Accordingly, histometabolic dysergia may cause reversible or lead to irreversible changes through pathergia and patoclysis.[134]

Miscellaneous Medico-Socio-Ecological Cofactors

Patients with hyperthyroidism may develop toxic conditions, even coma, after small doses of morphine. The opiate addict is often amenorrhoic, but may become pregnant, and there is a high incidence of obstetrical complications, including stillbirths.[135,136] Infant withdrawal symptoms shortly after birth are expressed by restlessness, crying, irritability, poor feeding, vomiting, yawning (a great deal), coryza, goose flesh, etc.[137]

Recent socio-epidemiologic studies have disclosed that the abuse of marihuana, amphetamines, barbiturates, hallucinogens, and other psychotropic substances has spread to all levels of society and from school children to young adults. Some difficulties in the evaluation of "drug reactions" in human pathologic material exist, since correlations are not synonymous with explanations. Although several "validation criteria" for drug reactions have been devised in accordance with several investigators,[138] still some difficulties are encountered in evaluating retrospective drug reactions in human cases such as (1) inadequate information about the dosage of the drug and the overall medico-biological conditions of the patient, (2) multiple drug intake, (3) uncertainties of the chemical identification and its temporal relationship to the adverse reaction, (4) existence of inborn or acquired "predisposing" or facilitating factors, (5) inadequate surveillance or follow-up of out-clinic patients, and (6) the body's limited means of reaction.

Significance of Animal Experimentation

To facilitate or recognize, at least, some fundamental "drug reaction profiles," animal experimentation may help to establish (1) the pharmacodynamics of drug administration, (2) the sites of drug distribution (body fluids and anatomical location), (3) the sequence of the physiological and toxicological reactions, (4) short and prolonged (chronic) effects of medications, (5) temporal relationship between drug administration and chemical, histometabolic, and structural examinations, (6) monitoring system, close surveillance, and direct observations of reaction patterns of the organism, (7) the role of age, sex, and race or strain variables, and (8) correlation of "in vivo" with "in vitro" experimentation, as well as controlled studies. However, although the animal model experiments may be informative, delayed effects are very little known and causal associations, which are an integral part of human life, are artificially excluded. Furthermore, no single animal may be adequate for all studies at all times and for all diseases.[139] A few human cases, at times, are more crucial than hundreds of experimental studies.[140] For instance, the analogy between the syphilitic chancre and the aortic aneurysms was observed long before the spirochete and the Wasserman reaction were discovered. And there are many similar observations which lead to the conclusion that animals are no substitute for humans. In summation, it appears, however, that as the human findings may serve a useful purpose

TABLE 2

Relative Tissue Reaction Patterns Resulting from the Interaction of the Pharmacodynamic Properties and Biological Cofactors

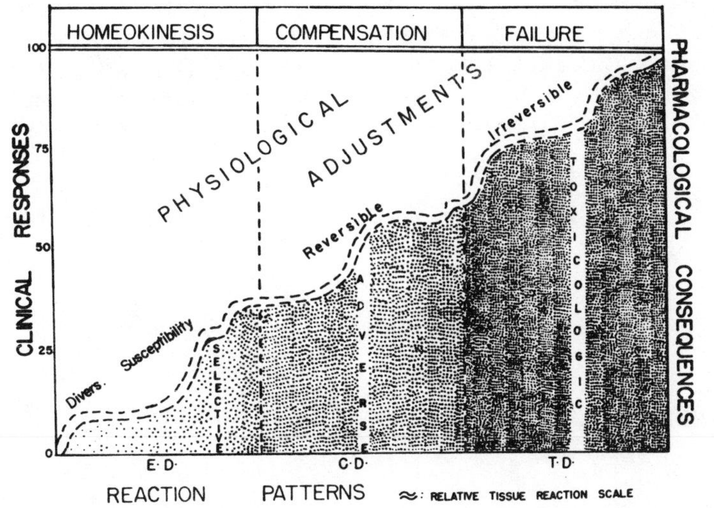

E = effective, C = concentrated or high, T = toxic, and D = dose

for "hypothesis generating," the preclinical animal experimentation is helpful for hypothesis testing (Jick[141]), and a wise clinician or research investigator must use both.

Comparative studies of human and experimental toxicology suggest that the tissue reaction patterns (tissue reaction scale, Table 2) are the result of the interplay between the overall histological cofactors of the reacting organism (inherited and acquired) and the pharmacodynamic properties of the chemical agents with the coparticipation of accessory or secondary cofactors (environmental, nutritional, stressors, and socioecological).

CONCLUDING REMARKS

Alcohol, multiple drug intake, and medical, behavioral, or psychiatric cofactors represent the most common potentiating and aggravating pathogenic effects of drug dependence. Therefore, drug-dependent patients should not be abandoned when they neglect to follow the detoxification or withdrawal treatment programs.

The significance of the cumulative effects of co-participating biological factors with drug pharmacodynamics, and the most common causes of death* in the heroin addicts treated with methadone strongly warn against the indiscriminate use of drugs in addiction by nonmedical and improperly trained professional personnel.

Histochemical and electron microscopic investigations reveal that the drugs are bound in the tissues in a diversified distribution and concentration and that adverse and toxic drug reactions are associated with changes of the (a) hydrolytic enzyme systems, (b) fine ultrastructural alterations of the ultracellular organelles, (c) communication or transport mechanisms in the CNS (particularly the synaptic complex and axonal flow), and (d) membrane permeability (including brain-blood barrier).

Almost one hundred years ago (1878), Bernard[2] remarked that "en ètudiant attentivement le mèchanisme de la mort dans les divers empoison-

*Respiratory depression or failure, pulmonary edema and pulmonary complications, liver damage (hepatitis and postnecrotic cirrhosis), secondary infections, trauma (violent deaths, accidents, etc.) and, in some instances, anaphylactic or allergic mechanisms.

ments, il s'instruit par voie indirect sur le mèchanisme physiologique de la vie."*

Currently clinical observations, biochemical examinations, and ultracellular studies show that the toxicologic effects and histochemical tissue reaction patterns induced by some psychotropic agents (particularly morphine and opiates) could be blocked or inhibited by antagonists (nalorphine, levallorphan, and naloxone). Thus, some of the reversible pathologic processes of the "biochemical lesions" could be turned "on and off."[142,143] Consequently, today we could amplify Cl. Bernard's[2] remarks with the emphasis that the present research of the pathogenic mechanisms of poisons offers new insights into the possible control and prevention of the toxicologic processes and even fatalities.

*In the careful study of the mechanism of death in various poisonings, one is taught indirectly the physiological mechanism of life.

REFERENCES

1. Belloni, L., in *Psychotropic Drugs*, Garattini, S. and Ghetti, V., Eds., Elsevier Publishing Co., Amsterdam, 1957, 5.

2. Bernard, C., La science experimentale, Bailliere, Paris 1878, 237, quoted by Stoner, H. B. and Magee, P. N., *Brit. Med. Bull.*, 13, 102, 1957.

3. Castiglioni, A., *A History of Medicine*, A. A. Knopf, New York, 1941.

4. Roizin, L., True, C., Knight, M., Structural effects of tranquilizers. The effect of pharmacologic agents on the nervous system, *Proc. Ass. Res. Nerv. Ment. Dis.*, 37, 285, 1959.

5. Courville, C., *Forensic Neuropathology*, Callaghan, Mundelein, I11., 1964, 153. Courville, C., Case studies in cerebral anoxia. VI. Typical anoxic alterations in cerebral gray matter overdosage of barbiturates, *Bull. Los Angeles Neurol. Soc.*, 20, 16, 1955.

6. Weimann, W. and von Marenholtz, F., Dappelseitige Linsenkerner weichung nach akuter Morphiumvergiftung, *Dtsch. Z. Gerichtl. Med.*, 12, 297, 1928.

7. Weimann, W., Gehirnveränderungen bei Akuter und Chronischer Morphiumvergiftung, *Ztschr. Neurol. Psychiat.*, 105, 704, 1926.

8. Cherbuin, C. E., The medical sequelae of narcotic addiction, *Ann. Intern. Med.*, 67, 23, 1967.

9. Helpern, M. and Strassman, G. S., Injury of the CNS by chemical agents, in *Neuropathology Methods and Diagnosis*, Tedeschi, C. G., Ed., Little, Brown and Co., Boston, 1970, 345.

10. Louria, D. B., Hensle, T., and Rose, J., The major medical complications of heroin addiction, *Ann. Intern. Med.*, 67, 1, 1967.

11. Mason, P., Mortality among young narcotic addicts, *J. Mount Sinai Hosp.*, 34, 4, 1967.

12. Baden. M. M., Methadone related death in New York City, in *Methadone Maintenance*, Einstein, S., Ed., Marcel Dekker, Inc., New York, 1971, 143.

13. Hameroff, S. B., Eckholdt, J. W., and Lindenberg, R., Cerebral phycomycosis in an heroin addict, *Neurology*, 20, 261, 1970.

14. Rodriguez, E., Smokvina, M., Sokolow, J., and Grynbaum, B. B., Encephalopathy and paraplegia occurring with use of heroin, *New York J. Med.*, 71, 2879, 1971.

15. Martin, W. R., Jasinski, D. R., Sapira, J. D., Flanary, H. G., Kelly, O. A., Thompson, A. K., and Logan, C. R., The respiratory effects of morphine during a cycle of dependence, *J. Pharmacol. Exp. Ther.*, 162, 182, 1968.

16. Martland, H. and Martland, H., Jr., Placental barrier in carbon monoxide, barbiturate and radium poisoning, *Amer. J. Surg.*, 50, 270, 1950.

17. Adelson, L., Pathologic findings in patients dead of common poisons, *Amer. J. Clin. Path.*, 22, 509, 1952.

18. Strassmann, G., Pathologic findings in poisonings, in *Legal Medicine*, Gradwohl, R. B. H., Ed., Mosby, St. Louis, 1954, 285.

19. Wintrobe, M., Adriani, J., Huguley, C., Hollister, L., Schreiner, G., Modell, W., Parera, G., Shirkey, N., Scidl, L., Friend, D., and Sadusk, J., The problem of adverse drug reactions, *J.A.M.A.*, 196, 404, 1966.

20. Mulé, S. J., Morphine and the incorporation of Pl^{32} into brain phospholipids of nontolerant, tolerant and abstinent guinea pigs, *J. Pharmacol. Exp. Ther.*, 156, 92, 1967.

21. Way, E. L., Distribution and metabolism of morphine and its surrogates, *Proc. Ass. Res. Nerv. Ment. Dis.*, 46, 13, 1968.

22. McIlwain, H., *Biochemistry and the Central Nervous System*, Churchill, London, 1955.

23. Schaumann, W., On the hypothesis of a cholinergic mechanism of action of morphine, *Naunyh Schmiedeberg Arch. Exp. Pat.*, 237, 229, 1959.

24. Hano, K., Kaneto, H., Kakunaga, T., and Moribayashi, N., The administration of morphine and changes in acetylcholine metabolism in mouse brain, *Biochem. Pharmacol.*, 13, 441, 1964.

25. Heinrich, M., Lichtensteiger, W., and Langeman, H., Effect of morphine on the catecholamine content of midbrain nerve cell groups in rat and mouse, *J. Pharmacol. Exp. Ther.*, 179, 259, 1971.

26. Eisenman, A. J., Sloan, J. W., Martin, W. R., Jasinski, D. R., and Brooks, J. W., Catecholamine and 17-hydroxycorticosteroid excretion during a cycle of morphine dependence in man, *J. Psychiat. Res.*, 7, 19, 1969.

27. Gearing, F., The evaluation of methadone maintenance treatment program, in *Methadone Maintenance*, Einstein, S., Ed., Marcel Dekker, Inc., New York, 1971, 179.

28. Craig, J. O. and Fraser, M. S., quoted in Medical Memoranda, *Brit. Med. J.*, 1, 1069, 1963.

29. Gardner, R., Methadone misuse and deaths by overdosage, *Brit. J. Addict.*, 65, 113, 1970.

30. Perkins, M. E., Perlman, N. D. and Bloch, H. I., A study of some failures in methadone treatment, *Amer. J. Psychiat.*, 128, 47, 1971.

31. Fraser, D. W., Methadone overdose. Illicit use of pharmaceutically prepared parenteral narcotics, *J.A.M.A.*, 217, 1387, 1971.

32. Dole, V. P., Foldes, F., Trigg, H., Robinson, J. W. and Blatman, S., Methadone poisoning, *New York J. Med.*, 71, 541, 1971.

33. Hoogerbeets, J., Methadone in Miami, in *Methadone Maintenance*, Einstein, S., Ed., Marcel Dekker, Inc., New York, 1971, 153.

34. Alha, A. R. and Ohela, K., Fatal cases of methadone-intoxication in Finland, 1951-54, established by forensic-medical examination, *Acta Pharmacol. Toxicol.*, 11, 156, 1955.

35. Bieter, R. N. and Hirsh, S. A., Methadone in internal medicine, *Ann. N.Y. Acad. Sci.*, 51, 137, 1948.

36. Petersohn F., Ein Fall von tödlicher Polamidon-Vergiftung Mit 3 Text-abbildungen, *Arch. Toxikol.*, 15, 403, 1955.

37. Schmidt, G., Zur Frage der letalen Dosis und des Nachweises von Polamidon. Zugleich ein Fall von tödlicher medizinaler Polamidonvergiftung, *Arch. Toxikol.*, 15, 178, 1954.

38. Wagner, H. J., Tödliche Vergiftung nach subletalen Alkoholund Polamidongaben, *Arch. Toxikol.*, 17, 159, 1958.

39. Naeve, W. and Körner, K. F., Tod durch Polamidonüberdosierung bei einem Kleinkinde, *Arch. Toxikol.*, 15, 96, 1954.

40. Martin, W. R., Commentary on the second National Conference on Methadone treatment, in *Methadone Maintenance*, Einstein, S., Ed., Marcel Dekker, Inc., New York, 1971, 199.

41. Cranley, W. R. and Haddow, J. E., Methadone overdosage in children, *New Eng. J. Med.*, 284, 792, 1971.

42. Sano, I., Nagasaka, Ueber chronische Weckaminsucht in Japan, *Fortschr. Neurol. Psychiat.*, 24, 391, 1956.

43. Greenwood, R. and Peachey, R. S., Acute amphetamine poisoning; an account of 3 cases, *Brit. Med. J.*, 1, 742, 1957.

44. Bartholomew, A. A. and Marley, E., Toxic response to 2-phenyl-3-methyltetrahydro-1, 4 oxazine hydrochloride, "Preludin" in human, *Psychopharmacologia* (Berlin), 1, 124, 1959.

45. Conrad, K., Die symptomatischen Psychosen, in *Psychiatrie Gegenwart, Band N*, Springer Verlag, Berlin, 1960, 369.

46. Silverman, M., Subacute delirious state due to "Preludin" addiction, *Brit. Med. J.*, 1, 696, 1959.

47. Tatetsu, S., Methamphetamine psychosis, *Folia Psychiat. Neurol. Jap. Suppl.*, 7, 377, 1963.

48. Van Praag, H. M., Abuse of, dependence on and psychoses from anorexigenic drugs, in *Drug Induced Diseases*, Vol. 3, Meyler, L. and Peck, H. M., Eds., Excerpta Med. Found., Amsterdam, 1968, 281.

49. Gonzales, T. A., Vance, M., Helpern, M., and Umberger, C. J., *Legal Medicine, Pathology and Toxicology*, 2nd ed., Appleton-Century-Crofts, New York, 1954.

50. Utena, H., Ezoe, T., Kato, N., and Hada, H., Effects of chronic administration of methamphetamine on enzyme patterns in brain tissue, *J. Neurochem.*, 4, 161, 1959.

51. Utena, H., Behavioral aberrations produced by long-term administration of methamphetamine in animals, *Folia Psychiat. Neurol. Jap. Suppl.*, 7, 285, 1963.

52. Sulser, F. and Sanders-Bush, E., Biochemical and metabolic considerations concerning the mechanism of action of amphetamine and related compounds, in *Psychotomimetic Drugs*, Efron, D. H., Ed., Raven Press, New York, 1970, 83.

53. Robison, G. A., Butcher, R. W., and Sutherland, E. W., Adenyl cyclase as an adrenergic receptor, *Ann. N. Y. Acad. Sci.*, 139, 703, 1967.

54. de Robertis, E., Arnaiz, G. R. D. L., Alberici, M., Butcher, R. W., and Sutherland, E. W., Subcellular distribution of adenyl cyclase and cyclic phosphodiesterase in rat brain cortex, *J. Biol. Chem.*, 242, 3487, 1967.

55. Weiss, B. and Costa, E., Adenyl cyclase activity in rat pineal gland: effects of chronic denervation and norepinephrine, *Science*, 156, 1750, 1967.

56. Miyakawa, T., Sumiyoski, S., Deshimaru, M., Murayama, E., and Tatetsu, S., Electron microscopic studies concerning the structural mechanisms of the development of mental disturbance in experimental chronic methamphetamine poisoning, *Acta Neuropath*, (Berlin), 14, 215, 1969.

57. Maier, H. W., *Der Kokainismus*, G. Theime, Leipzig, 1926.

58. Petri, E., Pathologische Anatomie and Histologie der Vergiftungen, *Handbuch der Speziellen Pathologisches Anatomie und Histologie*, Vol. 10, J. Springer, New York, 1930.

59. Pachomwow, Quoted by Petri, E. in Pathologische Anatomie and Histologie der Vergiftungen, *Handbuch der Speziellen Pathologisches Anatomie und Histologie*, Vol. 10, J. Springer, New York, 1930, 626.

60. Petri, E., Zur Kenntnis der pathologisch-anatomischen Gehirnschäden bei akuter Veronalvergiftung, *Virchows Arch. Path. Anat.*, 284, 84, 1932.

61. Slager, V. T., Reilly, E. B. and Brandt, R. A., Neuropathology of barbiturate intoxication, *J. Neuropath. Exp. Neurol.*, 25, 237, 1966.

62. Hassin, G. B., Cerebral changes in fatal cases following treatment with barbital, insulin and metrazol, *Arch. Neurol. Psychiat.*, 42, 679, 1939.

63. De Groat, A., Symmetric necrosis of the globus pallidus in barbiturate poisoning, *Arch. Path.*, 29, 271, 1940.

64. Scheidegger, S., Veränderungen des Zentralnervensystems bei Vergiftungen durch Schlafnittel (Barbitursäure-vergiftungen), *Schweiz. Arch. Neurol. Psychiat.*, 39, 388, 1937.

65. Lucas, B. G. B., Anoxia and anaesthesia, *Proc. Roy. Soc. Med.*, 43, 606, 1950.

66. Neuman, M. A., Encephalopathy following barbiturate intoxication. Report of a case, *J. Neuropath. Clin. Neurol.*, 1, 145, 1951.

67. Jervis, G. and Joyce, F., Barbiturate-opiate intoxication with necrosis of the basal ganglions of the brain, *Arch. Path.*, 45, 319, 1948.

68. Jetter, W. and McLean, R., Poisoning by the synergistic effect of phenobarbital and ethyl alcohol, *Arch. Path.*, 36, 112, 1943.

69. Hollister, L. E., Richards, R. K., and Gillespie, H. K., Comparison of tetrahydrocannabinol and synhexyl in man, *Clin. Pharmacol. Ther.*, 9, 783, 1968.

70. Holtzman, D., Lovell, R. A., Jaffe, J. H., and Freedman, D. X., 1-Δ^9-Tetrahydrocannabinol: Neurochemical and behavioral effects in the mouse, *Science*, 163, 1464, 1969.

71. Council on Mental Health and Committee on Alcoholism and Drug Dependence, Dependence on Cannabis (Marihuana), *J.A.M.A.*, 201, 108, 1967.

72. Patton, D., quoted in Marihuana Risk, *Amer. Med. News*, 12, 2, 1971.

73. King, A. B. and Cowen, D. L., Effect of intravenous infection of marihuana, *J.A.M.A.*, 210, 72, 1969.

74. Sterne, J. and Ducastaing, C., Arteritis caused by Cannabis indica, *Rev. Atheroscler* (Paris), 53, 143, 1960.

75. Richter, R. W. and Rosenberg, R. N., Transverse myelitis with heroin addiction, *J.A.M.A.*, 206, 1255, 1968.

76. Kew, M. C., Bersohn, I., and Siew, S., Possible hepatotoxicity of cannabis, *Lancet*, 1, 578, 1969.

77. Campbell, A. M. G., Evans, M., Thomson, J. L. G., and Williams, M. J., Cerebral atrophy in young cannabis smokers, *Lancet*, 7736, 1219, 1971.

78. Persaud, T. V. N. and Ellington, A. C., Teratogenic activity of cannabis resin, *Lancet,* 2, 406, 1968.

79. Geber, W. F. and Schramm, L. C., Effect of marihuana extract on fetal hamsters and rabbits, *Toxic. Appl. Pharmacol.*, 14, 276, 1969.

80. Ames, F., A clinical and metabolic study of acute intoxication with cannabis sativa and its role in model psychoses, *J. Ment. Sci.*, 104, 972, 1958.

81. Korte, F., Recent results in Hashish chemistry, in *The Botany and Chemistry of Cannabis*, Joyce, C. R. B. and Curry, S. H., Eds., 1970, 119.

82. Joyce, C. R. B. and Curry, S. H., *The Botany and Chemistry of Cannabis*, Proc. Conf. the Institute of Drug Dependence at the Ciba Found., April 9-10, 1969, J. and A. Churchilll, London, 1970.

83. Tennant, F. S., Preble, M., Prendergast, T. J., and Ventry, P., Medical manifestations assoicated with Hashish, *J.A.M.A.*, 216, 1965, 1971.

84. Henderson, A. H. and Pugsley, D. J., Collapse after intravenous infection of Hashish, *Brit. Med. J.*, 3, 229, 1968.

85. Constantinidis, J. and Miras, C. J., Effect of Hashish smoke sublimate on hypothalamic noradrenaline studied by the fluorescence method, *Psychopharmacologia*, 22, 80, 1971,

86. Deliyannakis, E., Panagopoulos, C., and Huott, A. D., The influence of Hashish on human EEG, *Clin. Electroenceph.*, 1, 128, 1970.

87. Abramson, H. A., Ed., *The Use of LSD in Psychotherapy*, Transactions of a conference on d-Lysergic acid diethylamide (LSD-25), Josiah Macy, Jr. Fund., New York, 1960.

88. Ditman, K. S., Tietz, W., Prince, B. S., Forgy, E., and Moss, T., Harmful aspects of the LSD experiences, *J. Nerv. Ment. Dis.*, 145, 464, 1968.

89. Evarts, E. V., A review of the neurophysiological effects of lysergic acid diethylamide and other psychotomimetic agents, *Ann. N.Y. Acad. Sci.*, 66, 479, 1957.

90. Hoffer, A., D-Lysergic acid diethylamide (LSD): A review of its present status, *Clin. Pharmacol. Ther.*, 6, 183, 1965.

91. Schwarz, C. J., The complications of LSD: a review of the literature, *J. Nerv. Ment. Dis.*, 146, 174, 1968.

92. Kleber, H. D., Prolonged adverse reactions from unsupervised use of hallucinogenic drugs, *J. Nerv. Ment. Dis.*, 144, 308, 1967.

93. Rothlin, E., Pharmacology of lysergic acid diethylamide (LSD) and some of its related compounds, in *Psychotropic Drugs*, Garattini, S. and Getti, V., Eds., Int. Symposium on Psychotropic Drugs, Elsevier, Amsterdam, 1957, 36.

94. Lasagna, L., The diseases drugs cause, *Perspect. Biol. Med.*, 7, 457, 1964.

95. Hassler, O., Circulatory effects of d-lysergic acid diethylamide (LSD-25), *Psychopharmacologia*, 6, 311, 1964.

96. Hollister, L. E. and Sjoberg, B. M., Clinical syndromes and biochemical alterations following mescaline, lysergic acid diethylamide, Psilocybin and a combination of the three psychotomimetic drugs, *Compr. Psychiat.*, 5, 170, 1964.

97. Krawczynski, J., The influence of serotoin, D-lysergic acid diethylamide and 2-brom LSD on the incorporation of (^{35}S) methionine into brain proteins and on the level of ATP in the brain, *J. Neurochem.*, 7, 1, 1961.

98. Pavlin, R., The effect of lysergic acid diethylamide on the acetylcholinesterase activity of single nerve cells from the reticular formation (of the rat brain), *J. Neurochem.*, 10, 195, 1963.

99. Sankar, D. V. S., Broer, H. H., Cates, N., and Sankar, D. B., Studies on biogenic amines and psychoactive drug actions, special reference to lysergic acid diethylamide, *Trans. N.Y. Acad. Sci.*, 26, 369, 1964.

100. Schwartz, A. S. and Cheney, C., Retinal effects of high doses of LSD in the cat, *Exp. Neurol.*, 13, 273, 1965.

101. Shanthaveerappa, T. R., Histochemical studies on the mechanism of action of the hallucinogens d-lysergic acid diethylamide tartrate (LSD-25) and d-2-bromo-lysergic acid tartrate (BOL-148) in rat brain, *Acta Neuropath.*, 3, 29, 1963.

102. Weltman, A. S. and Sackler, A. M., Metabolic and endocrine effects of lysergic acid diethylamide (LSD-25) on male rats, *J. Endocr.*, 34, 81, 1966.

103. Aghajanian, G. K., Foote, R., and Sheard, M. H., Lysergic acid diethylamide: Sensitive neuronal units in the mid-brain raphe, *Science*, 161, 706, 1968.

104. Ludwig, A. M. and Levine, J., Pattern of hallucinogenic drug abuse, *J.A.M.A.*, 191, 104, 1965.

105. Aghajanian, G. K., Sheard, M. H., and Foote, W. E., LSD and Mescaline: Comparison of effects on single units in the mid-brain raphe, in *Psychotomimetic Drugs*, Efron, D. H., Ed., Raven Press, New York, 1970, 165.

106. Aghajanian, G. K. and Freedman, D. X., Biochemical and morphological aspects of LSD pharmacology, in *Psychopharmacology: A Review of Progress 1957-1967*, Efron, D. H., Ed., Public Health Service Publication 1836, 1967.

107. Ginzel, K., Effect of LSD on autonomic reflexes, in *Psychotropic Drugs*, Garattini, S. and Getti, V., Eds., Elsevier, Amsterdam, 1957, 48.

108. Pierre, R. and Grisoni, R., Etude de l'action de differents corps sur les perturbations EEG du lapin induities par une intoxication chronique ou aigue par la diethylamide de l'acide lysergique, in *Psychotropic Drugs*, Garattini, S. and Getti, V., Eds., Elsevier, Amsterdam, 1957, 286.

109. Snyder, S. H. and Reivich, M., Regional localization of lysergic acid diethylamide in monkey brain, *Nature* (London), 209, 1093, 1966.

110. Aghajanian, G. K. and Bing, O. H. L., Persistence of lysergic acid diethylamide in the plasma of human subjects, *Clin. Pharmacol. Ther.*, 5, 611, 1964.

111. Diaz, J. L. and Huttunen, M. O., Persistent increase in brain serotonin turnover after chronic administration of LSD in the rat, *Science*, 174, 62, 1971.

112. Denber, H. C. B., Charipper, H., and Roizin, L., Cytological effects of LSD-25 in rat brain and liver, *Fed. Proc.*, 23, 147, 1964.

113. Buscaino, G. A. and Frongia, N., Modificazioni biochimiche, electroencephalografiche, istochimiche ed istologiche, in cani, durante l'intossicazione sperimentale acuta e cronica da dietilamide dell' acido lisergico, *Acta Neurol.* (Naples), 8, 641, 1953.

114. Geiger, R. S., Effects of LSD-25, serotonin and sera from schizophrenic patients on adult mammalian brain cultures, *J. Neuropsychiat.*, 1, 185, 1959.

115. Roizin, L., Gold, G., Alexander, G., Miles, B., Kaufman, M. A., and Lawler H. C., Prenatal effects of hallucinogens, *Amer. J. Psychiat.*, 124, 185, 1968.

116. Braceland, F. J., (Ed.), The effects of pharmacological agents on the nervous system, in *Res. Publ. Ass. Nerv. Ment. Dis.*, Vol. 37, The Williams and Wilkins Co., Baltimore, 1959.

117. Roizin, L., Lazar, M., and Gold, G., Prenatal effects of phenothiazines, *Fed. Proc.*, 25, 353, 1966.

118. Roizin, L., Kaufman, M. A., and Casselman, B., Structural changes induced by neuroleptics. Extrapyramidal system and neuroleptic, *Rev. Canad. Biol.*, 20, 221, 1961.

119. Roizin, L., Kaufman, M. A., Gold, G., Iyengar, V. K. S., Liu, J. C., and Koeseian, S., A multidisciplinary investigation of the phenothiazines, *Ment. Hyg.*, 50, 574, 1966.

120. Wechsler-Berger, M. and Roizin, L., Tissue levels of chlorpromazine in experimental animals, *J. Ment. Sci.*, 106, 1501, 1960.

121. Forrest, F. M., Forrest, I. S., and Roizin, L., Clinical, biochemical and postmortem studies on a patient treated with chlorpromazine, *Agressologie*, 4, 259, 1963.

122. Roizin, L., Wechsler-Berger, M., and Brock, D., Ultracellular, functional and pathogenic mechanisms. V. In vivo and in vitro C.N.S. and liver mitochondrial following administration of phenothiazines, *Trans. Amer. Neurol. Ass.*, 89, 247, 1964.

123. Cares, R., Alkaloids, antipyretics, analgesics and other pharmaceuticals, in *Pathology of the Nervous System*, Vol. II, Minckler, J., Ed., McGraw-Hill, 1971, 1685.

124. Goldberg, L. I., Monoamine oxidase inhibitors, adverse reactions and possible mechanisms, *J.A.M.A.*, 190, 456, 1964.

125. Roizin, L., Helpern, M., Baden, M., Kaufman, M. A., and Akai, K., Toxosynpathies (A Multifactor pathogenic concept), in *Drug Abuse - Current Concepts and Research,* Keup, W., Ed., Charles C Thomas, Springfield, Ill., in press.

126. Goldstein, A., Aronow, L., and Kalman, S., *Principles of Drug Action - The Basis of Pharmacology*, Harper and Row, New York, 1969.

127. Meyler, L. and Peck H. M., Eds., *Drug Induced Diseases*, Vol. 3, Excerpta Medica Found., Amsterdam, 1968.

128. Dubach, U. C., Studies of nephrotoxicity in relation to regular intake of analgesics, in *Int. Conf. on Adverse Reaction Reporting Systems*, Washington, D.C., Oct. 22-23, 1970.

129. Dunlop, D., Definition of the adverse reaction reporting problem, in, *Abstracts Int. Conf. on Adverse Reaction Reporting Systems*, Washington, D.C., Oct. 22-23, 1970.

130. Oates, J. A., Metabolic data in drug interactions, in *Int. Conf. On Adverse Reaction Reporting Systems*, Washington, D.C., Oct. 22-23, 1970.

131. Cannon, W. B., *The Way of an Investigator - A scientist's experience in medical research*, W. W. Norton and Co., New York, 1945.

132. Richter, C. P., Neurological basis of responses to stress, in *Neurological Basis of Behavior,* Ciba Fund. Symposium, Walstenhelme, G. E. W. and O'Connor, C. M., Eds., Little, Brown, and Co., Boston, Mass., 1958, 204.

133. Gellhorn, E., *Autonomic Imbalance and the Hypothalamus*, University of Minnesota Press, Minn., 1957.

134. Roizin, L., Introduction to metabolic diseases, in *Pathology of the Nervous System*, Minckler, J., Ed., Vol. 2, McGraw Hill Book Co., New York, 1971.

135. Sussman, S., Narcotic and amphetamine use during pregnancy, *Amer. J. Dis. Child.*, 106, 325, 1963.

136. Stern, R., The pregnant addict, *Am. J. Obstet. Gynec.*, 94, 253, 1966.

137. Van Leeuren, G., Guthrie, R., and Stange, F., Narcotic withdrawal reaction in newborn infant due to cocaine, *Pediatrics*, 36, 635, 1965.

138. Irey, N. S., Registry of tissue reactions to drugs, AFIP, in *Int. Conf. on Adverse Reaction Reporting Systems*, Washington, D.C., Oct. 22-23, 1970.

139. Inman, W. H. W., British experience with voluntary reporting systems, in *Int. Conf. on Adverse Reaction Reporting Systems*, Washington, D.C., Oct. 22-23, 1970.

140. Long, J. W., Problems related to the dissemination of drug adverse reaction information, in *Int. Conf. on Adverse Reaction Reporting Systems*, Washington, D.C., Oct. 22-23, 1970.

141. Jick, H., Intensive surveillance systems, in *Int. Conf. on Adverse Reaction Reporting Systems*, Washington, D.C., Oct. 22-23, 1970.

142. Peters, R. A., *Biochemical Lesions and Lethal Synthesis*, Macmillan & Sons, New York, 1963.

143. Farber, E., Biochemical pathology, in *Ann. Rev. Pharmacol.*, 11, 71, 1971.

TERATOGENICITY, EMBRYOLETHALITY, AND MUTAGENICITY OF DRUGS OF DEPENDENCE

H. Kalter

TABLE OF CONTENTS

INTRODUCTION

A great variety and a large number of chemical substances have been demonstrated to be teratogenic in experimental mammalian species.[1-5] So many of them have already been discovered to have damaged human products of conception, or are suspected of having done so,[6-11] that the possibility of many others being potentially teratogenic cannot be doubted.

The classes of chemicals that have been studied and found to have mutagenic potentials in mammals are still only few, and most are fairly exotic,[12] but again the likelihood of them affecting human beings similarly cannot be discounted.

DEFINITIONS

Teratology is the study of congenital malformations, their causes and development, and experimental teratology the science of the induction of congenital malformations by actions on embryos and fetuses. As used here, in reference to experimental animals, congenital malformations are abnormalities of structure present at about the time of birth and readily observable with the unaided senses or by low-power microscopy and teratogenesis indicates the production of congenital malformations by interference with events occurring after fertilization.

Ordinarily these terms have much more sweeping senses. Thus, teratology can refer to many forms of prenatal maldevelopment, not only structural; and congenital malformations are frequently the outcome of hereditary factors and, therefore, have prefertilization, as well as postfertilization origins. But the restricted meanings outlined above have been adopted for the sake of clearly delimiting the experimental areas discussed in this paper.

Mutations are changes of the hereditary material, either of genes (called point or gene mutations) or chromosomal number or structure (chromosomal aberrations). Therefore, if they occur in germ cells, they are capable of being transmitted from one generation to another. (Parenthetically, congenital malformations produced by interfering with embryological processes are merely modifications, and are not hereditary.)

Because chemicals may not produce these two types of nuclear changes (gene and chromosomal) in the same way and because the embryological and clinical effects of the two types of changes may be different, it is unsatisfactory to lump them and consider them together. For example, Shaw[13] refers to chromosome-breaking chemicals as clastogens and infers that all clastogens may not be mutagenic, i.e., have hereditary consequences. In this paper only studies done on the hereditary (i.e., embryological) sequelae of drug-induced nuclear changes will be noted.

In practice, the types of chemicals that have mostly been used so far in studies with mammals only infrequently produced gene mutations,[14-17] while they much more often produced chromosomal aberrations, especially breakage.[18-20]

HOW TERATOLOGICAL AND MUTAGENIC STUDIES ARE DONE

The experimental mammalian teratologist subjects pregnant animals to some chemical, physical, etc. procedure at a definite time (or times) during gestation and later examines the offspring to determine the morphological, chemical, or other effects of the manipulation.

Malformations have rarely been induced in embryos by treating pregnant females before the approximate time of uterine implantation, which occurs at about 4.5 days after fertilization in mice and hamsters, 6 days in rats, 7 in rabbits, 9 in rhesus monkeys, and, for comparison, 6.5 in human beings. The total length of gestation in these species is about 16 days in hamsters, 19 in mice, 22 in rats, 32 in rabbits, 164 in rhesus monkeys, and 267 in human beings.

The "sensitive period" for the production of most major malformations comes to an end when the majority of the organ systems are established, which is about day 9 in hamsters, 11 in mice, 12.5 in rats, 10 in rabbits, 28 in rhesus monkeys, and 36 in human beings.[20a] As embryos are transformed into fetuses, fewer and fewer parts remain that can be disturbed sufficiently to result in gross malformations; instead most apparent harm done to fetuses is histological or is associated with growth retardation.

The mammalian mutagenologist, studying the hereditary consequences of nuclear changes, administers chemicals or other noxae to nonpregnant females, or, more commonly, to males. The animals are then bred to untreated ones and the pregnant females are ordinarily killed a few days after uterine implantation occurs. As stated above, the preponderant nuclear effect of chemicals yet found in mammals is chromosomal aberrations; those produced in germ cells may be transferred to the young, in which the major consequence has been found to be prenatal death. (Parenthetically, again, teratogens can also cause prenatal death, but not generally because of chromosomal damage. Also, teratogen-induced death may occur at many different stages of gestation, whereas mutagen-induced death is most frequent around the time of implantation.)

Thus, the mutagenic potential of chemicals in mammals is most often detected and measured by the frequency of prenatal death or, putting it another way, by the induction of quasi-dominantly inherited semisterility in treated animals or their surviving progeny.

EXPERIMENTAL STUDIES

Mutagenicity

This will be a very short section because although the mutagenic and clastogenic potential of a vast number of chemicals[21] has been studied, the reproductive and embryological effects of relatively few of them have been tested in mammals;[12] and these have included only several drugs of dependence.[13]

The hereditary ramifications of chromosomal aberrations produced by chemicals are as yet only conjectural, since critical experiments to determine this are presently almost nonexistent. As yet only one drug of dependence – chlorpromazine, which was found to be clastogenic in human beings[13] – has been preliminarily tested in animals, and it produced no increased prenatal mortality in litters sired by treated males.[22] However, only a single dose level, 8.3 mg/kg, was used, and perhaps larger quantities would have different results.

Teratogenicity

A fairly large number of drugs falling into the category of drugs of dependence or psychoactive agents have been tested for teratogenicity and effects on reproduction.[23] Table 1 contains some relevant details of many of these studies; the text will be reserved for additional comments.

Narcotic analgesics – Up to the time of writing there have not been many studies of the effects of narcotic analgesics on mammalian reproduction and fetal development. Large doses of these agents caused prenatal death and in some experiments[25,26,28,29] were said to induce malformations. The reports of some of these experiments have appeared in preliminary form only and lack sufficient detail to be judged. In other studies[28,29] the malformations produced, exencephaly and rib and vertebral abnormalities, also occurred in control offspring and those of pregnant female mice deprived of food for 24 hours. The latter experiment was performed because drug treatment greatly decreased food intake. There have been other reports[31-33] of exencephaly appearing in controls of the same stock of mice (CF1) that was used in these experiments; and exencephaly and axial skeletal defects have been produced previously by depriving pregnant mice of food for a day during early embryogenesis.[34-36]

Hence, in my opinion, the malformations noted in the offspring of the morphine-treated female mice were not convincingly the result of the drug acting by itself. Possibly, they may have been due to interaction between the drug and reduced maternal food consumption or, indeed, to the latter alone. The question certainly deserves further investigation in well-designed and rigidly controlled studies, especially since some of the same malformations appeared in other studies mentioned above,[25,26] and because in one of these reports[26] it was said that the narcotic analgesic-induced malformations were blocked in a dose-dependent fashion by the prior administration of the antagonists nalorphine and cyclazocine.

Barbiturates – A fair number of relevant studies have been made with barbiturates. However, clear-cut malformations or any that were unequivocally attributable to the drugs occurred in very few of them. In several studies with mice there were low to moderate incidences of various malformations[40,44,53,59] and in one with rats[48] and another with rabbits[58] some skeletal anomalies occurred. On the other hand phenobarbital reduced the embryotoxicity of diphenylhydantoin[61] and cyclophosphamide[52] in mice, probably by inducing maternal microsomal enzymes for their metabolism, but did not influence the effect of the well-known teratogens cortisone and vincristine.[62]

Histological and physiological effects were also investigated. Barbital Na caused no ultrastructural changes in the rat fetal liver[63] and only minor shifts in fetal liver ascorbic acid concentration;[64] soon after birth, however, the latter was greatly increased.[64] Injecting rats with pentobarbital late in pregnancy depressed certain fetal adrenal responses.[65]

Switching from the end of the gestation period to its beginning, pentobarbital Na delays ovulation in rats[66] and thus introduces the possibility of producing developmental abnormalities through fertilization of "aged" ova. This was apparently confirmed by the appearance of various forms of deviation, including abnormal preimplantation stages, chromosomal aberrations, and fetal anomalies and death.[67-69] Some of these results were not confirmed in a subsequent study.[70]

CNS stimulants (amphetaminelike) – This class of drugs has been used in only a few studies, but even these revealed its potential for prenatal damage. Mouse and rabbit embryos were malformed or destroyed in most experiments. However, rats, rabbits, and rhesus monkeys were apparently unaffected in studies in which relatively low doses were used.

TABLE 1

Effects on Prenatal Development and Reproduction of Drugs of Dependence Administered to Pregnant Animals

Drug	Reference	Species	Dose (mg/kg/day)	Route of administration[1]	Day(s) of gestation treated[2]	Effects: Malformations	Effects: Other	Comments
Narcotic analgesics								
Dihydromorphine	24	Rat	2–28	sc	2–21	None	Prenatal death	
Heroin	25	Hamster	100–1000	sc	8	?%, CNS[3]	Prenatal death	Maternal behavior markedly affected for 15–30 hr
Hydromorphone	26	Hamster	150	sc	8	45%, CNS, etc.		
Methadone	26a	Hamster	40–200	sc	8	?	Prenatal death	
Methadone	26b	Rat	20–60	po	7–16	None attributable to treatment	Prenatal death at highest doses	
Methadone	26b	Rabbit	20–60	po	7–19	None attributable to treatment	Prenatal death at highest dose	
Morphine	27	Rat	30–70	sc	3.5–5 mo before breeding and throughout gestation	None	None	
Morphine sulfate	28	Mouse	100–500	sc	9 or 10	6% CNS, day 9; 24% axial skeleton, day 10	Prenatal death	Maternal food intake decreased for 1 day; same malformations in untreated and starved controls.
Morphine sulfate	29	Mouse	200–400	sc	9 or 10	2% CNS, day 9; 14% axial skeleton day 10		
Morphine	26	Hamster	300	sc	8	33%, CNS, etc.		

TABLE 1 (continued)

Drug	Reference	Species	Dose (mg/kg/day)	Route of administration[1]	Day(s) of gestation treated[2]	Effects: Malformations	Effects: Other	Comments
Propoxyphene napsylate	30	Rat	ca. 170, 340	po	1 wk before breeding and throughout gestation	None	Postnatal growth retardation and death	
Propoxyphene napsylate	30	Rat	100–400	po	7–16	None	Fertility affected by largest dose	
Propoxyphene napsylate	30	Rabbit	32, 80	po	7–19	None	None	
Barbiturates								
Barbital Na	37	Rat	25 – 40	?	20	None	Behavioral changes at 3 mo of age	Dose-response relation unclear
Barbital Na	38	Rat	25 – 100	ip	3, 4, 8, or 12	None attributable to treatment	None	
Barbital Na	39	Rat	200	sc	9–20	None mentioned	Prenatal death, reduced fetal weight	
Barbital Na	40	Mouse	65 –330	ip	2–7	60%, CNS, limb, etc.	Prenatal death, reduced fetal size	Dose response
Barbital Na	40	Rabbit	50, 200	iv	1–10, or 10	None	None	
Hexobarbital	38	Rat	50, 100	ip	3, 4, 5, or 8	None attributable to treatment	None	
Methylcyclohexenyl-methylbarbituric acid Na	41	Rabbit	30, 60	iv	13 and 14	None mentioned	Prenatal death, chromosomal aberrations	
Pentobarbital Na	37	Rat	6	?	20	None	Behavioral changes at 3 mo of age	

TABLE 1 (continued)

Drug	Reference	Species	Dose (mg/kg/day)	Route of administration[1]	Day(s) of gestation treated[2]	Effects: Malformations	Effects: Other	Comments
Pentobarbital Na	42	Rat	40	im	10	None	None	
Pentobarbital Na	43	Rat	10	ip	11–20	None mentioned	Decreased pentobarbital-induced sleeping time, early postnatal, transient	
Pentobarbital Na	44	Mouse	ca. 50–60	ip	1–4, or –15	?%, head, limb	Reduced fertility; stillbirth	Data not presented
Pentobarbital Na	45	Mouse	ca. 0.4–108	sc	3–6	None	None	
Pentobarbital Na	46	Guinea pig	28–40	iv	22, 42, or 63	None mentioned	Prenatal death, stillbirth, neuromuscular deficits in postnatal survivors of high doses	
Pentobarbital Na	47	Rabbit	40	iv	7, 8, 9, or 10	None attributable to treatment	Prenatal death	
Phenobarbital	48	Rat	(0.16%, in feed)	po	3 days before breeding and throughout gestation	?%, axial skeleton	Reduced litter size, stillbirth	
Phenobarbital	49	Rat	5	sc	5–8, or 17–20	None mentioned	Behavioral changes, after earlier treatment time	
Phenobarbital	50	Rat	50	ip	1–20	None mentioned	Prenatal death, impaired postnatal growth	
Phenobarbital	51	Mouse	1–4	ip	During 5–14	None	Prenatal death	
Phenobarbital	52	Mouse	50	ip	9–11	None	None	
Phenobarbital	53	Mouse	?	?	?	?% (low), cleft palate		
Phenobarbital	54, 55	Mouse	120	im	14	None attributable to treatment	None	

TABLE 1 (continued)

Drug	Reference	Species	Dose (mg/kg/day)	Route of administration[1]	Day(s) of gestation treated[2]	Effects: Malformations	Effects: Other	Comments
Phenobarbital	56	Mouse	?	?	During last week	None mentioned	Small litters, stillbirth, perinatal death; impaired postnatal growth	
Phenobarbital	57	Rabbit	15	sc	2–14 days during entire gestation period	None mentioned	Hepatic enzyme induction, when treatment ended not later than 4 days before term	
Phenobarbital	58	Rabbit	50	po	8–16	?%, cardiac, axial skeleton	Prenatal death	
Thiamylal Na	59	Mouse	60	ip	Once, on 8–15	?%(low), only after day-10 treatment	None mentioned	
Thiopental	38	Rat	50, 100	ip	4	None	None	
Thiopental Na	60	Mouse	25–150	ip	12	None	Prenatal death; reduced fetal weight	
Thiopental	45	Mouse	ca. 0.4–108	sc	3–6	None	None	
Amphetamines								
Amphetamine	71	Rat	10	im	5	None	None	
Amphetamine sulfate	72	Rat	1	sc	12–15	None mentioned	Reduced neonatal brain butylcholinesterase activity	
Amphetamine sulfate	73	Mouse	50	po	Throughout	None attributable to treatment		
Dexamphetamine sulfate	74	Mouse	50	ip	9	12%, cardiac, etc.	Prenatal death	
Dexamphetamine sulfate	75	Mouse	50	ip	9	11–13%, cardiac	Prenatal death	Strain-specific cardiac defects

TABLE 1 (continued)

Drug	Reference	Species	Dose (mg/kg/day)	Route of administration[1]	Day(s) of gestation treated[2]	Effects: Malformations	Effects: Other	Comments
Dexamphetamine sulfate	76	Rabbit	up to 10	?	?	None	None mentioned	
Methamphetamine HCl	77	Mouse	5, 10	iv	9–11, –12, or –15; or 12–15	14%, CNS, cleft palate, etc., after larger dose on days 9 – 15	Prenatal death, decreased fetal weight	
Methamphetamine HCl	77	Rabbit	1.5	iv	12–15 or –30; 15–20	16%, CNS, after day-12–30 treatment	Prenatal death, reduced fetal weight	
Methamphetamine HCl	78	Rhesus monkey	0.5	po	Implantation to term	None	Apparently none	
Tranquilizers								
Benzodiazepine derivatives								
Chlordiazepoxide	79	Rat	20, 80	po	18 wk. before breeding and throughout gestation	None	None	
Chlordiazepoxide	80	Mouse	?	ip	10	Apparently none	Apparently none	
Chlordiazepoxide	53	Mouse	?	?	?	None		
Diazepam	53	Mouse	?	?	?	None		

TABLE 1 (continued)

Drug	Reference	Species	Dose (mg/kg/day)	Route of administration[1]	Day(s) of gestation treated[2]	Effects		Comments
						Malformations	Other	
Dibenzazepine compounds								
Amitriptyline	81	Rat	10, 20	po	2–19	None attributable to treatment	Some prenatal mortality	
Amitriptyline	81a	Rat	5, 25	po	4–18	None	Apparently none	
Butriptyline	81a	Rat	5, 25	po	4–18	None	Apparently none	
Imipramine	82	Rat	40	po	4–12	Apparently none	None mentioned	Prevented fetal death when given in conjunction with nicotinamide-deficient diet.
Imipramine	83	Rat	5, 15	po	60 days before breeding and throughout gestation	None	Reduced litter size, postnatal death	No dose-response relation for postnatal death
Imipramine	81	Rat	10	po	2–19	None	Some prenatal mortality	
Imipramine	84	Rat	5–100	sc, po	7–16, or 8–12	?% (very low), cleft palate, axial skeleton	Reduced fertility, fetal death after largest doses	
Imipramine	83	Mouse	10–150	sc, po	6–17	None attributable to treatment		
Imipramine	85	Rabbit	5–30	sc	1–13, –17, or –20	?%, 3 grossly malformed	Fetal death	
Imipramine	83	Rabbit	5–30	sc, po	7–17	?%, CNS, kidney, etc.	Fetal death, reduced fetal weight	

TABLE 1 (continued)

Drug	Reference	Species	Dose (mg/kg/day)	Route of administration[1]	Day(s) of gestation treated[2]	Effects: Malformations	Effects: Other	Comments
Imipramine	84	Rabbit	10–50	sc	7–16	?% (low), CNS, skeleton, etc.	Fetal death	
Imipramine HCl, imipramine-*N*-oxide HCl	86	Rabbit	15, 25	sc	3–18	2%, tail, kidney		
Diphenylmethane derivatives								
Haloperidol	87	Rat	2.5–10	im, sc, po	Various, during wk 1 – 3	None attributable to treatment	Delayed implantation	
Haloperidol	88	Rat	ca. 0.5–19	im	Various, during wk 2	None attributable to treatment		
Haloperidol	89	Rat	3–12	po	Various, during days 1–10	Apparently none	Reduced fetal weight	
Haloperidol	88	Mouse	ca. 2–17	im	Various, during wk 2	53%, cleft palate, after largest dose, on days 10–13	Prenatal death	
Haloperidol	87	Mouse	1.5–16	po	Various during wk 1–2	None attributable to treatment	Prenatal death	
Haloperidol	87	Rabbit	3–25	po	Various, during wk 2	None	None	
Hydroxyzine HCl or pamoate	90	Rat	60–200	po	11–, or 13–16	15–100%, cleft palate, etc.	None mentioned	

TABLE 1 (continued)

Drug	Reference	Species	Dose (mg/kg/day)	Route of administration[1]	Day(s) of gestation treated[2]	Effects: Malformations	Effects: Other	Comments
Hydroxyzine	91	Rat	?	?	12–14	?%, cleft palate		
Methylphenidate	80	Mouse	200	ip	10	Apparently none	Prenatal death	
Pipradol	80	Mouse	?	ip	10	Apparently none		
Monoamine oxidase inhibitors								
Harmaline HCl	93	Mouse	ca. 16, 32	sc	1–6, 4–7, 6–11, or 11–16	None		
Harmine-Harmaline HCl (2:1)	92	Rat	105.5	sc	7–12, or 14–19	None mentioned	Prenatal death	
Heptylhydrazine	93	Mouse	ca. 20	sc	1–6, 6–11, or 11–16	None	Pregnancy interrupted after early treatment times	
HP 1275	94	Rat, Mouse	(0.1–0.5 mg/ml, in drinking water)	po	Throughout	None	Pregnancy interrupted	
HP 1325	93	Mouse	ca. 80, 200	sc, po	1–3, 1–6, 4–7, 6–11, or 11–16	None	Pregnancy interrupted after all but latest treatment time	
Iproclozide	95	Rat	60, 120	po	2–6, 7–11, or 12–16, or 7, 8, or 9	None	Prenatal death	
Iproniazid	96	Rat	10–50	ip	8–14	None mentioned	Reduced litter size and birth weight, stillbirth; postnatal death	

TABLE 1 (continued)

Drug	Reference	Species	Dose (mg/kg/day)	Route of administration[1]	Day(s) of gestation treated[2]	Effects: Malformations	Effects: Other	Comments
Iproniazid	97	Rat	2–8	ip	5–8, 11–14, or 17–20	None mentioned	Pregnancy interrupted, pre- and postnatal death, behavioral changes postnatally	No dose-response relations
Iproniazid	93, 98	Mouse	200–400	sc	1–6, 3–8, 6–11, or 11–16	None mentioned	Pregnancy interrupted after all but latest treatment time	
Isocarboxazid	96	Rat	1–4	ip	5–8, 11–14, or 17–20	None mentioned	Behavioral changes postnatally	
Isocarboxazid	91	Mouse	100	ip	10	Apparently none	Prenatal death	
MO 911	93	Mouse	ca. 80	sc	1–, or 11–16	None	Pregnancy interrupted after earlier time of treatment	
Nialamide	99	Rat	80	po	2 or 4 mo before breeding and throughout gestation	None	Pregnancy interrupted	
Nialamide	93	Mouse	ca. 160	sc	1–6, 6–11, or 11–16	None	Pregnancy interrupted after earlier treatment times	
Tranylcypromine sulfate	93	Mouse	ca. 4, 8	sc	1–6, 4–7, 6–11, or 11–16	None	None	
Phenelzine	100	Mouse	25	sc	1–6	None	Pregnancy interrupted	Antifertility effect probably not due to MAO inhibition

TABLE 1 (continued)

Drug	Reference	Species	Dose (mg/kg/day)	Route of administration[1]	Day(s) of gestation treated[2]	Effects		Comments
						Malformations	Other	
Phenelzine derivatives, miscellaneous	100	Mouse	5–250	sc, po	1–3, 1–6 6–11, or 11–16	None	Pregnancy interrupted	
WL 27	100	Mouse	10, 20	sc	4–6, or 7–11	¼, head, limbs		
Phenothiazine derivatives								
Chlorpromazine	101	Rat	10	sc	8–15	None mentioned		
Chlorpromazine	102	Rat	30	sc	3 days, during 6–13	None	Abortion, stillbirth, reduced fetal size	
Chlorpromazine	71	Rat	20	im	5	None mentioned	Abortion, prenatal death	
Chlorpromazine	103	Rat	12.5	sc	5 times/wk, for months before breeding and throughout gestation	None mentioned	Reduced litter size, stillbirth	
Chlorpromazine	104	Rat	5	sc	Throughout	None mentioned	Reduced postnatal survival	
Chlorpromazine	105, 106	Rat	6	sc	6–9, 12–15, or 18–20	None	Behavioral changes persistent throughout adulthood	Same result regardless of gestation stage treated
Chlorpromazine	107, 110	Rat	30	?	Throughout	None mentioned	Prenatal death	
Chlorpromazine	108	Rat	6	sc	5–8, 11–14, or 17–20			

TABLE 1 (continued)

Drug	Reference	Species	Dose (mg/kg/day)	Route of administration[1]	Day(s) of gestation treated[2]	Effects: Malformations	Effects: Other	Comments
Chlorpromazine	109	Rat	10	ip	4	38%, CNS, etc, in BD II rats, not increased in Wistar rats		6% malformation in controls; young examined early in gestation
Chlorpromazine	81	Rat	20	po	4–12	None mentioned		Chlorpromazine prevented fetal death due to micotinamide-deficient diet
Chlorpromazine	42	Rat	2	im	10	None	None	
Chlorpromazine	111	Rat	6	sc	5–8, 11–14, or 17–20	None mentioned	Postnatal behavioral changes after later 2 treatment times	
Chlorpromazine	112	Rat	6	sc	4–7	Apparently none	Stillbirth, behavioral changes, transient postnatal growth retardation	
Chlorpromazine	113	Rat	6	sc	5–18, or 17–20	None mentioned	Behavioral changes, after earlier treatment time	
Chlorpromazine	80a	Rat	20	po	2–19	None	None	
Chlorpromazine	114, 115	Rat	6	sc	5–8, 11–14, or 17–20	None mentioned	Behavioral changes	
Chlorpromazine	116	Rat	3	sc	12–15	None mentioned	Reduced neonatal brain butylcholinesterase activity	
Chlorpromazine	117, 118	Mouse	4, 16	po	Throughout	None mentioned	Reduced litter size, fetal weight and postnatal survival, behavioral and biochemical changes	
Chlorpromazine	45	Mouse	ca. 0.44–40	sc	3–6	None	None	

TABLE 1 (continued)

Drug	Reference	Species	Dose (mg/kg/day)	Route of administration[1]	Day(s) of gestation treated[2]	Effects: Malformations	Effects: Other	Comments
Chlorpromazine	53	Mouse	?	?	ca. 14–15	3/152, cleft palate		
Fluphenazine	119	Rat	ca. 0.7–0.8, 2	po	From 9 days before breeding throughout	None mentioned	Reduced conception and implantation rates; reduced litter size	
Prochlorperazine	120	Rat	ca. 8–80	parenteral	Various	Total, 3%, CNS, etc.;12% cleft palate after day-12 treatment	Pregnancy interrupted; prenatal death	
Prochlorperazine	121	Rat	10	iv	?	?%, eye		
Prochlorperazine	87	Rat	ca. 8–40	im	12–14, or 13	None attributable to treatment	Reduced litter size	
Prochlorperazine	120	Mouse	ca. 40	po	Various	?% (low)	Reduced litter size	
Prochlorperazine	91	Mouse	100	ip	10	None	Prenatal death	
Prochlorperazine	87	Mouse	ca. 0.4-108	im	12–14, or 13	6–39%, cleft palate	Prenatal death	
Promazine	104	Rat	5	sc	Throughout	None mentioned		
Thioridazine	104	Rat	5	sc	Throughout	None mentioned		
Trifluoperazine	45	Mouse	ca. 0.4–108	sc	3–6	None	Delayed implantation, beginning at about 10 mg/kg	
Rauwolfia derivatives								
Deserpidine	122	Rat	0.3, 0.45	?	6–16	6% tail, limb, etc.; after higher dose only	Reduced litter size	

TABLE 1 (continued)

Drug	Reference	Species	Dose (mg/kg/day)	Route of administration[1]	Day(s) of gestation treated[2]	Effects: Malformations	Effects: Other	Comments
Reserpine	123	Rat	0.05	sc	From up to 21 wk before mating and throughout gestation	None mentioned	Reduced litter size and offspring weight	
Reserpine	124	Rat	ca. 0.25	sc	1–10, 3–12, or 6–12	None	Abortion	
Reserpine	71	Rat	0.5, 2.5	im, po	5	None mentioned	Abortion, prenatal death	
Reserpine	97	Rat	0.1	ip	8–14	None mentioned	Prenatal death, behavioral changes	
Reserpine	105, 106, 108	Rat	0.1	sc	6–9, 12–15, or 18–21	None	Behavioral changes, persistent throughout adulthood	Same result regardless of gestation stage treated
Reserpine	107, 110	Rat	0.1–1	ip	Throughout	None mentioned	Prenatal death	
Reserpine	125	Rat	0.1–1.5	im	9 or 10	4%, CNS, eye, etc.	Prenatal death	
Reserpine	111	Rat	0.1	sc	5–8, 11–14, or 17–20	None mentioned		
Reserpine	112	Rat	0.1	sc	4–7	Apparently none		
Reserpine	113	Rat	0.1	sc	5–8, or 17–20	None mentioned	Behavioral changes, after earlier treatment time	
Reserpine	114, 115	Rat	0.1	sc	5–8, 11–14, or 17–20	None mentioned	Behavioral changes	Different test used than previously[111]
Reserpine	45	Mouse	ca. 0.08–2	sc	3–6	None	None	

TABLE 1 (continued)

Drug	Reference	Species	Dose (mg/kg/day)	Route of administration[1]	Day(s) of gestation treated[2]	Effects: Malformations	Effects: Other	Comments
Reserpine	126	Rabbit	0.15–0.2	im, po	2–13, 9–19, or 20–27	None mentioned	Implantation prevented, prenatal death	
Reserpine	127	Rabbit	ca. 0.1	parenteral	1–, 11–, or 21–30	None mentioned		
Sedatives and Hypnotics								
Ethinamate	91	Mouse	400	ip	10	4%, ?	Prenatal death	
Glutethimide	48	Rat	(0.4%, in diet)	po	From 3 days before mating throughout gestation	?% (low), axial skeleton	Stillbirth	
Glutethimide	128	Rat	50–500	po	1–, or 6–14	None	Reduced fertility	
Glutethimide	91	Mouse	100, 300	ip, po	8–14, or 10	16%, ?	Prenatal death	Only ip effective; maternal food intake greatly decreased for 1–2 days
Glutethimide	128	Mouse	50–500	po	6–14	None	Reduced fertility, prenatal death	
Glutethimide	128, 129	Rabbit	100–400	parenteral, po	6–12, or 8–14	None	Reduced fertility, prenatal death	
Glutethimide	58	Rabbit	150	po	8–16	None	None	
Meprobamate	130	Rat	(0.5–2%, in diet)	po	From 12 wk before breeding, throughout gestation	None mentioned	100% postnatal death, young from females fed 2%	
Meprobamate	131	Rat	100–500	po	Throughout	None	Pregnancy interrupted; prenatal death	

TABLE 1 (continued)

Drug	Reference	Species	Dose (mg/kg/day)	Route of administration[1]	Day(s) of gestation treated[2]	Effects: Malformations	Effects: Other	Comments
Meprobamate	105, 106, 108	Rat	60	sc	6–9, 12–15, or 18–21	None	Behavioral changes, persistent throughout adulthood	Same effects regardless of gestation stage treated
Meprobamate	132	Rat	32-128	po	Throughout	None mentioned	None	
Meprobamate	133	Rat	60	sc	5–9, 10–14, or 14–18	None mentioned	None	
Meprobamate	111	Rat	60	sc	5–8, 11–14, or 17–20	None mentioned	Reduced offspring weight	
Meprobamate	113	Rat	60	sc	5–8, or 17–20	None mentioned	Behavioral changes	
Meprobamate	114, 115	Rat	60	sc	5–8, 11–14, or 17–20	None mentioned	Behavioral changes, type varying with gestation stage treated	Different behavior tests used than previously
Meprobamate	134	Mouse	200, 400	sc	6–12	None attributable to treatment	None mentioned	
Meprobamate	135	Mouse	100–750	sc	8, 10, 12, or 14	Up to 44%, digits, etc.; highest after day-10 treatment	Prenatal death	Dose-related embryotoxicity; drug dissolved in 50% propylene glycol, which was itself embryolethal
Meprobamate	136	Mouse	180–280	po	From 4 mo before mating, throughout gestation	None	None	
Meprobamate	134	Rabbit	100–400	sc, po	6–10, 10–14, 8–19, or 15–19	None attributable to treatment	Pregnancy interrupted after largest dose	
Methaqualone	137	Rat	25–100	po	1–20	4%, cleft palate, etc.	Prenatal death	Only highest doses effective
Methaqualone	48	Rat	(0.8%, in diet)	po	From 3 days before mating throughout gestation	None	Stillbirth	

TABLE 1 (continued)

Drug	Reference	Species	Dose (mg/kg/day)	Route of administration[1]	Day(s) of gestation treated[2]	Effects: Malformations	Effects: Other	Comments
Methaqualone	138	Rat	200	ip	4	2%, ?	None mentioned	
Methaqualone	91	Mouse	150	ip	10	7%, ?	Prenatal death	
Methaqualone	137	Rabbit	100–400	po	8–15, 8–16, or 1–29	None attributable to treatment	None mentioned	
Methaqualone	58	Rabbit	100	po	8–16	None	None mentioned	
Nitromethaqualone	138	Rat	300	ip	4	None	None mentioned	
Sodium bromide	139, 140	Rat	40–120	po	3–20	None mentioned	Increased preweaning mortality; learning rate and other behavior impaired	
Valnoctamide	141	Rat	100–300	po	1–12, 6–12, or 7–9	None	None mentioned	
Valnoctamide	141	Mouse	100–400	po	1–12, 6–12, or 7–9	None attributable to treatment	None mentioned	
Valnoctamide	141	Rabbit	100–400	po	6–8, –9, or –12, or 7–9	None attributable to treatment	None mentioned	
Other psychotropics								
Fenpentadiol	142	Rat	50, 100	po	1–18	None attributable to treatment	None	
Fenpentadiol	142	Mouse	5–100	po	1–18	None attributable to treatment	None	
Flupenthixol	119	Rat	1–3	po	From 9 days before mating throughout gestation	None	None mentioned	

TABLE 1 (continued)

Drug	Reference	Species	Dose (mg/kg/day)	Route of administration[1]	Day(s) of gestation treated[2]	Effects: Malformations	Effects: Other	Comments
Pemoline	91	Mouse	10	ip	10	None mentioned	Prenatal death	
Cannabis								
Marihuana resin	144	Rat	4.2	ip	1–6	?% (high), limb, umbilical hernia	Prenatal death, reduced fetal size	
Marihuana resin	145	Mouse	16	ip	6, or 1–16	None	Reduced fertility	
Marihuana extract, 2 geographic samples	146	Hamster	25–300	sc	6–8	3–9%, CNS, limb, umbilical hernia, beginning at 100 mg/kg	None	
Marihuana extract, 2 geographic samples	146	Rabbit	130–500	sc	7–10	5–33%, CNS, limb, umbilical hernia, beginning at 250 mg/kg	Prenatal death, at highest doses	Samples different in degree of embryotoxicity
Hallucinogens								
2-Bromo-LSD	107	Rat	4	ip	Throughout	None	None	
2-Bromo-LSD	150	Rat	0.002–0.41	ip	4, 7, or 8	None	None	
2-Bromo-LSD	151	Hamster	0.002–0.4	sc	8	6 – 13%, CNS	Prenatal death, fetal retardation, dose related	Malformations not dose related
LSD	107	Rat	1	ip	Throughout	None	None	
LSD (dry powder, Sandoz)	152	Rat	0.005	sc	4, 7, 8, 10, 13, or 16	None attributable to treatment	Reduced litter size, stillbirth	

TABLE 1 (continued)

Drug	Reference	Species	Dose (mg/kg/day)	Route of administration[1]	Day(s) of gestation treated[2]	Effects: Malformations	Effects: Other	Comments
LSD(Delysid, Sandoz, lot 65002)	153	Rat	0.0016–0.4	ip, po	4, 5, 7, 8, or 9; or 7–12	None attributable to treatment	None	
LSD (Delysid, Sandoz)	150	Rat	0.005–0.05	ip	4, 7, or 8	None	None	
LSD (Delysid, Sandoz, lot 88601)	154	Rat	0.1	sc, po	4, 8, or 4–5	None attributable to treatment	None	
LSD (dry powder, Sandoz)	155	Rat	0.005–0.1	sc, po	Once, on 1–16	None	Reduced litter size, early postnatal death	
LSD	156	Rat	0.001–0.1	po	Various days	None	Decreased postnatal brain 5-hydroxy-tryptamine	
LSD (Sandoz)	157	Rat	0.005–0.5	sc	4, 7, 4–7, or 7–13	None attributable to treatment	None	
LSD (Sandoz, lot 88601)	158	Rat	0.0025–0.01	sc	4	None	None	
LSD (Sandoz, lot 88601)	159	Rat	2–6	sc	4	None	Pregnancy interrupted	
LSD (Sandoz, lot 88601)	160	Rat	0.05–0.2	sc	4, 6, or 8	None attributable to treatment	None	
LSD (Delysid, Sandoz, lot 65002)	161	Mouse	ca. 0.002–0.04	ip	7, 8, 9, or 10	44%, CNS, etc., after day-7 or -8 treatment		Poor dose-response relation; 8% malformed controls, examined early in gestation
LSD (Delysid, Sandoz, lot 65002)	162	Mouse	(ca. 0.016–1.2, total/mouse)	ip	Once, on 7–10; or multiple days	19%, facial; in A strain, none in another	None	3% facial defects in A controls

TABLE 1 (continued)

Drug	Reference	Species	Dose (mg/kg/day)	Route of administration[1]	Day(s) of gestation treated[2]	Effects		Comments
						Malformations	Other	
LSD	163	Mouse	ca. 0.2	ip	Once, on 4–9	None external; 67%, lens, after day-6 treatment	None mentioned	
LSD (Sandoz)	157	Mouse	0.008–0.24	sc	4–10, or 6–13	None	None	
LSD	157a	Mouse	ca. 0.04	ip	Once, on 4 or 7–13	None attributable to treatment	Possibly prenatal mortality	
LSD	151	Hamster	0.005–0.05	sc	8	5–8%, CNS	Prenatal death	Malformations not dose related
LSD (Delysid, Sandoz, lot 65002)	162	Hamster	ca. 0.1–3.0	ip	6, 7, or 8; or 7–9	None attributable to treatment	None	
LSD (Sandoz)	157	Hamster	0.05–0.5	sc	4–12, or 7–13	None	None	
LSD	164	Rabbit	0.02–0.1	po	4–7, 7–9, or 8–12	None	Reduced fetal weight	
LSD	165	Rhesus monkey	ca. 0.015–0.04	po	22, 25, 27, or 29, or 22, 24, and 26, or 24, 26, and 28	None	Apparently none	
LSD	166	Rhesus monkey	0.125–1.0	sc	4–11 injections/monkey during last 6 wk of gestation	2 with "facial deformities," not attributable to treatment	Stillbirth	Female monkeys were in 3rd or 4th mo of pregnancy when imported
Mescaline	151	Hamster	0.45–3.25	sc	8	9–28%, CNS	Prenatal death	Malformations not dose related
Methyllysergic acid butanolamide	107	Rat	4	ip	Throughout	None	None	

TABLE 1 (continued)

Drug	Reference	Species	Dose (mg/kg/day)	Route of administration[1]	Day(s) of gestation treated[2]	Effects: Malformations	Effects: Other	Comments
α-Methyltryptamine	167	Rat	5–40	po	1–3 days during 4–13; or 2–21, or 3–18	ca. 5–8%, skeleton, etc.		
Psilocin	168	Mouse	25	po	Throughout	None mentioned	None mentioned	

[1] Im, intramuscular; ip, intraperitoneal; iv, intravenous; po, oral; sc, subcutaneous

[2] Day following that on which sexes put together, or day vaginal plug or sperm seen in vaginal smear, called day 1 of gestation; where possible other systems were converted to this one. In some cases authors did not state their system of denoting gestation time.

[3] Central nervous system.

Tranquilizers, minor – Numerous tranquilizers and types of tranquilizers have been tested for their embryotoxic properties. Relatively few, however, appeared to be teratogenic. Those about whose teratogenicity, in one species or another, there seemed to be little question, were haloperidol, hydroxyzine, trifluperidol, and prochlorperazine. Others, e.g., imipramine and deserpidine, gave equivocal teratogenic results. The numerous studies reporting contradictory effects of meprobamate on postnatal behavior were recently critically summarized.[143]

Cannabis – The number of experimental studies made of the embryotoxic properties of products of marihuana plants is fewer than the fingers on a normal hand and the results of these are contestable and inconclusive. For example, in one study[144] malformations were said to be produced in rats by treatment with cannabis resin on days 1 to 6 of pregnancy, but this result is unusual since administration of agents before germ-layer formation (ca. day 8 in rats) rarely produces developmental abnormalities.[4,147]

Studies of the placental transfer of labeled tetrahydrocannabinol gave contradictory results. In one experiment the substance crossed the golden hamster placenta soon after ip or sc administration on the 11th day of pregnancy;[148] but in A/J mice, radioactivity was apparently not present in fetal tissues, but was present in the yolk sac 24 hours after iv administration on the 12th day.[149]

Hallucinogens – In response to its clamorous notoriety, LSD has been given fairly thorough attention to determine its embryotoxic potentialities. With few apparent exceptions[151,161-163] it proved to be nonteratogenic, and was embryolethal only at very large doses. In cases where it appeared to be teratogenic, no dose-response relations or gestation-stage differences were noted.

SPECIES AND DOSES

The widespread, chronic exposure, both voluntary and involuntary, of modern-day populations to chemicals of every conceivable type has, not surprisingly, aroused much anxiety about the possible detrimental biological effects these agents might be causing in human beings. Frequent concerns are for possible mutagenic and teratogenic effects. Since these biohazards may be either long in developing or long undiscovered, and probably affect only a portion of even the exposed populations, animal tests must be resorted to to indicate the harmful potentials of suspected agents.

Numerous problems arise at this point. I will confine myself to two of these here; others will be alluded to below. The first and most difficult is the question of relevance: are the tests meaningful for human beings? Can testing the mutagenicity of chemicals in lower forms, hamster cells in vitro, a host-mediated system, or by the dominant-lethal method reveal whether it will mutate genes or break chromosomes in people?[169] Can testing the teratogenicity of chemicals in pregnant rats, mice, hamsters, or macaque monkeys help in deciding the risk these chemicals pose for pregnant women?[170] These questions cannot be answered categorically or be gone into in detail here; but it should be recognized that attempts to probe the validity of mutagenicity tests will not necessarily contribute to untying the teratogenicity knot and vice versa.

The second difficulty confronting animal testing is knowing when to stop. How many species need to be tested and how high should the doses be before conclusions are reached? In time, as knowledge replaces ignorance, there will be more logical means of choosing test species; but, no doubt, it will always be necessary to plumb the limits of toxicity of chemicals by using far larger doses than people can imaginably experience.

This brings us to the fact, well known to teratologists, but perhaps not clearly enunciated, that although large doses of most chemicals will kill many, even all, conceptuses, it is not correct to infer from this that every chemical found to be embryolethal is also teratogenic. This misinterpretation must be guarded against, since invoking it would mean that in every instance a substance found experimentally to kill fetuses would be debarred from human use.

While the lethal effects of chemicals on embryos may lead to overinterpretation of their conceivable hazards, it is possible that faulty experimental procedures may conduce to too sanguine a view. One example will suffice. Since some drugs induce microsomal enzymes catalyzing their own metabolism, multiple administration of such agents to pregnant animals will decrease their concentration and thus mask some of their possible embryopathic effects. For this and other reasons it is recommended that each pregnant animal receive a single injection of or brief exposure to the agent in tests of teratogenicity.

PITFALLS

Individuals planning how the possible teratogenic effects of chemicals and other environmental agents may be detected in human beings should be aware of some of the lessons learned from experimental teratology about the pitfalls involved in interpreting their observations, whether positive or negative.

Many elements must conjoin for agents to produce malformations. Some of these are proper dose, effective mode of administration, susceptible gestation period and genotype, possible metabolic transformation and interaction, and various other less obvious parameters. Thus, only when a set of facilitating conditions exists will a potentially teratogenic agent be enabled to manifest its effects. It is to be deduced that establishing the teratogenicity of a substance for human beings will not be straightforward, because, fortunately, all instances of exposure of pregnant women to it will not lead to deformity, since in some, perhaps many, cases one or another of the necessary ingredients will be lacking. Where this is so, and a teratogenic agent only rarely or infrequently causes malformations, its identification may be further clouded by the induced defects' being indistinguishable from more common sporadic ones. And still other obscurities may be added by an agent producing variable syndromes of defects, or one type of defect being caused by various agents.

PROBLEMS OF INTERPRETATION: A SUMMARY

As noted above, there are many doubts about the adequacy of present-day mutagenicity and teratogenicity tests and their relevance for human beings. Thus, we must inquire about the significance of the studies of the drugs of dependence outlined above and in the table. It hardly needs to be said that these experimental results are difficult to interpret: the data were frequently sparse; the species and stocks of animals often varied; the experimental conditions usually diverse. That the results were sometimes contradictory is not surprising. What may be surprising is that the contradictions were so relatively few.

Although capable of killing fetuses when given in sufficiently large quantities, it appears that most of the drugs of dependence yet tested were not teratogenic. Although it is tempting to compare the doses used in these studies with those usually taken by people, and on this basis try to project the likelihood of these drugs' causing congenital malformations in infants, it would be dangerous to do so, for many reasons; first and foremost because of the quantitative and qualitative differences in pharmacological and metabolic patterns between (and within) human beings and species of test animals. For example, absolute dose may be an entirely unreliable index of resulting plasma and tissue concentrations, upon which a drug's consequences may more directly depend.

In conclusion, until information of this and other relevant sorts becomes available, or what is already known is applied to drug teratology testing, it will be possible to make only feeble estimates of the teratogenic risks human embryos suffer when exposed to drugs of dependence.

REFERENCES

1. Fave, A., Les embryopathies provoquées chez les mammifères, *Thérapie*, 19, 43, 1964.

2. Karnofsky, D. A., Drugs as teratogens in animals and man, *Ann. Rev. Pharmacol.*, 5, 447, 1965.

3. Robson, J. M., Sullivan, F. M., and Smith, R. L., *A Symposium on Embryopathic Activity of Drugs*, Little, Brown, and Co., Boston, 1965.

4. Kalter, H., *Teratology of the Central Nervous System. Induced and spontaneous malformations of laboratory, agricultural, and domestic mammals*, University of Chicago, Chicago, 1968.

5. Giroud, A., *The Nutrition of the Embryo*, Charles C Thomas, Springfield, Ill., 1970.

6. Cohlan, S. Q., Teratogenic agents and congenital malformations, *J. Pediat.*, 63, 650, 1963.

7. Lenz, W., Malformations caused by drugs in pregnancy, *Amer. J. Dis. Child.*, 112, 99, 1966.

8. Smithells, R. W., Drugs and human malformations, *Advances Terat.*, 1, 251, 1966.

9. Nora, J. J., Nora, A. H., Sommerville, R. J., Hill, R. M., and McNamara, D. G., Maternal exposure to potential teratogens, *J.A.M.A.*, 202, 1065, 1967.

10. Richards, I. D. G., Congenital malformations and environmental influences in pregnancy, *Brit. J. Prev. Soc. Med.*, 23, 218, 1969.

11. Warkany, J., *Congenital Malformations. Notes and comments*, Year Book Medical, Chicago, 1971.

12. Kalter, H., Correlation between teratogenic and mutagenic effects of chemicals in mammals, in *Chemical Mutagens. Principles and methods for their detection*, Vol. 1, Hollaender, A., Ed., Plenum Press, New York, 1971, 57.

13. Shaw, M. W., Human chromosome damage by chemical agents, *Ann. Rev. Med.*, 21, 409, 1970.

14. Cattanach, B. M., Chemically induced mutations in mice, *Mutat. Res.*, 3, 346, 1966.

15. Ehling, U. H., The multiple loci method, in *Chemical Mutagenesis in Mammals and Man*, Vogel, F. and Röhrborn, G. Eds., Springer-Verlag, New York, 1970, 156.

16. Cattanach, B. M., Specific locus mutation in mice, in *Chemical Mutagens. Principles and methods for their detection*, Vol. 2, Hollaender, A. Ed., Plenum Press, New York, 1971, 535.

17. Russell, W. L. and Cumming, R. B., Chemically induced specific-locus mutations in the mouse, *Environ. Mutag. Soc., 2nd Ann. Mtg.*, 8 abst., 1971.

18. Falconer, D. S., Slizynski, B. M., and Auerbach, C., Genetical effects of nitrogen mustard in the house mouse, *J. Genet.*, 51, 81, 1952.

19. Cattanach, B. M., Induction of translocations in mice by triethylenemelamine, *Nature*, 180 1364, 1957.

20. Datta, P. K., Frigger, H., and Schleiermacher, E., The effect of chemical mutagens on the mitotic chromosomes of the mouse, in vivo, in *Chemical Mutagenesis in Mammals and Man*, Vogel, F. and Röhrborn, G., Eds., Springer-Verlag, New York, 1970, 194.

20a. Witschi, E., Time variations in prenatal development, in *Growth, Including Reproduction and Morphological Development*, Altman, R. L. and Dittmer, D. S., Eds., FASEB, Washington, D.C., 1962, 272.

21. Fishbein, L., Flamm, W. G., and Falk, H. L., *Chemical Mutagens. Environmental effects on biological systems*, Academic Press, New York, 1970.

22. Epstein, S. S. and Shafner, H., Chemical mutagens in the human environment, *Nature*, 219, 385, 1968.

23. Kalter, H., Teratogenic hazards, in *Drugs of Abuse. Their genetic and other nonpsychiatric hazards*, Epstein, S. S., Lederberg, J., and Legator, M. S., Eds., M. I. T. Press, Cambridge, 1971, 93.

24. Yeh, S. Y. and Woods, L. A., Maternal and fetal distribution of H^3-dihydromorphine in the tolerant and nontolerant rat, *J. Pharmacol. Exp. Ther.*, 174, 9, 1970.

25. Geber, W. F. and Schramm, L., Heroin teratogenic and behavioral activity in hamsters, *Fed. Proc.*, 28, 262, abst., 1969.

26. Geber, W. F., Blockade of teratogenic effect of morphine and dihydromorphinone by nalorphine and cyclazocine, *Pharmacologist*, 12 296, abst., 1970.

26a. Geber, W. F. and Schramm, L. C., Comparative teratogenecity [*sic*] of morphine, heroin and methadone in the hamster, *Pharmacologist*, 11, 248, abst., 1969.

26b. Markham, J. K., Emmerson, J. L., and Owen, N. V., Teratogenicity studies of methadone HCl in rats and rabbits, *Nature*, 233, 342, 1971.

27. Myers, H. B., The effect of chronic morphine poisoning upon growth, the oestrous cycle and fertility of the white rat, *J. Pharmacol. Exp. Ther.*, 41, 317, 1931.

28. Harpel, H. S., Jr. and Gautieri, R. F., Morphine-induced fetal malformations. I. Exencephaly and axial skeletal fusions, *J. Pharm. Sci.*, 57, 1590, 1968.

29. Iuliucci, J. D. and Gautieri, R. F., Morphine-induced fetal malformations. II. Influence of histamine and diphenhydramine, *J. Pharm. Sci.*, 60, 420, 1971.

30. Emmerson, J. L., Owen, N. V., Koenig, G. R., Markham, J. K., and Anderson, R. C., Reproduction and teratology studies on propoxyphene napsylate, *Toxic. Appl. Pharmacol.*, 19, 471, 1971.

31. Flynn, R. J., Exencephalia: its occurrence in untreated mice, *Science*, 160, 898, 1968.

32. Rugh, R., Normal incidence of brain hernia in the mouse, *Science*, 163, 407, 1969.

33. Davis, R. H., Letter to editor, *Lab. Anim. Care*, 20, 289, 1970.

34. Runner, M. N., Inheritance of susceptibility to congenital deformity – embryonic instability, *J. Nat. Cancer Inst.*, 15, 637, 1954.

35. Runner, M. N. and Miller, J. R., Congenital deformity in the mouse as a consequence of fasting, *Anat. Rec.*, 124, 437, abst., 1956.

36. Runner, M. N., Inheritance of susceptibility to congenital deformity. Metabolic clues provided by experiments with teratogenic agents, *Pediatrics*, 23, 245, 1959.

37. Armitage, S. G., The effects of barbiturates on the behavior of rat offspring as measured in learning and reasoning situations, *J. Comp. Physiol. Psychol.*, 45, 146, 1952.

38. Persaud, T. V. N., Tierexperimentelle Untersuchungen zur Frage der teratogenen Wirkung von Barbituraten, *Acta Biol. Med. German.*, 14, 89, 1965.

39. Champakamalini, A. V. and Rao, M. A., Foetal resorption in barbital sodium treated pregnant rats, *Curr. Sci.*, 36, 3, 1967.

40. Persaud, T. V. N. and Henderson, W. M., The teratogenicity of barbital sodium in mice, *Arzneimittelforschung*, 19, 1309, 1969.

41. Grote, W., Kabarity, A., and Schade, H., Auswirkungen eines Barbitursäurederivates auf die Embryogenese von Kaninchen durch Mitosestörungen, *Humangenetik*, 8, 280, 1970.

42. Goldman, A. S. and Yakovac, W. C., Prevention of salicylate teratogenicity in immobilized rats by certain central nervous system depressants, *Proc. Soc. Exp. Biol. Med.*, 115, 693, 1964.

43. Mork, D. P. S., Kessler, W. V., and Shaw, S. M., Placental transfer of pentobarbital in the rat, *J. Pharm. Sci.*, 59, 803, 1970.

44. Setälä, K. and Nyyssönen, O., Hypnotic sodium pentobarbital as a teratogen for mice, *Naturwissenschaften*, 51, 413, 1964.

45. Bindon, B. M., The role of the pituitary gland in implantation in mice: delay of implantation by hypophysectomy and neurodepressive drugs, *J. Endocr.*, 43, 225, 1969.

46. Becker, R. F., Flannagan, E., and King, J. E., The fate of offspring from mothers receiving sodium pentobarbital before delivery. A study in the guinea pig, *Neurology*, 8, 776, 1958.

47. Johnson, W. E., Fetal loss from anesthesia and surgical trauma in the rabbit, *Toxic. Appl. Pharmacol.*, 18, 773, 1971.

48. McColl, J. D., Globus, M., and Robinson, S., Drug induced skeletal malformations in the rat, *Experientia*, 19, 183, 1963.

49. Murai, N., Effect of maternal medication during pregnancy upon behavioral development of offspring, *Tohoku J. Exp. Med.*, 89, 265, 1966.

50. Fahim, M. S., Hall, D. G., Jones, T. M., Fahim, Z., and Whitt, F. D., Drug-steroid interaction in the pregnant rat, fetus, and neonate, *Amer. J. Obstet. Gynec.*, 197, 1250, 1970.

51. Olivecrona, H., Embryo-destroying effect of injected phenobarbital in the mouse, *Acta Anat.*, 58, 217, 1964.

52. Gibson, J. E. and Becker, B. A., Effect of phenobarbital and SKF 525-A on the teratogenicity of cyclophosphamide in mice, *Teratology*, 1, 393, 1968.

53. Walker, B. E., Relation of embryonic movements to formation of cleft palate, *Teratology*, 2, 272, abst., 1969.

54. Jacobs, R. M., The effect of central nervous system depressants, general anesthetics and muscle relaxants on palate closure in two strains of mice, *Anat. Rec.*, 166, 323, abst.,1971.

55. Jacobs, R. M., Failure of muscle relaxants to produce cleft palate in mice, *Teratology*, 4, 25, 1971.

56. Manning, D. E., Stout, A. G., and Zemp, J. W., Effects of maternal phenobarbital administration on some aspects of neonatal brain development, *Fed. Proc.*, 30, 495, abst., 1971.

57. Hart, L. G., Adamson, R. H., Dixon, R. L., and Fouts, J. R., Stimulation of hepatic microsomal drug metabolism in the newborn and fetal rabbit, *J. Pharmacol. Exp. Ther.*, 137, 103, 1962.

58. McColl, J. D., Robinson, S., and Globus, M., Effect of some therapeutic agents on the rabbit fetus, *Toxic. Appl. Pharmacol.*, 10, 244, 1967.

59. Tanimura, T., Effects of administration of thiamylal sodium to pregnant mice upon the development of their offspring (in Japanese), *Acta Anat. Nippon.*, 40, 323, 1965.

60. Tanimura, T., Owaki, Y., and Nishimura, H., Effect of administration of thiopental sodium to pregnant mice upon the development of their offspring, *Okajima. Folia Anat. Jap.*, 43, 219, 1967.

61. Harbison, R. D. and Becker, B. A., Effect of phenobarbital and SKF 525-A pretreatment on diphenylhydantoin teratogenicity in mice, *J. Pharmacol. Exp. Ther.*, 175, 283, 1970.

62. Wilson, J. G., Fradkin, R., and Schumacher, H. J., Influence of drug pretreatment on the effectiveness of known teratogenic agents, *Teratology*, 3, 210, abst., 1970.

63. Franke, H. and Klinger, W., Untersuchungen zum Mechanismus der Enzyminduktion. IX. Die Wirkung von Barbital auf die Substruktur der Leberzellen gravider Ratten und ihrer Foeten, *Acta Biol. Med. German.*, 17, 507, 1966.

64. Klinger, W. and Heinrich, I., Untersuchungen zum Mechanismus der Enzyminduktion. XI. Die Wirkung von Barbital auf den *L*-Ascorbinsäuregehalt der Leber bei graviden Ratten, ihren Foeten und bei infantilen Ratten, *Acta Biol. Med. German.* 18, 493, 1967.

65. Cohen, A. and Pernot, J.-C., Réponse des surrénales foetales du rat à une agression dans differéntes conditions expérimentales; effet du nembutal, *C.R. Soc. Biol.*, 162, 1675, 1968.

66. Everett, J. W. and Sawyer, C. H., A 24-hour periodicity in the "LH-release apparatus" of female rats, disclosed by barbiturate sedation, *Endocrinology*, 47, 198, 1950.

67. Fugo, N. W. and Butcher, R. L., Overripeness and the mammalian ova. I. Overripeness and the early embryonic development, *Fertil. Steril.*, 17, 804, 1966.

68. Butcher, R. L. and Fugo, N. W., Overripeness and the mammalian ova. II. Delayed ovulation and chromosome anomalies, *Fertil. Steril.*, 18, 297, 1967.

69. Butcher, R. L., Blue, J. D., and Fugo, N. W., Overripeness and the mammalian ova. III. Fetal development at midgestation and at term, *Fertil. Steril.*, 20, 223, 1969.

70. Toyoda, Y. and Chang, M. C., Delayed ovulation and embryonic development in the rat treated with pentobarbital sodium, *Endocrinology*, 84, 1456, 1969.

71. Bovet-Nitti, F. and Bovet, D., Action of some sympatholytic agents on pregnancy in the rat, *Proc. Soc. Exp. Biol. Med.*, 100, 555, 1959.

72. Vernadakis, A. and Clark, C. V. H., Effects of prenatal administration of psychotropic drugs to rats on brain butylcholinesterase activity at birth, *Brain Res.*, 21, 460, 1970.

73. Yasuda, M., Ariyuki, F., and Nishimura, H., Effect of amphetamine on pregnancy in ICR-JCL mice, *Okajima. Folia Anat. Jap.*, 41, 227, 1965.

74. Nora, J. J., Trasler, D. G., and Fraser, F. C., Malformations in mice induced by dexamphetamine sulphate, *Lancet*, 2, 1021, 1965.

75. Nora, J. J., Sommerville, R. J., and Fraser, F. C., Homologies for congenital heart diseases: murine models, influenced by dextroamphetamine, *Teratology*, 1, 413, 1968.

76. Paget, G. E., Dexamphetamine sulphate in mice, *Lancet*, 2, 1129, 1965.

77. Kasirsky, G. and Tansy, M. F., Teratogenic effects of methamphetamine in mice and rabbits, *Teratology*, 4, 131, 1971.

78. Courtney, K. D. and Valerio, D. A., Teratology in the *Macaca mulatta*, *Teratology*, 1, 163, 1968.

79. Zbinden, G., Bagdon, R. E., Keith, E. F., Phillips, R. D., and Randall, L. O., Experimental and clinical toxicology of chlordiazepoxide (Librium®), *Toxic. Appl. Pharmacol.*, 3, 619, 1961.

80. Takano, K., Tanimura, T., and Nishimura, H., Effects of some psychoactive drugs administered to pregnant mice upon the development of their offspring, *Proc. Cong. Anom. Res. Ass. Jap.*, 3, 2, abst., 1963.

81. Jelinek, V., Zikmund, E., and Reichlova, R., L'influence de quelques médicaments psychotropes sur le développement du foetus chez le rat, *Thérapie*, 22, 1429, 1967.

81a. DiCarlo, R. and Pagnini, G., Comparative action of amitriptyline and butriptyline on skeletal development in rat embryo, *Teratology*, 4, 486, abst., 1971.

82. Fratta, I., Zak, S. B., Greengard, P., and Sigg, E. B., Fetal death from nicotinamide-deficient diet and its prevention by chlorpromazine and imipramine, *Science*, 145, 1429, 1964.

83. Harper, K. H., Palmer, A. K., and Davies, R. E., Effect of imipramine upon the pregnancy of laboratory animals, *Arzneimittelforschung*, 15, 1218, 1965.

84. Aeppli, L., Teratologische Studien mit Imipramin an Ratte und Kaninchen, *Arzneimittelforschung*, 19, 1617, 1969.

85. Robson, J. M. and Sullivan, F. M., The production of foetal abnormalities in rabbits by imipramine, *Lancet*, 1, 638, 1963.

86. Larsen, V., The teratogenic effects of thalidomide, imipramine HCl and imipramine-*N*-oxide HCl on white Danish rabbits, *Acta Pharmacol.*, 20, 186, 1963.

87. Bertelli, A., Polani, P. E., Spector, R., Seller, M. J., Tuchmann-Duplessis, H., and Mercier-Parot, L., Retentissement d'un neuroleptique, l'halopéridol, sur la gestation et le développement prénatal des rongeurs, *Arzneimittelforschung*, 18, 1420, 1968.

88. Vichi, F., Neuroleptic drugs in experimental teratogenesis, in *Teratology*, Bertelli, A. and Donati, L.,Eds., Excerpta Med., Amsterdam, 1969, 87.

89. Einer-Jensen, N. and Secher, N. J., Diminished weight of rat foetuses after treatment of pregnant rats with haloperidol, *J. Reprod. Fertil.*, 22, 591, 1970.

90. King, C. T. G. and Howell, J., Teratogenic effect of buclizine and hydroxyzine in the rat and chlorcyclizine in the mouse, *Amer. J. Obstet. Gyn.*, 95, 109, 1966.

91. Harris, J. W. S. and Morgan, P. R., Aetiology of cleft palate induced by meclozine, buclizine and hydroxyzine, in *3rd International Conference Congenital Malformations*, Fraser, F. C., Ed., Excerpta Med., Amsterdam, 1969, 47, abst.

92. Kamel, S. H., Ibrahim, T. M., and Hamza, S. M., Effect of harmine and harmaline hydrochloride on pregnancy in white rats, *Zbl. Veterinärmed*, 18, 230, 1971.

93. Poulson, E. and Robson, J. M., The effect of amine oxidase inhibitors on pregnancy, *J. Endocr.*, 27, 147, 1963.

94. Spector, W. G., Anti-fertility action of a monoamine oxidase inhibitor, *Nature*, 187, 514, 1960.

95. Lauro, V., Giornelli, C., and Fanelli, A., Inhibitori delle monoaminossidasi e fertilità: indagini sperimentali, *Arch. Ostet. Ginec.*, 71, 153, 1966.

96. Werboff, J., Gottlieb, J. S., Dembicki, E. L., and Havlena, J., Postnatal effect of antidepressant drugs administered during gestation, *Exp. Neurol.*, 3, 542, 1961.

97. Werboff, J., Gottlieb, J. S., Havlena, J., and Wood, T. J., Behavioral effects of prenatal drug administration in the white rat, *Pediatrics*, 27, 318, 1961.

98. Poulson, E., Botros, M., and Robson, J. M., Effect of 5-hyroxytryptamine and iproniazid on pregnancy, *Science*, 131, 1101, 1960.

99. Tuchmann-Duplessis, H. and Mercier-Parot, L., Diminution de la fertilité du rat soumis à un traitement chronique de niamide, *C.R. Acad. Sci.*, 253, 712, 1961.

100. Poulson, E. and Robson, J. M., Effect of phenelzine and some related compounds on pregnancy and on sexual development, *J. Endocr.*, 30, 205, 1964.

101. Courrier, R. and Marois, M., Action de l'hypothermia expérimentale sur la gestation chez le rat, *C.R. Soc. Biol.*, 147, 1922, 1953.

102. Chambon, Y., Action de la chlorpromazine sur l'évolution et l'avenir de la gestation chez la rate, *Ann. Endocr.*, 16, 912, 1955.

103. Roizin, L., True, C., and Knight, M., Structural effects of tranquilizers, *Res. Publ. Ass. Res. Nerv. Ment. Dis.*, 37, 285, 1959.

104. Murphree, O. D., Monroe, B. L., and Seager, L. D., Survival of offspring of rats administered phenothiazines during pregnancy, *J. Neuropsychiat.*, 3, 295, 1962.

105. Werboff, J. and Dembicki, E. L., Toxic effects of tranquilizers administered to gravid rats, *J. Neuropsychiat.*, 4, 87, 1962.

106. Werboff, J. and Havlena, J., Postnatal behavioral effects of tranquilizers administered to the gravid rat., *Exp. Neurol.*, 6, 263, 1962.

107. West, G. B., Drugs and rat pregnancy, *J. Pharm. Pharmacol.*, 14, 828, 1962.

108. Werboff, J. and Kesner, R., Learning deficits of offspring after administration of tranquillizing drugs to the mothers, *Nature*, 197, 106, 1963.

109. Brock, N. and von Kreybig, T., Experimenteller Beitrag zur Prüfung teratogener Wirkungen von Arzneimitteln an der Laboratoriumstratte, *Naunyn Schmiedeberg Arch. Exp. Path.*, 249, 117, 1964.

110. West, G. B., Teratogenic activity of drugs, *J. Pharm. Pharmacol.*, 16, 63, 1964.

111. Hoffeld, D. R. and Webster, R. L., Effect of injection of tranquillizing drugs during pregnancy on offspring, *Nature*, 205, 1070, 1965.

112. Jewett, R. E. and Norton, S., Effect of tranquilizing drugs on postnatal behavior, *Exp. Neurol.*, 14, 33, 1966.

113. Murai, N., Effect of maternal medication during pregnancy upon behavioral development of offspring, *Tohuk J. Exp. Med.*, 89, 265, 1966.

114. Hoffeld, D. R., Webster, R. L., and McNew, J., Adverse effects on offspring of tranquilizing drugs during pregnancy, *Nature*, 215, 182, 1967.

115. Hoffeld, D. R., McNew, J., and Webster, R. L., Effect of tranquilizing drugs during pregnancy on activity of rat offspring, *Nature*, 218, 357, 1968.

116. Vernadakis, A. and Clark, C. V. H., Effects of prenatal administration of psychotropic drugs to rats on brain butylcholinesterase activity at birth, *Brain Res.*, 21, 460, 1970.

117. Ordy, J. M., Latanick, A., Johnson, R., and Massopust, L. C., Chlorpromazine effects on pregnancy and offspring in mice, *Proc. Soc. Exp. Biol. Med.*, 113, 833, 1963.

118. Ordy, J. M., Samorajski, T., Collins, R. L., and Rolsten, C., Prenatal chlorpromazine effects on liver, survival and behavior of mice offspring, *J. Pharmacol. Exp. Ther.*, 151, 110, 1966.

119. Spieth, K. and Lorenz, D., Untersuchungen mit Fluphenazin und Flupenthixol über die Beeinflussung der Fertilität und uber die fetale Toxicität an der Ratte, *Nauyn Schmiedeberg Arch. Exp. Path.*, 257, 316, 1967.

120. Roux, C., Action tératogène de la prochlorpémazine, *Arch. Franc. Pédiat.*, 16, 968, 1959.

121. Roizin, L., Lazar, M., and Gold, G., Prenatal effects of phenothiazines, *Fed. Proc.*, 25, 252, abst., 1966.

122. Tuchmann-Duplessis, H. and Mercier-Parot, L., Malformations foetales chez le rat traité par de fortes doses de déserpidine, *C.R. Soc. Biol.*, 155, 2291, 1961.

123. Gaunt, R., Renzi, A. A., Antonchak, N., Miller, G. J., and Gilman, M., Endocrine aspects of the pharmacology of reserpine, *Ann. N.Y. Acad. Sci.*, 59, 22, 1954.

124. Tuchmann-Duplessis, H. and Mercier-Parot, L., Répercussions de la réserpine sur la gestation chez la ratte, *C.R. Acad. Sci.*, 243, 410, 1956.

125. Goldman, A. S. and Yakovac, W. C., Teratogenic action in rats of reserpine alone and in combination with salicylate and immobilization, *Proc. Soc. Exp. Biol. Med.*, 118, 857, 1965.

126. Kehl, R., Audibert, A., Gage, C., and Amarger, J., Action de la réserpine à différentes périodes de la gestation, chez la lapine, *C.R. Soc. Biol.*, 150, 2196, 1956.

127. Arnaud, G., Nouvelles recherches concernant l'influence de la réserpine sur la gestation de la lapine, *C.R. Soc. Biol.*, 157, 1585, 1963.

128. Tuchmann-Duplessis, H. and Mercier-Parot, L., Répercussion d'un somnifère, le glutéthimide, sur la gestation et le développement foetal du rat, de la souris et du lapin, *C.R. Acad. Sci.*, 256, 1841, 1963.

129. Tuchmann-Duplessis, H. and Mercier-Parot, L., Influence de doses croissantes de glutethimide (Doridène) sur la gestation et le développement foetal du lapin, *C.R. Soc. Biol.*, 157, 5, 1963.

130. Berger, F. M., The pharmacological properties of 2-methyl-2-*n*-propyl-1, 3-propanediol dicarbamate (Miltown®), a new interneuronal blocking agent, *J. Pharmacol. Exp. Ther.*, 112, 413, 1954.

131. Bertrand, M., Effets du méprobamate sur l'évolution de la gestation chez la ratte, *C.R. Soc. Biol.*, 154, 2309, 1960.

132. Caldwell, M. B. and Spille, D. F., Effect on rat progeny of daily administration of meprobamate during pregnancy and lactation, *Nature*, 202, 832, 1964.

133. Kletzkin, M., Wojciechowski, H., and Margolin, S., Postnatal behavioural effects of meprobamate injected into the gravid rat, *Nature*, 204, 1206, 1964.

134. Clavert, J., Etude de l'action du méprobamate sur la formation de l'embryon, *C.R. Soc. Biol.*, 157, 1481, 1963.

135. Nishikawa, M., Effect of the administration of meprobamate to pregnant mice on the development of the fetus. [In Japanese with Eng. summary.], *Acta Anat. Nippon.*, 38, 258, 1963.

136. Brar, B. S., The effect of meprobamate on fertility, gestation, and offspring viability and development of mice, *Arch. Int. Pharmacodyn.*, 177, 416, 1969.

137. Bough, R. G., Gurd, M. R., Hall, J. E., and Lessel, B., Effect of methaqualone hydrochloride in pregnant rabbits and rats, *Nature*, 200, 656, 1963.

138. Szirmai, E. A., Über die teratogene Untersuchung eines Nitromethaqualon des Parnox, *Aerztl. Forsch.*, 20, 47, 1966.

139. Harned, B. K., Hamilton, H. C., and Cole, V. V., The effect of the administration of sodium bromide to pregnant rats on the learning ability of the offspring. II. Maze-test, *J. Pharmacol. Exp. Ther.*, 82, 215, 1944.

140. Hamilton, H. C., The effect of the administration of sodium bromide on the behavior of the offspring: IV. Emotionality (timidity) and experimentally induced seizures, *J. Psychol.*, 19, 17, 1945.

141. Tuchmann-Duplessis, H. and Mercier-Parot, L., Difficultés d'interprétation rencontrées au cours de l'étude tératogène d'un neuro-sédatif, *C.R. Soc. Biol.*, 159, 6, 1965.

142. Kriegel, H., Untersuchungen zur Frage einer teratogenen Wirkung von Fenpentadiol bei Maus und Ratte, *Arzneimittelforschung*, 21, 13, 1971.

143. Kletzkin, M. and Berger, F. M., Influence of meprobamate on the fetus, fertility and post-natal development, in *Malformations Congénitales des Mammifères*, Tuchmann-Duplessis, H., Ed., Masson, Paris, 1971, 255.

144. Persuad, T. V. N. and Ellington, A. C., Teratogenic activity of cannabis resin, *Lancet*, 2, 406, 1968.

145. Persaud, T. V. N. and Ellington, A. C., Ganja (Cannabis sativa L.) in early pregnancy, *Lancet*, 2, 1306, 1967.

146. Geber, W. F. and Schramm, L. C., Effect of marihuana extract on fetal hamsters and rabbits, *Toxic. Appl. Pharmacol.*, 14, 276, 1969.

147. Wilson, J. G., Embryological considerations in teratology, *Ann. N.Y. Acad. Sci.*, 123, 219, 1965.

148. Idänpään-Heikkilä, J., Fritchie, G. E., Englert, L. F., Ho, B. T., and McIssac, W. M., Placental transfer of tritiated-1-Δ^9-tetrahydrocannabinol, *New Eng. J. Med.*, 281, 330, 1969.

149. Kennedy, J. S. and Waddell, W. J., Whole body autoradiography of the pregnant mouse after administration of C^{14}-Δ^9-tetrahydrocannabinol (Δ^9-THC), *Fed. Proc.*, 30, 279, abst., 1971.

150. Nosal, G., Complications et dangers des hallucinogénes aspects cytopharmacologiques, *Laval Med.*, 40, 48, 1969.

151. Geber, W. F., Congenital malformations induced by mescaline, lysergic acid diethylamide, and bromolysergic acid in the hamster, *Science*, 158, 265, 1967.

152. Alexander, G. J., Miles, B. E., Gold, G. M., and Alexander, R. B., LSD: injection early in pregnancy produces abnormalities in offspring of rats, *Science*; 157, 459, 1967.

153. Warkany, J. and Takacs, E., Lysergic acid diethylamide (LSD): no teratogenicity in rats, *Science*, 159, 731, 1968.

154. Sato, H., Pergament, E., and Nair, V., Lysergic acid diethylamide in pregnancy, *Fed. Proc.*, 28, 549, abst., 1969.

155. Alexander, G. J., Gold, G. M., Miles, B. E., and Alexander, R. B., Lysergic acid diethylamide intake in pregnancy: fetal damage in rats, *J. Pharmacol. Exp. Ther.*, 173, 48, 1970.

156. Nair, V., Bau, D., and Siegel, S., Effect of LSD in pregnancy on the biochemical development of brain and liver in the offspring, *Pharmacologist*, 12, 296, abst., 1970.

157. Roux, C., Dupuis, R., and Aubry, M., LSD: no teratogenic action in rats, mice, and hamsters, *Science*, 169, 588, 1970.

157a. Jensen, B. and Bro-Rasmussen, F., LSD's virkning på musefostre. [In Danish with Eng. summary.], *Ugeskr. Laeg.*, 133, 237, 1971.

158. Uyeno, T., Lysergic acid diethylamide in gravid rats, *Proc. West. Pharmacol. Soc.*, 13, 200, 1970.

159. Uyeno, E. T., Effects of prenatally administered lysergic acid diethylamide on the viability and behavioral development of rat offspring. Reported to the Committee on Problems of Drug Dependence, 32nd Annual Conference, NAS-NRC, Washington, D.C., Feb. 16-7, 1970.

160. Uyeno, E. T., Lysergic acid diethylamide administered to pregnant rats, *Hosp. Formul. Manag.*, 6, 15, 1971.

161. Auerbach, R. and Rugowski, J. A., Lysergic acid diethylamide: effect on embryos, *Science*, 157, 1325, 1967.

162. DiPaolo, J. A., Givelber, H. M., and Erwin, H., Evaluation of teratogenicity of lysergic acid diethylamide, *Nature*, 220, 490, 1968.

163. Hanaway, J. K., Lysergic acid diethylamide: effects on the developing mouse lens, *Science*, 164, 574, 1969.

164. Fabro, S. and Sieber, S. M., Is lysergide a teratogen?, *Lancet*, 1, 639, 1968.

165. Wilson, J. G., Teratological and reproductive studies in non-human primates, in *Methods for Teratological Studies in Experimental Animals and Man*, Nishimura, H. and Miller, J. R., Eds., Shoin, Tokyo, 1969, 16.

166. Kato, T., Jarvik, L. F., Roizin, L., and Moralishvili, E., Chromosome studies in pregnant rhesus macaque given LSD-25, *Dis. Nerv. Syst.*, 31, 245, 1970.

167. Yakovleva, A. I. and Sorakina, M. N., Effect of indopan on white rats and their progeny. [In Russian with Eng. summary.], *Farmakol. Toksik.*, 29, 224, 1966.

168. Rolsten, C., Effects of chlorpromazine and psilocin on pregnancy of C57BL/10 mice and their offspring at birth, *Anat. Rec.*, 157, 311, abst., 1967.

169. Vogel, F., and Röhrborn, G., Concluding remarks, in *Chemical Mutagenesis in Mammals and Man*, Vogel, R. and Röhrborn, G., Eds., Springer, New York, 1970, 453.

170. Tuchmann-Duplessis, H., Teratogenic drug screening – present procedures and requirements, *Teratology*, 5, in press.

BIOCHEMICAL ASPECTS OF DRUG DEPENDENCE

ENZYMES

S. T. Christian

TABLE OF CONTENTS

INTRODUCTION

This review is intended to summarize the effects of narcotic analgesics, psychotomimetics, barbiturates, and stimulants on isolated enzymes and enzyme systems. Desirable studies will be discussed that may not be directly related to the mechanism of drug action through enzyme inhibition, but certainly are related to the overall understanding of the properties of these compounds.

The discovery of enzymes per se and the ensuing knowledge concerning their biological function have inevitably allowed the pharmacologist to focus on these catalytic units as possible sites of drug action. Consequently, in the late 1940's and early 1950's, interest was generated in describing single enzyme systems that, if inhibited, could explain the mechanism of action of these drugs. This review begins with a discussion of the effect of narcotic analgesics on enzymes.

NARCOTIC ANALGESICS

Acetylcholine

Since the early observation by Richter and Crossland[1] that the amount of brain acetylcholine was increased considerably by the action of general depressants, many investigators studied the effects of narcotic drugs on the levels of this neurotransmitter in the brain. For example, Giarman and Pepeu[2] found that 50 mg/kg of morphine in rats resulted in a rise of 47% in total brain acetylcholine concentration. Later, Crossland and Slater[3] separated this increase in acetylcholine levels into its "free" and "bound" components. They found that anesthetics such as pentobarbital caused a rise in both free and bound brain acetylcholine, while morphine apparently raised the bound form and lowered the free form. These findings suggested that the effect of narcotic analgesics was to prevent acetylcholine release from the bound to the free form. This overall increase in total brain acetylcholine concentration could be accomplished by one of several mechanisms or by a combination of mechanisms. For example, a decrease in the rate of hydrolysis of acetylcholine by cholinesterase could explain the overall increase. Likewise, any stimulation of acetylcholine synthesis or inhibition of acetylcholine release could equally be invoked as an explanation. Each of these possibilities will be discussed further in this review.

Cholinesterases

The first demonstrable effects of a narcotic analgesic directly on an enzyme or enzyme system were reported by Bernheim and Bernheim[4] in 1936. These investigators found that the addition of morphine to crude brain homogenates containing cholinesterase inhibited the hydrolysis of acetylcholine to choline and acetic acid. This observation was later corroborated by other investigators.[5,6] It should be pointed out that crude brain homogenates contain at least two distinct types of cholinesterase, i.e., acetylcholinesterase (EC 3.1.1.7, acetylcholine acetylhydrolase) and butyrylcholinesterase (EC 3.1.1.8, acetylcholine acetylhydrolase). In many of these early studies no distinction was made between the inhibition of the two enzymes. Because acetylcholinesterase is found in the neuronal postsynaptic membrane, it is presumed to be the more relevant entity.[7] After these initial observations on brain homogenates Fraser[8] showed that both cholinesterases were inhibited by morphine, with butyrylcholinesterase being the more sensitive. In a comprehensive study by Young and co-workers[9] morphine and several morphinan derivatives were studied as inhibitors of cholinesterases derived from bovine erythrocytes, rat brains, and dog serum. This study was carried out using an inhibitor concentration of 10^{-3} molar and the results were reported in terms of % inhibition over control. With the erythrocyte enzyme (acetylcholinesterase) levorphanol was found to be the most potent inhibitor (95%) while codeine, levomethorphan, and dextromethorphan showed no inhibition at the 10^{-3} molar concentration. One important finding indicated that the narcotic antagonist nalorphine was also a moderately potent inhibitor. Using the enzyme from dog serum (butyrylcholinesterase), the authors reported no significant inhibition with the morphinan derivatives. Based on their findings that (1) no linear correlations existed between enzyme inhibition (for any of the cholinesterases studied) and analgesic potency and (2) the partial agonist levallorphan was one of the most potent inhibitors of acetylcholinesterase, the authors concluded that no correlation could be demonstrated between enzyme inhibition and analgesic potency. Unfortunately, this study as well as other early studies suffered from inadequate design. One of the problems, i.e., the lack of enzyme differentiation, has already been mentioned. Another and perhaps more serious problem has been the apparent lack of an efficient reproducible system. Hein and Powell[10] eliminated this latter criticism. Utilizing a purified acetylcholinesterase preparation and a technique described by Webb,[11] these investigators were able to reproducibly calculate both the type and magnitude of enzyme inhibition produced by a variety of narcotic drugs. A series of 13 substituted benzomorphans as well as morphine, nalorphine, and levallorphan were studied as inhibitors of the enzyme. The results of this study confirmed the earlier findings of Young and co-workers.[9] By utilizing the techniques discussed, the authors were unable to correlate analgesic activity with either magnitude of inhibition or nature of inhibition. In addition, these investigators also found that the partial-agonist levallorphan was a potent inhibitor of the enzyme.

In a recent study in our own laboratory, a series of methyl through dodecyl *N*-Alkyl substituted normeperidine congeners were studied as inhibitors of both acetyl and butyrylcholinesterase.[12] In this study attempts were also made to correlate the physical-chemical parameters of these compounds such as molecular parachors, hemolytic activity, alkyl chain length, and R_m values with both enzyme inhibition and analgesic potency. Like the benzomorphans, the normeperidine congeners were also found to be mixed inhibitors of acetylcholinesterase. In addition, they produced the same type of inhibition with butyrylcholinesterase when acetylcholine was used as substrate. Simple linear relationships were observed with butyrylcholinesterase when alkyl chain length, R_m values, and molecular parachors were plotted as a function of the logarithm of the enzyme inhibitor dissociation constants. More complex relationships were noted with acetylcholinesterase and these parameters. When analgesia was determined as a function of the alkyl chain substituent on the normeperidine molecule, a biphasic correlation was observed between chain length and ED_{50}. Analgesia increased until a chain length of about six carbons was reached and then decreased. These results suggest that the analgesic receptor possesses a definitive nonpolar geometric area that contributes to the binding of the analgesiophore through Van der Waal's interactions. Small changes in binding energies were reflected as significant increases in analgesic potency.

No linear correlation was found between analgesic activity and enzyme inhibition (with either enzyme). However, since both enzymes and the analgesic receptor display important nonpolar regions, the evidence indicates that the enzyme active center and the analgesic receptor have this property in common. The other physical-chemical parameters previously mentioned also exemplified this relationship.

In vivo studies concerning the nature of analgesic activity as a function of enzyme inhibition have also been reported. In a study by Johanesson[13] it was shown that the ratio of substrate concentration to enzyme (tissue) concentration was critical in determining inhibition. That is, the higher the substrate (acetylcholine) concentration, the more inhibitor had to be utilized to produce the same effect. This observation is to be expected in accordance with the concepts of enzyme saturation and basic Michaelis-Menton enzyme kinetics.[14] Johanesson[13] found brain concentrations in rats of 20 to 40 μg of morphine per gram of brain tissue 35 to 60 minutes after parenteral injection of 600 to 700 mg/kg of the drug. Using the in vivo data, sufficient morphine was added to brain homogenates to reproduce the actual in vivo drug concentration. Under these experimental conditions, substrate hydrolysis was inhibited 30 to 60%. No difference was noted in the levels of cholinesterase activity in brain homogenates of animals given morphine acutely or chronically under the same experimental conditions. In a recent study by Naik and Sheth[15] meperidine (24 mg/kg), codeine (50 mg/kg), and morphine (16 mg/kg) were injected intraperitoneally into rats and the animals sacrificed at the time of peak drug effect. Total cholinesterase activity was then determined in brain homogenates. Under these conditions only meperidine brought about decreased enzyme activity.

N-Demethylating Enzymes

In an attempt to invoke enzyme interactions in the explanation of the mechanism of tolerance to narcotic agents Axelrod[16] and later Axelrod and Cochin[17] studied an *N*-demethylating enzyme found in mammalian liver as a model system. These investigators found that the antagonist nalorphine inhibited the enzymatic *N*-demethylation of a variety of narcotic drugs. This blocking of the in vitro enzyme system is qualitatively similar to the antagonism of the pharmacological properties of these drugs. In enzyme preparations from animals chronically treated with morphine, substrates which showed the greatest degree of in vivo cross tolerance to morphine also showed the greatest inhibition (depression) of the *N*-demethylation process. In addition, this enzymatic process displays a high degree of stereospecificity toward both substrate (morphine, etc.) and inhibitor (nalorphine). This high degree of specificity represents a specific protein-drug interaction and, therefore, is considered a model of the receptors for narcotic drugs.[18] If the narcotic receptors in the brain were decreased with chronic exposure to these drugs, the reactivities of the specific neurons involved might diminish as an expression of tolerance. Unfortunately, these theories have since proven unfounded because they fail to account for physical dependence which seems to be integral with tolerance.

Protein Synthesis and Tolerance

Other theories which relate to an as yet unidentified protein moiety involved in the mechanism of narcotic tolerance development have arisen from the action of protein synthesis inhibitors in rats and mice.[19,20] In these experiments,[21-23] drugs such as actinomycin D, 8-azaguanine, puromycin, and cyclohexamide, administered with repeated doses of narcotics, appear to retard or impair the development of tolerance. However, if they are given alone to nontolerant animals, no change in the analgesic effect of morphine is seen. Similarly, if administered to tolerant animals, no change in tolerance is observed. These observations have been invoked as evidence for the synthesis of some specific protein necessary for the development of tolerance. Unfortunately, since metabolic protein synthesis inhibitors have such complex effects, it is nearly impossible to identify a specific protein involved.

Neuronal Metabolism

Neuronal metabolism itself, as reflected by studies on brain slices, appears to be unresponsive to the direct action of most narcotic drugs.[24] With various Krebs cycle substrates, brain slices respire at normal rates with morphine concentrations as high as 10^{-3} molar. This concentration is many times higher than that required for in vivo analgesia. If brain homogenates are likewise treated with these high drug concentrations, no changes are seen in the activity of various respiratory enzymes.[25,26] These findings indicate that the lack of response found with tissue slices is apparently not due to any cytoplasmic exclusion of the drug by cell membranes. Mulé[27,28] has shown that high concentrations of both morphine and nalorphine affect the overall turnover of various phospholipid fractions in brain slices. Since the drug concentrations are much higher than those found under physiological conditions, the meaning of these findings is difficult to interpret.

Cholinergic Transmission

Although it is doubtful that narcotics exert their effect directly on cholinesterase enzyme systems (since both agonist and antagonist are inhibitors of the enzymes), recent evidence reported using isolated strips of guinea pig ileum suggests that narcotics do directly affect cholinergic transmission.[29-31] Inhibition of ileum contractions and blockage of acetylcholine release occur at morphine concentrations as low as 10^{-7} molar. These effects are blocked by antagonists and are highly stereospecific.[32] Removal of the outer cellular layer from the gut strip destroys the ability of the ileum to respond to these drugs. This outer layer contains the nerve plexus.[33] Since Kosterlitz and Wallis[34] have shown that concentrations of morphine as high as 10^{-2} molar have no effect on axonal conduction, the most likely site of action appears to be at the synapse itself. Further evidence which supports this idea comes from experiments which show that impulse transmission is blocked at the synaptic junction when morphine is injected into the afferent artery of this superior cervical ganglion.[35,36] In addition, bathing brain tissue with 10^{-5} molar morphine through the ventricular or subarachnoid spaces diminishes the release of acetylcholine from synapses.[37,38] The relative importance of these findings is reflected in the fact that the concentration of drug required to inhibit acetylcholine release is low enough to be comparable with in vivo analgesic concentrations.

Acetylcholine Synthesis and Release

Even though the buildup of acetylcholine at the synapse has been interpreted as resulting from the inhibition of transmitter release, other mechanisms may be equally possible. For example, the buildup of acetylcholine may also be explained by a net increase in the synthesis of acetylcholine. In order to clarify this situation, the effect of narcotics on acetylcholine synthesis was studied. Morris[39] found that levorphanol, levallorphan, and dextrorphan stimulated the synthesis of acetylcholine in vitro. However, even at concentrations of 10^{-3} molar morphine showed no stimulation. In fact, it actually brought about a decrease in the rate of synthesis. These findings have been corroborated by De La Lande and Bentley.[40]

In more recent studies Sharkawi[41] and Datta et al.[42] have shown that the concentration of acetylcholine at the site of synthesis can also control the synthetic activity of choline acetyltransferase. That is, any decrease in the release of this neurotransmitter would be reflected as an inhibition of the enzyme. Consequently, the lowering of enzyme activity may be brought about by both enzyme inhibition and a negative feedback mechanism. In this latter study, choline acetyltransferase activity was depressed only in the caudate nucleus and not in the cortex or thalamus.

Even though these studies implicate acetylcholine in the mechanism of analgesic action, it is difficult to ascribe any exact function to this neurotransmitter. The overall brain concentration of this compound is quite large (about 10^{-5} molar) when compared to the theoretical number of analgesic receptors.[43] Moreover, the control of acetylcholine synthesis by a negative feedback system tends to stabilize its concentration except under exceptional cases.[44] The finding by Datta et al.[42] that choline acetyltransferase activity is most affected by morphine in the caudate nucleus and not in other areas of the brain may have further implications with regard to receptor localization, but to date no such data have been forthcoming.

In summary, it should be noted from this brief review that the narcotic drugs interact with several enzyme and enzyme related processes both in vivo and in vitro. However, a clear differentiation between these interactions and relevancy to pharmacological activity of narcotic drugs is difficult. It seems reasonable to assume that the mode of action of these compounds is much more complicated than the inhibition of a single enzyme specie. In fact, neuropharmacological and neurophysiological evidence will be presented in other sections of this book which implicate all four major neurotransmitters, i.e., 5-hydroxytryptamine, acetylcholine, norepinephrine, and dopamine in the mechanism of action of narcotic analgesics. Dole[45] has recently reviewed current theories regarding the biochemistry of addiction.

PSYCHOTOMIMETICS

Introduction

In recent years, the psychotomimetic agents (hallucinogens, psychoactive drugs) have become important not as therapeutic agents but primarily because of their abuse by a large segment of our society. The psychotomimetic drugs are unusual in that their major effect on behavior seems to be the direct result of a perceptual distortion of any sensory input. This characteristic is said to be similar to certain types of mental illness. Consequently, an understanding of the mechanism of action of these compounds may lead to a better understanding of the cellular and subcellular events involved in some types of mental disease.

Of the compounds which possess psychotomimetic activity, lysergic acid diethylamide (LSD-25) has been the most extensively studied. This compound has been chosen as a representative of this class of drugs with respect to its effects on enzymes and enzyme related systems.

LSD and Cholinesterases

Much attention has been paid to the inhibition of various cholinesterases by LSD. However, the results of these studies are somewhat contradictory. Thompson et al.[46,47] found that 10^{-6} molar LSD was the approximate I_{50} value for human plasma butyrylcholinesterase. The I_{50} value refers to the amount of inhibitor necessary to reduce the hydrolysis of substrate to 50% of a given control value. This amount of inhibition at 10^{-6} molar indicates that LSD is indeed a potent inhibitor of enzyme. However, when concentrations 10 times higher were incubated with acetylcholinesterase no inhibition could be detected. In a series of papers by Zsigmond and co-workers[48-50] the inhibitory properties of LSD were defined using cholinesterases from plasma, red cell, and gray matter. In these studies, LSD was found to be a true competitive inhibitor of all the enzymes tested. Results indicated that acetylcholinesterase was indeed inhibited by the drug, but its I_{50} value was nearly 100 times greater than with the plasma enzyme. Therefore, one must conclude that in earlier studies the concentration of LSD used was simply too low to observe any appreciable inhibition. A few investigators[51-53] have reported an activating effect of LSD on the cholinesterases derived from human serum and rat brain. This observation was made when the drug concentration was very low. These findings may be due to artifacts introduced with impure or mixed enzyme preparations.[54]

Goldenberg and Goldenberg[55] found that the nonpsychogenic drug 2-bromo-d-lysergic acid diethylamide (BOL) was equal in potency to LSD as an inhibitor of the plasma enzyme. This important finding was also confirmed for red cell acetylcholinesterase by Zsigmond and co-workers.[48]

Part of the confusion with regard to enzyme inhibition by LSD may be due to species differences. For example, Tabachnick and Grelis[56] reported that both LSD and BOL would inhibit the enzyme derived from mouse or human serum, but would not inhibit the enzyme when the source was dog, cat, or guinea pig serum. Even with these conflicting results, one important fact remains relatively clear. Since BOL (or morphine) is not a hallucinogenic agent but does inhibit both esterases, it is unlikely that any correlation exists between the psychotomimetic properties of LSD and enzyme inhibition. However, these conclusions are based on the inhibition of isolated in vitro enzyme systems. Using histochemical techniques, Goldberger[57] studied the inhibition of brain esterases by LSD in intact cells. Under these conditions the drug did not inhibit butyrylcholinesterase, but markedly inhibited acetylcholinesterase in brain sections. These findings contradict those reported in the isolated enzyme systems. Unfortunately, the effects of BOL were not determined in this study. These results seem to point out real differences between isolated systems and enzymes protected by cellular environments. Even though it seems unlikely, the possibility may still exist and a correlation between the two modes of action will be uncovered with further study.

LSD and Other Enzymes

Hoagland[58] reported that LSD was an inhibitor of the enzyme monoamine oxidase (MAO). In rat diaphragm preparations LSD also decreases oxygen consumption[59] and inhibits succinic dehydrogenase.[60] In a study by Clark and co-workers,[61] the drug inhibited alkaline phosphatase from rat brain. For further information on LSD and enzyme activity the reader is referred to a recent review by Giarman and Freedman.[62]

Selected Psychotomimetics

Interactions of other psychotomimetic drugs with various enzyme systems have also been described. For example, mescaline was found to inhibit the oxygen consumption of guinea pig cerebral cortex slices when the substrates were glucose, lactate, pyruvate, and glutamate.[63] Oxygen consumption was not inhibited with succinate as a substrate. Schueler[64] corroborated these findings, but found that respiration was inhibited only after prolonged preincubation without substrate. In electrically stimulated cortex slices both respiration and glycolysis are more sensitive to inhibition by mescaline than resting tissue.[65] Oxidative phosphorylation is not influenced by mescaline.[66]

Like LSD, bufotenin and psilocybin are inhibitors of both acetyl and butyrylcholinesterases[50,67] and *N*-diethyl (DET) and *N*-dimethyltryptamine (DMT) are inhibitors of monoamine oxidase.[68]

Studies on the mechanism of action of Δ1-tetrahydrocannabinol (THC) as a hallucinogenic drug at the enzyme level are as yet almost nonexistent. However, with the synthesis and release of this compound for scientific investigation intense experimentation in relation to enzymatic activity will surely ensue.

To date no enzyme studies have been reported which may be regarded as being specific for psychotomimetic drug action.

BARBITURATES

Oxygen Consumption and Oxidative Phosphorylation

Barbiturates as a pharmacological class of drugs have various properties or characteristics in common. The amount of oxygen consumed by the brain in situ per unit time decreases considerably during deep barbiturate coma. This decrease in oxygen consumption can be as great as 70%.[69] However, respiration in vitro of cerebral tissue obtained from animals pretreated with barbiturates is almost identical to control values.[70,71] The increase in brain oxygen consumption induced by electrical stimulation or 2, 4-dinitrophenol is apparently more sensitive to the depressing action of barbiturates than is normal respiration.[72] Barbiturates like phenobarbital exhibit a biphasic in vitro effect on oxygen uptake. At low concentrations the oxygen consumption of cerebral tissue is increased, while at high concentrations it is decreased.[73] Oxygen consumption and its subsequent inhibition are also direct consequences of the substrate being oxidized. For example, oxidation processes which involve the NAD (nicotinamide adenine dinucleotide)-linked substrates, are completely blocked by low concentrations of barbiturates (i.e., amobarbital) while the oxidation of succinate remains unaffected.[74] The explanation of this phenomenon lies in the fact that drugs like amobarbitol are specific inhibitors of NADH dehydrogenase.[75] Biochemists have taken advantage of this fact in elucidating the enzymatic steps involved in the mitochondrial respiratory chain.

Amobarbitol, along with other barbiturates, inhibits oxidative phosphorylation under in vitro conditions.[76-78] The uncoupling effect is usually accompanied by an inhibition of the inorganic phosphate-ATP exchange reaction.[79] Another barbiturate, thiopental, uncouples oxidative phosphorylation at concentrations as low as 2.5 x 10^{-4}M.[77] However, this effect does not effectively explain the mechanism whereby barbiturates exert their depressant effects.

Enzyme Induction

Barbiturates (such as phenobarbital) markedly increase the activity of liver enzymes which are responsible for the metabolism of various drugs.[80-83] This fact is of extreme importance when medical patients are being treated on any multiple drug therapy regime. A practical example is one of patients being treated simultaneously with barbiturates for sedation while on anticoagulant therapy. If a patient is receiving 75 mg/day of bishydroxycoumarin and is given an additional 60 mg/day of phenobarbital, a substantial decrease in plasma anticoagulant activity occurs. If the phenobarbital is discontinued, the plasma level of the anticoagulant and prothrombin time return to the pre-phenobarbital values.[84] This same phenomenon has been demonstrated with other sedative-hypnotics such as glutethimide, amobarbital, secobarbital, and with the minor tranquilizer, meprobamate.[85] The metabolism of other drugs is also stimulated by simultaneous barbiturate administration, e.g., diphenylhydantoin, griseofulvin, and digitoxin.[86] More recently, investigators have shown that ethanol, besides being metabolized by alcohol dehydrogenase, is also metabolized by microsomal enzymes. These enzymes are likewise induced by barbiturates.[87] The actual mechanism by which barbiturates stimulate drug metabolism may be twofold. Guarino et al.[88] found that in rats microsomal aniline hydroxylase activity was increased both quantitatively and qualitatively by treatment with phenobarbital. Not only did the barbiturate increase the relative amount of aniline hydroxylase, but it also produced an increase in Michaelis and binding constants for aniline.

Recent studies in several laboratories have shown that liver microsomes contain NADPH-dependent (reduced nicotinamide adenine dinucleotide phosphate) enzyme systems which hydroxylate steroids such as estradiol, testosterone, etc.[89-94] Therefore, prolonged treatment with barbiturates may be paralleled by increased metabolism and decreased phsyiologocal action of steroids in vivo.[95,96] Kuntzman[97] has thoroughly reviewed this subject recently.

Acetylation

Some barbiturates appear to have a direct action on acetylation processes. Pentobarbital has been extensively studied in this regard under in vitro conditions.[98-100] Results of these studies indicate that the drug inhibits aerobic acetylation, but has little if any effect on anaerobic acetylation. Therefore, the effect must be on the energy-yielding processes necessary for acetylation in the absence of added ATP. However, this effect is mimicked by many other drugs, particularly the convulsant barbiturates.[101]

Other Effects

Most barbiturates inhibit the incorporation of ^{32}P into erythrocytes[102] and other organs.[103] They also inhibit the incorporation of ^{35}S-methionine into cerebral proteins[104] but have no effect on ^{14}C-acetate incorporation into adipose tissue.[105] Barbiturates may furthermore inhibit the in vivo breakdown of high energy phosphate.[106] However, this point is somewhat unclear. Barbiturates like phenobarbital also increase the acetylcholine level in cerebral tissue.[1] Phenobarbital has no effect on cholinesterase activity.[4] Studies with amobarbital indicate that moderate concentrations of the drug almost completely inhibit the metabolism of sulfer in cerebral proteins and glutathione in vivo.[107] In addition, this drug apparently blocks the incorporation of labeled glycine into cerebral proteins.[108]

In the foregoing discussion it is evident that the barbiturate drugs affect various cellular and enzymatic processes. However, these effects, as well as others which were not discussed, do not appear to relate to any specific function which might be directly responsible for the depressant action of these compounds. For further details on the biochemical aspects of barbiturate action the reader is referred to several reviews.[109-113]

STIMULANTS

Monoamine Oxidase

Unlike the other classes of drugs of abuse

the stimulants have not been studied with regard to many diverse enzyme systems. However, d-amphetamine has been shown to inhibit mitochondrial monoamine oxidase in broken cells and other brain preparations.[114-116] Animals pretreated with amphetamines have demonstrated an inhibition of the oxidative deamination of intraventricularly injected ^{3}H-norepinephrine in rat brains.[117,118] Since amphetamines inhibit monoamine oxidase in vitro, investigators have speculated that the same phenomenon must occur in vivo. However, in a recent study by Rutlidge,[119] evidence was presented that indicated that the inhibition of the in vivo oxidative deamination of norepinephrine was primarily an indirect effect brought about by the inhibition of the neuronal uptake of norepinephrine. Conclusions were based on results demonstrating that pretreatment of rabbits with amphetamine caused an inhibition in the oxidative deamination of norepinephrine of isolated cortex slices and synaptosomes, but not in preparations without an intact neuronal membrane. These findings, coupled with the fact that various stereoisomers of amphetamine that exhibit a high degree of enzyme inhibition have the lowest pharmacological activity, thus appear to make any correlation unlikely.[120]

Other Interactions

Following the systemic administration of amphetamines, the in vitro consumption of oxygen by the brain is decreased. This observation has been corroborated in both humans[121] and monkeys.[122-124] In brain homogenates, however, with pyruvate as substrate no depression was observed in respiration or in oxidative phosphorylation with concentrations of 800 mg/ml.

Like the amphetamines, cocaine at a concentration of 5 x 10^{-5} molar caused a slight decrease in brain oxygen consumption. In electrically stimulated tissue the inhibition of both oxygen uptake and glycolysis was increased.[125,126]

The site of action at which cocaine inhibits respiration may be the first reaction in the Tricarboxylic acid cycle, that is, the condensation of acetic acid and coenzyme A. This reaction has been shown to be inhibited by the drug.[127]

A close quantitative relationship has been observed between the inhibitory action of local anesthetics on cellular respiration on the one hand and their local anesthetic potency on the other.[128,129]

Like many other CNS active drugs, cocaine also inhibits cholinesterase in erythrocytes, in *Electrophorus electricus,* and in plasma.[130,131] In plasma an enhancing action has also been observed when butyrylcholine was used as substrate.[132] The inhibitory action of cocaine on cholinesterase was about 5,000 times weaker than that of physostigmine.[131] At extremely high concentrations ($> 10^{-2}$ M) cocaine inhibits monoamine oxidase.[133,134]

CONCLUSION

Thus far in the evolution of our understanding with regard to the mechanism of action of those drugs that induce dependence, it appears unlikely that the inhibition of a single enzyme or enzyme system explains the activity of these compounds at the molecular or subcellular level. In fact, any interpretation of data relating to the effect of these drugs on the cellular metabolism of cerebral tissue, itself, is by and large more difficult than with any other organ. In part, this difficulty is due to the extreme complexity of such tissue. In most in vitro preparations the investigator must deal with complex nonuniform material composed of a mixture of neuronal and nonneuronal elements, each of which is composed of varying cell types. Unfortunately, under these conditions, the same overall effect can be produced by a variety of mechanisms. There is, however, little doubt that various enzymes are affected by those drugs and eventually with more data we may fully understand the role enzymes play in the mechanism of action of drugs inducing physical and/or psychic dependence.

REFERENCES

1. Richter, D. and Crossland, G., Variation in acetylcholine content of the brain with physiological state, *Amer. J. Physiol.,* 159, 247, 1949.

2. Giarman, N. J. and Pepeu, G., Drug-induced changes in brain acetylcholine, *Brit. J. Pharmacol.,* 19, 226, 1962.

3. Crossland, J. and Slater, P., The effect of some drugs on the "free" and "bound" acetylcholine of rat brain, *Brit. J. Pharmacol.,* 33, 42, 1968.

4. Bernheim, F. and Bernheim, M. L. C., Action of drugs on the choline esterases of the brain, *J. Pharmacol. Exp. Ther.,* 57, 427, 1936.

5. Wright, C. I., The inactivation of choline esterase by morphine and derivatives, *J. Pharmacol. Exp. Ther.,* 72, 45, 1941.

6. Herken, H., Maibauer, D., and Mueller, S., Acetylcholine content of brain and analgesic action of morphine and some 3-oxymorphinans, *Arch. Exp. Path. Pharmakol.,* 230, 313, 1951.

7. Nachmansohn, D., Proteins in excitable membranes, *Science,* 168, 1059, 1970.

8. Fraser, P. J., Acceleration of the enzymic hydrolysis of benzoylcholine, *Brit. J. Pharmacol.,* 11, 7, 1956.

9. Young, D. C., Vaude Ploeg, R. A., Featherstone, R. M., and Gross, E. G., The interrelationships among the central, peripheral, and anticholinesterase effects of some morphinan derivatives, *J. Pharmacol. Exp. Ther.,* 114, 33, 1955.

10. Hein, G. E. and Powell, K., Evaluation of kinetic constants for mixed inhibitors of cholinesterase, *Biochem. Pharmacol.,* 16, 567, 1967.

11. Webb, J. L., *Enzymes and Metabolic Inhibitors,* Vol. 1, Academic Press, New York, 1963, 58.

12. Christian, S. T., Gorodetzky, C. W., and Lewis, D. V., Structure-activity relationships of normeperidine congeners on cholinesterase systems *in vitro* and analgesia *in vivo, Biochem. Pharmacol.,* 20, 1167, 1971.

13. Johanesson, T., The concentration of morphine in the brains of rats receiving morphine and neostigmine, *Acta Pharmacol. Toxicol.,* 19, 23, 1962.

14. Dixon, M. and Webb, E. C., *Enzymes,* Longman's, Green and Co. Ltd., London, 1964, Chap. IV.

15. Naik, S. R. and Sheth, U. K., Studies on rat brain acetylcholine and cholinesterase. Part II. The influence of centrally acting drugs, *Indian J. Med. Res.,* 58, 480, 1970.

16. Axelrod, J., Possible mechanism of tolerance to narcotic drugs, *Science*, 124, 263, 1956.

17. Axelrod, J. and Cochin, J., The inhibitory action of nalorphine on the enzymatic *N*-demethylation of narcotic drugs, *J. Pharmacol. Exp. Ther.,* 121, 107, 1957.

18. Axelrod, J., The enzymatic *N*-demethylation of narcotic drugs, *J. Pharmacol. Exp. Ther.,* 117, 322, 1956.

19. Cohen, M., Keats, A. S., Krivoy, W., and Ungar, G., Effect of Actinomycin D on morphine tolerance, *Proc. Exp. Biol. Med.,* 119, 381, 1965.

20. Cox, B. M., Ginsburg, M., and Osman, O. H., Acute tolerance to narcotic analgesic drugs in rats, *Brit. J. Pharmacol.,* 33, 245, 1968.

21. Spoerlein, M. T. and Scrafani, J., The effect of various protein synthesis inhibitors on the development of narcotic tolerance, *Life Sci.,* 6, 1549, 1967.

22. Smith, A. A., Karmin, M., and Gavitt, J. A., Blocking effect of puromycin, ethanol, and chloroform on the development of tolerance to an opiate, *Biochem. Pharmacol.,* 15, 1877, 1966.

23. Way, E. L., Loh, H. H., and Shen, F. H., Morphine tolerance, physical dependence, and synthesis of brain 5-hydroxytryptamine, *Science*, 162, 1290, 1968.

24. Takemori, A. E., The effects of morphine, other opioids and their derivatives on the metabolism of cerebral cortex, in *The Addictive States,* Wickler, A., Ed., Williams and Wilkins, Baltimore, 1968, 53.

25. Seevers, M. H. and Shidemann, F. E., Effects of morphine and its deriv. on intermediary metabolism. I. The influence of morphine, codeine, and thebaine on the activity of several dehydrogenases and on the respiration of rat cerebrum, *J. Pharmacol. Exp. Ther.*, 71, 373, 1941.

26. Dodge, P. W. and Takemori, A. E., Effect of morphine on cerebral glycolytic intermediates and enzymes of rats *in vitro, Biochem. Pharmacol.,* 18, 1873, 1969.

27. Mulé, S. J., Effects of morphine and nalorphine on the metabolism of phospholipids in guinea pig cerebral cortex slices, *J. Pharmacol. Exp. Ther.,* 154, 370, 1966.

28. Mulé, S. J., Morphine and the incorporation of P_i^{32} into brain phospholipids of nontolerant, tolerant and abstinent guinea pigs, *J. Pharmacol. Exp. Ther.,* 156, 92, 1967.

29. Paton, W. D. M., The action of morphine and related substances on contractions and on acetylcholine output of co-axially stimulated guinea-pig ileum, *Brit. J. Pharmacol.,* 12, 119, 1957.

30. Cox, B. M. and Weinstock, M., The effects of analgesic drugs on the release of acetylcholine from electrically stimulated guinea-pig ileum, *Brit. J. Pharmacol.,* 27, 81, 1966.

31. De La Lande, I. S. and Porter, R. B., Factors influencing the action of morphine on acetylcholine release in the guinea-pig intestine, *Brit. J. Pharmacol.,* 29, 158, 1967.

32. Gyang, E. A., Kosterlitz, H. W., and Lees, G. M., The inhibition of autonomic neuroeffector transmission by morphine-like drugs and its use as a screening test for narcotic analgesic drugs, *Arch. Exp. Pathol. Pharmakol.,* 248, 231, 1964.

33. Paton, W. D. H. and Zar, M. A., The origin of acetylcholine released from guinea-pig intestine and longitudinal muscle strips, *J. Physiol.,* 194, 13, 1968.

34. Kosterlitz, H. W. and Wallis, D. I., The action of morphine-like drugs on impulse transmission in mammalian nerve fibers, *Brit. J. Pharmacol.,* 22, 499, 1964.

35. Pelikan, E. W., The mechanism of ganglionic blockade produced by nicotine, *Ann. N. Y. Acad. Sci.,* 90, 52, 1960.

36. Lewis, G. P. and Reit, E., Further studies on the action of peptides on the superior cervical ganglion and suprarenal medulla, *Brit. J. Pharmacol.,* 26, 444, 1966.

37. Beleslin, D. and Polak, R. L., Depression by morphine and chloralose of acetylcholine release from the cat's brain, *J. Physiol.,* 177, 411, 1965.

38. Beleslin, D., Polak, R. L., and Sproull, D. H., The release of acetylcholine into the subarachnoid space of anaesthetized cats, *J. Physiol.* (London), 177, 420, 1965.

39. Morris, R. W., Effects of drugs on the biosynthesis of acetylcholine; pentobarbital, morphine, and morphinan derivatives, *Arch. Int. Pharmacodyn.,* 133, 236, 1961.

40. De La Lande, I. S. and Bentley, G. A., The action of morphine and antagonists of the narcotic action of morphine on acetylcholine synthesis in brain, *Aust. J. Exp. Biol.,* 33, 555, 1955.

41. Sharkawi, M., Effects of morphine and pentobarbitone on acetylcholine synthesis by rat cerebral cortex, *Brit. J. Pharmacol.,* 40, 86, 1970.

42. Datta, K., Thal, L., and Wajda, I. J., Effects of morphine on choline acetyltransferase levels in the caudate nucleus of the rat, *Brit. J. Pharmacol.,* 41, 84, 1971.

43. Takahashi, R. and Aprison, M. H., Acetylcholine content of discrete areas of the brain obtained by a near-freezing method, *J. Neurochem.*, 11, 887, 1964.

44. Karczmar, A. G., Is the central cholinergic nervous system over-exploited?, *Fed. Proc.*, 28, 147, 1969.

45. Dole, V. P., Biochemistry of addiction, *Ann. Rev. Biochem.*, 39, 821, 1970.

46. Thompson, R. H. S., Tickner, A., and Webster, G. R., Cholinesterase inhibition by lysergic acid diethylamide, *Biochem. J.*, 58, 19, 1954.

47. Thompson, R. H. S., Tickner, A., and Webster, G. R., The action of lysergic acid diethylamide on mammalian cholinesterases, *Brit. J. Pharmacol.*, 10, 61, 1955.

48. Zsigmond, E. K., Foldes, F. F., and Foldes, V., The lack of correlation between the psychopharmacologic and acetylcholinesterase effect of LSD and its congeners, *Fed. Proc.*, 19, 266, 1960.

49. Zsigmond, E. K., Foldes, F. F., and Foldes, V., The *in vitro* inhibitory effect of LSD, its congeners and 5-hydroxytryptamine on human cholinesterases, *J. Neurochem.*, 8, 72, 1961.

50. Zsigmond, E. K., Foldes, F. F., and Foldes, V., The inhibitory effect of psilocybin and related compounds on human cholinesterase, *Fed. Proc.*, 20, 393, 1961.

51. Tonini, G., Particolari aspetti delle azioni centrali delle ammidi dell'acido lisergico e della 5-idrossitriptamina, *Boll. Soc. Ital. Biol. Sper.*, 31, 768, 1955.

52. Fried, G. H. and Antopol, W., The effect of psychotomimetic compounds on human cholinesterases, *Anat. Rec.*, 125, 610, 1956.

53. Fried, G. H. and Antopol, W., Effects of psychotomimetic compounds on human pseudocholinesterase, *J. Appl. Physiol.*, 11, 25, 1957.

54. Dixon, M. and Webb, E. C., *Enzymes*, 2nd ed., Longmans, Green and Co., London, 1964, 88.

55. Goldenberg, H. and Goldenberg, V., Inhibition of serum cholinesterases by lysergic acid derivatives. Submicro detection of LSD, *J. Hillside Hospt.*, 5, 246, 1956.

56. Tabachnick, I. I. A. and Grelis, M. E., Inhibition of cholinesterase hydrolysis of dihydromurexine by lysergic acid diethylamide and its 2-bromo derivative: a selective relationship, *Nature*, 182, 935, 1958.

57. Goldberger, M., The effects of lysergic acid diethylamide (LSD-25) upon the histochemical reactions for cholinesterases in the central nervous system, *Acta Anat.*, 46, 185, 1961.

58. Hoagland, H., A review of biochemical changes induced *in vivo* by lysergic acid diethylamide and similar drugs, *Ann. N. Y. Acad. Sci.*, 66, 445, 1957.

59. Ernsting, M. J. E., Kafoe, U. F., Nauta, W. Th., Oosterhais, H. K., and De Warrt, C., Biochemical studies on psychotropic drugs. I. The effect of psychotropic drugs on 2-aminobutyric acid and glutamic acid in brain tissue, *J. Neurochem.*, 5, 121, 1959.

60. Clark, L. C., Jr., Fox, R. P., Benington, F., and Morin, R., Effect of mescaline, lysergic acid diethylamide, and related compounds on the respiratory enzyme activity of brain homogenates, *Fed. Proc.*, 13, 27, 1954.

61. Clark, L. C., Jr., Fox, R. P., and Benington, F., Effects of psychotomimetic compounds on certain oxidative and hydrolytic enzymes in mammalian brain, *J. Nerv. Ment. Dis.*, 124, 466, 1956.

62. Giarman, N. J. and Freedman, D. X., Biochemical aspects of the actions of psychotomimetic drugs, *Pharmacol. Rev.*, 17, 1, 1965.

63. Quastel, J. H. and Wheatley, A. H. M., CCXIX. The effects of amines on oxidations of the brain, *Biochem. J.*, 27, 1609, 1933.

64. Schueler, F. W., The effect of succinate in mescaline hallucinations, *J. Lab. Clin. Med.*, 33, 1297, 1948.

65. Lewis, J. L. and McIlwain, H., The action of some ergot derivatives, mescaline and dibenamine on the metabolism of separated mammalian cerebral tissue, *Biochem. J.*, 57, 680, 1954.

66. Bain, J. A., A review on the biochemical effects *in vitro* of certain psychotomimetic agents, *Ann. N. Y. Acad. Sci.*, 66, 459, 1957.

67. Augustinsson, K. B., Cholinesterases. A study in comparative enzymology, *Acta Physiol. Scand.*, 15, Supp. 52, 1948.

68. Barlow, R. B., Effects on amine oxidase of substances which antagonize 5-hydroxytryptamine more than tryptamine on the rat fundus strip, *Brit. J. Pharmacol.*, 16, 153, 1961.

69. Bernheim, A. and Gottstein, Die sauerstoffaufnahme des menschlichen gehirns unter phenothiocinen, barbituraten und in der ischamie, *Pflügers Arch.*, 263, 102, 1956.

70. Wortis, S. B., Respiratory metabolism of excised brain tissue. II. The effect of some drugs on brain oxidation, *Arch. Neurol. Psychiatr.*, 33, 1022, 1935.

71. Grennell, R. G., Mendelson, J., and McElroy, W. D., Neuronal metabolism and ATP synthesis in narcosis, *J. Cell. Comp. Physiol.*, 46, 143, 1955.

72. Ghosh, J. J. and Quastel, J. H., Narcotics and brain respiration, *Nature*, 174, 28, 1954.

73. Westfall, B. A., Effects of phenobarbital on oxygen consumption of brain slices, *J. Pharmacol. Exp. Ther.*, 96, 193, 1949.

74. Low, H., Ernster, L., and Lindberg, O., Yield of oxidative phosphorylation in the succinate oxidase system, *Acta Chem. Scand.*, 9, 199, 1955.

75. Karlson, P., *Introduction to Modern Biochemistry*, Academic Press, New York, 1968, 208.

76. Kini, M. M., Methanol poisoning. I. Phosphorylation coupled to the mitochondrial oxidation of formaldehyde, *Biochim. Biophs. Acta*, 44, 599, 1960.

77. Brody, T. M. and Bain, J. A., Effect of barbiturates on acetylation, *Proc. Soc. Exp. Biol.*, 77, 50, 1951.

78. Aldridge, W. N. and Parker, V. H., Barbiturates and oxidative phosphorylation, *Biochem. J.*, 76, 47, 1960.

79. Jalling, O., Low, H., Ernester, L., and Lindberg, O., The relation of the site of action of amytal to oxidative phosphorylation, *Biochim. Biophys. Acta*, 26, 231, 1959.

80. Remmer, H., Die beschleunigung von enzymatischen oxydationen in dem lebermikrosomen unter dem einflub von barbituraten, *Arch. Exp. Pathol. Pharmakol.*, 236, 7, 1959.

81. Conney, A. H. and Burns, J. J., Biochemical pharmacological considerations of Zoxazolamine and Chlorzoxazone, *Ann. N. Y. Acad. Sci.*, 86, 167, 1960.

82. Kato, R., Induced increase of meprobamate metabolism in rats treated with phenobarbital or phenaglycodol, *Med. Exp.*, 3, 95, 1960.

83. Remmer, H. and Siegert, M., Beschleunigung des abbaus und adaptation des ZNS während der gewohnung or barbituraten, *Arch. Exp. Path. Pharmakol.*, 240, 22, 1960.

84. Cucinell, S., Conney, S. A., Sansur, A. H., and Burnes, M., Drug interactions in man. I. Lowering effect of phenobarbital on plasma levels of bishydroxycoumarin (Dicumarol®) and diphenylhydantoin (Dilantin®), *J. Clin. Pharmacol. Ther.*, 6, 420, 1965.

85. Hunningshake, D. B. and Azarnoff, D. L., Drug interactions with Warfarin, *Arch. Intern. Med.*, 121, 349, 1968.

86. Conney, A. H., Pharmacological implications of microsomal enzyme induction, *Pharmacol. Rev.*, 19, 317, 1967.

87. Mezey, F., Effect of phenobarbital administration on ethanol oxidizing enzymes and rates of ethanol degradation, *Biochem. Pharmacol.,* 20, 508, 1971.

88. Guarino, A. M., Gram, T. E., Gigon, P. L., Green, F. E., and Gillette, J. R., Changes in Michaelis and spectral constants for analine in hepatic microsomes from phenobarbital treated rats, *Molec. Pharmacol.,* 5, 131, 1969.

89. Kuntzman, R., Jacobson, M., Schneidman, K., and Conney, A. H., Similarities between oxidative drug-metabolizing enzymes and steroid hydroxylases in liver microsomes, *J. Pharmacol. Exp. Ther.,* 146, 280, 1964.

90. Kuntzman, R., Welch, R., and Conney, A. H., Factors influencing steroid hydroxylases in liver mitochondria, *Advances Enzyme Regulat.,* 4, 149, 1966.

91. Conney, A. H. and Klutch, A., Increased activity of androgen hydrolases in liver microsomes of rats pretreated with phenobarbital and other drugs, *J. Biol. Chem.,* 238, 1611, 1963.

92. Garren, L. D., Conney, A. H., and Thompkins, G. M., Stimulatory effect of phenobarbital on steroid metabolism, *J. Clin. Invest.,* 40, 1041, 1961.

93. Conney, A. H., Jacobson, M., Levin, W., Schneidman, K., and Kuntzman, R., Decreased central depressant effect of progesterone and other steroids in rats pretreated with drugs and insecticides, *J. Pharmacol. Exp. Ther.,* 154, 310, 1969.

94. Conney, A. H., Jacobson, M., Levin, W., Schneidman, K., and Kuntzman, R., Induction of liver microsomal 6 β-hydroxylase by diphenylhydantoin or phenobarbital: an explanation for the increased excretion of 6-hydroxycontisol in humans treated with these drugs, *Life Sci.,* 4, 1091, 1965.

95. Conney, A. H. and Schneidman, K., Enhanced androgen hydroxylase activity in liver microsomes of rats and dogs treated with phenylbutazone, *J. Pharmacol. Exp. Ther.,* 146, 225, 1964.

96. Kuntzman, R., Sansur, M., and Conney, A. H., Effects of drugs and insecticides on the anesthetic action of steroids, *Endocrinology,* 77, 952, 1965.

97. Kuntzman, R., Drugs and enzyme induction, *Ann. Rev. Pharmacol.,* 9, 21, 1969.

98. Johnson, W. J. and Quastel, J. H., Narcotics and biological acetylations, *Nature,* 171, 602, 1953.

99. Govier, W. M. and Gibbons, A. J., Phenobarbital inhibition of sulfanilamide acetylation in pigeon liver extracts, *Science,* 119, 185, 1954.

100. Mendelson, J. and Grenell, R. G., Effects of narcotics on coenzyme-A activity in acetylation, *Science,* 120, 802, 1954.

101. Marks, B. H., Effects of barbiturates on acetylation, *Science,* 123, 332, 1965.

102. Laity, J. L. H., The action of certain drugs on the uptake of ^{32}P by human erythrocytes, *Biochem. J.,* 71, 528, 1959.

103. Lingjaerde, P., Malm, O. J., Natrig, R. A., Skaug, O. E., Effect of pentobarbital on the uptake of ^{32}P by the rat, *Acta Pharmacol. Toxicol.,* 14, 214, 1958.

104. Gaitonde, M. K. and Richter, D., Metabolic activity of the proteins in the brain, *Proc. Roy. Soc.,* 145, 83, 1956.

105. Williams, W. R. and Van Bruggen, J. T., Acetate metabolism and nembutal anesthesia, *Biochim. Biophys. Acta,* 21, 172, 1956.

106. Lepage, G. A., Biological energy transformations during shock as shown by tissue analysis, *Amer. J. Physiol.,* 146, 267, 1964.

107. Nechaeve, G. A., Sulfur metabolism of protein, glutathione, and sulfatides, of the cerebrum of rats in narcosis and stimulation of the central nervous system, *Biochimija,* 22, 546, 1957.

108. Viadimirou, G. E. and Urinson, A. P., Glycine metabolism of brain tissue of rats in the normal state and in amytal narcosis, *Biochimija,* 22, 707, 1957.

109. Brody, T. M. and Bain, J. A., Effect of barbiturates on acetylation, *Proc. Soc. Exp. Biol.,* 77, 50, 1951.

110. Brody, T. M. and Bain, J. A., Barbiturates and oxidative phosphorylation, *J. Pharmacol. Exp. Ther.,* 110, 148, 1954.

111. Bain, J. A., Enzymatic aspects of barbiturate action, *Fed. Proc.,* 11, 653, 1952.

112. Aldridge, W. N., Action of barbiturates on respiratory enzymes, in *Ciba Foundation Symposia on Enzymes and Drug Action,* Monger, J. L. and de Reuck, A. V. S., Eds., J. and A. Churchill Ltd., London, 1962, 155.

113. Krebs, H. A. and Eggleston, L. V., The effect of dinitrophenol and amytal on the reduction of acetoacetate in the presence of succinate, *Biochem. J.,* 82, 134, 1962.

114. Blaschko, H., Richter, D., and Schlossmann, H., The oxidation of adrenaline and other amines, *Biochem. J.,* 31, 2187, 1937.

115. Mann, P. J. G. and Quastel, J. H., Benzedrine (B-phenylisopropylamine) and brain metabolism, *Biochem. J.,* 34, 414, 1940.

116. Pratesi, P. and Blaschko, H., Specificity of amine oxidase for optically active substrates and inhibitors, *Brit. J. Pharm.,* 14, 256, 1959.

117. Glowinski, J. and Axelrod, J., Effect of drugs on the uptake, release, and metabolism of ^{3}H-norepinephrine in the rat brain, *J. Pharmacol. Exp. Ther.,* 149, 43, 1965.

118. Glowinski, J., Axelrod, J., and Iverson, L. L., Regional studies of catecholamines in the rat brain. IV. Effects of drugs on the disposition and metabolism of ^{3}H-norepinephrine and ^{3}H-dopamine, *J. Pharmacol. Exp. Ther.,* 153, 30, 1966.

119. Rutledge, C., The mechanisms by which amphetamine inhibits oxidative deamination of morepinephrine in brain, *J. Pharmacol. Exp. Ther.,* 171, 188, 1970.

120. Grana, E. and Lilla, L., The inhibition of amine oxidase and the central stimulating action of the stereoisomeric amphetamines and l-phenylethylamines, *Brit. J. Pharmacol.,* 14, 501, 1959.

121. Abreu, B. E., Liddle, G. W., Burks, A. L., Shuterland, V., Elliott, H. W., Simon, A., and Margolis, L., *J. Amer. Pharm. Ass. Sci. Ed.,* 38, 186, 1949.

122. Dunke, P. R. and Schmidt, D. F., Quantitative measurements of cerebral blood flow in the Macaque monkey, *Amer. J. Physiol.,* 138, 421, 1942.

123. Schmidt, D. F., Kety, S. S., and Pennes, H. H., The gaseous metabolism of the brain of the monkey, *Amer. J. Physiol.,* 143, 33, 1945.

124. Desci, L., Uber die kombinerte wirkungs von luminal-Na und analeptica auf die phosphatesterbildung bzw. atmungskettenphosphorylierung von rattengehirnhomogenaten, *Arch. Exp. Path. Pharmakol.,* 230, 547, 1957.

125. Bollard, B. M. and McIlwain, H., Cocaine and procaine on the electrically stimulated metabolism of cerebral tissue, *Biochem. Pharmacol.,* 2, 81, 1959.

126. Decsi, L., Biochemical effects of drugs, in *Progress in Drug Research,* Jucker, E., Ed., Birkhaüser Verlag, Basel, 1965, 53.

127. Ryman, B. E. and Walsch, E., Site of inhibitory action of cocaine on cellular respiration, *Biochem. J.,* 58, 111, 1954.

128. Geddes, I. C. and Quastel, J. H., Effects of local anesthetics on respiration of rat brain cortex *in vitro, Anesthesiology,* 17, 666, 1956.

129. Watts, D. T., The effect of local anesthetics on the respiration of brain homogenates, *J. Pharmacol. Exp. Ther.*, 96, 325, 1949.

130. Skou, J. C., Local anesthetics. VIII. local anesthetic potency and inhibition of acetylcholinesterase in erythrocytes, *Acta Pharmacol. Toxicol.*, 12, 115, 1956.

131. Skou, J. C., Local anesthetics. VII. local anesthetic potency and inhibition of acetylcholinesterase, *Acta Pharmacol. Toxicol.*, 12, 109, 1956.

132. Fraser, P. J., Acceleration of the enzymic hydrolysis of benzoylcholine, *Brit. J. Pharmacol.*, 11, 7, 1956.

133. Mead, J. A. P., Shore, H., Weissbach, L., Leeper, L., and Brodie, B. B., Analgesic action of a series of substituted benzylic acid esters, *J. Pharmacol. Exp. Ther.*, 122, 51A, 1958.

134. Pletscher, A. and Gey, K. F., Pharmakologische beeinflussung des 5-hydroxytryptamin-stoffwechsels im gehirn und monoaminoxydasehenung *in vitro, Helv. Physiol. Pharmacol. Acta,* 17, C35, 1959.

PROTEINS AND NUCLEIC ACIDS

M. Ginsburg and B. M. Cox

TABLE OF CONTENTS

INTRODUCTION

Recent advances in the field of molecular biology have demonstrated the close interrelationship between nucleic acid and protein metabolism, and the overriding importance of these substances in the control of cell function has become apparent. Genetic information has been shown to be encoded in deoxyribonucleic acid (DNA), while ribonucleic acids (RNA), in various forms whose structure is determined by DNA, are concerned in translating this information into a functionally more useful form by specifying the sequence of amino acids in the synthesis of protein molecules. Proteins, as enzymes or structural proteins, control the reactions taking place within the cell. This information encoded in DNA will thus determine the cell's repertoire of possible responses, and in particular specify the nature of the adaptive response to a changed environment (for review see Reference 1). Therefore, it is not improbable that chronic drug administration could lead to metabolic changes involving this system.

The possible functions of nucleic acids and proteins in the phenomena of dependence on and tolerance to narcotic analgesic drugs have recently received some attention. Much less work has been directed to similar studies of ethanol and the barbiturates (except in relation to the metabolism of these substances), while this aspect of amphetamine pharmacology seems to have been entirely neglected. In this review we have confined ourselves to a discussion of studies directly related to protein and nucleic acids. Changes in degradative enzymes, and effects on neurohumonal transmission, which might well be initially directed by altered nucleic acid metabolism, are considered in other chapters.

NARCOTIC ANALGESIC DRUGS

Nucleic Acids

Experiments with Inhibitors of Nucleic Acid Metabolism

Actinomycin D – Actinomycin D has been shown to be a potent inhibitor of RNA transcription.[2] Cohen, Keats, Krivoy, and Ungar[3] reported that the administration of actinomycin D together with morphine to rats or mice over a period of days prevented or reduced the development of tolerance to the analgesic effects of morphine. These results have been confirmed by Cox, Ginsburg, and Osman,[4] who used a continuous intravenous infusion of morphine in rats to produce tolerance rapidly; a technique which thus allowed the effects of actinomycin D to be demonstrated during a treatment period as short as six hours. Actinomycin D was also shown to reduce the rate of development of tolerance to the analgesic effects of heroin, pethidine, etorphine, and dihydromorphine.[5] Rats, in which the acquisition of tolerance had been prevented by actinomycin D at a first exposure to morphine, showed at a second test infusion of morphine, started 24 hours after the start of the first, an analgesic response almost identical to that given by rats which had not previously been exposed to morphine.[6] Smith, Karmin, and Gavitt[7] have shown that the tolerance which develops to the lenticular opacity-producing effects of levorphanol in mice was significantly reduced by giving a large dose of actinomycin D with the levorphanol. The effects of actinomycin D on tolerance to other actions of morphine do not appear to have been studied quantitatively, but qualitative observation suggests that the development of tolerance to the respiratory depression, and the reduction of motor activity produced by morphine in rats is also delayed.

When rats were made tolerant by several exposures to morphine, or by a long intravenous infusion of morphine, the administration of actinomycin D, together with morphine, did not restore the analgesic response to the nontolerant level, but prevented the further development of tolerance. The actinomycin D also exposed the slow decay of the tolerant state, in that there was a gradual recovery of the analgesic response during the actinomycin infusion.[4]

Effects of actinomycin D on the development of physical dependence on narcotic analgesics have not been conclusively established. Cox[8] has shown that concurrent administration of actinomycin D with morphine will reduce the frequency with which morphine-dependent mice exhibit the characteristic jumping response elicited by naloxone. These results may be caused by the debilitating effects of the combined treatment, rendering the mice physically incapable of jumping with the same frequency as mice receiving morphine alone. It is not clear whether actinomycin D was affecting the processes responsible for physical dependence.

In reducing the rate of development of tolerance to analgesic drugs, actinomycin D appears to be acting in the central nervous system, rather than at peripheral sites. Actinomycin D administered intracerebrally to rats was effective at lower doses than required by the intravenous route; the dose ratio, intravenous/intracerebral was about 10:1.[5] Loh, Shen, and Way[9] have shown that actinomycin D at a dose of 0.5 mg/kg i.p. increases the amount of morphine that penetrates from the blood to the brain. However, it seems unlikely that this is responsible for the observed effects of actinomycin D on tolerance development, since Loh et al. found that the penetration of heroin into the brain was unaffected by actinomycin D, although the development of tolerance to this drug can also be impaired by actinomycin D.[4] Furthermore, in experiments with ^{3}H-labelled dihydromorphine, a lower dose of actinomycin D than used by Loh et al. has been shown to prevent tolerance development without affecting the brain concentration of the analgesic drug.[5]

It is possible that the action of actinomycin D on tolerance development is unrelated to inhibition of RNA transcription. However, Cox and Osman[6] have demonstrated that a dose of actinomycin D, which prevented the development of tolerance, significantly reduced the incorporation of ^{14}C-lysine into brain protein. These measurements were made between two and three hours after the start of administration of actinomycin D and morphine, when tolerance development, and its inhibition by the antibiotic were only just becoming apparent. At later times the inhibition of RNA and protein synthesis is likely to have been greater.[10]

Purine and pyrimidine analogues – The administration of certain purine and pyrimidine analogues has been reported to reduce the degree of tolerance developed to morphine. Spoerlin and Scrafani[11] gave mice 8-azaguanine together with morphine over a period of five days. On the fifth day they determined the LD_{50} for morphine in one group of rats, and measured the dose of morphine required to give a standard increase in reaction time in another group. Using both measures of the action of morphine, they found that 8-azaguanine reduced the increase in effective dose produced by the five-day treatment with the analgesic drug.

During the course of an intravenous infusion of morphine in rats 6-mercaptopurine and 5-fluorouracil have been shown to reduce the rate of tolerance development to morphine analgesia. In both cases the drugs were ineffective after systemic administration, but inhibited tolerance development when given by intracerebral injection. The two drugs were also more effective when administered in three doses divided over the 2 days prior to the morphine infusion.[2] Those treatments which inhibited the acquisition of tolerance were shown to produce significant reductions in the incorporation of ^{14}C-orotic acid into brain RNA.[6]

Nucleic Acid Metabolism During Morphine Treatment

An analogue of morphine, levorphanol, has been shown to inhibit the synthesis of RNA in *E. coli*, ribosomal RNA synthesis being more sensitive to this inhibitory action than mRNA or tRNA.[12] However, the concentrations employed in these experiments (of the order of 10^{-3} M) are much higher than those likely to be encountered by intact mammals during the development of tolerance and dependence.

There have been very few reported studies of the effects of morphine treatment on nucleic acid metabolism in higher animals. Cox and Osman[6] measured the effect of a three-hour morphine intravenous infusion in rats on the incorporation of ^{14}C-orotic acid, injected intracerebrally, into total brain RNA. The morphine treatment produced no effect on RNA synthesis in these experiments. Clouet[13] reports that narcotic drug administration did not affect the levels of messenger RNA, brain ribonuclease, or ribonuclease inhibitor in rat brain, but gives no experimental details.

In a histochemical study, Nosal, Radouco-Thomas, Garcin, and Radouco-Thomas[14] measured the effects of morphine treatment on the staining by toluidine blue-molybdate of structures in Purkinje cells of the rat cerebellum. This stain is selective for nucleoproteins and permits the differentiation of desoxyribonucleoproteins and ribonucleoproteins. Doses of 2 to 10 mg/kg i.p. of morphine lead to a less dense and more diffuse appearance of the cells studied. Larger doses produced a more consistant effect. When increasing doses were given over several days, similar changes occurred which became stabilized around the fourteenth day, despite the continued increase in morphine dosage. Other ribonucleoprotein-containing structures in the nucleus, cytoplasm, and desoxyribonucleoprotein in the nucleus were not affected by these morphine treatments. The functional significance of these changes in the cell body is uncertain. Since actinomycin D (10 mg/kg i.p.) treatment was shown to produce rather similar effects, it might be concluded that they are a consequence of reduced RNA synthesis. However, Koenig et al.[10] have shown that under certain circumstances actinomycin D can cause an increase in cytoplasmic (but not nuclear) RNA synthesis.

Nosal et al.[14] also investigated the effects of incubating morphine in vitro with human buccal cancer cells in culture, recording the fluorescence produced by the nucleic acids after exposure to acridine orange. A morphine concentration of 10^{-3} M was required to produce significant effect. The principal effect was an increase in fluorescence, attributable to cytoplasmic RNA after a one-hour exposure to morphine, but after 24 hours the cytoplasmic RNA fluorescence was less than in control cultures. The relevance of these studies, with very high concentrations of analgesic drug, to the action of morphine on the nervous system remains to be demonstrated.

Interactions Between Narcotic Analgesics and Nucleic Acids

Mellet and Woods[15] injected N-^{14}C-methyl levorphanol into rats and showed, after subcellular fractionation of the brain, liver, and kidney, that there was a relatively high concentration of radioactivity in the fraction containing nuclei. They did not, however, attempt to determine whether the drug was bound to nucleic acid or protein (Mulé, Redman, and Flesher[16] did not find a similar distribution for ^{3}H-morphine). Clouet and Williams,[13,17] have studied the interaction between analgesic drugs and nucleic acids of the central nervous system in more detail. ^{3}H-dihydromorphine injected into the cisterna magna of the rat was found in fractions containing RNA isolated from the brains of animals killed from 30 minutes to 4 hours after injection of the drug. After separation by sucrose density gradient centrifugation, most of the radioactivity was associated with heavy RNA (285 and over), although all RNA fractions contained some label. The binding was firm enough to withstand a second fractionation in the presence of unlabelled RNA, but the dihydromorphine could be removed by exhaustive dialysis. It is not clear whether this binding is responsible for the general reduction in protein synthesis seen after morphine treatment (see overleaf).

An in vitro reaction between narcotic antagonists nalorphine and levallorphan and sRNA has been demonstrated.[13] Addition of concentrations of 10^{-3}M levallorphan and 10^{-2}M nalorphine, to an amino acid incorporating system containing rat brain ribosomes leads to the coprecipitation of the analgesic antagonist and sRNA. Similar concentrations of morphine, pethidine, and levorphanol were ineffective.

Protein

Experiments with Inhibitors of Protein Synthesis

Two drugs which inhibit protein synthesis directly, namely cycloheximide and puromycin, have been used in studies of morphine tolerance and dependence. Cycloheximide acts at the ribosome to inhibit peptidyl transferase,[18,19] while puromycin appears to behave as an analogue of a tRNA-amino acid complex.[20]

Way, Loh, and Shen[21,22] have shown that the administration of cycloheximide (20 mg/kg i.p. per day) together with increasing doses of morphine over a period of three weeks prevented the development of tolerance to the analgesic effect of morphine that was observed in mice receiving morphine alone. These experiments may be criticized on the grounds that three weeks is a very long period to administer such a potentially toxic drug, and indeed these workers report a cumulative mortality of 85% produced by the combined cycloheximide morphine treatment over this period. However, they claim that the response to the painful test stimulus employed (application of heat to the tail) was not impaired despite the considerable loss of weight of the survivors. In a second experiment carried out over five days, the smaller development of tolerance produced by attenuated morphine treatment was also prevented by concurrent cycloheximide treatment.

The ability of cycloheximide to impair the development of tolerance to the analgesic effects of morphine has also been demonstrated in rats.[5,6] In these experiments, the morphine was given by intravenous infusion over a period of seven hours, and the decline in analgesic response over the last five hours of the infusion as tolerance developed was prevented or slowed by the simultaneous administration of cycloheximide. When tolerance development was prevented in this way, a second infusion of morphine alone on the following day produced a much greater analgesic response than in animals which simply received two consecutive morphine infusions in the absence of cycloheximide. Tolerance development was also suppressed when cycloheximide was administered by intracerebral administration.

Using the same technique, the development of tolerance to the analgesic effects of morphine in rats has also been inhibited by puromycin.[5,6] The drug was administered intracerebrally in these experiments, and in doses of 100 μg or 200 μg produced approximately an 80% inhibition of the tolerance developed during the course of the morphine infusion. Effective doses of both cycloheximide and puromycin were shown to cause a large reduction in the incorporation of ^{14}C-lysine into brain protein, under similar experimental conditions.

The effects of cycloheximide on the development of physical dependence in mice have been described by Way and co-workers[21,22] who showed that characteristic jumping response elicited in morphine-dependent mice by injection of naloxone did not occur if the mice were treated with cycloheximide throughout their period of exposure to morphine. These results are supported by essentially similar experiments in which a much larger dose of morphine was administered as pellet subcutaneously,[8] and in which concurrent administration of cycloheximide approximately halved the frequency of jumping following naloxone challenge. As in the parallel experiments with actinomycin D (described previously), it is not certain that these effects of the metabolic inhibitor on a particular characteristic of the withdrawal syndrome are necessarily due to a direct effect on the processes responsible for the development of physical dependence. The debilitating effects of protein synthesis inhibitor may prevent the mice from jumping as vigorously as animals receiving morphine alone. Measurement of other aspects of the withdrawal syndrome less athletic in character would be more appropriate in animals given drugs such as cycloheximide.

Protein Metabolism During Morphine Treatment

The rate of synthesis of protein is conventionally estimated, after the injection of a radioactively-labelled amino acid, by measuring the specific activity of the protein and expressing this relative to the specific activity of the free amino acid pool. Studies of the effect of morphine treatment on the rate of protein synthesis in vivo are complicated by the effects of morphine on the rate of decline of radioactivity in the free amino acid pool. Clouet and Neidle[23] have shown that a very large dose of morphine (60 mg/kg as sulphate) in rats results in the retention in the brain for a longer period of time of ^{14}C-leucine injected intracisternally, although the conversion of leucine to other amino acids was not impaired. The effect of morphine on amino acid efflux was not confined to the naturally occurring *l*-isomer, since the efflux of *d*-leucine was also reduced by morphine.[23]

In any particular animal, the specific activity of the free amino acid pool can only be estimated at the end of the experiment, and not at the time that incorporation into protein actually occurs. Radioactivity in amino acid metabolites of the injected labelled amino acid becomes increasingly significant in incorporation studies as the period over which incorporation is measured is increased, and may be different in drug-treated and control groups. When attempts are made to estimate the rate of synthesis of proteins of subcellular fractions, a further complication is introduced by the improbability that the precursor amino acid pool for protein synthesis is the same for all subcellular fractions. This problem is particularly relevant to studies of the synaptosomal fraction, where some of the protein present will have been transported down the axon while other protein will probably have been synthesised locally. With these complications in mind, it is apparent that the effects of morphine on protein synthesis can only be described in a qualitative or comparative manner.

Clouet and Ratner[24] found that the incorporation into brain protein of ^{14}C-leucine injected intracisternally in rats was reduced by pretreatment of the rats following 60 mg/kg i.p. dose of morphine. This reduction was apparent in the nuclear, crude mitochondrial (i.e., containing, presumably, mitochondria, synaptosomes, and myelin), microsomal, and soluble fractions of brain homogenates. The reduction was maximal three to four hours after the morphine dose. Concurrent administration of a dose of nalorphine, which completely prevented the analgesic action of this dose of morphine, only partially reduced the fall in amino acid incorporation. After five daily injections of morphine, rats showed tolerance to the analgesic effects of morphine although the inhibition of leucine incorporation into brain proteins still occurred. It is unfortunate that in these experiments such a large dose of morphine was used since tolerance to the depressant effects on protein synthesis may have become apparent at lower morphine dose levels. Some of the effects on protein synthesis might also be attributed to the general depressant effects of the drug with concomitant reduction in neuronal activity. However, Clouet and Ratner were able to show that hypothermia produced by this morphine treatment did not contribute to the observed decline in amino acid incorporation. Ribosomes isolated from both the brain and liver of rats showed reduced ability to incorporate amino acids into protein after morphine treatment.[25]

Cox and Franklin[26] have compared the relative distribution of intracerebrally injected ^{14}C-lysine incorporated in protein, between the mitochondrial, synaptosomal, myelin, microsomal, and soluble fractions of rat brain homogenates, in control and morphine treated animals. Acute or chronic treatment with morphine did not alter the relative distribution of radioactive protein between the subcellular fractions, suggesting that morphine treatment did not have a selective effect on protein synthesis in any particular subcellular fraction.

In view of these results it is probable that any increased synthesis of (a) protein that might be presumed, from experiments with inhibitors of protein synthesis, must take place against a background of an overall reduction in amino acid incorporation. In such circumstances it may be necessary to study amino acid incorporation into individual proteins or protein fractions in order to correlate changes in protein synthesis with drug treatment and the onset of tolerance.

Morphine and related drugs have been shown to inhibit transmitter release at certain peripheral synapses[27,28] and it is possible that a similar action at certain central synapses may be responsible for some of the effects of these drugs. The synapse may also be the locus of adaptive changes brought about in response to prolonged reductions in the efficiency of synaptic transmission.[29] Cox[8] has investigated the effects of morphine on the incorporation of radioactivity-labeled lysine into proteins of the synaptic plasma membrane (SPM) fraction (consisting of paired thickened synaptic membranes, together with some single membranes, and a little myelin) isolated from the hypothalamus, pons, and medulla of the rabbit. Preliminary experiments indicated that a three hour intravenous infusion of morphine did not alter the incorporation of lysine into the SPM fraction.

In subsequent experiments the SPM fraction was solubilised in phenol; acetic acid (2:1, w/v) containing 5M urea, and the protein constituents fractionated by polyacrylamide gel electrophoresis. Morphine treated rabbits received four doses over a period of 48 hours, each dose being followed by an injection into the cerebral ventricles (aqueduct) of ^{3}H-lysine after 30 minutes. This dose regimen was shown to produce almost complete tolerance to the analgesic effects of a test dose of morphine. Control rabbits received saline in place of the morphine and ^{14}C-lysine in place of the tritium isotope. At the end of the treatment period the hypothalamus, pons, and medulla taken from one morphine treated and one control rabbit were homogenised and fractionated together. Measurement of the relative levels of ^{3}H to ^{14}C in serial slices of the polyacrylamide gels failed to demonstrate any difference in amino acid incorporation caused by the morphine administration.

These experiments suggest that large-scale changes in the turnover of particular proteins in the synaptic membranes do not occur following this morphine treatment. However, smaller scale changes, for example, the postulated increase in transmitter receptor population,[29] would not in all probability have been detected by the techniques employed.

Interactions Between Narcotic Analgesics and Proteins

Binding of morphine to dog serum proteins was demonstrated by Blaney and Woods[30] who found in their in vitro experiments that approximately 20 to 30% of the morphine added to the serum was bound. When the serum was obtained from morphine-tolerant dogs, a similar degree of binding was observed.

In a study of the subcellular distribution of ^{3}H-morphine in guinea pig brain tissue after subcutaneous administration, Mulé, Redman, and Flesher[16] found that the morphine was primarily located in the soluble fraction, and that less than 2% of the morphine in this fraction was protein bound. They reported no significant accumulation of morphine in the synaptosomal fraction. However, in contrast, Scrafani, Williams, and Clouet[31] have found that ^{3}H-dihydromorphine was accumulated by the synaptosomal fraction of rat brain homogenates. Similar results were obtained after both in vivo in vitro studies. Binding was reduced if the drug and brain homogenate were incubated at 0°C, and increased in the presence of oxygen and added ATP, suggesting that it was partially dependent on metabolic energy. These experiments involved only a single centrifugation step, and it is possible that the failure of Mulé et al.[16] to observe accumulation in the synaptosomes was due to redistribution of the drug occurring during the repeated centrifugation steps employed in their experiments.

Accumulation of drug by particulate fractions of cell homogenates, or binding of drug to protein is not necessarily of pharmacological significance. In a preliminary report, Pal, Goldstein, and Lowney[32] have described experiments in which the observation that morphine-like activity resides only in the D-(-) isomer of isomeric pairs of analgesic drugs has been employed in an attempt to identify pharmacologically significant interactions between analgesic drugs and constituents of brain homogenates. They have attempted to locate stereoselective binding sites, measured as the difference in binding of radioactive levorphanol in two experimental situations: (1) in the presence of a large excess of nonradioactive dextrorphan and (2) in the presence of a large excess of nonradioactive levorphanol. Significant stereoselective binding was found only in a membrane fraction which initially separated with the crude nuclear pellet, but subsequently floated on 2M sucrose. The chemical nature of this binding site has not so far been determined, but it was not extracted from the membranes by surface active agents although 70% of the membrane protein could be solubilised in this way. The morphological nature of this membrane fraction, and the significance of this binding remain to be established.

Transferable Factors Claimed to Affect the Sensitivity of Animals to Morphine

There are several reports of experiments in which serum or tissue extracts from tolerant animals modified the response of recipient animals to a subsequent dose of morphine. Kornetsky and Kiplinger[33] injected serum from morphine-tolerant dogs into rats, and measured the effect of a standard dose of morphine given 48 hours later on the time taken to swim a measured distance.

Rats receiving serum from tolerant dogs took significantly longer than rats receiving serum from untreated dogs, when tested 30 and 60 min after the morphine dose, although at later times there was no difference. Kiplinger and Clift[34] subsequently showed that interperitoneal injection of morphine-tolerant dog serum potentiated the analgesic effects of morphine in mice, as measured by the hot plate test. In contrast, when serum was taken from rabbits 24 hours or one week after withdrawal of morphine, the analgesic effect of a test dose in mice was reduced and not potentiated.[35] In a subsequent review of this work Cochin and Kornetsky[36] indicated that they were unable to confirm the results reported by Kiplinger and Clift,[34] or their own experimental work with rabbits. Their original experiments with rats suggested that serum obtained from morphine-withdrawn rats reduced the analgesic effects of morphine in mice, but again in subsequent experiments they were unable to confirm these results. Cochin and Kornetsky[36] were unwilling to consider that errors of experimental design or procedure had been responsible for the earlier positive results, and suggest that a very unstable active factor in the serum may have been unwittingly destroyed in subsequent attempts to replicate the experiments.

Shortly after the publication of the early reports implying the existence of factors in serum of morphine-treated animals which modified the response to morphine in recipient animals, Ungar and Cohen[37] claimed that extracts of morphine-tolerant rat brain injected into mice, reduced analgesic response to subsequent test doses of morphine. The responsible factor was reported to be soluble in water, insoluble in ethanol or acetone, and dialysable. Incubation with chymotrypsin caused loss of activity, and it was suggested that the active material might be a small protein or peptide. Tirri[38] attempted to demonstrate the existence of a transferable factor in morphine-tolerant mouse brains, but failed to observe any reduction of response to morphine in treated mice. Failure to transfer tolerance from rats to mice by injection of brain extracts from tolerant animals has also been reported by Smits and Takemori[39] and Cox and Ginsburg.[5] Nevertheless, Ungar and Galvan[40] have confirmed their ability to reduce the sensitivity of recipient animals to morphine by injecting extracts of tolerant rat brain, although, like Tirri,[38] they were unable to transfer tolerance from mice to mice. They suggest that failure to observe transfer from rats to mice may occur if inadequate amounts of brain extract are administered, or if the recipient animals are tested at too short a time interval after treatment with brain extracts. Successful transfer of morphine tolerance from rats to rats has been described by Tulunay, Kiran, and Kaymakcalan.[41]

It seems appropriate to refer here to the analogous experiments in which transfer of learned behavior has been attempted by the injection into recipient animals of brain extracts from trained animals.[42,43] In this field also, some workers have been unable to demonstrate significant transfer,[44] but in a recent summary, Ungar[45] has pointed out that successful transfer has now been claimed by groups in many different laboratories.

In all these experiments the transferred material has been injected into the peritoneal cavity of the recipient animals. One difficulty that must be overcome in accepting the claims of successful transfer is the difficulty of conceiving how material with high molecular weight claimed to be RNA or protein,[41,46] could pass from the peritoneal cavity to the central nervous system without being subjected to extensive metabolic degradation. If, as Ungar[45] claims, the active material is a polypeptide, then its passage across membrane barriers may be conceded more readily, but its escape from possible inactivation processes (not to mention its actions in the CNS, should it reach there) remains difficult to conceive. However, if the transfer factor is sufficiently stable to survive this passage, it becomes inappropriate to ascribe failure to demonstrate transfer to the high lability of the active material.

ETHANOL AND BARBITURATES

The function of nucleic acids and proteins in the increased metabolic degradation of ethanol and certain barbiturate drugs during their chronic administration is discussed elsewhere. The possible significance of nucleic acids and proteins in the altered sensitivity of the central nervous system has received little attention.

Short-term administration of ethanol to mice as a 10% solution in their drinking water does not alter the ability of cell-free brain preparations to incorporate amino acids into protein.[47] However, when ethanol was administered in this way for 10 days or longer, the brain preparations showed a reduced ability to synthesize protein in vitro. Homogenates from brains of chronically-treated animals showed a reduced ability to synthesise amino-acyl-tRNA, and the ribosomes were less functionally active than ribosomes from untreated mice brain. Perhaps in compensation for this reduction in efficiency, there was an increase in the number of ribosomes obtained from the brains of the mice after several days of ethanol ingestion. Tewari and Noble[47] have pointed out that these effects were produced by a lower daily ethanol consumption than has been shown, in the same strain of mice, to impair shock avoidance learning.[48]

A single dose of pentobarbitone has been found to reduce incorporation of ^{3}H-histidine into mouse brain proteins,[49] and ^{35}S-methionine into rat brain proteins.[50] In both cases this inhibition was primarily caused by the hypothermic effects of the drug, since the reduction in incorporation was very much less when body temperature was maintained.

Iida, Kanno, and Nakamura[51] have claimed that a factor contained in the microsomal fraction obtained from brain homogenates prepared from untreated rabbits increases the sensitivity of recipient rabbits to a subsequent dose of ethanol. The brain extracts were administered by intraperitoneal injection and the rabbits challenged with a single intravenous dose of ethanol after which the time for reappearance of the corneal reflex was measured. Maximum increases in the time for recovery of the reflex occurred around one week after injection of the brain extract. However, in untreated animals the reflex reappeared within about 25 seconds after ethanol injection, and it is not clear that this is a valid index of central nervous system depression. Severe cardiovascular disturbance following the intravenous ethanol injection might well cause such symptoms.

Turnbull and Stevenson[52] have attempted to transfer tolerance to barbiturates by injecting brain extracts from barbitone tolerant rats into untreated rats, and measuring the sleeping time following a challenge dose of hexobarbitone or barbitone given 24 hours later. Sensitivity to barbitone was unchanged, but there was a slight reduction in the sensitivity to hexobarbitone, which might have been produced by the barbitione present in the brain extract increasing the liver enzyme activity.

DISCUSSION

The experimental evidence that is available concerning the functions of nucleic acids and proteins in the reduced sensitivity of the central nervous system to ethanol or barbiturate, and in physical dependence on these drugs following chronic administration, is inadequate to permit any conclusions to be drawn.

In experiments with narcotic analgesic drugs the only evidence which clearly seems to implicate nucleic acid and proteins in the phenomena of tolerance and physical dependence is the inhibition of the development of these states by drugs which modify RNA or protein synthesis. The effectiveness of these chemically unrelated substances with different primary modes of action on protein synthesis, together with the observation that doses which inhibited tolerance development also reduced RNA or protein synthesis, appears to indicate unambiguously that synthesis of protein is essential to the development of the tolerant state.

However, experiments in which protein synthesis has been measured directly during morphine treatment suggest that while morphine may have little effect on RNA synthesis, incorporation of amino acids into protein tends to be reduced by the drug. Certain protein fractions, particularly those thought to be relevant to synaptic transmission, have been studied in more detail. Thus, the activities of enzymes concerned in the synthesis and degradation of putative neurotransmitters have been measured, but increases in activity of any such enzyme have not been consistently reported (see chapter by C. B. Smith). In experiments described above morphine treatment did not appear to alter the incorporation of amino acids into proteins of the synaptic membrane complex. The effects of morphine treatment on the synthesis of other brain protein fractions, isolated in a relatively pure state, do not appear to have been studied. Thus, at the present state of knowledge there appears to be a discrepancy between predictions from experiments using inhibitors of RNA and protein synthesis and the experiments in which direct measurement of protein synthesis has been attempted.

A possible explanation for this discrepancy is that the synthesis of relevant protein fractions has not been examined. Because of the effects of morphine on transmission at peripheral synapses, a study of protein involved in synaptic transmission in the central nervous system seemed worthwhile. However, other isolated protein fractions are less clearly indicated as possible sites of morphine action. It is also probable that any morphine induced increase in protein synthesis will be of small magnitude compared with the overall ongoing synthesis of protein, and hence not detectable by the relatively crude techniques currently available.

The prediction based on experiments with inhibitors may well be incorrect. Inhibition of protein synthesis will inevitably have numerous secondary consequences for cell function. It is quite possible that such secondary effects may account for the ability of these substances to inhibit the development of tolerance to, and physical dependence on narcotic analgesic drugs.

REFERENCES

1. Munro, H. N., A general survey of mechanisms regulating protein metabolism in mammals, in *Mammalian Protein Metabolism,* Munro, H. N., Ed., Academic Press, New York, 1970.

2. Reich, E. and Goldberg, I. H., Actinomycin and nucleic acid function, *Progr. Nucl. Acid Res.,* 3, 183, 1964.

3. Cohen, M., Keats, A. S., Krivoy, W., and Ungar, G., Effects of actinomycin D on morphine tolerance, *Proc. Soc. Exp. Biol. Med.,* 119, 381, 1965.

4. Cox, B. M., Ginsburg, M., and Osman, O. H., Acute tolerance to narcotic analgesic drugs in rats, *Brit. J. Pharmacol. Chemother.,* 33, 245, 1968.

5. Cox, B. M. and Ginsburg, M., Is there any relationship between protein synthesis and tolerance to analgesic drugs?, in *Scientific Basis of Drug Dependence,* Steinberg, H., Ed., Churchill, London, 1969, 77.

6. Cox, B. M. and Osman, O. H., Inhibition of the development of tolerance to morphine in rats by drugs which inhibit ribonucleic acid or protein synthesis, *Brit. J. Pharmacol.,* 38, 157, 1970.

7. Smith, A. A., Karmin, M., and Gavitt, J., Blocking effect of puromycin ethanol and diloroform on the development of tolerance to an opiate, *Biochem. Pharmacol.,* 15, 1877, 1966.

8. Cox, B. M., Effects of inhibitions of protein synthesis in morphine tolerance and dependence, *Symposium on agonist and antagonist actions of narcotic analgesic drugs,* Aberdeen, 1971, in press.

9. Loh, H. H., Shen, F-H., and Way, E. L., Effect of dactinomycin on the acute toxicity and brain uptake of morphine, *J. Pharmacol. Exp. Ther.,* 177, 326, 1971.

10. Koenig, H., Lu, C. Y., Jacobsen, S., Sanghavi, P., and Nayyar, R., Effects of actinomycin D on RNA transcription, protein synthesis and nuclear structure, in *Protein Metabolism of the Nervous System,* Lajtha, A., Ed., Plenum Press, New York, 1970, 491.

11. Spoerlin, M. T. and Scrafani, J., Effects of time and 8-azaguamine on the development of morphine tolerance, *Life Sci.,* 6, 1549, 1967.

12. Simon, E. J. and Van Praag, D., Selective inhibition of synthesis of ribosomal RNA in *Escherichia coli* by levorphanol, *Proc. Nat. Acad. Sci. U S A,* 51, 1151, 1964.

13. Clouet, D. H., The effects of drugs on protein synthesis in the nervous system, in *Protein Metabolism of the Nervous System,* Lajtha, A., Ed., Plenum Press, New York, 1970, 699.

14. Nosal, G., Radouco-Thomas, S., Garcin, F., and Radouco-Thomas, C., Effects de la morphine et de la dactinomycine sur les ribonucleoproteines des neurones du systeme nerveux central, *Arch. Biol. Med. Exp.*, 4, 72, 1967.

15. Mellet, L. B. and Woods, L. A., The intracellular distribution of N-^{14}C-methyl levorphanol in brain, liver and kidney tissue of rat, *J. Pharmacol. Exp. Ther.*, 125, 97, 1959.

16. Mule, S. J., Redman, C. M., and Flesher, J. W., Intracellular disposition of ^{3}H-morphine in the brain and liver of non-tolerant and tolerant guinea pigs, *J. Pharmacol. Exp. Ther.*, 157, 459, 1967.

17. Clouet, D. H. and Williams, N., The binding of narcotic analgesic drugs to nucleic acids in the central nervous system, *Abstracts of the Fourth International Congress on Pharmacology*, Basel, 1969, 412.

18. Colombo, B., Felicetti, L., and Baglioni, C., Inhibition of protein synthesis by cycloheximide in rabbit reticulocytes, *Biochem. Biophys. Res. Commun.*, 18, 389, 1965.

19. Munro, H. N., Baliga, B. S., and Pronczuk, A. W., *In vitro* inhibition of peptide synthesis and GTP hydrolysis by cycloheximide and prevention of inhibition by glutathione, *Nature* (London), 219, 914, 1968.

20. Yarmolinsky, M. B. and De la Haba, G., Inhibition by puromycin of amino acid incorporation into protein, *Proc. Nat. Acad. Sci. USA*, 45, 1721, 1959.

21. Way, E. L., Loh, H. H., and Shen, F-H., Morphine tolerance, physical dependence and synthesis of brain 5-hydroxytryptamine, *Science*, 162, 1290, 1968.

22. Loh, H. H., Shen, F.-H, and Way, E. L., Inhibition of morphine tolerance and physical dependence development and brain serotonin synthesis by cycloheximide, *Biochem. Pharmacol.*, 18, 2711, 1969.

23. Clouet, D. H. and Neidle, A., The effect of morphine on the transport and metabolism of intracisternally injected leucine in the rat, *J. Neurochem.*, 17, 1069, 1970.

24. Clouet, D. H. and Ratner, M., The effect of the administration of morphine on the incorporation of (^{14}C)-leucine into the proteins of rat brain *in vivo, Brain Res.*, 4, 33, 1967.

25. Clouet, D. H. and Ratner, M., The effect of the administration of morphine administration on the incorporation of (^{14}C)-leucine into protein in cell-free systems from rat brain and liver, *J. Neurochem.*, 15, 17, 1968.

26. Cox, B. M. and Franklin, G. I., unpublished observations.

27. Paton, W. D. M., The action of morphine and related substances on the contraction and on acetylcholine output of co-axially stimulated guinea pig ileum, *Brit. J. Pharmacol. Chemother.*, 12, 119, 1957.

28. Cairnie, A. B., Kosterlitz, H. W., and Taylor, D. W., Effect of morphine on some sympathetically innervated effectors, *Brit. J. Pharmacol. Chemother.*, 17, 539, 1961.

29. Collier, H. O. J., Tolerance, physical dependence and receptors: a theory of the genesis of tolerance and physical dependence through drug-induced changes in the number of receptors, *Advances Drug Res.*, 3, 171, 1966.

30. Blaney, D. J. and Woods, L. A., Plasma protein binding of morphine, 116, 7, 1956.

31. Scrafani, J. T., Williams, N., and Clouet, D. H., Binding of dihydromorphine to subcellular fractions of rat brain, *Pharmacologist*, 11, 256, 1969.

32. Pal, B. K., Goldstein, A., and Lowney, L. I., Stereospecific binding of the morphine congener levorphanol in mouse brain preparations, *Fed. Proc.*, 30, 272(Abs), 1971.

33. Kornetsky, C. and Kiplinger, G. F., Potentiation of an effect of morphine in the rat by sera from morphine-tolerant and abstinent dogs and monkeys, *Psychopharmacologia*, 4, 66, 1963.

34. Kiplinger, G. F. and Clift, J. W., Pharmacological properties of morphine-potentiating serum obtained from morphine-tolerant dogs and men, *J. Pharmacol. Exp. Ther.*, 146, 139, 1964.

35. Kornetsky, C. and Cochin, J., Evidence of tolerance to morphine in the mouse after injection of serum from morphine-tolerant rabbits, *Fed. Proc.*, 23, 283, 1964.

36. Cochin, J. and Kornetsky, C., Factors on blood of morphine-tolerant animals that alternate or enhance the effects of morphine in nontolerant animals, *Res. Publ. Ass. Res. Nerv. Ment. Dis.*, 46, 268, 1968.

37. Ungar, G. and Cohen, M., Indication of morphine tolerance by material extracted from brain of tolerant animals, *Int. J. Neuropharmacol.*, 5, 183, 1966.

38. Tirri, R., Transfer of induced tolerance to morphine and promazine by brain homogenate, *Experientia*, 23, 278, 1967.

39. Smits, S. E. and Takemori, A. E., Lack of transfer of morphine tolerance by administration of rat cerebral homogenates, *Proc. Soc. Exp. Biol. Med.*, 130, 287, 1969.

40. Ungar, G. and Galvan, L., Conditions for transfer of morphine tolerance by brain extracts, *Proc. Soc. Exp. Biol. Med.*, 130, 287, 1969.

41. Tulunay, F. C., Kiran, B. D., and Kaymakcalan, S., Transfer of morphine tolerance in rats by brain extracts, *J. Pharm. Pharmacol.*, 22, 870, 1970.

42. Rosenblatt, F., Farrow, J. T., and Rhine, S., The transfer of learned behaviour from trained to untrained rats by means of brain extracts, *Proc. Nat. Acad. Sci. USA*, 55, 548, 1966.

43. Ungar, G. and Oceguera-Navarro, C., Transfer of habituation by material extracted from brain, *Nature* (London), 207, 301, 1965.

44. Byrne, W. L. et al., Memory transfer, *Science*, 155, 849, 1966.

45. Ungar, G., Molecular mechanisms in information processing, *Int. Rev. Neurobiol.*, 13, 223, 1970.

46. Faiszt, J. and Adam, G., Role of different RNA fractions from the brain in the transfer effect, *Nature* (London), 220, 367, 1968.

47. Tewari, S. and Noble, E. P., Ethanol and brain protein synthesis, *Brain Res.*, 26, 469, 1971.

48. Freund, G., Impairment of shock avoidance learning after long-term alcohol ingestion in mice, *Science*, 168, 1599, 1970.

49. Shuster, L. and Hannam, R. V., The indirect inhibition of protein synthesis *in vivo*, by chlorpromazine, *J. Biol. Chem.*, 239, 3401, 1964.

50. Gaitonde, M. K. and Richter, D., The metabolic activity of the proteins of the brain, *Proc. Roy. Soc., Ser. B.*, 145, 83, 1965.

51. Iida, S., Kanno, M., and Nakamura, K., An increased sensitivity to alcohol in rabbits treated with a certain factor contained in a microsomal subfraction of the brain, *Jap. J. Pharmacol.*, 19, 409, 1969.

52. Turnbull, M. J. and Stevenson, I. H., Tolerance experiments with barbitone dependent rats, *J. Pharm. Pharmacol.*, 20, 884, 1968.

CARBOHYDRATES

E. O'F. Walsh

TABLE OF CONTENTS

INTRODUCTION

Early indications that narcotics affected carbohydrate metabolism were the common observations that they depressed respiration and that hyperglycemia, hyperlactemia, and sometimes glycosuria followed their administration. These factors alone were not necessarily indicative of a direct action on the cellular metabolism of carbohydrates. Diminished availability of oxygen to the tissues resulting from depression of the respiratory center, for example, could in theory account for all these effects. Such an explanation was indeed advanced by Underhill as early as 1905 to account for the action of nicotine in provoking hyperglycemia and glycosuria.[1] These effects of nicotine were not abolished by oxygen administration as they were when provoked by piperidine which, it was concluded, had a more direct action on the oxidation of carbohydrate.

Evidence that morphine-hyperglycemia is central in origin was obtained by Brooks and others who found that only by massive injury to the posterior portion of the hypothalamus could the hyperglycemic action in the cat be completely abolished.[2]

Effects on other aspects of carbohydrate metabolism in the whole animal could, of course, also be induced by a drug having no direct action on intracellular respiratory oxidation of carbohydrate. This was often assumed to be the case with morphine. The Bernheims, for example, attributed the depressant effect of morphine on respiration to inhibition of acetylcholine esterase.[3] On the other hand, with a drug having a direct effect on tissue oxidation, the nervous system would probably be the most susceptible tissue. Therefore, depression of the respiratory metabolism of nerve would be the major factor influencing general metabolism in the whole animal. Niwa's claim in 1919 that cocaine in sufficient concentration to anesthetize the sciatic nerve of frog inhibited respiration of the isolated nerve would place cocaine within this category.[4]

Interpretation of whole animal experiments is further complicated by the participation of hormones in the control of carbohydrate metabolism. Attention was drawn to this factor in 1922 by the observation that adrenalectomy reduced, though it did not completely abolish, morphine-hyperglycemia.[5] The hyperglycemic effect of both nicotine and smoking tobacco has also been attributed to hormonal disturbance following action on the nervous system.[6] Cocaine has been observed to potentiate the hyperglycemic action of epinephrine in rabbits.[7]

Studies of the effects of opium in diabetes[8] and on sugar distribution in the body of insulin, epinephrine, and morphine[9] showed the liver to be the source of additional sugar in morphine-hyperglycemia and glycosuria. Depletion of liver glycogen by morphine and an abnormally low glycogen content of liver in chronically morphinized rats was observed by Horning.[10] Such depletion was shown to be a result of increased glycolysis in liver by Abood and co-workers, who found that even in rats tolerant to very high doses of morphine (250 mg/kg), the ability to synthesize glycogen from glucose was unchanged, while lactate production was much increased.[11,12] The abnormally high alkaline phosphatase activity that has been observed in liver of chronically morphinized rats with depleted glycogen stores could account for the hyperglycemia.[13] A morphine-induced change in the balance between carbohydrate and fat metabolism in liver is indicated by Kyo's observation in the rabbit that the increased lactate level in blood is accompanied by a decrease in the acetone bodies.[14] Kyo commented that morphine here shows an action similar to that of adrenaline, to which comparison we might add the above mentioned effect on liver phosphatase activity. Kyo also noted that injections of phenobarbitone tended to decrease both acetone bodies and lactate, but the effects were very small.

In disagreement with the general conception that narcotics depressed respiration and the oxidation of carbohydrate, in 1930 Barbour and others reported that morphine actually increased carbohydrate metabolism and its action was essentially that of a stimulant.[15] This assertion was based on experiments with dogs whose R.Q. and B.M.R. were raised by chronic administration of the drug. It was also suggested that the calorigenic effect of single doses of morphine in the dog had previously escaped attention because it was masked by the neuromuscular depression. Morphine was known to excite cats and, as early as 1874, von Boeck and Bauer claimed that oxidations were much increased by a single dose of morphine in the cat, but that the reverse occurred in the dog.[16] Barbour et al. argued that the increased oxidation in the cat was simply a result of increased muscular activity in the morphine-excited animal and the real effect on respiratory oxidation could be assessed only when metabolic rate was basal.[15] It has been established that morphine lowers the B.M.R. in man.[17] That of the rabbit is also depressed: the keto-derivatives; dihydromorphinone and dihydrocodeinone having ten times the potency of morphine and dihydromorphine in this respect.[18]

A more direct approach to the study of the effects of narcotics on metabolic processes is the use of tissue preparations and cell suspensions in vitro. One might have expected more consistent results and better agreement between the conclusions of different workers employing such techniques than was likely with interpretations based on experiments with whole animals, but with the earlier work this was certainly not the case. The techniques employed still had to be perfected, controls were often inadequate, and there was insufficient knowledge of the metabolic processes that were apparently affected by the drug under test. The result was a variety of contradictory reports, some making exaggerated claims later to be refuted. Techniques improved, however, and biochemical methods now have much to contribute to the detailed understanding of the modes of action of drugs.

An advantage of the in vitro techniques with tissue preparations is that the complications of nervous and hormonal factors are avoided. The use of such techniques has revealed that some narcotics have, in addition to and independently of any effect on nervous activity and transmission, a direct effect, usually inhibitory, on specific steps in the pathways of carbohydrate metabolism.

They have also revealed, though nervous and hormonal factors are not excluded here, that characteristic changes in the properties of a tissue, in skeletal muscle for example, may be induced in an animal by chronic administration of a drug; changes of a type that could be a major factor contributing to a state of physical dependence on the drug.[19] The details of such findings and of the more specific effects of narcotics on cellular metabolism are discussed below under the headings indicative of the type of drug.

MORPHINE AND RELATED DRUGS

Effects on Nervous Tissue

In 1928 Kumagai reported that subcutaneous injections of morphine (30 mg/kg) did not depress oxygen uptake by the central nervous system in the rabbit, and only after lethal doses was a slight reduction in respiration of the cerebral cortex observed.[20] A similar result was obtained in later work with brain from deeply narcotized rats by Wortis who reported that morphine did not affect either the Q_{O_2} or R.Q.[21] Meanwhile, Quastel and Wheatley found oxygen uptake of minced rat brain in vitro to be depressed by morphine (0.12%) with either glucose, pyruvate, lactate, or glutamate, but not with succinate as added substrate.[22] On the basis of this and similar findings with other narcotics they proposed that depression of cerebral respiration might be the basis of narcosis.[23] Other work for a time lent support to this idea.[24,25]

Quastel and Wheatley's work implied that morphine specifically inhibited an early stage in carbohydrate metabolism in brain, but not the final stages in cellular respiration involving electron-transfer since succinate oxidation was not affected. Reports conflicting with this interpretation then began to appear. The more detailed investigations of Seevers and Shideman were in part agreement: the Q_{O_2} of rat cerebrum without added substrate or with added succinate, fumarate, or malate was not affected by morphine, but though lactate and pyruvate oxidations were inhibited, that of added glucose was not![26] Elliott confirmed that morphine (0.12%) had no effect on Q_{O_2} of cerebral cortex slices in glucose-Ringer, but he reported depression by methadone and by pethidine.[27] Further evidence that electron transport in brain respiration was not affected was obtained by Mayer and McCawley who observed no effect of morphine or nalorphine (3 to 15 mM) on respiration of cerebral cortex slices with either succinate or *p*-phenylenediamine, a substrate for cytochrome oxidase.[28] Meanwhile, further work of Shideman and Seevers with various tissue preparations of rat, rabbit, and cat led them to conclude that the effects of morphine differed not only with different tissues, but with the methods of preparation.[29]

Surprising results, for their implication was quite different from that of earlier workers, were claimed by Watts in 1949 who reported a 50% inhibition of oxygen uptake of an ox-brain homogenate with succinate as substrate by morphine or meperidine (20 mM), by codeine (30 mM), and by methadone (6 mM).[30] Watts concluded that the drugs interfered with electron transport, mainly with reduction of cytochrome c and cytochrome oxidase, to a lesser extent. This conclusion was supported by Wang and Bain who reported a 60% inhibition of NAD-cytochrome c reductase and a 20% inhibition of cytochrome oxidase by morphine (1 mM) in preparations of brain and liver from dog and rat.[31,32]

Later work, including that in the author's laboratory, has confirmed that though morphine (1 mM) may depress the oxygen uptake of homogenates by 10 to 30%, it has no significant effect on the Q_{O_2} of cerebral cortex slices respiring in oxygenated, buffered saline media containing glucose, although the intracellular concentration of the drug may reach 2.5 mM.[33-35] Therefore, the lack of effect on the respiration of brain slices cannot be attributed to failure of the drug to enter the cells. Sensitivity of homogenates towards the drug, on the other hand, may be associated with the lowered concentration of cofactors resulting from dilution of ruptured cell contents by the incubating media. Such effects cannot be regarded as being of real pharmacological significance.

Pharmacological interest in the effects of morphine on respiration of brain was revived by the suggestion of Ghosh and Quastel in 1954, that narcotics inhibited the increased Q_{O_2} of brain that is produced in vitro either by electrical stimulation or by raising the potassium concentration of a physiologically normal incubating medium.[36] A 50% inhibition by morphine (1 mM) of the increased Q_{O_2} produced in cerebral cortex slices by electrical pulses was recorded in McIlwain's laboratory.[33] When stimulated by increase of potassium in the medium, or by addition of glutamate which has a similar effect, work in the author's laboratory showed morphine (1 mM) to be without effect, provided that the tissue slices were undamaged and had not suffered diminution in sensitivity to the stimulant.[34] Later, however, Takemori claimed that morphine depressed the potassium-stimulated respiration of cerebral cortex slices from normal, but not from chronically morphinized rats; this change being reversed by injection of the chronically morphinized rat with nalorphine.[37] If such change does occur, it is unlikely to be a major factor contributing directly to a state of physical dependence on the drug since it is so easily reversed by nalorphine, which does not immediately abolish an established physical dependence. By antagonizing the acute effects of morphine, nalorphine brings on withdrawal symptoms in the addict.

Achor and Geiling found that morphine decreased the permeability of brain cells to glucose and nalorphine antagonized this effect.[38] Takemori, however, found that morphine (1 mM) increased glucose utilization by cerebral cortex slices without affecting oxygen uptake or lactate formation, and the rate of glucose utilization was greater in slices of brain from chronically morphinized rats.[39] This could not be attributed to a permeability effect, since glucose utilization was also increased by morphine in homogenates. It was suggested that metabolism by the pentose phosphate pathway might be encouraged by morphine. A lag period of 30 min was found to be associated with the stimulation of cerebral glucose utilization and carbon dioxide production by morphine.[40] Further work in Takemori's laboratory indicated that morphine stimulates glycolysis in brain, an increased ratio of ATP to AMP facilitating 3-phosphoglyceral dehydrogenase and phosphofructokinase activities.[41]

In summary of this profusion of contradictory findings concerning the action of morphine on carbohydrate metabolism in brain, the writer concludes that morphine has no pharmacologically significant direct effect on the enzymes concerned with the respiratory oxidation of glucose in intact nerve. The variety of effects that has been observed on nerve preparations in vitro, apart from any that may have been due to faulty technique, such as inadequate control of pH, are probably a consequence of differences in the proportions of intact cells in the preparations and of effects on respiratory metabolism of these with variations in activity of their membranes upon which the drug appears to have a direct effect.

Effects on Muscles

In 1940 Shideman and Seevers reported that respiration of minced skeletal muscle of rabbit was increased by morphine and thebaine (0.12%), especially with pyruvate as added substrate, and the drugs apparently antagonized the stimulatory effect of added thiamine.[25] With pigeon breast muscle, on the other hand, the drugs had no significant effect. The same workers also studied the effects of narcotics on dehydrogenase activity in a heart muscle preparation using the Thunberg methylene blue technique. They found that morphine (0.06 to 0.24%) inhibited with either glucose, citrate, or lactate, but not with succinate or alcohol as substrate; codeine and thebaine were without effect.[26] The respiration of heart muscle was not affected, however.[29] In work with rats they found that the Q_{O_2} of skeletal muscle from chronically morphinized animals (20 → 240 mg/kg up to 15 weeks) was markedly higher than normal.[42-44] A severe thiamine deficiency was apparently induced in the rat concurrently with chronic morphine poisoning though the cocarboxylase content of the brain, liver, and muscle was not changed. Morphine and pyruvate were found to have a synergistic effect in raising the Q_{O_2} of normal but not of chronically morphinized muscle.[43]

In a study of the effects of morphine on the hormonal control of metabolism, excised diaphragm was used in the writer's laboratory to compare the acute effects in vitro of morphine (0.4 to 0.8 mM) and adrenal hormones in similar concentration on glucose uptake, net glycogen synthesis, lactate accumulation, and oxygen uptake in muscle of normal and chronically morphinized (30 mg/kg for 6 weeks) rats.[45-49] This study was inspired by the intriguing realization that the chemical structure of morphine, which is synthesized in the poppy from two molecules of tyrosine, embodies both a steroid-like and an epinephrine-like component and would therefore be expected to interfere with, and possibly mimic, some of the effects of adrenal hormones at their target sites.[19,46] Morphine stimulated glucose uptake of normal diaphragm but had the opposite effect on diaphragm from chronically morphinized animals.[45] The drug had no significant effect in vitro on the rate of net glycogen synthesis, lactate accumulation, or respiration. No significant difference between normal and chronically morphinized diaphragm was detected in the basic rates of glucose uptake and metabolism. The glycogen content of muscle from chronically morphinized animals was significantly higher than normal, however. That morphine stimulates glucose uptake by normal muscle is not in itself of great significance since almost any means of poisoning the tissue, depriving it of oxygen, or uncoupling oxidative phosphorylation has this effect. It is a specialized property of skeletal muscle to keep the rate of entry under control and breakdown of such control permits a more rapid entry of the sugar. The fact that morphine depresses the rate of glucose uptake by muscle from a chronically morphinized animal is of much greater significance, for in this respect the drug mimics the action of adrenal hormones.

These findings implied that morphine has no significant, direct effect on the intracellular metabolism of carbohydrate in intact muscle, and that the site of action of the drug is the cell membrane in which the hormone-sensitive system that controls glucose uptake is located. Experiments with hormones supported this conclusion. Addition of cortisol (0.4 mM) in vitro, for example, depressed glucose uptake by normal muscle, but stimulated that of chronically morphinized muscle. Epinephrine (0.4 mM) also depressed glucose uptake by normal muscle, but had little or no effect on the chronically morphinized.[47-49] The effects of these hormones on respiration and intracellular metabolism remained unchanged by chronic morphinization.

Extension of the work to include other hormones has revealed that the in vitro sensitivity of the glucose uptake system of muscle to insulin (0.1 unit/ml) is lost by chronic morphinization, but restored by addition of morphine to the medium.[50] The effects on the system of aldosterone (0.0035 mM) which depressed, and of thyroxine (0.04 mM) which stimulated glucose uptake by normal muscle were, like cortisol, reversed by chronic morphinization.[51] The effects on a common metabolic process of several hormones of different type are changed, not simply abolished, by chronic morphinization. This implies that specific hormone receptors, if they exist, have survived, and that the drug-induced change in the membrane directly affects a regulatory mechanism that is commonly involved in responses to hormones and other factors that influence glucose uptake.

A study of the effects of changes in the ionic composition of the incubating medium has indicated that probably a magnesium-potassium sensitive and calcium-dependent system is affected.[52-55]

The standard incubating medium used in the study of the effects of morphine and hormones on glucose metabolism in rat diaphragm contained sodium (130 mM), potassium (5 mM), magnesium (1.25 mM), calcium (2.8 mM), and glucose (0.15%). The rate of glucose uptake from the oxygenated standard medium at pH 7.4 and 37° by hemidiaphragms from either normal or chronically morphinized rats is about half-maximal. The maximal rate is reached with normal diaphragm when insulin is added; when the glucose concentration is raised above 0.4%, when the magnesium concentration is doubled, when the potassium concentration is trebled, or when calcium is omitted from the medium.[53-55] Chronically morphinized diaphragm, on the other hand, shows no such sensitivity to variation in extracellular concentrations of metal ions. Neither increase of potassium or magnesium, nor omission of calcium has significant effect on the rate of glucose uptake but, as with normal diaphragm, the rate of uptake is depressed by increase of extracellular calcium.

The acute effects of both morphine and hormones on glucose uptake by normal diaphragm are modified or changed by variations in the ionic composition of the medium. For example, the stimulant effect of morphine appears to be a direct antagonism to the depressant effect of calcium and is also dependent on the presence of magnesium in the medium. In normal diaphragm, the potassium-stimulated, not the magnesium-stimulated uptake is particularly sensitive to epinephrine; the action of which is also magnesium-dependent and maximal in media containing the standard concentration of magnesium (1.25 mM). On the other hand, with chronically morphinized diaphragm, the acute effects of morphine and of hormones are not significantly affected by variations in extracellular potassium or magnesium concentration, but some sensitivity to calcium concentration is retained. In the presence of high calcium concentrations, the membrane is much less stable than that of normal diaphragm, for it readily breaks down, releasing free glucose into the medium. Cortisol (0.4 mM) has this effect and the stimulant effect of the hormone in lower concentration (0.004 mM) is dependent upon the presence of calcium.

Such evidence suggested that the change in membrane properties resulting from chronic morphinization might involve a change in the ratios and concentrations of metal ions in membranes. A variety of observations have indicated that morphine interferes with both magnesium and calcium metabolsim.[56-60] In the present context, Mulé's finding that morphine inhibits the binding of calcium to phospholipids is especially interesting.[60] Analysis of subcellular fractions of normal and chronically morphinized muscle confirm that abnormal concentrations of metal ions are associated with the drug-induced changes in membranes. Normal concentrations of potassium, magnesium, and calcium were found in the nuclear and mitochondrial fractions, but in the microsomal fraction of chronically morphinized muscle the potassium concentration was 200%, the magnesium concentration 100%, and the calcium concentration about 40% higher than in that of normal muscle.[61] This is indeed a drastic change, for it involves a system that is concerned not only with glucose uptake, but with the hormonal control of the body's metabolism including salt and water balance.

COCAINE AND RELATED DRUGS

While the effect of morphine on cellular respiration has been a matter of controversy, cocaine has provoked no dispute. Cocaine appears to be toxic to living cells in general, certainly to all animal cells, inhibiting both respiration and fermentation. In 1891 Araki found that unusually large amounts of lactate appeared in urine following cocaine injections.[62] Underhill and Black observed that daily injections of the drug impaired fat utilization in the dog.[63] As discussed below, this is an inevitable consequence of the manner in which cocaine inhibits cellular oxidations.

Niwa first studied the action of cocaine on isolated nerve and found that production of carbon dioxide was depressed.[4] Wortis reported that both R.Q. and Q_{O_2} of brain suspensions in vitro were depressed by cocaine.[21] It is not clear why R.Q. should have been depressed in brain, but in this respect cocaine apparently differed from other respiratory inhibitors such as the barbiturates which did not affect the R.Q. of the tissue. Felloni observed that cocaine depressed the oxygen uptake of blood.[64] Cook and McDevitt showed that cocaine inhibited respiration of yeast which was a property shared with other local anesthetics.[65] Bach and Lambert reported that cocaine inhibited dehydrogenases in suspensions of a *Staphylococcus.*[66]

In a comparative study of the acute and chronic effects of narcotics on the metabolism and growth of unicellular organisms, it was observed in the writer's laboratory that cocaine (5 mM) completely inhibited fermentation and growth of *Saccharomyces cerevisiae* in a nutrient medium of pH 7.0 containing glucose, but growth continued in the presence of 4 mM cocaine.[67] In acid media, even at pH 6.0, the drug had little or no effect on the yeast; an observation in agreement with Travell's conclusion that usually the free, unionised base is absorbed with alkaloids.[68] For this reason and to facilitate comparison with effects on animal tissues, cultures were grown and studied in neutral media, although in common with most fungi yeasts prefer an acid medium. A pure strain of fermenting yeast was chosen for this preliminary study in order to observe effects on glycolysis independently of respiration and nervous or hormonal influence.

The inhibition of yeast fermentation by cocaine was traced to a specific inhibition of carboxylase which the drug in 1 mM concentration inhibited by about 50%. No difference between normal and chronically cocainized yeast (a twin culture grown in the presence of the drug) was found in the specific activity of this enzyme, nor could any hint of biological dependence on the drug be detected, but a striking difference was revealed in the effect of added thiamine.[67,69] Addition of thiamine (4 mM) to an acid-washed suspension of the yeast in phosphate buffer at pH 7.0 containing glucose (2%) stimulated production of carbon dioxide, but it had the opposite and stronger effect on similar suspensions of the chronically cocainized yeast. The nature of this drug-induced change has yet to be explained.

For preliminary study of effects on respiration,

a pure strain of a respiring yeast, *Torulopsis utilis*, was used. Cocaine (2 mM) inhibited by about 50% the oxidation of pyruvate both in a suspension of this yeast and in a homogenate of rat brain.[70,71] Inhibition of respiration in the yeast was much higher with either acetate or pyruvate as substrate than with glucose, which implied that the drug inhibited oxidation via the citric acid cycle. The synthesis of citrate was found to be most strongly inhibited, cocaine (2 mM) effecting a 90 to 100% inhibition of citrate synthesis from acetate in a suspension of washed and starved baker's yeast in magnesium acetate solution, and 100% inhibition of synthesis from pyruvate and oxaloacetate in a brain homogenate. Degradation of pyruvate to acetate by the pyruvic dehydrogenase system in a dialysed pigeon brain homogenate by cocaine (2 mM) was inhibited only by about 15% as measured by acetate production and oxygen consumption. Acetylations with acetate as acetyl donor of sulphanilamide in a pigeon liver extract and of choline in a choline acetylase preparation of guinea pig brain were not affected by cocaine. The drug therefore did not inhibit the formation of active acetate, but its incorporation into the citric acid cycle. The incorporation of acetate into the glyoxylate cycle in bacteria was later found to be similarly inhibited by cocaine, which in 1 mM concentration inhibited malate synthesis in *Escherichia coli* by about 80%.[72]

The ability to inhibit carboxylase and to block oxidations via the citric acid and glyoxylate cycles can account for the toxicity of cocaine to living cells of animals and microorganisms in general. Obviously, it cannot account for cocaine's exceptional narcotic properties, however, since the ability to inhibit respiration in nerve by blocking oxidation via the citric acid cycle is a property shared with other local anesthetics, toxic and potent ones, such as cinchochaine and amethocaine, being the most strongly inhibiting.[73]

NICOTINE

Nicotine is much less potent than cocaine in its direct effects on cellular metabolism. By comparison it is a mild inhibitor of cellular respiration and a stimulator of fermentation and anaerobic glycolysis. It is, however, peculiarly toxic to nerve cells. This was realized as early as 1890 by Langley and Dickinson who studied its action on mammalian nerve,[74-76] and by Greenwood who concluded from its action on various invertebrates that the toxicity of nicotine to any organism is determined mainly by the degree of development of the nervous system.[77] The possibility that respiration of nervous tissue might be specifically inhibited by nicotine was raised by McIndoo's observation in 1916 that structural changes in nerve cells like those resulting from oxygen deprivation were apparent in nicotine-poisoned insects.[78] In 1928 Wilson suggested that nicotine was readily absorbed by the nitrogenous fatty components of nerve and that this prevented absorption of oxygen.[79]

Effects on Glycolysis and Cellular Respiration

In 1935 Himwich and Fazekas reported that nicotine (14 mM) reduced the "no substrate" respiration of minced brain of rat, cat and dog and inhibited by 60% the increased oxygen uptake with added lactate, but it had no effect on the increase with added glucose or pyruvate.[80,81] It was concluded that lactic dehydrogenase was inhibited. Oxidation of succinate was also inhibited. These observations led Himwich and Fazekas to suggest that glucose oxidation in brain might proceed directly without previous glycolysis, a suggestion based on the assumption that lactate was an intermediate in the oxidation of glucose via the glycolytic pathway of metabolism. The precise role of lactate in carbohydrate metabolism was a matter of debate at that time, and it was not then commonly realized that pyruvate is reduced to lactate in quantity only when there is insufficient oxygen for its complete oxidation. Nor was it always appreciated that an inhibitor of lactic dehydrogenase would inhibit the formation of lactate to the same extent that it inhibits its oxidation. It is however of interest that it was this early work with nicotine that inspired later research leading to the discovery of alternative metabolic pathways for the oxidation of glucose.

In subsequent work, Baker, Fazekas, and Himwich found that nicotine (30 mM) inhibited respiration of slices of rat brain by 49% with glucose, 76% with pyruvate, and 91% with lactate.[82] Higher concentrations of nicotine were required to give the same effect in a cat brain preparation, while in preparations of testes and kidney, glucose and lactate oxidations were equally inhibited. It was also observed that lactate production was increased, from which it was concluded that nicotine stimulated glycolysis. Such increase could of course be a result simply of depressed respiration, but Quastel and Wheatley reported that anaerobic glycolysis in brain is stimulated by nicotine.[83] It is not clear why this should be so if a major effect of nicotine is to inhibit lactic dehydrogenase.

Inhibitions as high as those reported by Baker et al. were not obtained in the writer's laboratory in experiments with homogenates of rat cerebral cortex, but it was confirmed that nicotine (7.5 to 30 mM) depressed oxidation of pyruvate more strongly than that of glucose. From this it was inferred that the drug depressed respiration by inhibiting the pyruvic oxidase system.[84] This inference was encouraged by various reports of physiological antagonism between nicotine and thiamine.[85-87] The synthesis of citrate from pyruvate and oxaloacetate in both rat brain and kidney was inhibited by 20 to 40% by nicotine (7.5 to 30 mM) but, unlike cocaine, the drug had no appreciable effect on citrate synthesis from acetate in yeast. This implied that pyruvate dehydrogenase was the enzyme most directly affected and was confirmed as follows.

Production of acetate by oxidative decarboxylation of pyruvate in a dialysed pigeon brain homogenate was inhibited by nicotine (7.5 to 30 mM) to the same extent as citrate synthesis in rat brain and kidney. Enzymes in the citric acid cycle were less affected, the most sensitive being α-ketoglutarate dehydrogenase which was inhibited by 5 to 16%. Succinic dehydrogenase of muscle and succinoxidase system of brain were equally inhibited by 5 to 8%. This implies that the electron transport system is not affected. Oxidation of fumarate to oxaloacetate in kidney was inhibited by 0 to 12%.[84]

While inhibition of pyruvic dehydrogenase fully accounts for the inhibitory effect of nicotine on cellular respiration, this effect is insufficient to account for the high toxicity to nerve. Such inhibition would result in a tendency for pyruvate to be raised above the normal level, especially if glycolysis is increased and the conversion of pyruvate to lactate is retarded. Inhibition of coupled oxidative phosphorylation would contribute to this effect by lowering the ATP/ADP ratio and thus facilitating conversion of phosphoenolpyruvate to free pyruvate. Such inhibition has been found to occur in brain preparations.[85] Also, it has been shown that pyruvate in a concentration only slightly higher than that normally present in nerve is a powerful inhibitor of choline acetylase.[89] Other inhibitors of pyruvate oxidation, cocaine for example which has no direct action on purified choline acetylase, have been found to inhibit acetylcholine synthesis in a respiring brain homogenate. Nicotine, however, is itself a direct inhibitor of choline acetylase.[90]

Alternative metabolic pathways for the oxidation of glucose are also mildly affected by nicotine. Glucose dehydrogenase of liver is inhibited by about 16% of the drug in 7.5 mM concentration.[91] Glucose dehydrogenase in *Saccharomyces cerevisiae* and *Torulopsis utilis* is inhibited to a similar extent, a factor which led to discovery of this enzyme in yeasts.[92] Glucose-6-phosphate dehydrogenase, on the other hand, is activated; nicotine (10 mM) activating this enzyme by 40%. The hexokinase reaction was shown not to be affected by nicotine.

Effects on Fermentation

Early work on the effects of nicotine on microorganisms has been reviewed by Enders and Windisch who investigated the ability of various yeasts to decompose nicotine and use it as a sole nitrogen source.[93] They and previous workers agreed that while nicotine is poisonous to aerobic growth, it stimulates fermentation and may even accelerate anaerobic growth. Dickens observed that nicotine inhibits the Pasteur effect.[94] In relation to this McIlwain studied the effect of nicotine on the enzymic degradation of cozymase (NAD) which was found to be inhibited 50% by nicotine (1 mM).[95] Niacinamide also inhibited and to a similar extent. In the writer's laboratory after growth in a nutrient medium containing nicotine, a niacin-dependent strain of *Lactobacillus* was stimulated in lactic fermentation and growth by nicotine in a niacin-deficient culture medium but, disappointingly, no specific physical dependence on nicotine could be demonstrated, for the organism still preferred the natural vitamin.

In a comparison of the effects of nicotine on various dehydrogenases it appeared that only those which required a pyridine nucleotide as coenzyme were appreciably affected. Not all such enzymes were sensitive; isocitric dehydrogenase, for example, was unaffected by nicotine (30 mM). Glucose, lactic, pyruvic, and malic dehydrogenases were inhibited and addition of coenzyme did not reverse the inhibition. Alcohol dehydrogenase of yeast which is NAD-dependent, like glucose-6-phosphate dehydrogenase which is NADP-dependent, was activated (30%) by nicotine (7.5 mM).[91] Such activation could account for the stimulant action of nicotine on alcoholic fermentation.

BARBITURATES AND ALCOHOL

While it is well established that barbiturates inhibit respiration, there has been much controversy concerning the manner in which they do so and to what extent such action may be related to their narcotic properties. Kyo, who observed that morphine increased lactate and depressed acetone bodies in blood, found that phenobarbitone tended to decrease both only slightly.[14] This would imply a mild, general depression of energy-yielding metabolism in the body as a whole. However, it has been claimed that in brain tissue, stimulation of glycolysis accompanies barbiturate-depression of respiration.[96] In a study of the effects of barbiturates on respiration of perfused brain in the living cat, Geiger and Magnes observed that when the Q_{O_2} was reduced from 4.70 ml O_2/100 g brain/min to 2.85 ml by sodium amytal (20 mg %), all reflexes were abolished.[97]

Disturbances of carbohydrate metabolism by barbiturates and alcohol, as revealed by glucose-tolerance and pyruvate-metabolism tests, have been described in detailed reports by Hunter and others.[98,99]

As a narcotic, alcohol is exceptional for it is metabolized as a food of high calorific value with acetaldehyde, which is toxic, as its immediate oxidation product. It has been suggested that the synergism between alcohol and barbiturates may be associated with a barbiturate-enhanced tendency for the free aldelyde to accumulate in brain.[100] Ethanol as an end product of anaerobic glycolysis in plant cells is analogous to lactate in mammalian tissues. Yeasts, used in producing alcohol from carbohydrate, continue to ferment and to grow anaerobically until the alcohol concentration reaches that of an unfortified wine, which may approach 14%. With the possible exception of pyruvic and lactic dehydrogenases, one would not therefore expect alcohol in concentrations tolerated in the tissue fluids of man to interfere with enzymes involved in glycolysis.

Aloholic depression of brain respiration in vivo was observed by Dewan in 1943,[101] but others have since shown that such depression can be accounted for by the lowered rate of blood flow to the brain.[102]

Effects of Barbiturates on Cellular Respiration

In 1935 Wortis reported that phenobarbitone depressed respiration of brain suspensions in vitro but, unlike cocaine, it did not affect the R.Q.[21]

In an attempt to discover the site of action of narcotics on brain metabolism, Greig compared effects on brain with those of a barbiturate on the lactic dehydrogenase system of yeast, which differs from the mammalian enzyme in that it does not require NAD.[103] She found that "nembutal" (0.01%) inhibited the oxidation of lactate in yeast by oxygen, but not the anaerobic reduction of methylene blue. Therefore, she concluded that the drug interferred with electron transfer and not with hydrogen transfer. She argued that since succinate oxidations were inhibited the narcotic-sensitive region in the electron transfer chain must be between flavoprotein and cytochrome b. This contention was refuted by Persky and others who found no inhibition of oxidation of the flavoproteins, *d*-amino acid oxidase and cytochrome reductase.[104]

Johnson and Quastel have suggested that pentobarbitone and other narcotics inhibit oxidative steps in cell respiration which are concerned with ATP synthesis.[105] Eiler and McEwen, however, reported that pentobarbitone (0.16 to 10 mM) does not affect the P/O ratio of a respiring brain homogenate; generation of high energy phosphate being depressed to the same extent as respiration.[106] In agreement with this, Aldridge and Parker found that the oxybarbiturates, phenobarbitone, amylobarbitone, and hexobarbitone did not affect the P/O ratio of liver mitochondria, but thiobarbiturates depressed the P/O ratio.[107] Others have suggested that barbiturates uncouple oxidative phosphorylation in brain and liver mitochondria. A large number of barbiturates were tested, but it was pointed out that the most potent agent in this respect, 1:3-dimethylbutylethylbarbiturate, is not a depressant in the intact animal, but a convulsant in relatively small doses.[108,109] It has been suggested that depression of P/O ratio might be a result of increased activity of an ATP-ase, rather than an uncoupling action.[107] This aspect has been discussed by Aldridge and by McIlwain.[110,111]

The site of barbiturate inhibition of carbohydrate oxidation in cells was discovered by Persky, Goldstein, and Levine.[104] They found, in agreement with Davies and Quastel,[112] that respiration of a rat brain homogenate with either glucose or pyruvate as substrate was inhibited; pyruvate oxidation being completely blocked by pentobarbitone (4 mM) and glycolysis also being inhibited. Hexokinase and lactic dehydrogenase were not affected. In experiments with a respiring, washed liver homogenate containing malonate, in which citrate and acetoacetate accumulate, they found stronger inhibitions with pyruvate as substrate than with fumarate and concluded that pyruvic dehydrogenase was inhibited. A conclusion from this evidence alone could be disputed, but they found supporting evidence in the observation that the oxidative decarboxylation of pyruvate to acetate in a suspension of *Gonococcus* was likewise inhibited, and α-ketoglutaric dehydrogenase was also, but less strongly inhibited.

Greig had found that ascorbic acid relieved barbiturate-blocked respiration of brain in vitro. Since ascorbic acid was known to be an activator of -SH enzymes and from the known chemical analogy between barbiturates and alloxan, which reacts with thiol groups, Persky et al. concluded that the NAD-dependent oxidation of acetaldehyde in the second stage of the reaction, $CH_3.CO.COOH \rightarrow CH_3.CHO \rightarrow CH_3.COOH$, is catalysed by an -SH enzyme. The role of coenzyme A and thioctic acid in the pyruvic-dehydrogenase complex had not then been elucidated. It is of interest to compare this inhibition with that of nicotine which probably interferes with the first, thiamine-dependent stage of the reaction.

Inhibition of pyruvic dehydrogenase by barbiturates, like that by nicotine, could fully account for the drug's depressant effect on cellular respiration with carbohydrate as substrate. Such inhibition may contribute to pharmacological properties, nerve being especially sensitive to interference with pyruvate oxidation.

It has been observed, however, that sedation by barbiturates could be achieved without depression of cerebral respiration, though at anesthetic levels of dosage respiration was much reduced.[113] Also, depression of synaptic transmission by "nembutal" has been observed without depression of the resting Q_{O_2}.[114] Others have reported that pentobarbitone (0.5 mM) inhibits oxidation of glucose more than that of pyruvate in rat brain slices with low concentrations (0.05 to 0.2%) of substrate, and that the drug in a concentration (0.2 mM) which corresponds to the anesthetic dose for rats (48 mg/kg) has negligible effect on glucose or pyruvate oxidation.[115]

In support of their contention that narcotics inhibit the stimulated respiration of brain, Ghosh and Quastel stated that pentobarbitone (1 mM) inhibited the resting Q_{O_2} of cortex slices only by 9% and the potassium-stimulated by 37%.[36] With phenobarbitone (3.3 mM), however, the difference was much less, the inhibitions being 40 and 55%, respectively. McIlwain found greater differences with the drugs in lower concentrations: phenobarbitone (0.68 to 1.7 mM), butobarbitone (0.64 mM), and allobarbitone (0.64 mM), which had negligible effect on the resting Q_{O_2} of cerebral cortex slices but inhibited the electrically (20 v) stimulated Q_{O_2} by 14 to 30%.[116]

It has been observed that injections of glucose and some other sugars cause a return to deep narcosis in animals coming round from barbiturate-anesthesia.[117] The injections were strongly hypertonic; however, others have observed the same effect with strongly hypertonic saline injections and have suggested that dehydration prolongs anesthesia.[118] This raises the question: is the synergistic effect of alcohol in part due to its properties as a dehydrating agent?

Effects of Alcohol on Cellular Respiration

In 1938 Jowett noted that alcohol behaved differently from other narcotics in that it inhibited brain respiration in vitro progressively with time and that such inhibition was apparently irreversible.[119] Others have observed that alcoholic inhibition of brain respiration had a high temperature coefficient.[120] At 37.7°, low concentrations of alcohol stimulated brain respiration with glucose as substrate, depression of Q_{O_2} beginning with a concentration of 2.5%, rising to an inhibition of about 90% with 9.5% ethanol, while complete inhibition required 47.5% ethanol! Beer and Quastel found the potassium-stimulated respiration of cortex slices to be more strongly inhibited than the resting respiration by the lower alcohols, pentanol having the greatest effect.[121] They commented that the membrane of cells was the likely site of action and this has not been challenged by any evidence that alcohol has any direct inhibitory action of significance on the enzymes involved in carbohydrate metabolism.

Wallgren, who compared the effect of alcohol on brain respiration in vitro with that of malonate, reported that ethanol (87 mM) increased Q_{O_2} by 8%, Q glucose by 23%, and had no effect on lactate in unstimulated cerebral cortex slices of rat. However, it depressed the electrically stimulated Q_{O_2} by 9.5%, Q glucose by 11%, and increased lactate accumulation by 12.5%.[122,123] The lower alcohols have been shown to have no direct effect on the activity of lactic dehydrogenase fractions prepared from heart homogenates.[124] A nonspecific inhibition by the lower alcohols of a sodium-stimulated, microsomal ATP-ase of brain has been reported.[125]

Taken in quantity, alcohol is a ketogenic substitute for carbohydrate and other energy-yielding foods in the diet and is oxidized, mainly in the liver, to acetyl derivatives and ultimately to CO_2 and water without accumulation of the toxic intermediate, acetaldehyde. Tissues of highest aqueous content, eye and nonmedullated nerve, are especially sensitive to the toxic properties of the lower alcohols, especially methanol. In relation to this, Kini and Cooper's findings are of special interest.[126] They found that while formaldehyde (< 1 mM) is rapidly oxidized by liver mitochondria with a P/O ratio of 2, retinal mitochondria cannot effect such oxidation.

AMPHETAMINES AND HALLUCINOGENS

In general, amphetamines, unlike narcotics, tend to stimulate respiration and glucose utilization in the body. Such effects would appear to be a result of stimulation of the respiratory center and of increased blood flow to muscle, rather than to a direct action on cellular oxidation of carbohydrate. Mann and Quastel in 1940 showed that amphetamine had no effect on respiration of cerebral cortex in vitro and did not antagonize depression of respiration by narcotics.[127] More recently, using ^{14}C-labeled substrates, an increased utilization of glucose with increased glycolysis and a depressed utilization of acetate by amphetamine (0.01 to 10 μM) without increased citric acid cycle activity have been detected in brain of a snail, *Helix aspersa.*[128]

An increase of blood glucose and liver glycogen after dosage with amphetamine has been observed in the rat, but only in animals subjected to severe food restriction.[129] A fenfluramine derivative, S992, which is exceptional in having a mild sedative action, did not have this effect but, like amphetamine, it apparently possessed adipokinetic activity. Adipokinetic activity by amphetamines, including fenfluramine, had been previously described.[130] Others have observed that fenfluramine and methamphetamine (1 mM) do not affect lipolysis and apparently do not interfere with glucose metabolism in epididymal fat cells of the rat, but they reduce incorporation of labeled carbon from glucose into CO_2 and total lipid, fenfluramine in higher concentration (10 mM) apparently preventing glucose metabolism.[131] Fenfluramine increases tolerance to carbohydrates and it has been demonstrated that small doses (0.4 μg/min) infused intra-arterially into one arm increase both glucose uptake and blood flow above that of the other arm.[132,133]

Moore found that methylamphetamine (even 10 mg/kg) did not affect the resting blood lactate level in mice.[134] This has been confirmed by others, with the further observation that the drug (1 to 3 mg/kg) prevented a rise in blood lactate in the rat following exercise, but 5 mg/kg had the reverse effect.[135] Stimulation of the respiratory center was noted.

McIlwain in 1950 found LSD (0.3 mM) to be without effect on carbohydrate metabolism in brain preparations.[95] Mescaline is known to produce hypoglycemia which prior injection of epinephrine prevents.[136] Generally it would appear that LSD and other hallucinogens which are potent in very small doses have no appreciable effects on carbohydrate metabolism.

REFERENCES

1. Underhill, F. P., Certain aspects of experimental diabetes, *J. Biol. Chem.*, 1, 113, 1905.

2. Brooks, C. M., Goodwin, R., and Willard, H. N., The effect of various brain lesions on morphine-induced hyperglycemia and excitement in the cat, *Amer. J. Physiol.*, 133, 226, 1941.

3. Bernheim, F. and Bernheim, M. L. C., Action of drugs on the choline esterase of the brain, *J. Pharmacol. Exp. Ther.*, 57, 427, 1936.

4. Niwa, S., The effect of cocaine hydrochloride on the CO_2 production of the mixed nerve fibre, *J. Pharmacol. Exp. Ther.*, 12, 323, 1919.

5. Stewart, G. N. and Rogoff, J. M., Morphine hyperglycemia and the adrenals, *Amer. J. Physiol.*, 61, 93, 1922.

6. Burn, J. H., Truelove, L. H., and Burn, I., The antidiuretic action of nicotine and of smoking, *Brit. Med. J.*, 1, 403, 1945.

7. Moller, K. O. and Stefansson, K., Effect of cocaine and procaine on hyperglycaemic action of adrenaline, *Arch. Int. Pharmacodyn.*, 57, 35, 1937.

8. Chopra, R. N. and Bose, J. P., The action of opium in diabetes, *Indian J. Med. Res.*, 18, 15, 1930.

9. Kochneva, N. P., The action of insulin, adrenaline and morphine on the distribution of sugar in the organism, *Ark. Biol. Nauk.*, 30, 45, and *C. A.*, 24, 4860, 1930.

10. Horning, E. S., Cytopathological studies of morphine poisoning and chronic morphinism in the albino rat, with reference to subsequent lecithin treatment, *Amer. J. Path.*, 10, 219, 1934.

11. Abood, L. G., Effect of morphine *in vivo* and *in vitro* on glycolysis of rat tissues, *Fed. Proc.*, 9, 252, 1950.

12. Abood, L. G., Kun, E., and Geiling, E. M. K., Phosphorylated intermediates of chronically and acutely morphinized rats, *J. Pharmacol. Exp. Ther.*, 98, 373, 1950.

13. Duckworth, M. W. and Ryman, B. E., Metabolic changes in tissues of the rat in acute and chronic morphinisation, *Arch. Int. Pharmacodyn.*, 113, 127, 1957.

14. Kyo, S., The influence of morphine and phenobarbital on the blood content of acetone-bodies in normal rabbits, *Jap. J. Pharmacol.*, 1, 79, 1952.

15. Barbour, H. G., Gregg, D. E., and Hunter, L. G., The calorigenic action of morphine as revealed by addiction studies, *J. Pharmacol. Exp. Ther.*, 40, 433, 1930.

16. von Boeck, H. and Bauer, J., Ueber den Einfluss einiger Arzneimittel auf den Gasaustausch bei Thieren 1. Einfluss des Morphiums auf den Gaswechsel, *Zschr. Biol.*, X, 336, 1874.

17. Williams, E. C. and Oberst, F. W., Cycle of morphine addiction; biological and psychological studies; biological investigations, *Public Health Rep.*, 61, 1, 1946.

18. Wright, C. J. and Barbour, F. A., The respiratory effects of morphine, codeine and related substances. III. The effect of morphine, dihydromorphine, dihydromorphinone and dihydrocodeinone on the respiratory activity of the rabbit, *J. Pharmacol. Exp. Ther.*, 53, 34, 1935.

19. Walsh, E. O'F., The hormonal basis of drug addiction, *Med. News,* London, 136, 13, 1965.

20. Kumagai, K., Experimental studies on the oxidase reaction of normal tissue and its significance, *Jap. Med. World,* 8, 508, 1928.

21. Wortis, S. B., Respiratory metabolism of excised brain tissue. II. Effects of some drugs on brain oxidations, *Arch. Neurol. Psychiat.*, 33, 1022, 1935.

22. Quastel, J. H. and Wheatley, A. H. M., Narcosis and oxidations of brain, *Proc. Roy. Soc.*, London, B, 112, 60, 1932.

23. Quastel, J. H. and Wheatley, A. H. M., The effects of amines on oxidations of the brain, *Biochem. J.*, 27, 1609, 1933.

24. Gross, E. G. and Pierce, I. H., Effect of morphine on the oxygen consumption of brain tissue in the rat, *J. Pharmacol. Exp. Ther.*, 53, 156, 1935.

25. Shideman, F. E. and Seevers, M. H., Some effects of morphine on the respiration of brain, spinal cord, and skeletal muscle *in vitro*, *J. Pharmacol. Exp. Ther.*, 69, 301, 1940.

26. Seevers, M. H. and Shideman, F. E., Effects of morphine and its derivatives on intermediary metabolism. I. On dehydrogenase activity and respiration of rat cerebrum, *J. Pharmacol. Exp. Ther.*, 71, 373, 1941.

27. Elliott, H. W., Comparative effects of 1:1-diphenyl-1-(dimethylamino-isopropyl)-butanone-2 (10820), demerol, and morphine on the respiration of rat cerebral cortex slices, *Fed. Proc.*, 6, 327, 1947.

28. Mayer, N. and McCawley, E. L., Comparison of the influence of morphine and a morphine antagonist, *N*-allylnormorphine, on the respiration of rat cerebrum, *Fed. Proc.*, 4, 129, 1945.

29. Shideman, F. E. and Seevers, M. H., Some in vitro effects of morphine on the respiratory metabolism of skeletal muscle, *J. Pharmacol. Exp. Ther.*, 72, 36, 1941.

30. Watts, D. T., Inhibition of succinoxidase system by meperidine, methadon, morphine and codeine, *J. Pharmacol. Exp. Ther.*, 95, 117, 1949.

31. Wang, R. I. H. and Bain, J. A., Cytochrome enzymes in the brain and liver of the chronically morphinized rat, *J. Pharmacol. Exp. Ther.*, 108, 349, 1953.

32. Wang, R. I. H. and Bain, J. A., Analgesics and enzymes of the cytochrome chain, *J. Pharmacol. Exp. Ther.*, 108, 354, 1953.

33. Lewis, J. L., Tissue distribution and metabolic effects of some analgesics and other agents affecting the CNS, Ph. D. Thesis, University of London, London, 1955.

34. Davidson, M., Some effects of morphine upon the respiration of rat cerebrum, M. Sc. Thesis, University of London, London, 1958.

35. Bell, J. L., Concentration of some analgesic compounds and their analogues in tissues surviving *in vitro*: relation to *in vitro* metabolism and *in vivo* effects, *J. Neurochem.*, 2, 265, 1958.

36. Ghosh, J. J. and Quastel, J. H., Narcotics and brain respiration, *Nature*, London, 174, 28, 1954.

37. Takemori, A. E., Studies on cellular adaptation to morphine and its reversal by nalorphine in cerebral cortical slices of rats, *J. Pharmacol. Exp. Ther.*, 135, 89, 1962.

38. Achor, L. B. and Geiling, E. M. K., Morphine and N-allylnormorphine: effects on brain C-14 levels following tracer doses of glucose-C-14, *Arch. Int. Pharmacodyn.*, 105, 313, 1956.

39. Takemori, A. E., The influence of morphine on glucose utilization in cerebral preparations of rats, *J. Pharmacol. Exp. Ther.*, 145, 20, 1964.

40. Takemori, A. E., The lag period associated with the stimulation of cerebral glucose utilization and CO_2 formation by morphine *in vitro*, *J. Pharmacol. Exp. Ther.*, 6, 87, 1967.

41. Dodge, P. W. and Takemori, A. E., Effect of morphine on cerebral glycolytic intermediates and enzymes of rats *in vitro*, *Biochem. Pharmacol.*, 18, 1873, 1969.

42. Seevers, M. H. and Shideman, F. E., On the oxidative metabolism of skeletal muscle from chronically morphinized rats, *J. Pharmacol. Exp. Ther.*, 72, 35, 1941.

43. Shideman, F. E. and Seevers, M. H., Effects of morphine and its derivatives on intermediary metabolism. III. The influence of chronic morphine poisoning on the oxygen consumption of rat skeletal muscle, *J. Pharmacol. Exp. Ther.*, 74, 88, 1942.

44. Shideman, F. E. and Seevers, M. H., Effects of morphine and its derivatives on intermediary metabolism. II. The influence of thiamine deficiency on the respiration of skeletal muscle and cocarboxylase content of tissues of normal and chronically morphinized rats, *J. Pharmacol. Exp. Ther.*, 71, 383, 1941.

45. Lee Peng, C. H. and Walsh, E. O'F., Effects of morphine on uptake of glucose and synthesis of glycogen in muscle of normal and chronically morphinized rats, *Nature,* London, 196, 171, 1962.

46. Lee Peng, C. H. and Walsh, E. O'F., Effects of morphine on the hormonal control of metabolism. I. *In vitro* effects of morphine and hydrocortisone on utilization of glucose by muscle of normal and chronically morphinized rats, *Biochem. Pharmacol.*, 12, 921, 1963.

47. Walsh, E. O'F., Lee Peng, C. H. and Ng, M. L., Reversal of hormonal effects as a result of chronic morphinization, *Nature,* London, 204, 698, 1964.

48. Ng, M. L. and Walsh, E. O'F., Effects of morphine on the hormonal control of metabolism. II. *In vitro* effects of adrenaline and hydrocortisone on utilization of glucose by muscle of normal and chronically morphinized rats, *Biochem. Pharmacol.*, 14, 1003, 1965.

49. Ng, M. L. and Walsh, E. O'F., Effects of morphine on the hormonal control of metabolism. III. Effects *in vitro* of morphine and adrenaline on utilization of glucose by muscle of normal and chronically morphinized rats, *Biochem. Pharmacol.*, 15, 1867, 1966.

50. Walsh, E. O'F., Lee Peng, C. H., and Wong, S. C., Sensitivity to insulin is morphine-dependent in muscle of chronically morphinized rats, *Biochem. Pharmacol.*, 18, 1529, 1969.

51. Wong, S. C. and Walsh, E. O'F., Effects of morphine on the hormonal control of metabolism.VI. Effects *in vitro* of thyroxine and aldosterone on uptake of glucose by muscle of normal and chronically morphinized rats, *Biochem. Pharmacol.*, 20, 417, 1971.

52. Poon, M. W. and Walsh, E. O'F., Morphine cancels effect of magnesium on hormone-sensitive uptake of glucose by muscle, *Nature,* London, 215, 525, 1967.

53. Ng, M. L., Poon, M. W., and Walsh, E. O'F., Effects of morphine on the hormonal control of metabolism. IV. Morphine-induced changes in sensitivity of the glucose-uptake system of muscle to extracellular magnesium, *Biochem. Pharmacol.*, 17, 1575, 1968.

54. Wong, S. C. and Walsh, E. O'F., Effects of morphine on the hormonal control of metabolism. V. Morphine-induced changes in sensitivity of the glucose-uptake system of muscle to extracellular potassium, *Biochem. Pharmacol.*, 18, 1979, 1969.

55. Fong, Y. Y. and Walsh, E. O'F., Effects of morphine on the hormonal control of metabolism. VII. Morphine-induced changes in sensitivity of the glucose-uptake system of muscle to extracellular calcium, *Biochem. Pharmacol.*, 20, 619, 1971.

56. Krueger, H., Eddy, N. B. and Sumwalt, M., The pharmacology of the opium alkaloids, *Public Health Rep.*, 165, Suppl. part 1, 666, 1941.

57. Vachon, M. and Marchand, C., The influence of morphine on magnesium metabolism in rats, *J. Pharmacol. Exp. Ther.*, 172, 122, 1970.

58. Kakunaga, T., Kaneto, H., and Hano, K., Pharmacologic studies on analgesics. VII. Significance of the calcium ion in morphine analgesia, *J. Pharmacol. Exp. Ther.*, 153, 134, 1966.

59. Marchand, C. and Denis, G., Diuretic effect of chronic morphine treatment in rats, *J. Pharmacol. Exp. Ther.*, 162, 331, 1968.

60. Mulé, S. J., Inhibition of phospholipid-facilitated calcium-transport by central nervous system acting drugs, *Biochem. Pharmacol.*, 18, 339, 1969.

61. Fong, Y. Y., Walsh, E. O'F., and Wong, S. C., Changes in intracellular distribution of potassium, magnesium, and calcium in skeletal muscle as a result of chronic morphinization, *Biochem. Pharmacol.*, in press.

62. Araki, T., Ueber die Bildung von Milchsaüre und Glycose im Organismus bei Saurestoffmangel, *Z. Physiol Chem.*, 15, 335, 1891.

63. Underhill, F. P. and Black, C. L., The influence of cocaine upon metabolism with special reference to the elimination of lactic acid, *J. Biol. Chem.*, 11, 235, 1912.

64. Felloni, G., L'action de la cocaine sur la fonction respiratoire du sang, *Arch. Ital Biol.*, 89, 69, 1935.

65. Cook, E. S. and McDevitt, M., Depression of tissue and yeast respiration by local anesthetics, *Stud. Inst. Divi Thomae*, 4, 107, 1945.

66. Bach, M. D. and Lambert, J., Action des anesthétiques et des hypnotiques sur les déshydrogénases du *Staphylocoque doré*, *Bull. Soc. Chim. Biol.*, 20, 818, 1938.

67. Ryman, B. E. and Walsh, E. O'F., Some effects of cocaine on the metabolism of *Saccharomyces cerevisiae*, *Biochem. J.*, 50, 570, 1952.

68. Travell, J., The influence of hydrogen ion concentration on the absorption of alkaloids from the stomach, *J. Pharmacol. Exp. Ther.*, 69, 21, 1940.

69. Ryman, B. E. and Walsh, E. O'F., Reversal of the effect of vitamin B_1 on yeast fermentation as a result of growth in the presence of cocaine, *Nature*, London, 167, 770, 1951.

70. Ryman, B. E. and Walsh, E. O'F., Inhibitory action of cocaine, *Nature*, London, 172, 679, 1953.

71. Ryman, B. E. and Walsh, E. O'F., Site of inhibitory action of cocaine in cellular respiration., *Biochem. J.*, 58, 111, 1954.

72. Kalyanpur, S. G. and Walsh, E. O'F., Malic acid synthesis in *Escherichia coli* and its inhibition by cocaine, *Nature*, London, 188, 99, 1960.

73. Ryman, B. E. and Walsh, E. O'F., Local anaesthetics as inhibitors of citrate synthesis, *J. Pharmacol.*, London, 7, 341, 1955.

74. Langley, J. N. and Dickinson, W. L., On the local paralysis of the peripheral ganglia, and on the connection of different classes of nerve fibres with them, *Proc. Roy. Soc.*, 46, 423, 1889; 47, 379, 1890.

75. Langley, J. N. and Dickinson, W. L., Actions of various poisons upon nerve fibres and peripheral nerve-cells, *J. Physiol.*, 11, 509, 1890.

76. Langley, J. N. and Dickinson, W. L., Pituri and Nicotin, *J. Physiol.*, 11, 265, 1890.

77. Greenwood, M., On the action of nicotin upon certain invertebrates, *J. Physiol.*, 11, 573, 1890.

78. McIndoo, N. E., Effects of nicotine as an insecticide, *J. Agr. Res.*, 7, 89, 1916.

79. Wilson, G. F., Nicotine as an insecticide, *Amer. J. Pharmacol.*, 100, 403, 1928.

80. Himwich, H. E. and Fazekas, J. F., Effect of nicotine on oxidations in the brain, *Amer. J. Physiol.*, 113, 63, 1935.

81. Himwich, H. E. and Fazekas, J. F., Effect of nicotine on the oxidations of diabetic brain, *Amer. J. Physiol.*, 116, 46, 1936.

82. Baker, Z., Fazekas, J. F., and Himwich, H. E., Carbohydrate oxidation in normal and diabetic cerebral tissues, *J. Biol. Chem.*, 125, 545, 1938.

83. Quastel, J. H. and Wheatley, A. H. M., Observations on anaerobic glycolysis in brain, *J. Biol. Chem.*, 119, 1xxx, 1937.

84. Fahmy, A. R. and Walsh, E. O'F., Effects of nicotine on the pyruvic oxidase system in brain, *Biochem. J.*, 58, 231, 1954.

85. Unna, K. and Pick, E. P., Inhibition of nervous transmission in synapses and end plates by thiamine, *J. Pharmacol. Exp. Ther.*, 81, 294, 1944.

86. Pick, E. P. and Unna, K., Blockade of the nicotine action on the blood pressure by thiazole compounds (sulphathiazole and thiamine), *J. Pharmacol. Exp. Ther.*, 87, 138, 1946.

87. Haimovici, H. and Pick, E. P., Inhibitory effect of thiamine on vasoconstrictor action of nicotine tested in the Laewen-Trendelenburg preparation, *Proc. Soc. Exp. Biol. Med.*, 62, 234, 1946.

88. Case, E. M. and McIlwain, H., Respiration and phosphorylation in preparations from mammalian brain, *Biochem. J.*, 48, 1, 1951.

89. Nachmansohn, D. and John, H. M., Inhibition of choline acetylase by α-keto-acids, *Proc. Soc. Exp. Biol. Med.*, 57, 361, 1944.

90. Fahmy, A. R., Ryman, B. E., and Walsh, E. O'F., Inhibition of choline acetylase by nicotine, *J. Pharmacol.*, London, 6, 607, 1954.

91. Fahmy, A. R. and Walsh, E. O'F., Some effects of nicotine on various dehydrogenase systems, *J. Pharmacol.*, London, 7, 107, 1955.

92. Fahmy, A. R. and Walsh, E. O'F., Evidence for the occurrence of glucose dehydrogenase in yeast, *Nature*, London, 173, 872, 1954.

93. Enders, C. and Windisch, Untersuchung über den Abbau von Nicotin durch Hefen, *Biochem. Z.*, 318, 54, 1947.

94. Dickens, F., The metabolism of normal and tumour tissue. XVII. The action of some derivatives of phenazine, quinoline and pyridine on the Pasteur reaction, *Biochem. J.*, 30, 1233, 1936.

95. McIlwain, H., Properties of preparations from the central nervous system which degrade coenzyme I and II: their connection with carbohydrate metabolism, *Biochem. J.*, 46, 612, 1950.

96. Greig, M. E., The effect of ascorbic acid in reducing the inhibition of brain metabolism produced by pentobarbital in vitro, *J. Pharmacol. Exp. Ther.*, 91, 317, 1947.

97. Geiger, A. and Magnes, J., The isolation of the cerebral circulation and the perfusion of the brain in the living cat, *Amer. J. Physiol.*, 149, 517, 1947.

98. Merivale, W. H. H. and Hunter, R. A., Abnormal glucose-tolerence tests in patients treated with sedative drugs (mainly barbiturates), *Lancet*, London, 2, 939, 1954.

99. Hunter, R. A., Merivale, W. H. H., and Smith, A. J., Disturbances of carbohydrate metabolism caused by barbiturates and alcohol, *Lancet*, London, 2, 1353, 1955.

100. Sutherland, V. C., Hine, C. H., and Burbridge, T. N., The effect of ethanol on cerebral cortex metabolism *in vitro*, *J. Pharmacol. Exp. Ther.*, 116, 469, 1956.

101. Dewan, J. G., Alcohol detoxication mechanism in central nervous system, *Amer. J. Psychiat.*, 99, 565, 1943.

102. Hine, C. H., Shick, A. F., Margolis, L., Burbridge, T. N., and Simon, A., Effects of alcohol in small doses and tetraethylthiuramdisulphide (antabus) on the cerebral blood flow and cerebral metabolism, *J. Pharmacol. Exp. Ther.*, 106, 253, 1952.

103. Greig, M. E., The site of action of narcotics on brain metabolism, *J. Pharmacol. Exp. Ther.*, 87, 185, 1946.

104. Persky, H., Goldstein, M. S., and Levine, R., The enzymatic mechanism of barbiturate action, *J. Pharmacol. Exp. Ther.*, 100, 273, 1950.

105. Johnson, W. J. and Quastel, J. H., Narcotics and biological acetylation, *Nature*, London, 171, 602, 1953.

106. Eiler, J. J. and McEwen, W. K., The effect of pentobarbital on aerobic phosphorylation in brain homogenates, *Arch. Biochem.*, 20, 163, 1949.

107. Aldridge, W. N. and Parker, V. H., Barbiturates and oxidative phosphorylation, *Biochem. J.*, 76, 47, 1960.

108. Bain, J. A., Enzymatic aspects of barbiturate action, *Fed. Proc.*, 11, 653, 1952.

109. Brody, T. M. and Bain, J. A., Barbiturates and oxidative phosphorylation, *J. Pharmacol. Exp. Ther.*, 110, 148, 1954.

110. Aldridge, W. N., Action of barbiturates upon respiratory enzymes, in *Enzymes and Drug Action,* J. and A. Churchill Ltd., London, 1962, 155.

111. McIlwain, H., Appraising enzymic actions of central depressants by examining cerebral tissues, in *Enzymes and Drug Action,* J. and A. Churchill Ltd., London, 1962, 170.

112. Davies, D. R. and Quastel, J. H., Dehydrogenations by brain tissue. Effects of narcotics, *Biochem. J.*, 26, 1672, 1932.

113. Himwich, W. A., Homburger, E., Maresca, R., and Himwich, A. E., Brain metabolism in man: unanesthetized and in pentothal narcosis, *Amer. J. Psychiat.*, 103, 689, 1947.

114. Larrabee, M. G., Ramos, J. G., and Bülbring, E., Do anesthetics depress nerve cells by depressing oxygen consumption? *Fed. Proc.*, 9, 75, 1950.

115. Karlsson, J. L., Sutherland, V. C., and Elliot, H. W., Delayed arrest of rat-brain slice respiration caused by pentobarbitone during glucose metabolism, *J. Pharmacol. Exp. Ther.*, 103, 1, 1951.

116. McIlwain, H., The effect of depressants on the metabolism of stimulated cerebral tissues, *Biochem. J.*, 53, 403, 1953.

117. Lamson, P. D., Greig, M. E., and Hobdy, C. J., Potentiation of barbiturate anesthesia by certain brain metabolites, *Trans. Ass. Amer. Physicians,* 64, 237, 1951.

118. Kaufmann, M. J., Water metabolism and narcosis, *Arch. Int. Pharmacodyn.*, 103, 167, 1955.

119. Jowett, M., The action of narcotics on brain respiration, *J. Physiol.*, 92, 322, 1938.

120. Fuhrman, F. A. and Field, J., Inhibition of brain respiration by ethyl alcohol at varied temperature levels, *Proc. Soc. Exp. Biol. Med.*, 69, 331, 1948.

121. Beer, C. T. and Quastel, J. H., The effects of aliphatic alcohols on the respiration of rat brain cortex slices and rat brain mitochondria, *Canad. J. Biochem. Physiol.*, 36, 543, 1958.

122. Wallgren, H., Comparison of effect of ethanol and malonate on respiration of rat brain cortex slices, *Acta Physiol. Scand.*, 49, 216, 1960.

123. Wallgren, H. and Kulonen, E., Effect of ethanol on respiration of rat-brain-cortex slices, *Biochem. J.*, 75, 150, 1960.

124. Conklin, J. L., Duvey, M. M., and May, B., On heterogeneity of lactic dehydrogenase, *J. Histochem. Cytochem.*, 10, 365, 1962.

125. Järnefelt, J., Properties of sodium-stimulated ATP-ase in microsomes from rat brain, *Exp. Cell. Res.*, 21, 214, 1960.

126. Kini, M. M. and Cooper, J. R., Biochemistry of methanol poisoning 1. Phosphorylation coupled to mitochondrial oxidation of formaldehyde, *Biochim. Biophys. Acta,* 44, 599, 1960.

127. Mann, P. J. G. and Quastel, J. H., Benzedrine (β-phenylisopropylamine) and brain metabolism, *Biochem. J.*, 34, 414, 1940.

128. Kerkut, G. A., Rick, J. T., and Huggins, A. K., The intermediary metabolism *in vitro* of glucose and acetate by ganglia from *Helix aspersa,* and the effects of amphetamine, *Comp. Biochem. Physiol.*, 28, 765, 1969.

129. Duhault, J. and Malen, C., Effect of a fenfluramine derivative (S992) on lipid and sugar metabolism, *International Symposium on Amphetamines and Related Compounds,* Costa, E. and Garattini, S., Eds., Raven Press, New York, 1970, 619.

130. Duhault, J. and Boulanger, M., Actions de l'amphétamines et de certains de ses dérivés halogénés sur les métabolismes lipidique et glucidique, *Journées Annuelles de Diabétologie de l'Hôtel Dieu,* Médicales Flammarion, Paris, 1966.

131. Dannenburg, W. N. and Kardian, B. C., Metabolic effects of fenfluoramine and methamphetamine on free fatty acid release and glucose utilisation in epididymal fat cells of the rat, *International Symposium on Amphetamines and Related Compounds,* Costa, E. and Garattini, S., Eds., Raven Press, New York, 1970, 597.

132. Butterfield, W. J. H. and Whichelow, M. J., Fenfluoramine and muscle glucose uptake in man, *Lancet,* London, 13, 109, 1968.

133. Whichelow, M. J. and Butterfield, W. J. H., Effects of fenfluoramine on peripheral glucose metabolism in man, *International Symposium on Amphetamine and Related Compounds,* Costa, E. and Garattini, S., Eds., Raven Press, New York, 1970, 611.

134. Moore, K. E., Effects of (+)-amphetamine on lactic acid concentrations in the tissues of aggregated mice, *J. Pharmacol.,* London, 18, 196, 1966.

135. Chatterjee, A. K., Jacob, S. A., Srivastava, R. H., Pabrai, P. R., and Ghose, A., Influence of methylamphetamine on blood lactic acid following exercise, *Jap. J. Pharmacol.,* 20, 170, 1970.

136. Downing, D. F., Psychotomimetic compounds, *Psychopharmacological Agents,* Vol. 1, Gordon, M., Ed., Academic Press, New York, 1964, 598.

NEUROTRANSMITTERS AND THE NARCOTIC ANALGESICS

C. B. Smith

TABLE OF CONTENTS

INTRODUCTION

In recent years, considerable attention has been focused upon the relationship between neurotransmitter substances in the brain and various peripheral tissues and certain specific pharmacological actions of the narcotic analgesics and other dependence-producing drugs. The first evidence that the narcotic analgesics affected neurotransmitters was provided by Vogt who found that morphine decreased the catecholamine content of the brain and adrenal medulla of the cat.[1] Subsequently, norepinephrine, dopamine, serotonin (5-hydroxytryptamine), and acetylcholine have been implicated with regard to certain specific actions of the narcotic analgesics. One approach to the study of the relationship between neurotransmitters and the narcotic analgesics has been to use drugs which alter the synthesis, storage, release, and metabolism of various neurotransmitters. Such drugs cause complex changes in certain specific effects of the narcotic analgesics. These drug interactions have been reviewed extensively and will not be discussed in this chapter.[2-7]

In order to relate the effects of the narcotic analgesics upon neurotransmitters to other specific actions of these drugs, the specificity of the effects of these drugs upon the synthesis, storage, release, and metabolism of various neurotransmitters must be established. Seevers and Deneau describe three features of the pharmacological actions of the narcotic analgesics which are characteristic of the specific effects of all such drugs.[8] First, when these drugs are administered repeatedly, tolerance develops to their specific effects. Second, once tolerance develops to a specific effect of any narcotic analgesic, tolerance (cross tolerance) exists to that effect produced by all other drugs of this class. The degree of tolerance and the rate of development of tolerance depend upon the specific effect being studied, species, drug dosage, and frequency and duration of drug administration. Third, antagonists such as nalorphine, levallorphan, and naloxone block the specific effects of the narcotic analgesics. Seevers and Deneau suggest that tolerance develops only to the depressant effects of this class of drugs upon the central nervous system.[8] Such depressant effects include analgesia, hypothermia, respiratory depression, and narcosis. However, tolerance and cross tolerance also develop to the stimulant effects of the narcotic analgesics upon the locomotor activity of mice.[9] Naloxone also blocks the effects of various narcotic analgesics upon mouse locomotor activity.

In the present chapter, the effects of the narcotic analgesics upon the synthesis, storage, release, and metabolism of norepinephrine, dopamine, serotonin, and acetylcholine will be discussed. An attempt will be made to determine whether the actions of these drugs represent specific effects as defined by Seevers and Deneau.[8] Finally, the relationship between the ability of the narcotic analgesics to produce physical dependence and their ability to alter neurotransmitter function will be evaluated.

CATECHOLAMINES – NOREPINEPHRINE AND DOPAMINE

Brain Catecholamine Content

The acute administration of morphine reduced the adrenal catecholamine content of rats and cats and the brain catecholamine content of mice, rats, and cats.[1,9-15] Levorphanol, *l*-methadone, and ketobemidone were more potent, and meperidine less potent than morphine in depleting catecholamines from the mouse brain. A good correlation was found between the ability of a narcotic analgesic to increase the locomotor activity of the mouse and its ability to deplete brain catecholamines.[9]

The effect of morphine and related drugs upon brain catecholamine content appears to be a specific effect as defined by Seevers and Deneau.[8] After the repeated administration of morphine to mice, tolerance developed to the catecholamine-depleting effect of this drug upon the mouse brain.[9] Similar tolerance developed to the effects of levorphanol upon brain catecholamine content after repeated administration of levorphanol. Chronic administration of levorphanol to mice resulted in cross tolerance to the catecholamine-depleting effect of morphine, ketobemidone, *l*-methadone, and meperidine.[9] Naloxone, which is devoid of morphine-like activity, is a specific antagonist of many specific effects of morphine.[16] Naloxone prevented the catecholamine-depleting effect in the mouse brain of morphine, levorphanol, *l*-methadone, and ketobemidone.[9] Thebaine, *d*-methadone, and dextrorphan, drugs structurally related to the narcotic analgesics, are devoid of analgesic and dependence-producing activity. Thebaine and *d*-methadone did not affect the catecholamine content of the mouse brain.[9] Dextrorphan resembles *d*-amphetamine in that it increases the locomotor activity of mice and decreases brain catecholamine content. However, cross tolerance to the activity-increasing and catecholamine-depleting effects of these drugs did not develop after the repeated administration of morphine. Also, naloxone did not antagonize either effect of dextrorphan or *d*-amphetamine.[9] Therefore, the effect of the narcotic analgesics upon brain catecholamine content appears to be a specific effect.

Release of Catecholamines

Acute administration of morphine increases the release and turnover of catecholamines from the adrenal medulla and the brain. The intravenous injection of morphine, 2 mg/kg, to the anesthetized dog caused a release of adrenal catecholamines.[17] During the primary phase of addiction to morphine in man, the urinary excretion of epinephrine, norepinephrine, dopamine, and their metabolites was increased.[18] These observations indicate that morphine also releases adrenal catecholamines in man. After inhibition of catecholamine biosynthesis by *a*-methyltyrosine, the depletion of dopamine from the rat brain caused by the acute administration of morphine was markedly accelerated.[19] This observation suggests that morphine releases dopamine from neurons in the brain. Therefore, a plausible explanation of the catecholamine-depleting effect of morphine is that this drug releases catecholamines from neurons and increases the rate of catecholamine turnover. Increases in the rate of catecholamine turnover should be reflected by increases in the rate of catecholamine synthesis.

Synthesis of Catecholamines

After the acute administration of either morphine or levorphanol, the conversion of ^{14}C-tyrosine in vivo into ^{14}C-catecholamines was nearly doubled in mouse brain and adrenals.[20-22] Morphine also increased the incorporation of ^{14}C-tyrosine into ^{14}C-dopamine in the hypothalamus and striatum of the rat brain.[23] Levorphanol was about ten times more potent than morphine in its effect upon ^{14}C-catecholamine synthesis in the mouse brain.[21,22] The effects of the narcotic analgesics are specific to the brain and adrenals and do not occur in other tissues containing adrenergic neurons such as the heart or spleen. The increases in incorporation of ^{14}C-tyrosine into ^{14}C-catecholamines in the mouse brain are not merely a consequence of either drug-induced increases in locomotor activity or decreases in brain catecholamine content. Moreover, *d*-amphetamine and dextrorphan, which both increase locomotor activity and decrease brain catecholamine content, do not increase incorporation of ^{14}C-tyrosine into ^{14}C-catecholamines in the mouse brain.[21,22]

Clouet and Ratner found morphine-induced increases in incorporation of ^{14}C-tyrosine into ^{14}C-dopamine in the hypothalamus and striatum, but not in other areas of the rat brain.[23] In contrast, Smith and his colleagues observed that the synthesis of ^{14}C-dopamine was increased in the striatum, cerebral cortex, diencephalon, brainstem, and cerebellum of the mouse brain.[21] Similar increases in ^{14}C-norepinephrine synthesis were seen in the diencephalon, cerebral cortex, brainstem and cerebellum, but not in the striatum of the mouse brain.[21] The differences between these two studies are probably due to the fact that Clouet and Ratner injected ^{14}C-tyrosine intracisternally, whereas Smith et al. injected the labeled amino acid intravenously.

The increase in ^{14}C-catecholamine synthesis in the mouse brain produced by both morphine and levorphanol is an effect which possesses those features characteristic of the other specific effects of the narcotic analgesics. With repeated administration of these drugs, tolerance developed to their effect upon the incorporation of ^{14}C-tyrosine into ^{14}C-catecholamines in the mouse brain.[20-22] Tolerance was manifested by a shift to the right in the dose-response curves for morphine and levorphanol. Clouet and Ratner reported that tolerance did not develop to the effect of a large dose of morphine, 60 mg/kg, upon the incorporation of ^{14}C-tyrosine into ^{14}C-dopamine in the rat brain.[23] In that study, however, only one dose of morphine was studied which apparently produced a maximum effect upon ^{14}C-dopamine synthesis in both tolerant and nontolerant rats. In a similar study, Reis et al. suggested that tolerance to morphine was associated with increased tyrosine hydroxylase activity in rat brain.[24] The differences among these various studies indicate the necessity of determining complete dose-response relationships when evaluating the development of tolerance to a drug. Mice made tolerant to the effect of levorphanol upon brain ^{14}C-catecholamine synthesis were also tolerant (cross tolerant) to the effect of morphine upon ^{14}C-catecholamine synthesis.[21] Finally, naloxone blocked the effect of morphine upon the incorporation of ^{14}C-tyrosine into ^{14}C-catecholamines in the mouse brain.[20,21]

Dependence

A recent study suggests that once mice are made tolerant to the effects of morphine upon catecholamine synthesis, the brain becomes dependent upon morphine to maintain normal rates of catecholamine synthesis (S. J. Rosenman and C. B. Smith, unpublished observations). Mice were made tolerant by injections of morphine, 100 mg/kg, at six-hour intervals for about three days. Once complete tolerance had developed, abrupt withdrawal from morphine resulted in decreased incorporation of ^{14}C-tyrosine into ^{14}C-dopamine and ^{14}C-norepinephrine in the mouse brain below levels of incorporation observed in tolerant mice prior to withdrawal or in control mice never exposed to morphine. The maximum decrease in catecholamine synthesis occurred about 36 hours after the last injection of morphine. These observations suggest that the catecholamines might play an important role in the mechanisms by which morphine-like drugs produce physical dependence.

ACETYLCHOLINE

Brain Acetylcholine Content

In contrast to the decrease in brain catecholamine content caused by the narcotic analgesics, the acetylcholine content of whole brain is increased in several species by the acute administration of morphine and related drugs. Morphine increased the acetylcholine content of the mouse brain and of the rat brain.[25-31] Crossland and Slater reported that morphine increased "bound" acetylcholine but decreased "free" acetylcholine in the rat brain.[30] Richter and Goldstein,[27] however, found that both morphine and levorphanol increased the acetylcholine content of all fractions, including the "free" acetylcholine defined operationally by Crossland and Slater. Free acetylcholine may be an artifact resulting from the means by which various fractions are prepared and probably does not represent any known anatomical compartment of acetylcholine.

In addition to the narcotic analgesics, other drugs with central nervous system depressant effects increase the acetylcholine content of whole brain. Phenothiazines, barbiturates, and the Rauwolfia alkaloids increase the acetylcholine content of the rat brain.[31,32] Nevertheless, the effect of the narcotic analgesics upon brain acetylcholine content appears to be a specific effect of this class of drugs. Repeated administration of narcotic analgesics over prolonged periods of time results in the development of tolerance to the effect of these drugs upon brain acetylcholine content. The development of tolerance depends upon the dosage of the narcotic, the daily schedule of administration, and the duration of pretreatment. Rats treated with morphine, 100 mg/kg, twice daily for nine days showed tolerance to the behavioral and analgesic effects of this drug. However, the final dose of morphine caused nearly as large an increase in brain acetylcholine content as did the first dose.[29] In contrast, when morphine, 100 mg/kg, was administered to rats twice daily for periods of six to ten weeks, complete tolerance developed to the effects of morphine upon brain acetylcholine content.[33] Tolerance also developed to the effects of morphine upon the acetylcholine content of mouse brain.[25] A similar development of tolerance to the effects of levorphanol upon the acetylcholine content of the mouse brain occurred when levorphanol, 50 mg/kg, was administered twice daily for two to three weeks.[27] In this study, the development of tolerance to the effects of levorphanol upon acetylcholine content appeared to be correlated with the development of tolerance to the analgesic effect of this drug as tested by the hot plate technique. Maynert reported that nalorphine had little antagonistic effect against morphine-induced increases in brain acetylcholine content of the rat.[29] Nalorphine is a partial agonist, however, and the large doses used alone might have increased brain acetylcholine content, thus masking any antagonistic action. The relationship between morphine-induced changes in brain acetylcholine content and other specific effects of the narcotic analgesics remains obscure.

Synthesis and Metabolism of Acetylcholine

Among the explanations of the morphine-induced increases in brain acetylcholine content are the possibilities that the narcotic analgesics either increase acetylcholine synthesis or inhibit cholinesterases to prevent the enzymatic destruction of acetylcholine. Rather than increase synthesis, morphine and its antagonists, nalorphine, naloxone, and pentazocine, actually inhibited the synthesis of acetylcholine by mouse cerebral cortex slices in vitro.[34] Morphine also inhibited the synthesis of ^{14}C-acetylcholine from ^{14}C-glucose by rat brain slices in vitro.[35,36] Morphine probably does not have prominent direct effects upon choline acetylase, the enzyme responsible for the conversion of choline to acetylcholine.[37-40] Thus, the observed decreases in ^{14}C-acetylcholine synthesis may result from a feedback inhibition secondary to the morphine-induced accumulation of acetylcholine. Pharmacologically effective doses of morphine also do not inhibit cholinesterases.[31,41]

Release of Acetylcholine

An alternative explanation of the morphine-induced increases in brain acetylcholine content is the possibility that the narcotic analgesics prevent release of acetylcholine from neurons. Morphine and related narcotic analgesics inhibit the release of acetylcholine from the coaxially stimulated guinea pig ileum.[42-44] Dihydromorphinone, methadone, heroin, and levorphanol were more effective, and codeine less effective than morphine in inhibiting acetylcholine release.[42,45,46] Nalorphine was equipotent to morphine in inhibiting release of acetylcholine from the isolated guinea pig ileum.[46] It is of interest that in man nalorphine is equipotent to morphine as an analgesic.[47] In the rat and rabbit, morphine diminished the effect of vagal stimulation upon the heart which suggested an inhibition of acetylcholine release.[48] Morphine also produced a relatively specific inhibition of acetylcholine release from cardiac postganglionic cholinergic fibers in isolated rabbit sino-atrial node-right atrial preparations.[49] In general, there is a good correlation between the analgesic potency of a morphine-like drug and the ability of the drug to inhibit acetylcholine release.

The narcotic analgesics also inhibit the release of acetylcholine from cholinergic neurons within the central nervous system. Beleslin and Polack showed that morphine depressed the release of acetylcholine into perfusates of the lateral ventricle of the cat brain.[50] Recently, morphine, meperidine, and methadone were found to be equipotent in preventing the spontaneous release of acetylcholine from the perfused surface of the sensorimotor cortex of the cat.[51,52] Codeine had a similar effect but was much less potent than morphine. The partial agonists, levallorphan and nalorphine, also reduced the spontaneous release of acetylcholine from this preparation.[52] Naloxone did not alter the spontaneous release of acetylcholine. Pentazocine and propoxyphene, analgesics with little morphine-like potential to produce physical dependence, also decreased the spontaneous release of acetylcholine.[52] Chlorpromazine resembled the narcotic analgesics in that this drug reduced spontaneous release of acetylcholine from the perfused cortex. Naloxone, however, did not antagonize the effects of chlorpromazine upon the release of acetylcholine.[52] In addition, the inhibitory effects of pentazocine and propoxyphine were antagonized only poorly by naloxone. In contrast, naloxone, nalorphine, and levallorphan were very effective in antagonizing the inhibitory effect of morphine upon the release of acetylcholine from the perfused sensorimotor cortex of the cat.[52] The antagonistic effect of naloxone was overcome by large doses of morphine. Naloxone is considered to be a competitive inhibitor of morphine. Drugs with central nervous system depressant activity, like chlorpromazine, appear to decrease the spontaneous release of acetylcholine from the perfused cat cortex. However, the inhibitory action of the narcotic analgesics apparently is a specific effect since it is antagonized by drugs which block other specific effects of morphine-like drugs. Inhibition of release of acetylcholine from cholinergic neurons in the brain seems to be the basis for the increases in brain acetylcholine content which occur after the acute administration of the narcotic analgesics.

Dependence

Tolerance to morphine-induced changes in the release and turnover of acetylcholine in the brain may be related to the dependent state. In rats made tolerant by the injection of morphine, 100 mg/kg, twice daily for a period of 6 to 10 weeks, morphine caused no increases in brain acetylcholine content. Nalorphine, 50 mg/kg, caused a marked increase in the brain acetylcholine content of these tolerant rats.[33] Nalorphine precipitates a withdrawal syndrome in animals physically dependent upon morphine. Abrupt withdrawal of morphine from the tolerant rat also caused an increase in brain acetylcholine content which reached a peak between 39 and 46 hours after the final administration of morphine.[33] It is of interest that in the brains of the morphine-tolerant mouse, abrupt withdrawal of morphine resulted in changes in ^{14}C-catecholamine synthesis which had a time course similar to that of the changes in brain acetylcholine content in the withdrawn rat. The relationship between morphine-induced changes in brain catecholamine synthesis and turnover and changes in brain acetylcholine content remains to be studied.

SEROTONIN

Brain Serotonin Content

Acute administration of morphine has neither pronounced nor consistent effects upon brain serotonin content. Bonnycastle et al. found that morphine, meperidine, numerous barbiturates, and ethyl alcohol caused a slight increase in the serotonin content of the rat brain.[53] In contrast,

Lee and Fennessy reported that morphine caused a transient decrease in the serotonin content of the rat brain.[13] Most investigators, however, find that morphine has little effect upon brain serotonin content when administered either acutely or over prolonged periods of time to a variety of species.[54-57]

Dependence

Recently, considerable controversy has arisen over the possibility that serotonin turnover is increased in the brains of animals treated chronically with morphine. In one study, mice were injected with morphine, 40 mg/kg, every 8 hours for 3 weeks.[58] Tolerance was determined by measuring the increase in the median analgesic dose of morphine in response to a thermal stimulus (the tail-flick method). Dependence was considered to be present when the mice demonstrated marked jumping behavior after the administration of naloxone. In these studies, the rate of accumulation of serotonin in the brain was measured after inhibition of monoamine oxidase by pargyline. In the brains of mice considered to be both tolerant to the analgesic effects of morphine and physically dependent, the rate of accumulation of serotonin was increased.[58] Maruyama et al. also observed an increased rate of accumulation of serotonin after inhibition of monoamine oxidase by pargyline in the brains of mice 3 days after implantation with morphine pellets.[59] In similar studies, the accumulation of 5-hydroxyindoleacetic acid (5-HIAA), a major metabolite of serotonin, was measured after its egress from the brain was blocked by probenecid.[60] The rate of accumulation of 5-HIAA was greater in the brains of mice made tolerant to the analgesic actions of morphine than in control mice. Chronic administration of methadone also resulted in increased rates of accumulation of 5-HIAA in the mouse brain.[61] In contrast, when mice were treated with high doses of morphine for 4 days, no changes from saline control values were detected for the rate of accumulation of serotonin in the brain after administration of the monoamine oxidase inhibitor tranylcypromine.[62] These mice were considered to be dependent on the basis of naloxone-induced jumping. Azmitia et al. reported increased tryptophan hydroxylase activity in the brains of rats treated chronically with morphine.[63] This observation is consistent with an increase in the rate of turnover of serotonin in the morphine-dependent rat. Recently, a technique was described for determining rates of synthesis of ^{3}H-serotonin from ^{3}H-tryptophan in vivo.[64] Using this technique, Cheney et al. found no increase in the synthesis of ^{3}H-serotonin in the brains of mice rendered tolerant to the analgesic effects of morphine and dependent as determined by the naloxone-induced jumping test.[65] These differences among the various studies of the effects of the narcotic analgesics upon serotonin turnover in tolerant and dependent animals remain to be resolved.

CONCLUSIONS

Among the drugs which produce dependence, the narcotic analgesics have specific effects upon the content and turnover of various neurotransmitters in the brain. Acute administration of these drugs prevents the release of acetylcholine and causes an accumulation of this substance in the brains of various species. Tolerance to these effects develops when the narcotic analgesics are administered over prolonged periods of time. These effects of the narcotic analgesics are specifically blocked by narcotic antagonists. Acute administration of the narcotic analgesics also causes decreases in brain catecholamine content and increases in the synthesis and turnover of both dopamine and norepinephrine in the brain. Tolerance develops to morphine-induced changes in brain catecholamine turnover when narcotic analgesics are administered chronically. Specific narcotic antagonists block the effects of the narcotic analgesics upon catecholamine turnover in the brain. The acute administration of the narcotic analgesics does not have pronounced effects upon brain serotonin content. Changes in the rates of turnover of acetylcholine, dopamine, norepinephrine, and serotonin have been related to the dependent state produced by chronic administration of the narcotic analgesics.

REFERENCES

1. Vogt, M., The concentration of sympathin in different parts of the central nervous system under normal conditions and after the administration of drugs, *J. Physiol.* (London), 123, 451, 1954.

2. Cochin, J., Possible mechanisms in development of tolerance, *Fed. Proc.*, 29, 19, 1970.

3. Dole, V., Biochemistry of addiction, *Ann. Rev. Biochem.*, 39, 821, 1970.

4. Harris, L. S., Central neurohumoral systems involved with narcotic agonists and antagonists, *Fed. Proc.*, 29, 28, 1970.

5. Weinstock, M., Acetylcholine and cholinesterase, in *Narcotic Drugs: Biochemical Pharmacology*, Clouet, D., Ed., Plenum Press, New York, 1971, 254.

6. Way, E. L. and Shen, F., The effect of narcotic analgesic drugs on specific systems: catecholamines and 5-hydroxytryptamine, in *Narcotic Drugs: Biochemical Pharmacology*, Clouet, D., Ed., Plenum Press, New York, 1971, 229.

7. Way, E. L., Role of serotonin in morphine effects, *Fed. Proc.*, 31, 113, 1972.

8. Seevers, M. H. and Deneau, G. A., Physiological aspects of tolerance and physical dependence, in *Physiological Pharmacology*, Root, W. J. and Hoffman, F. G., Eds., Academic Press, New York, 1963, 565.

9. Rethy, C. R., Smith, C. B., and Villarreal, J. E., Effects of narcotic analgesics upon the locomotor activity and brain catecholamine content of the mouse, *J. Pharmacol. Exp. Ther.*, 176, 472, 1971.

10. Gunne, L-M., Catecholamines and 5-hydroxytryptamine in morphine tolerance and withdrawal, *Acta Physiol. Scand.*, 58, 5, 1963.

11. Ray, A. K., Mukherji, M., and Ghosh, J. J., Adrenal catecholamines and related changes during different phases of morphine administration – a histochemical study, *J. Neurochem.*, 15, 875, 1968.

12. Takagi, H. and Nakama, M., Effect of morphine and nalorphine on the content of dopamine in mouse brain, *Jap. J. Pharmacol.*, 16, 483, 1966.

13. Lee, J. R. and Fennessy, M. R., The relationship between morphine analgesia and the levels of biogenic amines in the mouse brain, *Europ. J. Pharmacol.*, 12, 65, 1970.

14. Maynert, E. W. and Klingman, G. I., Tolerance to morphine. I. Effects on catecholamines in the brain and adrenal glands, *J. Pharmacol. Exp. Ther.*, 135, 285, 1962.

15. Reis, D. J., Rifkin, M., and Corvelli, A., Effects of morphine on cat brain norepinephrine in regions with daily monoamine rhythms, *Europ. J. Pharmacol.*, 9, 149, 1969.

16. Blumberg, H., Dayton, H. B., and Wolf, P. S., Counteraction of narcotic antagonist analgesics by the narcotic antagonist naloxone, *Proc. Soc. Exp. Biol. Med.*, 123, 755, 1966.

17. Kayaalp, S. O. and Kaymakcalan, S., Studies on the morphine-induced release of catecholamines from the adrenal glands in the dog, *Arch. Intern. Pharmacodyn.*, 172, 139, 1968.

18. Weil-Malherbe, H., Smith, E. R. B., Eisenman, A. J., and Fraser, H. F., Plasma catecholamine levels and urinary excretion of catecholamines and metabolites in two human subjects during a cycle of morphine addiction and withdrawal, *Biochem. Pharmacol.*, 14, 1621, 1965.

19. Gunne, L-M., Jonsson, J., and Fuxe, K., Effects of morphine intoxication on brain catecholamine neurons, *Europ. J. Pharmacol.*, 5, 338, 1969.

20. Smith, C. B., Villarreal, J. E., Bednarczyk, J. H., and Sheldon, M. I., Tolerance to morphine-induced increases in [^{14}C] catecholamine synthesis in mouse brain, *Science*, 170, 1106, 1970.

21. Smith, C. B., Sheldon, M. I., Bednarczyk, J. H., and Villarreal, J. E., Morphine-induced increases in the incorporation of ^{14}C-tyrosine into ^{14}C-dopamine and ^{14}C-norepinephrine in the mouse brain: antagonism by naloxone and tolerance, *J. Pharmacol. Exp. Ther.*, 180, 547, 1972.

22. Smith, C. B. and Sheldon, M. I., Effects of narcotic analgesic drugs on brain noradrenergic mechanisms, in *The Pharmacology of Morphine Agonists and Antagonists,* Kosterlitz, H. W., Villarreal, J. E., and Collier, H. O. J., Eds., McMillan Co., London, 1972, in press.

23. Clouet, D. H. and Ratner, M., Catecholamine biosynthesis in brains of rats treated with morphine, *Science,* 168, 854, 1970.

24. Reis, D. J., Hess, P., and Azmitia, E. C., Changes in enzymes subserving catecholamine metabolism in morphine tolerance and withdrawal in rat, *Brain Res.,* 20, 309, 1970.

25. Hano, K., Kaneto, H., Kakunaga, T., and Moribayashi, N., Pharmacological studies of analgesics. VI. The administration of morphine and changes in acetylcholine metabolism in mouse brain, *Biochem. Pharmacol.,* 13, 441, 1964.

26. Howes, J. F., Harris, L. S., Dewey, W. L., and Voyda, C. A., Brain acetylcholine levels and inhibition of the tail-flick reflex in mice, *J. Pharmacol. Exp. Ther.,* 169, 23, 1969.

27. Richter, J. A. and Goldstein, A., Effects of morphine and levorphanol on brain acetylcholine content in mice, *J. Pharmacol. Exp. Ther.,* 175, 685, 1970.

28. Giarman, N. J. and Pepeu, G., Drug-induced changes in brain acetylcholine, *Brit. J. Pharmacol.,* 19, 226, 1962.

29. Maynert, E. W., Effects of morphine on acetylcholine and certain other transmitters, *Arch. Biol. Med. Exp.,* 4, 36, 1967.

30. Crossland, J. and Slater, P., The effect of some drugs on the "free" and "bound" acetylcholine content of rat brain, *Brit. J. Pharmacol.,* 33, 42, 1968.

31. Naik, S. R. and Sheth, U. K., Studies on rat brain acetylcholine and cholinesterase. Part II. The influence of centrally acting drugs, *Indian J. Med. Res.,* 58, 480, 1970.

32. Naik, S. R., Anjaria, R. K., and Sheth, U. K., Studies on rat brain acetylcholine and cholinesterase. Part I. Effect of body weight, sex, stress and C.N.S. depressant drugs, *Indian J. Med. Res.,* 58, 473, 1970.

33. Large, W. A. and Milton, A. S., The effect of acute and chronic morphine administration on brain acetylcholine levels in the rat, *Brit. J. Pharmacol.,* 38, 451, 1970.

34. Howes, J. F., Harris, L. S., and Dewey, W. L., The effect of morphine, pentazocine, cyclazocine and oxotremorine on the synthesis and release of acetylcholine by mouse cerebral cortex slices in vitro, *Arch. Intern. Pharmacodyn.,* 184, 267, 1970.

35. Sharkawi, M. and Schulman, M. P., Inhibition by morphine of the release of [^{14}C]acetylcholine from rat brain cortex slices, *J. Pharm. Pharmacol.,* 21, 546, 1969.

36. Sharkawi, M., Effects of morphine and pentobarbitone on acetylcholine synthesis by rat cerebral cortex, *Brit. J. Pharmacol.,* 40, 86, 1970.

37. Torda, C. and Wolff, H. G., Effect of convulsant and anticonvulsant agents on acetylcholine metabolsim (activity of choline acetylase and cholinesterase) and on sensitivity to acetylcholine of effector organs, *Amer. J. Physiol.,* 151, 345, 1947.

38. De La Lande, I. S. and Bentley, G. A., The action of morphine and antagonists of the narcotic action of morphine on acetyl choline synthesis in brain, *Aust. J. Exp. Biol. Med. Sci.,* 33, 555, 1955.

39. Kumagai, H., Ebashi, S., and Takeda, F., Studies on choline acetylase (1), *Jap. J. Pharmacol.,* 4, 24, 1954.

40. Morris, R. W., Effects of drugs on the biosynthesis of acetylcholine: pentobarbital, morphine, and morphinan derivatives, *Arch. Int. Pharmacodyn. Ther.,* 133, 236, 1961.

41. Jóhannesson, T., Morphine as an inhibitor of brain cholinesterases in morphine-tolerant and non-tolerant rats, *Acta Pharmacol. Toxicol.*, 19, 23, 1962.

42. Paton, W. D., The action of morphine and related substances on contraction and on acetylcholine output of co-axially stimulated guinea-pig ileum, *Brit. J. Pharmacol.*, 12, 119, 1957.

43. Schaumann, W., Inhibition by morphine of the release of acetylcholine from the intestine of the guinea-pig, *Brit. J. Pharmacol.*, 12, 115, 1957.

44. Cowie, A. L., Kosterlitz, H. W., and Watt, A. J., Mode of action of morphine-like drugs on autonomic neuro-effectors, *Nature* (London), 220, 1040, 1968.

45. Cox, B. M. and Weinstock, M., The effect of analgesic drugs on the release of acetylcholine from electrically stimulated guinea-pig ileum, *Brit. J. Pharmacol.*, 27, 81, 1966.

46. Gyang, E. A. and Kosterlitz, H. W., Agonist and antagonist actions of morphine-like drugs on the guinea-pig isolated ileum, *Brit. J. Pharmacol.*, 27, 514, 1966.

47. Lasagna, L. and Beecher, H. K., The analgesic effectiveness of nalorphine and nalorphine-morphine combinations in man, *J. Pharmacol. Exp. Ther.*, 112, 356, 1954.

48. Kosterlitz, H. W. and Taylor, D. W., The effect of morphine on vagal inhibition of the heart, *Brit. J. Pharmacol.*, 14, 209, 1959.

49. Kennedy, B. L. and West, T. C., Effect of morphine on electrically-induced release of autonomic mediators in the rabbit sinoatrial node, *J. Pharmacol. Exp. Ther.*, 157, 149, 1967.

50. Beleslin, D. and Polak, L., Depression by morphine and chloralose of acetylcholine release from the cat's brain, *J. Physiol.* (London), 177, 411, 1965.

51. Jhamandas, K., Pinsky, C., and Phillis, J. W., Effects of morphine and its antagonists on release of cerebral cortical acetylcholine, *Nature*, 228, 176, 1970.

52. Jhamandas, K., Phillis, J. W., and Pinsky, C., Effects of narcotic analgesics and antagonists on the *in vivo* release of acetylcholine from the cerebral cortex of the cat, *Brit. J. Pharmacol.*, 43, 53, 1971.

53. Bonnycastle, D., Bonnycastle, M. F., and Anderson, E. G., The effect of a number of central depressant drugs upon brain 5-hydroxytryptamine levels in the rat, *J. Pharmacol. Exp. Ther.*, 135, 17, 1962.

54. Brodie, B. B., Shore, P. A., and Pletscher, A., Serotonin-releasing activity limited to rauwolfia alkaloids with tranquilizing action, *Science*, 123, 992, 1956.

55. Maynert, E. W., Klingman, G. I., and Kaji, H. K., Tolerance to morphine. II. Lack of effects on brain 5-hydroxytryptamine and γ-aminobutyric acid, *J. Pharmacol. Exp. Ther.*, 135, 296, 1962.

56. Bartlett, A. L., The 5-hydroxytryptamine content of mouse brain and whole mice after treatment with some drugs affecting the central nervous system, *Brit. J. Pharmacol.*, 15, 140, 1960.

57. Sloan, J. W., Brooks, J. W., Eisenman, A. J., and Martin, W. R., The effect of addiction to and abstinence from morphine on rat tissue catecholamine and serotonin levels, *Psychopharmacologia*, 4, 261, 1963.

58. Loh, H. H., Shen, F., and Way, E. L., Inhibition of morphine tolerance and physical dependence development and brain serotonin synthesis by cycloheximide, *Biochem. Pharmacol.*, 18, 2711, 1969.

59. Maruyama, Y., Hayashi, G., Smits, S. E., and Takemori, A. E., Studies on the relationship between 5-hydroxytryptamine turnover in brain and tolerance and physical dependence in mice, *J. Pharmacol. Exp. Ther.*, 178, 29, 1971.

60. Shen, F. H., Loh, H. H., and Way, E. L., Brain serotonin turnover in morphine tolerant and dependent mice, *J. Pharmacol. Exp. Ther.*, 175, 427, 1970.

61. Bowers, M. R. and Kleber, H. D., Methadone increases mouse brain 5-hydroxyindoleacetic acid, *Nature*, 229, 134, 1971.

62. Marshall, I. and Grahame-Smith, D. G., Unchanged rate of brain serotonin synthesis during chronic morphine treatment and failure of parachlorophenylalanine to attenuate withdrawal syndrome in mice, *Nature*, 228, 1206, 1970.

63. Azmitia, E. C., Hess, P., and Reiss, D., Tryptophan hydroxylase changes in midbrain of the rat after chronic morphine administration, *Life Sci.*, 9, 633, 1970.

64. Neff, N. H., Spano, P. F., Groppetti, A., Wang, C. T., and Costa, E., A simple procedure for calculating the synthesis rate of norepinephrine, dopamine and serotonin in rat brain, *J. Pharmacol. Exp. Ther.*, 176, 701, 1971.

65. Cheney, D. L., Goldstein, A., Algeri, S., and Costa, E., Narcotic tolerance and dependence: lack of relationship with serotonin turnover in the brain, *Science,* 171, 1169, 1971.

LIPIDS

E. J. Simon

TABLE OF CONTENTS

INTRODUCTION

This chapter is devoted to a review of the most important studies of interactions with cellular lipids of drugs which produce dependence. The cell membrane has been shown to be of great importance for conduction and transmission of impulses in the nervous system and recent studies from a number of laboratories have revealed that various dependence-producing drugs affect the structure and function of the cell membrane. Some of these studies will be briefly cited, where appropriate, and special emphasis will be placed on the effect of the drugs on the metabolism of phospholipids. These are found almost exclusively in cell membranes and are thought to have great importance in membrane function and structural integrity. The importance of lipids in biological systems has been even further enhanced in recent years by the discovery of the group of compounds known as prostaglandins. These molecules exhibit a variety of physiological effects. They are synthesized in the cell by modification of fatty acids and evidence is available that they are made on cell membranes.

It will be evident from this review that numerous reports have appeared on the effects of dependence-causing drugs on the metabolism of lipids and, in particular, phospholipids in a variety of biological systems. While no clear-cut relationship between these effects and the pharmacological actions of the drugs has been established, it is hoped that a summary of the various results in this area will stimulate investigators to pursue those aspects which appear to offer some promise of further insight into the mode of action of the drugs and the process by which dependence is established.

MORPHINE AND RELATED DRUGS

In Brain

The effect of morphine on phospholipid synthesis in rat cerebral cortex slices was first reported in a brief note by Brossard and Quastel[1] in 1963. Incubation of the cortical slices in the presence of 5 or 10 mM morphine resulted in a 40% increase in the incorporation of ^{32}P into

TABLE 1

The Incorporation of P_i^{32} into Phospholipids of Guinea Pig Cerebral Cortex Slices in the Presence of Morphine

Phospholipid	Control[a] cpm/100 mg[d]	Morphine[b] (10^{-2} M) cpm/100 mg	Change[c] %	Morphine (5×10^{-3} M) cpm/100 mg	Change %
Lysophosphatidylinositol	2,775 ± 182 (30)	5,445 ± 703[e] (9)	+96	3,937 ± 778[f] (6)	+42
Phosphatidylinositol	5,785 ± 432 (30)	15,852 ± 1542[e] (9)	+174	8,297 ± 1112[f] (6)	+44
Phosphatidylcholine	11,708 ± 1008 (34)	5,200 ± 1033[e] (8)	−56	5,528 ± 1248[f] (5)	−53
Phosphatidylserine	3,167 ± 315 (28)	5,817 ± 953[g] (9)	+84	3,378 ± 651 (6)	+7
Phosphatidylethanolamine	2,752 ± 268 (31)	5,663 ± 997[e] (8)	+106	4,056 ± 650[f] (6)	+47
Phosphatidic Acid	3,647 ± 156 (32)	12,259 ± 1775[e] (9)	+236	4,583 ± 387[f] (6)	+26
Diphosphoinositide	4,337 ± 321 (32)	9,349 ± 1568[e] (9)	+115	6,679 ± 1096[f] (6)	+54
Triphosphoinositide	13,263 ± 1399 (30)	14,273 ± 2640 (7)	+8	11,768 ± 3694 (6)	+11

a) Control values given are means ± S.E.M. with the number of observations in parentheses. Samples from 14 animals were used in these experiments.
b) Experimental values given are means ± S.E.M. with the number of observations in parentheses. Samples from four to eight animals were used to provide the data obtained at each concentration of morphine.
c) Percentage difference between the mean values obtained with morphine and the mean control values.
d) Fresh tissue. All radioactivity was corrected to a specific activity of 10^5 cpm/μg of phosphorus for the orthophosphate of the medium.
e) $P < .001$ as compared to the control value.
f) $P < .05$ as compared to the control value.
g) $P < .01$ as compared to the control value.

(Reprinted from Mulé[2] by courtesy of *J. Pharmacol. Exp. Ther.*)

phospholipids. This stimulation was due largely to increased labeling of phosphatidic acid and phosphoinositide and to a lesser extent of phosphatidyl serine and "unidentified spot 1."

More recently, a detailed study of the effect of morphine on phospholipid metabolism in guinea pig brain has been carried out by Mulé. In vitro studies[2] were carried out with cerebral cortex slices which were incubated in Krebs-Henseleit buffer with radioactive phospholipid precursors such as $^{32}P_i$ and ^{14}C-glycerol. The phospholipids were isolated and separated by chromatographic techniques and the effects of drugs on the incorporation of radioactivity into various phosphatides were determined.

Table 1 shows that addition of morphine to the cortical slices, at the very high concentration of 10 mM, resulted in stimulation of ^{32}P incorporation into all of the major phospholipids except phosphatidyl choline, for which a 56% inhibition was observed. The most striking stimulation was seen with phosphatidyl inositol (174%) and phosphatidic acid (236%). The latter showed a statistically significant stimulation (24%) even at 10^{-6}M morphine, but the significance of this result is doubtful since no such stimulation was seen at intermediate concentrations of morphine. Comparable results were obtained using other labeled phospholipid precursors such as glycerol-1, 3-^{14}C, myo-inositol-^{14}C and choline-methyl-^{14}C. These results indicate that morphine does not merely stimulate turnover of the phosphate

TABLE 1 (continued)

Morphine (10^{-3} M) cpm/100 mg	Change %	Morphine (10^{-4} M) cpm/100 mg	Change %	Morphine (10^{-6} M) cpm/100 mg	Change %
2,626 ± 382 (7)	+5	3,232 ± 345 (11)	+16	4,131 ± 746[g] (5)	+49
10,009 ± 1330[e] (8)	+73	7,282 ± 932 (12)	+26	6,861 ± 1228 (10)	+19
6,327 ± 1317[g] (10)	−46	9,704 ± 1044 (10)	−17	11,011 ± 1965 (10)	−6
3,225 ± 1250 (6)	+2	3,551 ± 579 (7)	+12	3,209 ± 583 (7)	+1
2,369 ± 677 (10)	−14	2,752 ± 450 (10)	0	2,929 ± 663 (10)	+6
3,958 ± 475 (10)	+8	3,924 ± 376 (10)	+8	4,512 ± 374[f] (9)	+24
4,722 ± 888 (4)	+9	3,960 ± 531 (4)	−9	6,062 ± 1195 (5)	+40
6,122 ± 1226[f] (8)	−54	5,857 ± 820[g] (10)	−56	11,959 ± 3039 (9)	+10

a) Control values given are means ± S.E.M. with the number of observations in parentheses. Samples from 14 animals were used in these experiments.
b) Experimental values given are means ± S.E.M. with the number of observations in parentheses. Samples from four to eight animals were used to provide the data obtained at each concentration of morphine.
c) Percentage difference between the mean values obtained with morphine and the mean control values.
d) Fresh tissue. All radioactivity was corrected to a specific activity of 10^5 cpm/μg of phosphorus for the orthophosphate of the medium.
e) P <.001 as compared to the control value.
f) P <.05 as compared to the control value.
g) P <.01 as compared to the control value.

(Reprinted from Mulé[2] by courtesy of *J. Pharmacol. Exp. Ther.*)

moiety, but affects turnover of the entire phospholipid molecule.

The morphine antagonist nalorphine gave results very similar to those obtained with morphine. When added with morphine it did not alter the morphine effect in a consistent manner.

Mulé suggests that the most likely explanation of these results is a direct effect on phospholipid biosynthesis, since no effects on the concentration and specific activity of the acid-soluble pool were observed, nor did there seem to be any change in overall energy metabolism.

Experiments were also carried out in which morphine was administered in vivo and phospholipid metabolism was examined in cerebral cortex slices prepared from the brains of such guinea pigs.[3] A single dose of 40 mg/kg (calculated as free base) of morphine sulfate was administered to guinea pigs by subcutaneous injection. The animals were sacrificed 1, 4, and 10 hours later. Cerebral cortex slices from injected and control animals were incubated in the presence and absence of morphine as described for the all-in vitro experiments. Table 2 shows that significant stimulation of ^{32}P incorporation into all phospholipids except diphosphoinositide was achieved by the level of morphine present in the brains of injected guinea pigs. The addition to the slices of 10 mM morphine resulted in a highly significant further stimulation of incorporation. No change beyond that caused by the in vivo level of morphine resulted from in vitro additions of lower concentrations of the drug. Incorporation of ^{32}P into phosphatidyl choline was stimulated in injected animals but when 10 mM morphine was present during the incubation, this phospholipid again exhibited inhibition. All of the in vivo effects were clear-cut one hour after injection of morphine, more variable at four hours, and largely absent after ten hours.

Of considerable interest is the finding depicted in Table 3 that in vivo morphine exerted no significant effect on phospholipid metabolism in brain slices from guinea pigs previously made tolerant to morphine. In vitro addition of 10 mM morphine to cortical slices from tolerant animals caused significant stimulation, but lower concentrations were without effect. The guinea pig brain thus appeared to have adapted completely to the in vivo level of morphine and to be sensitive only to the highest in vitro level.

More recently, Mulé[4] has been able to demonstrate an effect of morphine administration on phospholipid metabolism in the whole animal. Figure 1 shows that the subcutaneous injection of 40 mg of morphine per kg body weight into a guinea pig markedly increased incorporation of ^{32}P into total cerebral cortex phospholipids at 16 and 24 hours after injection of ^{32}P. No statistically significant effect was seen either at 4 or 48 hours post-injection. When individual phospholipids were examined, significant stimulation was seen in a number of them even 48 hours after ^{32}P administration. The greatest stimulatory changes were seen in phosphatidyl choline, the major brain phospholipid, which represents 25 to 40% of total brain lipid phosphorus. Subfractionation of cells showed similar alterations in phospholipid metabolism in each cell fraction. Experiments carried out with liver and its subfractions yielded rather similar results to those seen in cerebral cortex.

In Single Cells

Bacteria

A number of laboratories have reported effects of morphine and its congeners on membrane function and phospholipid metabolism in bacteria. The discussion of phospholipid metabolism will be preceded by a brief enumeration of some of the effects on cell membranes which led investigators to study effects on phospholipid metabolism.

Morphine and related drugs were found to alter the membrane transport of various molecules and ions. Simon et al.[5] reported a rapid efflux of the polyamine putrescine into the growth medium when cultures of *E. coli* were treated with 1 mM levorphanol. Gale[6] reported inhibition of accumulation in the free amino acid pool of certain amino acids (lysine and proline) by *S. aureus*, while that of others was stimulated. The drugs used in these experiments and their concentrations were heroin (30 to 60 mM), levallorphan (2 mM), and levorphanol (2 mM). In a more detailed study of putrescine transport in the presence of levorphanol, Simon et al.[7] demonstrated that levorphanol exerts two separate effects. It blocks putrescine uptake and it stimulates putrescine efflux. In the same report evidence was presented for altered transport of a number of amino acids, of spermidine, and of potassium ions. Greene and Magasanik[8] found a disappearance of accumulated β-galactoside upon treatment of *E. coli* with 5 mM levallorphan or 10 mM levorphanol. They also

TABLE 2

The Incorporation of P_i^{32} into Phospholipids of Cerebral Cortex Slices from Nontolerant Guinea Pigs[a]

Phospholipid	Control[c]	None[d]	Change[e] %	Additions of Morphine in vitro[b] 10⁻² M	Change %	10⁻⁴ M	Change %	10⁻⁶ M	Change %
Lysophosphatidyl-inositol	294 ± 49 (6)	419 ± 37[f] (4)	+42	698 ± 40[h] (4)	+137	433 ± 29[f] (4)	+47	443 ± 77[f] (4)	+51
Phosphatidyl-inositol	542 ± 68 (8)	867 ± 106[f] (6)	+60	1858 ± 39[h] (5)	+243	939 ± 144[f] (6)	+73	782 ± 128[f] (60	+44
Phosphatidyl-choline	1718 ± 279 (8)	2808 ± 216[g] (6)	+63	945 ± 130[f] (6)	–45	2758 ± 313[f] (6)	+60	2586 ± 178[f] (6)	+50
Phosphatidylserine + phosphatidyl-ethanolamine	395 ± 64 (8)	692 ± 118[f] (6)	+75	592 ± 44[f] (4)	+50	663 ± 43[g] (6)	+68	629 ± 85[f] (6)	+59
Phosphatidic acid	770 ± 99 (8)	1150 ± 162[f] (6)	+49	2095 ± 231[h] (5)	+172	1168 ± 99[f] (6)	+52	1076 ± 144[f] (6)	+40
Diphosphoinositide	696 ± 216 (8)	757 ± 66 (6)	+9	1184 ± 137[f] (5)	+70	798 ± 71 (6)	+15	795 ± 81 (6)	+14
Triphosphoinositide	1135 ± 107 (8)	2442 ± 377[h] (6)	+115	1479 ± 106[f] (5)	+30	1852 ± 111[g] (6)	+63	2089 ± 377[f] (6)	+84

a) Nontolerant guinea pigs were sacrificed 1 hour after a 40 mg/kg s.c. injection of morphine.
b) Results given as cpm/μmol of phosphorus/100 mg of fresh tissue. All radioactivity was corrected to a specific activity of 10^5 cpm/μg of phosphorus for the orthophosphate of the medium.
c) Control values given are means ± S.E.M. with the number of observations in parentheses. Samples from three saline-treated animals were used in these experiments.
d) Values given are means ± S.E.M. with the number of observations in parentheses. Samples from four morphine-treated animals were used in these experiments.
e) Percentage difference between the mean control value and the mean experimental value.
f) $P < .05$ as compared to the control value.
g) $P < .01$ as compared to the control value.
h) $P < .001$ as compared to the control value.

(Reprinted from Mule[3] by courtesy of *J. Pharmacol. Exp. Ther.*)

TABLE 3

The Incorporation of P_i^{32} into Phospholipids of Cerebral Cortex Slices from Chronically Morphine-treated Guinea pigs[a]

Additions of Morphine in vitro[b]

Phospholipid	Control[c]	None[d]	Change[e] %	10^{-2} M	Change %	10^{-4} M	Change %	10^{-6} M	Change %
Lysophosphatidyl-inositol	666 ± 133 (8)	487 ± 97 (6)	−27	914 ± 165 (6)	+37	433 ± 44 (6)	−35	468 ± 69 (6)	−30
Phosphatidyl-inositol	1009 ± 245 (12)	723 ± 140 (9)	−28	1623 ± 320 (9)	+61	808 ± 109 (9)	−20	902 ± 114 (9)	−11
Phosphatidyl-choline	1771 ± 339 (12)	1424 ± 198 (9)	−19	943 ± 122[f] (9)	−47	1865 ± 204 (9)	+ 5	2089 ± 202 (9)	+18
Phosphatidyl-serine	367 ± 55 (12)	357 ± 54 (9)	− 3	446 ± 45 (9)	+21	340 ±59 (9)	− 7	311 ± 29 (9)	−15
Phosphatidyletha-nolamine	364 ± 51 (12)	318 ± 54 (9)	−13	477 ± 38 (9)	+23	400± 58 (9)	+10	341± 32 (9)	− 6
Phosphatidic Acid	979 ± 90 (12)	918 ± 142 (9)	− 6	2350 ± 71[g] (9)	+ 140	1155 ± 153 (9)	+18	1200 ± 100 (9)	+22
Diphospho-inositide	626 ± 95 (12)	525 ± 55 (9)	−16	1049 ± 80[g] (9)	+67	621 ± 50 (9)	− 1	629 ± 28 (9)	0
Triphospho-inositide	1367 ± 169 (11)	1435 ± 261 (9)	+ 5	1902 ± 178[f] (9)	+39	1881 ± 222 (9)	+38	1722 ± 161 (9)	+26

a) Morphine-tolerant guinea pigs were sacrificed 1 hour after the last 40 mg/kg s.c. injection.

b) Results given as cpm/μmol of phosphorus/100 mg of fresh tissue. All radioactivity was corrected to a specific activity of 10^5 cpm/μg of phosphorus for the orthophosphate of the medium.

c) Control values given are means ± S.E.M. with the number of observations in parentheses. Samples from four saline-treated animals were used in these experiments.

d) Values given are means ± S.E.M. with the number of observations in parentheses. Samples from six chronically morphine-treated animals were used in these experiments.

e) Percentage difference between the mean control value and the mean experimental values.

f) $P < .05$ as compared to the control value.

g) $P < .001$ as compared to the control value.

(Reprinted from Mulé[3] by courtesy of *J. Pharmacol. Exp. Ther.*)

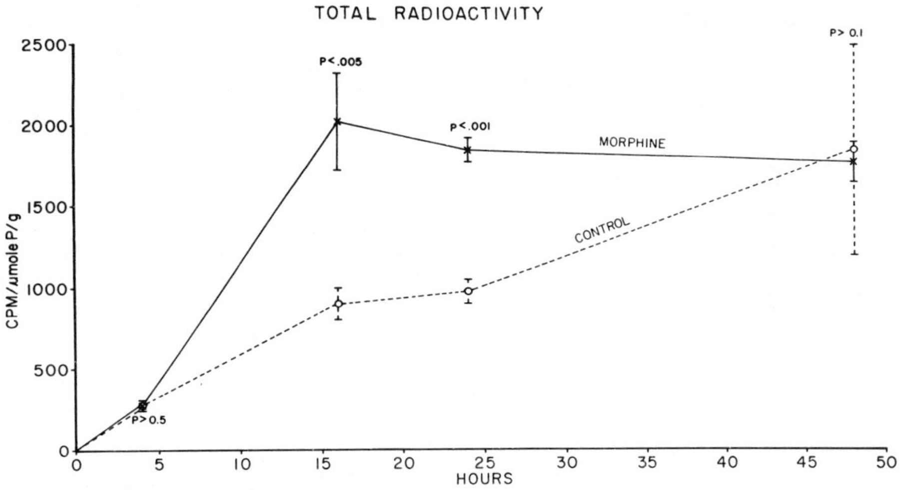

FIGURE 1. Morphine and the incorporation of $^{32}P_i$ in vivo into phospholipids of the whole cerebral cortex. Total radioactivities in the phospholipids extracted from the cerebral cortex after a $^{32}P_i$ (150 µc/100 g) i.p. injection to two to four guinea pigs. The time intervals of 4, 16, 24, and 48 hours represent time after $^{32}P_i$ administration. Morphine was administered s.c. (40 mg/kg, as free base) 1 hour prior to sacrifice. The control guinea pigs received a comparable volume of 0.9% saline s.c. 1 hour prior to sacrifice. Each value represents the mean obtained from four to eight determinations ±S.E. (Reprinted from Mulé, S. J.[4] by courtesy of *Biochem. Pharmacol.*)

observed a striking breakdown of ATP and leakage of hydrolysis products out of the cells. This ATP breakdown is not detectable at the 1 mM concentration used in our laboratory. Very recently Boquet et al.[9] reported effects of levallorphan on magnesium transport in *E. coli*.

These changes in membrane function in bacteria led investigators to examine effects of the drugs on phospholipid metabolism. Gale[10] reported the isolation of complexes of heroin (and of levorphanol or levallorphan) with *S. aureus* phospholipids, primarily phosphatidyl glycerol which is the major phospholipid of this organism (more than 90% of total phospholipid). He also found that concentrations of drugs which inhibit lysine uptake by 50% caused a drastic increase in the incorporation of labeled precursors into phospholipids. Interestingly, the stimulation was observed with ^{32}P and ^{14}C-glycerol, while incorporation of ^{14}C-acetate was inhibited (Figure 2). The stimulation of labeling with glycerol or ^{32}P was most striking in the minor phospholipid component, cardiolipin, which achieved levels of radioactivity as high as 60% of the total phospholipid label. Gale attributes this phenomenon to increased turnover of phosphatidyl glycerol which is an intermediate in the synthesis of cardiolipin.

A similar study was carried out in our laboratory[11] in the gram-negative bacteria, *E. coli*, which differ greatly from *S. aureus* in phospholipid composition. In logarithmically growing *E. coli*, the phospholipid composition is 60 to 70% phosphatidyl ethanolamine, 20 to 25% phosphatidyl glycerol, and 2 to 5% cardiolipin. Treatment of cultures with 1 mM levorphanol resulted in the following changes: 1. A reduction in incorporation of radioactive precursors into the total lipid fraction. In contrast to the results in *S. aureus*, even the incorporation of ^{32}P and ^{14}C-glycerol was diminished, though incorporation of glycerol tended to be decreased only slightly. 2. Incorporation of precursors into phosphatidyl ethanolamine was markedly reduced. The turnover of phosphatidyl glycerol was accelerated and phosphatidyl ethanolamine, normally stable in *E. coli*, exhibited turnover in the presence of levorphanol. 3. There was a gradual rise in the proportion of radioactivity present in cardiolipin, from 5% in untreated or very briefly treated cells to 55 to 70% of phospholipid radioactivity after 60 minutes of incubation in the presence of levorphanol. Most of these changes can be seen in the experiment depicted in Figure 3. It was of considerable interest that these labeling changes were accompanied by striking changes in phospholipid composition as deter-

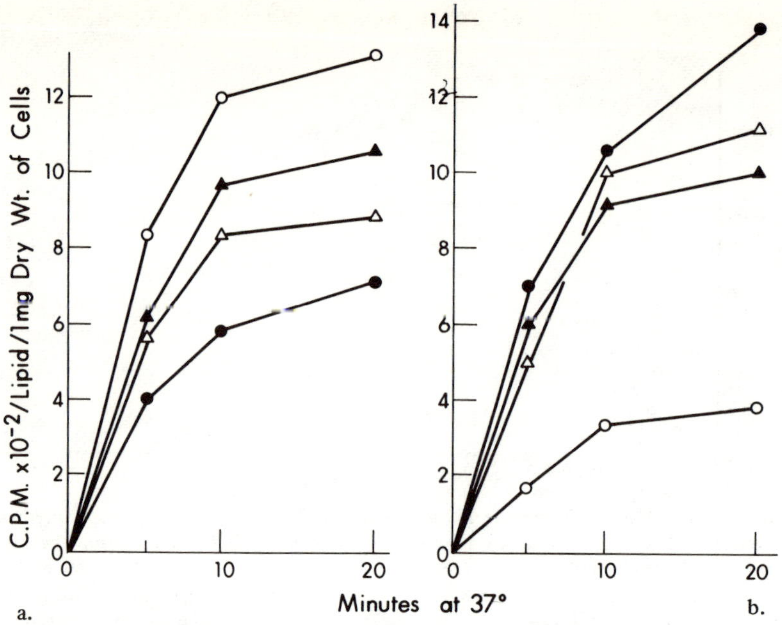

FIGURE 2. Effect of drugs on the incorporation of (1-^{14}C)-glycerol and (1-^{14}C)- acetate (b) into the lipid fraction of *S. aureus.* Cells were incubated at 0.2 mg dry weight per ml in buffered salts solution containing 0.3 mM glucose, 0.1 mM glycerol-(1-^{14}C) (specific activity, 1.57 mCi/mmol) in part a (unlabeled glycerol in part b), and 0.05 mM sodium acetate-(1-^{14}C) (specific activity, 2.9 mCi/mmol) in part b (unlabeled acetate in part a) with the drugs shown. Reaction stopped by rapid cooling, and lipid was extracted and counted. ●, no drug; 0, 30 mM heroin; ▲, 2 mM levorphanol; Δ, 2 mM levallorphan. (Reprinted with permission from Gale, E. F., *Molec. Pharmacol.*, 6, 134, 1970.)

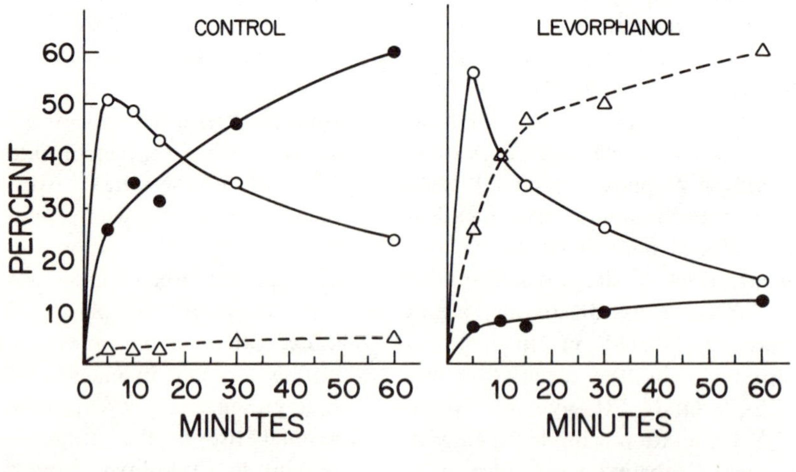

FIGURE 3. Effect of levorphanol on the percent distribution of radioactivity among the three major phospholipids of *E. coli* as a function of time. Cultures of *E. coli* B were incubated with (^{14}C) glycerol (0.4 μC/ml, 48 μM) and in the presence and absence of levorphanol (1.35 mM). Aliquots of the cultures were removed at the indicated intervals and extracted, chromatographed and counted as described in materials and methods. The ordinate represents the percent of total phospholipid radioactivity present in the individual phospholipids. ●-●, phosphatidyl ethanolamine; 0-0, phosphatidyl glycerol; Δ - Δ, cardiolipin. (Reprinted from Wurster et al.[11] by courtesy of *Biochim. Biophys. Acta.*)

mined by phosphorus analysis of the phospholipids separated by thin-layer chromatography. As shown in Table 4, after 1 hour of incubation with levorphanol, the phospholipid composition was 45% phosphatidyl ethanolamine, 10% phosphatidyl glycerol, and 45% cardiolipin, as compared to 68, 25, and 7%, respectively, in the control culture. As in *S. aureus*, all the observed changes slowly reverted towards normal after removal of the drug.

Two differences between the results of Gale in *S. aureus* and ours in *E. coli* require some comment. Whereas Gale found that heroin and the morphinans readily formed complexes with phospholipids, no evidence for such complexes was obtained with *E. coli*. The reason for this discrepancy is not clear but may be the result of the different separation procedures employed in the two laboratories.

As mentioned above, ^{14}C-glycerol incorporation was stimulated, while ^{14}C-acetate incorporation was reduced by the morphine congeners in *S. aureus*. The stimulation of glycerol incorporation was not seen in *E. coli*, but the inhibition of glycerol incorporation was considerably less than that of acetate incorporation. This lead the authors[11] to suggest that the explanation for both systems may be a stimulation of the independent turnover of the nonacylated glycerol of phosphatidyl glycerol. The independent turnover of this moiety has been reported by White and Tucker[12] for *Hemophilus parainfluenzae*. The much larger discrepancy seen in *S. aureus* is to be expected, since phosphatidyl glycerol represents a much larger proportion of its phospholipids.

The marked changes in phospholipid metabolism and composition in bacteria treated with drugs related to morphine may be responsible for the changes in cell membrane permeability produced by these drugs.

Leukocytes

Changes in membrane function and phospholipid metabolism have also been seen in levorphanol-treated mammalian cells.[13] Rabbit polymorphonuclear leukocytes were chosen for this study since they exhibit the easily measurable membrane function of phagocytosis. Levorphanol (1 to 2 mM) inhibits phagocytosis as shown by reduced killing of *E. coli* and a marked decrease in the uptake of latex particles and *E. coli* observed by electron microscopy.[14]

The major change in phospholipid metabolism observed during phagocytosis was a stimulation of the acylation of lysophosphatides.[15] This stimulation was completely abolished by levorphanol and there was a slight reduction in the level of acylation in resting granulocytes as shown for lysolecithin in Table 5. Levorphanol also caused a stimulation of incorporation of fatty acids into phosphatides. In contrast, incorporation of fatty acids into triglycerides was markedly reduced. Attempts to demonstrate complexes between levorphanol and phospholipids were unsuccessful. All effects of levorphanol were readily reversed upon removal of the drug.

Inhibition of phagocytosis and of the acylation

TABLE 4

Effect of Levorphanol on Phospholipid Labeling (^{32}P) and Composition in *E. Coli*

	Counts/minute x 10^{-3}		P(μg)		Counts/minute x 10^{-4} per μg P	
	Control	Levorphanol	Control	Levorphanol	Control	Levorphanol
Phosphatidyl ethanolamine	484 (69)	96 (19)	4.6 (68)	3.3 (45)	10	3
Phosphatidyl glycerol	180 (26)	72 (14)	1.7 (25)	0.7 (10)	10	10
Cardiolipin	36 (5)	345 (67)	0.5 (7)	3.2 (45)	7	11

Cultures (100 ml) were incubated with $^{32}P_i$ (0.8 μC/ml, 1 mM) in the absence and presence of levorphanol (1.3 mM) for 60 minutes. Cultures were extracted and extracts chromatographed and assayed for phosphorus and radioactivity as described in materials and methods. The figures in parentheses represent the percent distribution of counts and phosphorus among the three major phospholipids listed.
(Reprinted from Wurster et al.[11] by courtesy of *Biochim. Biophys. Acta*.)

TABLE 5

Effect of Levorphanol on the Acylation of Lysolecithin-^{32}P by Granulocytes

	–Polystyrene		+Polystyrene	
Control	100	(15)	241 ± 28	(15)
2 mM levorphanol	57 ± 4.5	(15)	91 ± 7.1	(15)
2 mM levorphanol preincubation*	63 ± 8.3	(4)	84 ± 6.2	(4)
Levorphanol removed	110 ± 16	(7)	208 ± 33	(7)

Granulocytes were incubated for 30 minutes in the presence or absence of polystyrene latex particles. LPC-^{32}P complexed to albumin was added in a concentration ranging from 15 to 100 μmol/l. in different experiments. In experiments in which recovery from the effect of levorphanol was examined, the cell suspension was divided into two portions incubated with or without levorphanol for 30 minutes, after which the cells were centrifuged at 200 g, resuspended twice in fresh medium, and reincubated for 30 minutes, with or without levorphanol as shown. Assay of PC-^{32}P formation was carried out as described in the section on methods. Results are expressed as percent of control values without polystyrene and are given as mean ±SE of the indicated number of experiments (n).

*Levorphanol added 30 minutes before addition of LPC-^{32}P and particles or saline.

(Reprinted from Wurster et al.[13] by courtesy of *J. Clin. Invest.*)

of lysocompounds could result from reduction in energy metabolism. However, levorphanol had no effect on glycolysis, the major energy-producing pathway in leukocytes, and a decrease in ATP level was not observed. Moreover, the stimulation of fatty acid incorporation into phospholipids was not compatible with this suggestion. It is, therefore, considered probable that the observed effects of levorphanol on phagocytosis and its biochemical concomitants are the results of alterations in the cell membrane, as has been postulated in the case of bacteria.

Giant Axon of Squid

It was of great interest to see whether morphine congeners exhibited membrane effects on nerve fibers, which have cell membranes specialized for the conduction of electrical impulses. For this purpose the well-studied giant axon of the squid *Loligo pealii* was used.[16]

When an excised giant axon was bathed in sea water (pH 8) containing 0.5 to 1 mM levorphanol, there was inhibition of the action potential which became complete in 20 to 30 minutes. Figure 4 shows this inhibition and its ready reversal by lowering the pH of the sea water. Similar effects

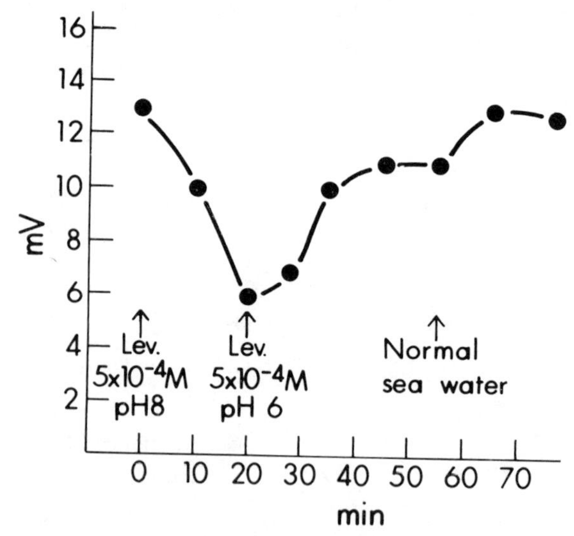

FIGURE 4. Effect of pH on potency of levorphanol (Lev.). The ordinate represents the height of action potentials recorded with extracellular electrodes. At 0 minutes the axon was treated with levorphanol (5 x 10^{-4} M) dissolved in sea water buffered with 10^{-3} M-tris at pH 8.0. At 20 minutes the drug solution was removed and replaced by sea water adjusted to pH 6.0 and containing the same concentration of levorphanol. At 55 minutes the axon was washed with and immersed in drug-free, normal sea water. (Reprinted from Simon, E. J. and Rosenberg, P.[16] by courtesy of *J. Neurochem.*)

were seen with levallorphan, dextrorphan, and morphine.

The effects on phospholipid metabolism of concentrations of levorphanol which block conduction were examined.[17] Squid giant axons (15 to 20) were excised and incubated for various periods in sea water buffered with Tris at pH 8, containing $^{32}P_i$. Phospholipids were extracted from homogenized axons and separated by two-dimensional thin-layer chromatography. Spots were visualized by autoradiography, scraped, and analyzed for radioactivity and phosphorus. A stimulation of ^{32}P incorporation into the total phospholipid fraction was observed which increased with time of incubation from 6% at 45 minutes to 55% at 135 minutes. Examination of individual phospholipids showed that in the presence of levorphanol (1 mM) there was reduced radioactivity in the major phospholipid components of squid axons, phosphatidyl choline, and phosphatidyl ethanolamine, and a dramatic increase in the labeling of two minor constituents, one of which has been identified as phosphatidic acid, while the other is as yet unidentified. The meaning of these changes in phospholipid metabolism is not clear, but they bear a striking resemblance to those seen by Mulé in guinea pig brain slices and they point once again to effects of morphine derivatives on cell membrane structure.

BARBITURATES

The observed effects of barbiturates on lipid metabolism are all related to the ability of these drugs to stimulate the activity of drug-metabolizing enzymes in liver microsomes. The effects of barbiturates on brain lipids have not been studied.

The ability of barbiturates to induce liver microsomal enzymes was discovered independently by Remmer et al. during their investigations of the mechanism of barbiturate tolerance[18,19] and by Conney et al. during their studies on the effects of drugs on ascorbic acid biosynthesis.[20,21] Maximum induction requires repeated administration of barbiturates. Thus, after daily administration of phenobarbital to rats, the maximum increase in enzyme levels (three to tenfold) is reached after 3 to 4 days. This stimulation is referred to as induction since evidence has been provided that the increase in enzyme activity represents an increase in enzyme protein. Induction is blocked by inhibitors of protein and RNA synthesis.

The effects of barbiturates on lipid metabolism stem from two characteristics of the induction phenomenon. 1) It is accompanied by considerable proliferation of the membranes of the smooth endoplasmic reticulum; and 2) many of the induced drug-metabolizing enzymes metabolize a variety of natural cell constituents including various lipid materials.

Remmer and Merker[22,23] and Fouts and Rogers[24] found that treatment of animals with phenobarbital and other inducers caused marked proliferation of smooth-surfaced membranes of the endoplasmic reticulum (ER) of the liver cell. Little or no change was seen in the rough-surfaced ER. Remmer and Merker[25] showed that treatment of rabbits with phenobarbital for several days increased drug-metabolizing enzymes, protein, and lipid in both rough and smooth ER, but the increases were greatest in smooth ER. Orrenius et al.[26] confirmed these results and found that the phenobarbital markedly increased the rate of incorporation of $^{32}P_i$ into the phospholipids of both smooth and rough vesicle fractions of liver microsomes. They suggested that enhanced phospholipid synthesis was an early step in the phenobarbital-induced proliferation of smooth ER. Holtzman and Gillette,[27] however, did not confirm these results, but found instead that phenobarbital increased hepatic microsomal phospholipids by inhibiting their catabolism. This controversy is still unresolved. The high level of membranes and phospholipid induced by phenobarbital treatment persists in the cytoplasm of rat hepatocytes for 15 days after the last of a series of 5 daily injections.

A number of normal body constituents have been shown to be substrates and in some cases probably the normal substrates of liver microsomal drug-metabolizing enzymes. Those which are classified as lipids will be discussed briefly.

Several enzymes necessary for the biosynthesis of cholesterol are localized in liver microsomes.[28] Administration of phenobarbital to hamsters and rats increased activity of hepatic enzymes that incorporate ^{14}C-acetate into cholesterol.[29] Recently, the stimulation of ^{14}C-acetate incorporation into cholesterol was also reported for slices of small intestine from rats treated with phenobarbital.[30]

Wada et al.[31] treated mice for three days with

phenobarbital and found increased incorporation of ^{14}C-acetate into liver cholesterol in vitro and in vivo. Surprisingly, they found that the serum cholesterol level was decreased 20% by this treatment. A similar observation was reported by Salvador et al.[32] More detailed studies are clearly required to explain those results.

An enzyme system which catalyzes the ω-oxidation of fatty acids is present in liver microsomes. Treatment of rats and rabbits with phenobarbital increased the activity of an enzyme which ω-hydroxylates lauric acid.[33,34] Phenobarbital did not stimulate the ω-oxidation of stearic acid,[35] which suggests that the ω-oxidation of these fatty acids may be catalyzed by different enzymes.

It is clear that barbiturates exert a variety of effects on lipid metabolism in liver. Whether similar effects occur in the brain and to what extent these effects are related to the pharmacological action of and the development of dependence to barbiturates remain to be answered by future investigations.

PHENOTHIAZINE TRANQUILIZERS

Phenothiazine tranquilizers and, in particular, their prototype, chlorpromazine, have been reported to manifest a variety of effects on cell membranes. Concentrations of chlorpromazine as low as 10^{-6}M prevent swelling in vitro of subcellular membranes in rat liver and brain mitochondria,[36,37] presumably by altering membrane permeability. Chlorpromazine has also been shown to prevent uptake of ^{3}H-norepinephrine[38-40] by various tissues including the brain. Effects of phenothiazine drugs on the permeability of mammalian erythrocyte membranes have been reported and these were found to correlate well with the clinical therapeutic activity of these compounds.[41,42] Guth and Spirtes[43] have proposed that a major mode of action of chlorpromazine may be through modification of membrane properties. It is, therefore, not surprising that the effect of this drug on brain phospholipid metabolism has been studied in a number of laboratories.

Ansell and Dohmen[44] studied the incorporation of $^{32}P_i$ into the brain phospholipids of young rats (50 g) 30 minutes after intramuscular administration of chlorpromazine (20 mg/kg). Since there was no consistent change in the concentration of labeling of the acid-soluble phosphorus pool, they used the ratio of phospholipid specific activity/acid soluble P specific activity as a measure of phospholipid synthesis. Table 6 shows that chlorpromazine-treated rats exhibit a depression of total brain phospholipid synthesis (44% of control). Phosphatidyl choline labeling was reduced to 37% and that of phosphatidyl ethanolamine to 50% of control. The depression of synthesis was observed uniformly in different parts of rat brain.

Magee et al.[45] carried out in vitro experiments with guinea pig brain slices. The addition of chlorpromazine or azacyclonol to the slices at 0.01 to 0.1 mM concentrations caused a considerable increase in the labeling of phospholipids by $^{32}P_i$.

TABLE 6

Effect of Chlorpromazine on Phospholipid Turnover in Whole Rat Brain

	Specific radioactivity ratios X 1000		
	Total phospholipid P / Acid-soluble P	Phosphatidylcholine / Acid-soluble P	Phosphatidylethanolamine P / Acid-soluble P
Normal	39.4 ± 1.7 (6)	49.8 ± 2.8 (6)	26.0 ± 2.2 (6)
Chlorpromazine	17.4 ± 3.1 (6)	18.3 ± 5.1 (6)	12.9 ± 2.4 (6)

These results were obtained on two separate litters of six animals, in each of which three were normal and three were treated with chlorpromazine.
Means are given ± standard deviations.
(Reprinted from Ansell, G. B. and Dohmen, H.[44] by courtesy of *J. Neurochem.*)

The increased specific activity of the phosphatides was not accompanied by any significant change in the concentration or specific activity of acid-soluble phosphorus compounds such as creatine phosphate or ATP. Among the individual phospholipids, stimulation of labeling was seen with diphosphoinositide and phosphatidyl serine, while incorporation into phosphatidyl choline and phosphatidyl enthanolamine was reduced. Higher drug concentrations of 1 mM and more caused a decrease in oxygen consumption followed by inhibition of phospholipid biosynthesis. Similar results were obtained with several other lipid precursors[46] such as glycerol-1-^{14}C and serine-3-^{14}C, but not with choline-1:2-^{14}C nor acetate-1-^{14}C.

These results are not in agreement with those reported by Christensen and Wase,[47] since under their experimental conditions chlorpromazine at 0.1 mM inhibited incorporation of fatty acids into phospholipid in vitro, preventing fatty acid esterification with α-glycerolphosphate. It inhibited incorporation of $^{32}P_i$ into the phospholipids of brain and liver homogenates even at 0.01 mM.

These conflicting reports led Grossi et al.[48] to investigate the effects of chlorpromazine on phospholipid synthesis in vitro and in vivo. These authors found, in agreement with Magee et al., that incorporation of acetate-1-C^{14} into the phospholipids of rat brain slices was stimulated 2 to 2.5-fold by chlorpromazine at 0.01 to 0.1 mM. This stimulatory effect exhibited some specificity in as much as it was not observed in liver slices. At 1 mM chlorpromazine there was strong inhibition of phospholipid synthesis in both brain and liver slices. These data are presented in Table 7. Similar effects were observed in vivo after administration of chlorpromazine (3.5 mg/kg). Maximum stimulation was seen between 1 and 4 hours after treatment.

A study by Ansell and Marshall[49] of the inhibition by chlorpromazine of the biosynthesis of choline and enthanolamine-containing phospholipids of rat brain cortex slices and dispersions led to the interesting conclusion that chlorpromazine may act by inhibiting the enzyme phosphorylcholinecytidyl transferase.

In summary, it is evident that phenothiazine tranquilizers exert effects on cell membranes and, in particular, on phospholipid metabolism. It is likely that these effects bear some relation to the therapeutic properties of these tranquilizers. This

TABLE 7

The in vitro Effect of Chlorpromazine on Acetate-1-^{14}C Incorporation into Lipids of Growing Rats

No. of animals	Treatment	$^{14}CO_2$ *	Cholesterol$^+$	Fatty acids‡: Acetone-soluble fraction	Fatty acids‡: Phospholipid
			Brain Lipids		
5	Controls	300.71 ± 17.10	13.15 ± 1.16	1.73± 0.38	0.42 ± 0.14
6	CPZ 10^{-3} M	29.69 ± 4.27‡	1.54 ± 0.26‡	0.38 ± 0.06‡	0.09 ± 0.01‡
6	CPZ 10^{-4} M	364.37 ± 15.67	14.70 ± 1.16	2.09 ± 0.26	0.90 ± 0.07‡
6	CPZ 10^{-5} M	390.45 ± 18.76 §	14.03 ± 1.35	2.20 ± 0.33	1.03 ± 0.16‡
			Liver Lipids		
6	Controls	163.42 ± 18.52	2.54 ± 0.15	0.08 ± 0.005	0.02 ± 0.002
6	CPZ 10^{-3} M	98.33 ± 8.78‡	0.62 ± 0.05‡	0.03 ± 0.002‡	0.01± 0.001‡
6	CPZ 10^{-4} M	187.64 ± 16.41	2.85 ± 0.21	0.08 ± 0.005	0.02 ± 0.002
6	CPZ 10^{-5} M	157.05 ± 6.41	2.42 ± 0.11	0.09 ± 0.009	0.02 ± 0.001

Sodium acetate-1-^{14}C added at a concentration 1.06 μmol/g tissue.

*) 1 x 10^{-3} μmol acetate oxidised per g tissue ± S.E.

+) 1 x 10^{-3} μmol acetate incorporated per mg of cholesterol or fatty acids ± S.E.

‡) $P < 0.01$ in comparison with controls.

§) $P < 0.05$ in comparison with controls.

(Reprinted with permission from Grossi, E., Paoletti, P., and Palotetti, R., *J. Neurochem.*, 6, 73, 1970.)

should, therefore, be a fruitful field for future investigation.

ALCOHOL

The situation with alcohol is similar to that with barbiturates. Effects of alcohol ingestion on lipid metabolism have been known for a long time, but no work has been done on the relationship of these effects to alcohol dependence. There is, in fact, no study known to this reviewer on the effects of alcohol on brain lipids.

An excellent review on the effects of acute and chronic alcohol administration on lipid metabolism was published recently in a chapter by Lieber, Rubin, and DeCarli in *The Biology of Alcoholism.*[50] Only a very brief summary is, therefore, included here.

Hyperlipemia associated with alcoholism was described as early as 1918 by Feigl.[51] This observation has been widely confirmed and the biochemical mechanisms involved have been studied. The rise in circulating free fatty acids (FFA) is thought to be due to enhanced peripheral fat mobilization and decreased utilization of fatty acids by the liver.[52,53] Serum phospholipids and cholesterol increase somewhat upon alcohol administration, but the main rise occurs in circulating glycerides, which is consistent with the finding that the most striking change takes place in the very low density lipoprotein fraction.[54] Studies showing enhanced incorporation of palmitate-^{3}H and lysine-^{14}C into lipoproteins suggest that ethanol-induced hyperlipemia may result from increased lipoprotein production in the liver.

Another well-known concomitant of alcoholism is the accumulation of lipids in the liver referred to as alcoholic fatty liver. Lieber et al.[55] demonstrated that alcohol has a greater capacity to generate a fatty liver than dietary fat itself. Fat accumulation was also obtained in normal nonalcoholic volunteers after periods of alcohol ingestion of two days or more.[56] It is interesting to note that liver fat accumulation was seen with amounts of alcohol which did not cause inebriation and which are commonly consumed by many so-called social drinkers.

It has been reported that in rats hepatic steatosis due to one large dose of alcohol is derived largely from adipose tissue fatty acids,[57-59] whereas fatty livers in both man and rats, which develop as a result of prolonged alcohol consumption, accumulate fats largely from dietary origin,[59,60] and from endogenously synthesized FA when the diet is low in fat.[59,60] Regardless of origin, fats will accumulate in the liver because of a decrease in lipid oxidation produced by alcohol. The relationship of liver cirrhosis to fatty liver is still unclear. Many alcoholics never develop cirrhosis, but alcoholic cirrhosis is almost always preceded by a stage of fatty liver.

CENTRAL NERVOUS SYSTEM STIMULANTS AND HALLUCINOGENS

A reasonably exhaustive search of the literature has revealed little information on the effects of amphetamines, LSD, or marijuana on lipid metabolism.

CONCLUSIONS

It is clear from this review that effects of dependence-producing drugs on lipid metabolism have been observed in every instance where they have been looked for. The meaning of these effects and their relation to drug action or dependence is by no means clear. In some cases they may, in fact, represent secondary changes or changes quite unrelated to the pharmacological action of the drug.

The importance of the cell membrane in nerve function, together with the finding that so many of these chemically unrelated compounds have been found to affect the membrane, makes it appear to this reviewer that much more work in this area is desirable. The recent reports by several laboratories indicating that receptors for neurotransmitters[61] and, perhaps, for drugs[62] may be proteolipids located in the neuronal membrane provide further impetus for studies of the effects of dependence-causing drugs on membranes and phospholipids. It is hoped that a future review of this topic will be able to discuss the relationship between lipid metabolism and drug dependence, or, at least, will be able to state with certainty whether a direct relationship exists.

REFERENCES

1. Brossard, M. and Quastel, J. H., Effects of morphine and tofranil on the incorporation of phosphate (^{32}P) into phospholipids of rat brain slices, *Biochem. Pharmacol.*, 12, 766, 1963.

2. Mulé, S. J., Effect of morphine and nalorphine on the metabolism of phospholipids in guinea pig cerebral cortex slices, *J. Pharmacol. Exp. Ther.*, 154, 370, 1966.

3. Mulé, S. J., Morphine and the incorporation of P^{32} into brain phospholipids of nontolerant, tolerant and abstinent guinea pigs, *J. Pharmacol. Exp. Ther.*, 156, 92, 1966.

4. Mulé, S. J., Morphine and the incorporation of ^{32}orthophosphate *in vivo* into phospholipids of the guinea pig cerebral cortex, liver and subcellular fractions, *Biochem. Pharmacol.*, 19, 581, 1970.

5. Simon, E. J., Cohen, S. S., and Raina, A., Polyamines and inhibition of RNA synthesis in *E. coli* by levorphanol, *Biochem. Biophys. Res. Commun.*, 24, 482, 1966.

6. Gale, E. F., Effects of diacetylmorphine and related morphinans on some biochemical activities of *Staphylococcus aureus, Molec. Pharmacol.*, 6, 128, 1970.

7. Simon, E. J., Schapira, L, and Wurster, N., Effect of levorphanol on putrescine transport in *Escherichia coli, Molec. Pharmacol.*, 6, 577, 1970.

8. Greene, R. and Magasanik, B., The mode of action of levallorphan as an inhibitor of cell growth, *Molec. Pharmacol.*, 3, 453, 1967.

9. Boquet, P. L., Devynck, M. A., Fromageot, P., and Simon, E. J., On the mode of action of levallorphan on *Escherichia coli*: effects on cellular magnesium, *Molec. Pharmacol.*, in press.

10. Gale, E. F., Effect of morphine derivatives on lipid metabolism in *Staphylococcus aureus, Molec. Pharmacol.*, 6, 134, 1970.

11. Wurster, N., Elsbach, P., Rand, J., and Simon, E. J., Effects of levorphanol on phospholipid metabolism in *E. coli, Biochim. Biophys. Acta*, 248, 282, 1971.

12. White, D. C. and Tucker, A. N., Phospholipid metabolism during bacterial growth, *J. Lipid Res.*, 10, 220, 1969.

13. Wurster, N., Elsbach, P., Simon, E. J., Pettis, P., and Lebow, S., The effects of the morphine analogue levorphanol on leukocytes–metabolic effects at rest and during phagocytosis, *J. Clin. Invest.*, 50, 1091, 1971.

14. Zucker-Franklin, D., Elsbach, P., and Simon, E. J., The effect of the morphine analog, levorphanol, on phagocytizing leukocytes - an electron microscope study, *Lab. Invest.*, 25, 415, 1971.

15. Elsbach, P., Increased synthesis of phospholipid during phagocytosis, *J. Clin. Invest.*, 47, 2217, 1968.

16. Simon, E. J. and Rosenberg, P., Effects of narcotics on the giant axon of the squid, *J. Neurochem.*, 17, 881, 1970.

17. Dole, W. and Simon, E. J., unpublished observations.

18. Remmer, H., Die Beschleunigung des Eripanabbaues unter der Wirkung von Barbituraten, *Naturwissenschaften*, 45, 189, 1958.

19. Remmer, H. and Alsleben, B., Die Aktivierung der Entgiftung in den Lebermikrosomen während der Gewöhnung, *Klin. Wschr.*, 36, 332, 1958.

20. Conney, A. H. and Burns, J. J., Stimulating effects of foreign compounds on ascorbic acid synthesis and on drug-metabolizing enzymes, *Nature*, 184, 363, 1959.

21. Conney, A. H., Davison, C., Gastel, R., and Burns, J. J., Adaption increases in drug-metabolizing enzymes induced by phenobarbital and other drugs, *J. Pharmacol. Exp. Ther.*, 130, 1, 1960.

22. Remmer, H. and Merker, H. J., Enzyminduktion und Vermehrung von endoplasmatschen Reticulum in der Leberzelle während der Behandlung mit Phenobarbital (Luminal), *Klin. Wschr.*, 41, 276, 1963.

23. Remmer, H. and Merker, H. J., Effects of drugs on the formation of smooth endoplasmic reticulum and drug-metabolizing enzymes, *Ann. N.Y. Acad. Sci.*, 123, 79, 1965.

24. Fouts, J. R. and Rogers, L. A., Morphological changes in the liver accompanying stimulation of microsomal drug metabolizing enzyme activity by phenobarbital, chlordane, benzpyrene or methylcholanthrene in rats, *J. Pharmacol. Exp. Ther.*, 147, 112, 1965.

25. Remmer, H. and Merker, H. J., Drug-induced changes in the liver endoplasmic reticulum: association with drug-metabolizing enzymes, *Science*, 142, 1657, 1963.

26. Orrenius, S., Ericsson, J. L. E., and Ernster, L., Phenobarbital-induced synthesis of the microsomal drug-metabolizing enzyme system and its relationship to the proliferation of endoplasmic membranes. A morphological and biochemical study, *J. Cell Biol.*, 25, 627, 1965.

27. Holtzman, D. R. and Gillette, J. R., The effect of phenobarbital on the synthesis of microsomal phospholipid in female and male rats, *Biochem. Biophys. Res. Commun.*, 24, 639, 1966.

28. Block, K., The biological synthesis of cholesterol, *Science*, 150, 19, 1965.

29. Jones, A. L. and Armstrong, D. T., Increased cholesterol biosynthesis following phenobarbital induced hypertrophy of agranular endoplasmic reticulum in liver, *Proc. Soc. Exp. Biol. Med.*, 119, 1136, 1965.

30. Middleton, W. R. J. and Isselbacher, K. J., The stimulation of intestinal cholestero-genesis in the rat by phenobarbital, *Proc. Soc. Exp. Biol. Med.*, 131, 1435, 1969.

31. Wada, O., Toyokawa, K., Uraba, G., Yano, Y., and Nakao, K., Cholesterol biosynthesis in the liver of experimentally induced porphyric mice, *Biochem. Pharmacol.*, 18, 1533, 1969.

32. Salvador, R. A., Atkins, C., Haber, S., and Conney, A. H., Changes in the serum concentration of cholesterol, triglycerides and phospholipids in the mouse and rat after administration of either chlorcyclizine or phenobarbital, *Biochem. Pharmacol.*, 19, 1463, 1970.

33. Lu, A. Y. H. and Coon, M. J., Role of hemoprotein P-450 in fatty acid ω-hydroxylation in a soluble enzyme system from liver microsomes, *J. Biol. Chem.*, 243, 1331, 1968.

34. Das, M. L., Orrenius, S., and Ernster, L., On the fatty acid and hydrocarbon hydroxylation in rat liver microsomes, *Europ. J. Biochem.*, 4, 519, 1968.

35. Wada, F., Shibata, H., Groto, M., and Sakamoto, Y., Participation of the microsomal electron transport system involving cytochrome P-450 in ω-oxidation of fatty acids, *Biochim. Biophys. Acta*, 162, 518, 1968.

36. Spirtes, M. A. and Guth, P. S., An effect of chlorpromazine on rat mitochondrial membranes, *Nature*, 190, 274, 1961.

37. Spirtes, M. A. and Guth, P. S., Effects of chlorpromazine on biological membranes. I. Chlorpromazine-induced changes in liver mitochondria, *Biochem. Pharmacol.*, 12, 37, 1963.

38. Axelrod, J., Whitby, G., Hertling, G., and Kopin, I. L., Studies on the metabolism of catecholamines, *Circ. Res.*, 9, 715, 1961.

39. Axelrod, J., Whitby, L. G., and Hertling, G., Effect of psychotropic drugs on the uptake of ^{3}H-norepinephrine by tissues, *Science*, 133, 383, 1961.

40. Dengler, H. J. and Titus, E. O., The effect of drugs on the uptake of isotopic norepinephrine in various tissues, *Biochem. Pharmacol.*, 8, 64, 1961.

41. Freeman, A. R. and Spirtes, M. A., Effect of some phenothiazine derivatives on the hemolysis of red blood cells *in vitro*, *Biochem. Pharmacol.*, 11, 161, 1962.

42. Freeman, A. R. and Spirtes, M. A., Further effects of chlorpromazine on the human erythrocyte membrane, *Biochem. Pharmacol.*, 12, 1235, 1963.

43. Guth, P. S. and Spirtes, M. A., The phenothiazine tranquilizers: biochemical and biophysical actions, *Int. Rev. Neurobiol.*, 7, 231, 1964.

44. Ansell, G. B. and Dohmen, H., The depression of phospholipid turnover in brain tissue by chlorpromazine, *J. Neurochem.*, 1, 150, 1956.

45. Magee, W. L., Berry, J. F., and Rossiter, R. J., Effect of chlorpromazine and azacyclonol on the labeling of phosphatides in brain slices, *Biochim. Biophys. Acta*, 21, 402, 1956.

46. Magee, W. L., Pritchard, E. J., and Strickland, K. P., Chlorpromazine and azacyclonol and the *in vitro* labeling of phosphatides in brain preparations, *Fed. Proc.*, 16, 215, 1957.

47. Christensen, J. A. and Wase, A., Further studies of the effect of chlorpromazine on phospholipid synthesis, *Fed. Proc.*, 18, 204, 1959.

48. Grossi, E., Paoletti, P., and Paoletti, R., The *in vitro* and *in vivo* effects of chlorpromazine on brain lipid synthesis, *J. Neurochem.*, 6, 73, 1960.

49. Ansell, G. B. and Marshall, E. F., Some effects of chlorpromazine on brain phospholipid metabolism. II. Labeling of choline- and ethanolamine-containing phospholipids, by radioactive precursors *in vitro, J. Neurochem.*, 10, 883, 1963.

50. Lieber, C. S., Rubin, E., and DeCarli, L. M., Effects of ethanol on lipid, uric acid, intermediary, and drug metabolism, including the pathogenesis of the alcoholic fatty liver, in *The Biology of Alcoholism*, Vol. 1, Kissin, B. and Begleiter, H., Eds., Plenum Press, New York, 1971, 263.

51. Feigl, J., Neue Untersuchungen zur Chemie des Blutes bei akuter Alkohol Intoxikation und bei chronishem Alkoholismus mit besonderer Berücksichtigung der Fette und Lipoide, *Biochem. Ztschr.*, 92, 282, 1918.

52. Lieber, C. S., Jones, D. P., Mendelson, J., and DeCarli, L. M., Fatty liver, hyperlipemia and hyperuricemia produced by prolonged alcohol consumption, despite adequate dietary intake, *Trans. Ass. Amer. Physicians*, 76, 289, 1963.

53. Schapiro, R. H., Scheig, R. L., Drummey, G. D., Mendelson, J. H., and Isselbacher, K. J., Effect of prolonged ethanol ingestion on the transport and metabolism of lipids in man, *New Eng. J. Med.*, 272, 610, 1965.

54. Baraona, E. and Lieber, C. S., Effects of chronic ethanol feeding on serum lipoprotein metabolism in the rat, *J. Clin. Invest.*, 49, 769, 1970.

55. Lieber, C. S., Jones, D. P., and DeCarli, L. M., Effects of prolonged ethanol intake: Production of fatty liver despite adequate diets, *J. Clin. Invest.*, 44, 1009, 1965.

56. Rubin, E. and Lieber, C. S., Alcohol-induced hepatic injury in non-alcoholic volunteers, *New Eng. J. Med.*, 278, 869, 1968.

57. Brodie, B. B., Butler, W. M., Horning, M. G., Maickel, R. P., and Maling, H. M., Alcohol-induced triglyceride deposition in liver through derangement of fat transport, *Amer. J. Clin. Nutr.*, 9, 432, 1961.

58. Scheig, R. and Isselbacher, K. L., Pathogenesis of ethanol-induced fatty liver. III. In vivo and in vitro effects of ethanol on hepatic fatty acid metabolism in rats, *J. Lipid Res.*, 6, 269, 1965.

59. Lieber, C. S., Spritz, N., and DeCarli, L. M., Role of dietary, adipose and endogenously synthesized fatty acids in the pathogenesis of the alcoholic fatty liver, *J. Clin. Invest.*, 45, 51, 1966.

60. Lieber, C. S. and Spritz, N., Effects of prolonged ethanol intake in man: Role of dietary, adipose, and endogenously synthesized fatty acids in the pathogenesis of the alcoholic fatty liver, *J. Clin. Invest.*, 45, 1400, 1966.

61. De Robertis, E., Molecular biology of synaptic receptors, *Science*, 171, 963, 1971.

62. Goldstein, A., Lowney, L. I., and Pal, B. K., Stereospecific and nonspecific interactions of the morphine congener levorphanol in subcellular fractions of mouse brain, *Proc. Nat. Acad. Sci., USA*, 68, 1742, 1971.

HORMONES

R. George and P. Lomax

TABLE OF CONTENTS

INTRODUCTION

The effects on endocrine function of drugs which induce physical and/or psychic dependence have scarcely been studied. Only the opiates and tranquilizers have received some degree of attention in relation to their effects on endocrine activity. With our present knowledge of endocrine physiology, it is apparent that the central nervous system (CNS) plays an essential role in the regulation of hormonal secretion.

It is now generally agreed that the hypothalamus acts as a 'final common pathway' for the integration of neural activity affecting anterior pituitary function. The link between the hypothalamus and the anterior lobe of the pituitary is by way of the hypophyseal portal system of blood vessels, not by nerve fibers, and the classical studies of Green and Harris,[1] which suggested that a neurohumoral mechanism controlled anterior pituitary function, have been abundantly supported by subsequent investigations. The presence of transmitter substances in the hypothalamus was first reported by Saffran and Schally[2] who demonstrated the existence of corticotropin-releasing factor (CRF). Since then, hypothalamic extracts have been shown to contain at least six substances that alter pituitary secretions: corticotropin-releasing factor (CRF), thyrotropin-releasing factor (TRF), growth hormone-releasing factor (GH-RF), follicle-stimulating hormone-releasing factor (FSH-RF), luteinizing hormone-releasing factor (LH-RF), and prolactin-inhibiting factor (PIF). These factors, which are short-chain polypeptides with molecular weights up to 2500, are synthesized in the hypothalamus and stored in the median eminence. The releasing factors are transported to the anterior lobe by the vessels passing down the pituitary stalk. Their release is modulated by neural inputs to the hypothalamus and by hormonal feedback from either the pituitary gland ('short feedback loop') or from the several target endocrine glands ('long feedback loop'). Centrally acting drugs can modify hypothalamic-pituitary function by affecting neuronal input to the hypothalamus or by altering the sensitivity of the neurosecretory cells to neural or hormonal activation. Either of these effects could be mediated by the drug acting directly on the effector neurons or by an indirect action of the drug due to modification of release of transmitter substances at central synapses.

The mammillary bodies of the hypothalamus can be considered as part of the limbic system and other hypothalamic regions, including the preoptic nuclei, receive many projections from the various limbic nuclei.[3] On the basis of experimental data and the case histories of patients with psychomotor epilepsy, MacLean[4] has suggested that the symptoms observed in toxic and endogenous psychoses may be due to neural perturbations of the limbic brain. These symptoms include disturbances of mood and emotion, feelings of depersonalization, distortions of sensory perception, and paranoia. It is striking that many of these symptoms are similar to those resulting from intoxication with drugs causing psychic or physical dependence and that these same drugs may, in certain instances, precipitate psychoses. These actions of the drugs could be due to interference with the metabolism of cerebral amines, and the data could be interpreted as indicating that this is occurring at the level of the limbic system. In view of the close relationship between the limbic nuclei and those regions of the hypothalamus subserving neuroendocrine systems, it would not be surprising if disturbances of activity in the former should cause marked changes in endocrine function. It is also to be expected that endocrine activity would be markedly influenced by drugs acting on the limbic system, as well as those having a direct effect on the hypothalamus.

In the following sections, much of the data concerning the effects of drugs on endocrine function have been based upon morphological and cytological changes, biochemical changes, and secretory changes observed in the target glands.

NARCOTIC ANALGESICS AND ANTAGONISTS

Alterations in endocrine activity following the acute or chronic administration of narcotics were first noted a half century ago. Since then, numerous reports have appeared in the literature which indicate that narcotics may exert profound effects on endocrine secretions via the hypothalamo-hypophysial target gland axes. Since the effects of narcotics on endocrine function have been reviewed recently,[5,6] they will be summarized briefly in this chapter.

The opioids have been shown to exert effects on the rates of secretion of all hormones of the anterior pituitary gland. Although most of the data point to alterations in target gland function, it can be assumed that these changes are a reflection of modified anterior pituitary activity induced by the drugs.

Pituitary-adrenal Axis

In considering the effects of narcotics on pituitary-adrenal function, one must determine if one or more of the following mechanisms has been interfered with: 1) basal secretion of ACTH; 2) ACTH release in response to stress; and 3) circadian rhythm of ACTH secretion.

Evidence will be cited below which indicates that all of these may be altered by either acute or chronic administration of narcotic analgesics.

Acute Administration

Using the depletion of adrenal ascorbic acid as a measure of ACTH release, several investigators[7-12] have reported that a single injection of morphine enhances the secretion of ACTH in the unanesthetized rat. Similar findings have been reported following acute administration of (+) and (−) methadone.[7] Preadministration of nalorphine in smaller doses (1/8 to 1/4 the morphine dose) inhibits the adrenal ascorbic acid depletion effect of both morphine[7,13] and the isomers of methadone,[7] suggesting that the ACTH releasing effect of these drugs is mediated via specific neural pathways and/or neuronal receptors. This ascorbic acid depleting effect of morphine and methadone is dependent upon an intact pituitary-adrenal axis since it is abolished by hypophysectomy.[7]

A more direct measure of pituitary-adrenal activity is reflected by changes in the plasma level of corticosteroids. The effect of acute morphine administration on adrenal cortical hormone secretion appears to be species dependent. Several reports have clearly shown that a single injection of morphine is capable of elevating plasma corticosterone levels in conscious rats[11,12,14,15] and plasma 17-hydroxycorticosterone levels in dogs.[16] However, this has not been confirmed in studies on the guinea pig[17] and man.[18]

Although it is evident that a single injection of morphine in the conscious rat stimulates ACTH secretion, this effect of the narcotic agent is blocked by an anesthetic dose of sodium pentobarbital.[19] In addition, the combination of pentobarbital and morphine prevents the ascorbic acid depletion or the rise in plasma corticosterone that normally follows a variety of stresses (laparotomy, Pitressin®, and histamine), but an increase in the intensity of the stress may override this blockade.[19] In man, this combination of drugs blocks the diurnal rise of cortisol.[20] When morphine is administered alone, it has been shown to prevent the late afternoon diurnal elevation of plasma corticosterone in the conscious rat[15] and to reduce the pituitary-adrenal response to vasopressin in man.[20]

In summary, it appears that the acute administration of morphine may:

1. produce a stress-like response by depletion of adrenal ascorbic acid or elevation of plasma corticosteroids,
2. inhibit ACTH release in response to a stress, or

3. block the diurnal rise of plasma corticosteroids.

Although the mechanism(s) by which morphine may exert these effects is not clear, it is evident that it is centrally-mediated. The studies of George and Way[22] in rats with hypothalamic lesions that were challenged with morphine and those of Lotti et al.[12] in which rats were injected intrahypothalamically with microquantities of morphine, have indicated that the integrity of the hypothalamic-pituitary axis is essential for these actions of morphine. It was found that hypothalamic lesions, primarily in the anterior median eminence where CRF is presumably synthesized and released, blocked the ascorbic acid depleting effect of morphine. Conversely, injection of microgram amounts of morphine into this hypothalamic region reduced adrenal ascorbic acid while elevating plasma corticosterone levels.

Chronic Administration

The chronic administration of morphine to rats produces a marked adrenal cortical hypertrophy. This observation, first made in 1926 by McKay and McKay,[21] has since been confirmed by others.[22-25] Investigations in which different parameters of pituitary-adrenal activity were studied seem to indicate an opposite effect, i.e., chronic administration of morphine depresses the basal level of adrenal cortical secretion. The injection of morphine into guinea pigs for 12 days was found to reduce the basal level of urinary 17-hydroxysteroids.[17] Similar findings have been observed in the rat and in man. Paroli and Melchiorri[26] injected rats for periods ranging between 10 to 40 days and 40 to 100 days and noted a decrease in the urinary levels of hydroxysteroids. In a study on human addicts Eisenman et al.[27] found that two-to-four month cycles of morphine addiction reduced both plasma and urinary 17-hydroxycorticosteroid levels. They showed that this reduction in the basal secretory rate of adrenal cortical hormones was due chiefly to a decrease in production of 17-OHCS, rather than an increase in their degradation. Furthermore, this reduction was not the result of the adrenal cortex becoming insensitive to ACTH, since the injection of ACTH during the addiction cycles produced an increase in 17-OHCS which was comparable to the response obtained during the preaddiction period.

Chronic administration of morphine may also depress the pituitary-adrenal response to a variety of stresses. In rats treated with morphine for a five day period, the response to several stresses (laparotomy, histamine, and Pitressin®) was blocked.[19] In other investigations on rats injected with morphine for 25 days[26] and guinea pigs injected for 12 days,[17] it was reported that the increase in urinary hydroxysteroids in response to cold stress was inhibited. On the basis of these findings it would appear that chronic morphine administration produces a depression in the basal secretion of adrenal cortical hormones and prevents pituitary-adrenal activation in response to numerous stresses. However, in a recent study on methadone-treated heroin addicts, Cushman et al.[28] found no differences in basal plasma 17-OHCS levels of the addicts from normal control values; also, chronic methadone treatment did not interfere with the metyrapone test, which produces an increase in urinary 17-ketogenic steroids, or to the stress of insulin hypoglycemia, as reflected by elevated plasma 17-OHCS levels.

The normal diurnal pattern of 17-OHCS also may be altered by the chronic administration of morphine and methadone. Eisenman et al.[27] found that morphine interfered with the early morning rise of plasma 17-OHCS; they also noted the presence of a midday increase of plasma 17-OHCS during the period of morphine administration. The results of Cushman et al.[28] in general, corroborate these findings. They were able to show that chronic methadone treatment in a group of 16 heroin addicts altered the normal diurnal variation of plasma 17-OHCS in 10 of the 16 subjects. In 6 of these subjects, the 4 p.m. plasma corticosteroid values exceeded the 9 a.m. control levels, indicating a reversal of the normal diurnal pattern.

Withdrawal Effects

In both the rat and man, abrupt withdrawal of morphine results in increased adrenal cortical activity. Rats given morphine chronically and then abruptly withdrawn from the drug or administered nalorphine show an increase in levels of urinary 17-hydroxycorticosteroids, 17-ketosteroids, and aldosterone.[26] In man, also, the abrupt withdrawal of morphine produces a marked increase in plasma and urinary 17-OHCS and an elevation in urinary 17-ketosteroids.[27] The maximal rise in adrenal cortical levels correlates well with the peak physiological effects of the abstinence syndrome, approximately 48 hours after withdrawal.

Pituitary-thyroid Axis

Nearly all of the studies regarding the effects of narcotic analgesics on pituitary-thyroid function indicate that these agents inhibit basal thyroid secretion. Single intravenous injections of morphine, meperidine, levorphanol, dextrorphan, and dihydromorphinone have been reported to stimulate TSH release, as measured by the release of thyroidal ^{131}I; codeine injected in the same dose was ineffective. The chronic injection of all of these compounds for a period of five days inhibited thyroid activity.[29] Codeine (approximately 5 mg/kg) administered to rats for 14 days has been found to lower basal thyroid function; however, codeine did not prevent hypersecretion of TSH since it did not block the thyroid hypertrophy induced by methylthiouracil.[30]

Chronic administration of morphine for three weeks (30 and 60 mg/kg twice daily) also decreases pituitary TSH content and prevents the appearance of pituitary thyroidectomy cells.[31] Injection of morphine for periods of three or five days inhibits release of ^{131}I-labeled thyroid hormone,[32] depresses ^{131}I uptake by the thyroid, and reduces thyroid and pituitary weights.[33]

These data show that morphine may have a dual action on the pituitary-thyroid axis. A single injection of morphine accelerates the release of ^{131}I-labeled thyroid hormone in mice, whereas administration of morphine for a period of three days or longer inhibits several parameters of thyroid activity in rats.

Although the mechanism through which this inhibition occurs is not clear, there are several lines of evidence which implicate hypothalamo-hypophysial involvement. It has been well documented that the hypothalamus controls TSH secretion. Anterior hypothalamic lesions block the goitrogenic effect of propylthiouracil,[34] whereas electrical stimulation of this area enhances TSH secretion.[35] On the basis of these findings, Lomax and George[36] studied the effect of morphine on thyroid activity in rats with hypothalamic lesions. They noted that lesions in the caudal regions of the hypothalamus completely blocked the morphine-induced thyroidal inhibition, but animals with lesions in the anterior hypothalamus displayed normal ^{131}I thyroidal release rates. These results suggested that morphine might be activating an inhibitory hypothalamic area rather than depressing a facilitatory one for TSH secretion. In a subsequent study Lomax et al.[37] found that intrahypothalamic administration of microquantities of morphine (5 μg) produced inhibition of thyroid activity when the drug was injected into both rostral and caudal regions of the hypothalamus. However, the degree of inhibition varied with the injection site. Injections of morphine into the caudal hypothalamus inhibited release of ^{131}I-labeled thyroid hormone throughout the period of drug administration, while injection of morphine into the rostral site produced a transient inhibition, suggesting the development of tolerance in this area. Since there is some evidence that electrical stimulation of the caudal hypothalamus may inhibit TSH secretion[38] and since injection of morphine into the caudal hypothalamus produces hyperactivity and hyperthermia,[39] Lomax et al.[37] suggested that morphine was producing its thyroid inhibiting effect primarily via stimulation of inhibitory neurons in the caudal hypothalamus.

Pituitary-gonad Axis

In contrast to its dual effects on the pituitary-adrenal and pituitary-thyroid axes, morphine appears to inhibit gonadotropin hormone secretion after either acute or chronic administration. Barraclough and Sawyer[40] found that acute administration of morphine (50 mg/kg) between 12 and 2 p.m. on the day of proestrus in rats prevents the spontaneous ovulation which normally occurs during the same night. Daily injections of morphine between 12 and 2 p.m. over periods ranging between 13 to 52 days inhibit ovulation for as long as 25 days. The failure of continuous inhibition of ovulation for the 52 days in these studies was probably due to the usage of the same daily dose so that tolerance probably occurred. However, even with the one dose level, all of their animals showed irregular estrus cycles for the entire 52 days. In subsequent investigations using the rabbit, Sawyer[41] reported that morphine, as well as atropine and pentobarbital, prevented ovulation in response to electrical stimulation of the posterior tuberal region of the hypothalamus. Electrical stimulation of the median eminence overcame the blockade of these agents, indicating the site of blockade was proximal to the median eminence.

Other studies in human females and male rats

support these findings. Menninger-Lerchenthal[42] found that morphine addiction produced amenorrhea sterility, and decreased libido. Withdrawal of morphine resulted in normal menstrual cycles in many of the subjects, but sterility was still evident. Chronic administration of morphine (3 week period) to male rats has been shown to produce atrophic changes in their seminal vesicles and prostates. Although these data are indicative of an LH suppressing effect of morphine, there is also some evidence in favor of an FSH-inhibiting action of morphine. Rennels[43] found that two weeks of morphine administration produced changes in pituitary cytology and gonadotropin content which were indicative of FSH suppression and without effect on LH secretion. In summary, it is apparent that morphine administration, either acute or chronic, inhibits gonadotropin secretion. Although there is evidence for a morphine inhibitory effect on both FSH and LH secretion, most of the evidence points to an interference with LH release.

Growth Hormone

The acute administration of morphine (20 to 40 mg/kg) to rats produces a marked increase in plasma radioimmunoassayable growth hormone (Kokka, Garcia, and George, unpublished data). This response to morphine is associated with an increase in plasma corticosterone and appears to be a specific one, since most of the pharmacologic agents or stimuli which increase corticosteroid secretion in the rat (Kokka et al., unpublished data) and cat[44] simultaneously inhibit growth hormone secretion. The investigations of Müller and Pecile[45] also suggest that morphine enhances growth hormone secretion. Using a bioassay method, they found that acute morphine administration slightly reduced the pituitary content of growth hormone.

Although the effects of chronic administration of morphine on growth hormone secretion have not yet been studied, there is some indication that long-term injections may inhibit its release. Tanabe and Cafruny[23] found that administration of morphine to rats for 3 weeks reduced their body weights to 30% below the controls. In hypophysectomized rats, the difference between morphinized and control groups was only 8%. However, the groups (normal and hypophysectomized) were not pair-fed, so it is difficult to interpret the significance of these data. In general, it would seem that acute administration of morphine stimulates the release of growth hormone, while chronic administration inhibits its secretion. Thus, it is obvious that more long-term studies on the effect of morphine on plasma levels of growth hormone are necessary.

Prolactin

Acute administration of morphine has been reported to stimulate lactation,[46] an index of increased prolactin secretion. Furthermore, it is well established that prolactin secretion increases in conjunction with increased ACTH secretion, while it varies inversely with FSH and LH secretion. Since acute morphine administration increases lactation and ACTH secretion while inhibiting FSH and LH secretion, it seems valid to assume that acute administration facilitates release of prolactin.

BARBITURATES

The effects of barbiturates on endocrine function have been studied from two general directions: changes in pituitary activity resulting from altered central nervous function and changes in hormone metabolism as a result of induction of hepatic microsomal enzyme systems. These effects of the barbiturates appear to be relatively nonspecific and chronic administration of the drugs might be expected to give rise to multiple changes in endocrine function.

Pituitary-adrenal Axis

Barbiturates have been reported to stimulate or inhibit ACTH secretion in many species. In general, small doses of the various drugs inhibit stress induced ACTH secretion, provided the stress is relatively mild. The responses to strong stimuli, such as those occurring during surgery, remain intact. Gold and Ganong[47] reviewed the literature up to 1967 and gave references to the different barbiturates and various species investigated. Some later studies are mentioned here.

Pentobarbital anesthesia did not significantly alter the resting plasma corticosterone levels of rats, whereas ether anesthesia caused a fivefold increase. Premedication with pentobarbital abolished the response to ether, but did not prevent the increased ACTH release produced by traumatic stress.[48] When the neural connections to the basal hypothalamus were severed (using the basal hypothalamic-pituitary island preparation), high resting cortisone levels were seen which were elevated further by ether, but not by traumatic stress. Pentobarbital lowered the resting levels and blocked the rise in response to ether in this preparation. It appears that ACTH release can be activated by different hypothalamic mechanisms which exhibit different sensitivities to barbiturates.[48]

Barbiturates appear to be able to cross the placental barrier and effect ACTH release in the fetal rat, since administration of pentobarbital into the maternal circulation prevented the fall in adrenal ascorbic acid in the fetus induced by chemical stress.[49]

The depletion of adrenal ascorbic acid in rats subjected to centrifugal stress was blocked by barbiturates, chlorpromazine, and chlordiazepoxide administered 60 minutes before the stress. Smaller doses of phenobarbital (0.5 mg/kg) were more effective than larger doses (10 mg/kg).[50]

The compensatory hypertrophy of the remaining adrenal after unilateral adrenalectomy in rats was enhanced by phenobarbital and by administration of propylthiouracil (PTU). The greatest increase in compensatory growth of the residual adrenal gland was obtained when the barbiturate and PTU were injected simultaneously. These data suggested that PTU has a stressful influence, releasing additional ACTH; the effect of the barbiturate might reflect accelerated catabolism of adrenal corticoids due to enzyme induction.[51]

The metabolism of endogenous and exogenous cortisol is increased by both acute and chronic administration of barbiturates in several species including the guinea pig,[52] the rat,[53] and man.[54-56] This increased catabolism appears to be due to stimulation of hepatic microsomal hydroxylase activity. On the other hand, Kröner and his associates[57] have reported that the induction of both tyrosine-2-oxo-glutarate transaminase and tryptophan pyrrolase in rat liver by cortisol is inhibited by sodium barbital. Barbital also inhibited cortisol gluconeogenesis in these animals.

Thyroid

Administration of phenobarbital results in marked alterations in the distribution and metabolism of thyroxine in rats.[58,59] There is a net increase in thyroxine turnover due to an increase in hepatocellular binding and augmented hepatic deiodination and biliary secretion.[60] Hyperthyroidism, induced by administration of triiodothyronine, increased the mortality to a number of barbiturates in rats; thyroidectomy did not significantly change the mortality, except in the case of thiopental where a decrease was found.[61]

Rats given phenobarbital in their drinking water for ten days had significantly higher thyroxine secretion rates than control animals receiving plain water.[62]

Pituitary-gonad Axis

General anesthetics and central nervous system depressants, including barbiturates, inhibit ovulation not only in rabbits, which ovulate reflexly in response to copulation, but also in spontaneously ovulating species, such as rats.[47] Daily administration of phenobarbital to female rats completely blocked ovulation induced by pregnant mare's serum. Omission of any injection of the barbiturate resulted in 100% ovulation. The barbiturate block of ovulation was overcome if the animals copulated during the period of administration.[63] The barbiturate block could also be prevented by progesterone.[64] These results were postulated to be due to either an alteration in the metabolism of steroids essential for ovulation, or to changes in the threshold of excitability of hypothalamic control of release of ovulating hormone.

When ovulation was delayed for one to two days in rats by appropriately timed doses of pentobarbital, the proportion of fertilized eggs and their morphology were not affected. Delay for one day did not affect fertility; delay for two days was accompanied by a slight reduction in the number of implantation sites and viable fetuses.[65]

Injection of pentobarbital at diestrus does not appear to prevent the release of gonadotropin responsible for estrogen secretion and the delayed ovulation may be due to interference with the normal effects of estrogen on the hypothalamo-hypophyseal system.[66]

Using a differential radioimmunoassay system Doane and Parlow[67] showed that serum LH concentration was elevated only on the late afternoon of proestrus and serum FSH, undetectable during diestrus, also began to rise on the late afternoon of proestrus and attained a maximum at

20:00 to 21:00 hour. Administration of pentobarbital on the afternoon of proestrus was highly effective in inhibiting the surge of LH, but was only partly effective in inhibiting FSH release. These results were interpreted as suggesting that LH and FSH do not share a common regulating mechanism.

When rats, in which advancement of ovulation was prevented by pentobarbital, were injected with ovine gonadotropin releasing factor, ovulation was restored in 50% of the animals.[68] These data were taken to indicate that ovulatory release of gonadotropins is dependent on neural stimulation which can be blocked by barbiturates.

Increased hydroxylation of estrogens in man[69] and of hepatic metabolism of androgens in the rat[70] after phenobarbital administration has been described.

Serum prolactin and LH values which increased markedly on the afternoon of proestrus, failed to exhibit this rise during pentobarbital anesthesia, although there was a significant increase in prolactin levels 10 to 30 min after injecting the drug. Ether anesthesia did not modify the normal increases in hormone levels.[71]

Growth Hormone

When rats were pretreated with growth hormone the metabolism of hexobarbital by their liver slices in vitro was significantly decreased[72] due to a decrease in hepatic microsomal drug-metabolizing enzymes. An alteration of normal postnatal development of these enzymes in young rats was observed after a single injection of growth hormone.[73]

Plasma growth hormone levels were studied in rats that had been handled daily and in unattended animals. Pentobarbital anesthesia caused a significant rise in growth hormone levels and a decline in plasma corticosterone in both groups.[74] In these studies, pentobarbital anesthesia did not block the suppression of growth hormone levels caused by surgical stress. Stimulation of plasma growth hormone levels in rats injected with pentobarbital has also been seen in the studies of Kokka, Garcia, and George.[75]

ALCOHOL

Pituitary-adrenal Axis

Ethanol has been reported to increase ACTH release in several species including rats, mice, and guinea pigs.[47] In man, inhibition of ACTH has been reported after ethanol,[76] whereas increased secretion was seen after combined ethanol plus antabuse treatment.[77] Adrenocorticotrophic hormone deficiency has been reported in patients exhibiting clinical alcohol hypoglycemia.[78] Oral intake of alcohol, in doses leading to a moderate degree of intoxication increased plasma 11-hydroxycorticoid levels in normal subjects.[79] In chronic alcoholics, ethanol does not stimulate cortisol release[80] and adrenocortical function is impaired.[81]

Pituitary-gonad Axis

Administration of ethanol to rats at 13:00 hour on the day of proestrus inhibited ovulation which lasted for at least 2 nights. If the administration was delayed until 18:00 hour, ovulation was not affected. The blockade by ethanol could be overcome by injection of HCG or LH. It was concluded that ethanol inhibits ovulation primarily by blocking the ovulating surge of LH.[82]

Antidiuretic Activity

It is well established that ethyl alcohol inhibits vasopressin secretion in most animal species investigated.[47]

TRANQUILIZERS

Phenothiazines

The phenothiazines, particularly chlorpromazine (CPZ), are known to produce profound effects on endocrine activity, and these effects are probably mediated via limbic-hypothalamic-midbrain neural circuits. Since this group of compounds has been used extensively in psychotherapy, a great deal of data has accumulated regarding their neuroendocrine effects. The neuroendocrine effects of these agents have recently been compiled and exhaustively reviewed in an excellent 1967 article by De Wied.[83] Therefore, it is the purpose of this review to summarize briefly the data reported prior to 1967 and to supplement these data with some current findings.

Pituitary-adrenal Axis

Although there are numerous reports regarding the effect of chlorpromazine on pituitary-adrenal function, it is not clear whether CPZ stimulates or inhibits ACTH secretion. The discrepancies could arise from a number of factors: the dose of CPZ used; the time CPZ was administered prior to stress challenge; the core temperature of the stressed animal; the parameter of pituitary-adrenal activation employed.

In general, numerous studies in rats have indicated that small doses of CPZ (2.5 to 3.0 mg/kg) do not alter adrenal ascorbic levels to an appreciable degree; larger doses (5 to 100 mg/kg) deplete adrenal ascorbic acid. Both small and large doses of CPZ have been reported to have no effect, a partial blocking effect, or complete blocking effect on the ascorbic acid depletion response to several stresses (surgical stress, histamine, morphine, epinephrine, heat, cold, ether).[83] However, in a recent study Marks et al.[84] showed that a single injection of CPZ (25 mg/kg) was capable of lowering hypothalamic CRF, while simultaneously elevating plasma corticosterone levels. When the CRF content of the ventral hypothalamus returned to control levels it was found to be closely related to return of normal adrenal corticosterone levels.

Marks et al.[84] interpret the blockade of stresses following CPZ administration as being due to the possibility that CRF secretion has become maximal, and this maximal secretion is the result of removal of inhibitory neural influences by CPZ.

The results obtained from other species are much more consistent. Using plasma 17-OHCS as an index of pituitary-adrenal activity, it has been shown that CPZ increases ACTH secretion in the guinea pig,[85] dog,[86,87] and monkey.[88] This effect of chlorpromazine is abolished by hypophysectomy,[86] thereby placing the site of action at the pituitary or hypothalamus.

As was the case with morphine, pretreatment of rats with pentobarbital blocks the ACTH releasing effect of CPZ. Although pentobarbital by itself is capable of inhibiting ACTH secretion in response to relatively mild stresses, in combination with CPZ pentobarbital blocks the pituitary adrenal response to numerous severe stresses.[83] The adrenals of such blocked animals still respond normally to injected ACTH.[89]

Chronic administration of CPZ, like morphine, produces adrenal cortical hypertrophy, but, unlike morphine, does not consistently prevent adrenal activation in response to stress.[83] In patients treated with chlorpromazine, the ACTH response to the stresses of insulin[90] and typhoid vaccine[91] is inhibited. Additionally, several reports indicate a reduction in urinary excretion of 17-hydroxysteroids during chronic CPZ treatment.[83]

Pituitary-thyroid Axis

Although it is quite evident that the phenothiazines may modify pituitary-thyroid activity, the mechanism is not yet known. Furthermore, the many contradictory reports regarding the actions of CPZ on this system render it difficult to draw definitive conclusions.

It is unfortunate that most of the data derived from these studies have involved the ^{131}I thyroidal uptake method; thus when large doses of CPZ have been used, alterations in hemodynamics and renal function may have yielded erroneous results and conclusions.

Generally, in acute animal experiments, low doses (less than 10 mg/kg) of CPZ do not affect thyroid activity, whereas higher doses inhibit ^{131}I uptake by the thyroid.[83]

Several workers using the rate of release of thyroid ^{131}I, a more reliable index of TSH secretion, have shown that CPZ, even in low doses, inhibits normal thyroid activity. The inhibitory effect appeared to be at a higher level than the thyroid since the effect of exogenous TSH on ^{131}I release was not inhibited.[83]

Chronic administration of CPZ reduces both the uptake and the release of ^{131}I in rats.[83] However, other studies[83,92,93] have shown a biphasic effect on ^{131}I uptake by the thyroid after long-term administration of high doses of chlorpromazine; initially, during the first two to three days, there is inhibition of ^{131}I uptake which is then followed nine to ten days later, by an increased uptake of ^{131}I. Long-term administration of CPZ also has been noted to produce goiter in the rat[94] although CPZ paradoxically, partly inhibits the goitrogenic effect of thiouracil derivatives.[95,96]

The effects of chronic CPZ administration in man are extremely difficult to interpret since most patients receiving CPZ have psychiatric disorders. Most of the studies in man have failed to show changes in thyroid activity,[83] although it has been reported that CPZ may increase thyroidal ^{131}I uptake without interfering with other parameters of thyroid function.[97]

Recently in vitro studies using whole thyroid, thyroid slices, and homogenates from a variety of species have contributed a great deal towards the elucidation of the mechanism of action of TSH. It now appears that TSH rapidly stimulates the adenylcyclase-cyclic AMP system. Also, the effects of TSH on thyroid activity can be mimicked by cyclic AMP and its derivative dibutyryl cyclic AMP. Although the mechanism by which CPZ interferes with the action of TSH on thyroid tissue has not clearly been established, there is some evidence which favors an interference at the adenyl cyclase-cyclic AMP level,[98,99] as well as the lysosomal membrane level.[100,101]

In summary, there is evidence that acute administration of the phenothiazines may inhibit both the uptake and release of thyroid ^{131}I, indicative of reduced TSH secretion, but that chronic administration reverses these effects. In vitro experiments suggest that CPZ interferes with thyroid function by interfering with the action of TSH on the thyroid.

Pituitary-gonad Axis

The endocrine system most uniformly affected by the phenothiazines is the pituitary-gonad axis. Numerous investigators studying a variety of species have shown that either acute or chronic administration of phenothiazines inhibits secretion of pituitary FSH and LH. Phenothiazines have produced some of the following effects which are indirect indices of depressed FSH and LH secretion: failure of ovulation, delayed sexual maturation, reduction in weight of ovaries, uteri and vaginae, reduction in size of sex organs in the male, and inhibition of compensatory ovarian hypertrophy.[83]

While most of the evidence points to an inhibitory effect of CPZ on hypothalamic-pituitary function, there are data that suggest the possibility of a blocking action of CPZ at the target gland.

In large doses CPZ has been found to block the action of gonadotropins on target glands in both sexes.[96,102-104] However, data contrary to these findings raise doubts regarding the target gland as the site of CPZ action.[83]

The results reported from animal studies have also been observed in the human female. Chlorpromazine administered one to three days prior to ovulation delays menstruation for a period of eight to sixteen days.[105] Also, many reports show that CPZ treatment may produce menstrual irregularities and amenorrhea.[83]

Prolactin

An increase in prolactin secretion is associated with a concomitant reduction in FSH and LH secretion. Phenomena such as lactation, pseudopregnancy, and mammary growth are generally the result of prolactin secretion.

Chlorpromazine stimulates mammary growth in normal rats[106,107] and milk secretion in estrogen primed rats.[83] CPZ also produces pseudopregnancy in all rats when it is administered on the first day of diestrus.[108] Other phenothiazines, perphenazine and acepromazine, have been shown to increase plasma prolactin levels in the rat and rabbit,[109] in sheep,[110] and in goats[111] following acute administration. This increase in prolactin secretion induced by phenothiazines appears to be due to an inhibition of the release of a prolactin-inhibiting factor in the hypothalamus.[112]

Growth Hormone

The effect of CPZ on growth hormone appears to be variable and depends largely on the species studied. This is not surprising in view of the fact that factors controlling growth hormone secretion in primates differ from those controlling growth hormone secretion in nonprimates. For example, several stresses, particularly insulin hypoglycemia, which increase radioimmunoassayable plasma growth hormone in primates, do not alter plasma growth hormone levels in several nonprimate species.[113,114] Thus, chronic CPZ administration has been reported to have no effect on body growth in rats[96] or to inhibit growth in mice,[115] whereas acute administration of CPZ in monkeys produces a marked increase in plasma radioimmunoassayable growth hormone.[116] Also, CPZ has been reported to inhibit release of growth hormone in response to insulin hypoglycemia in rats, as measured by the tibia test.[45] The latter finding is incompatible with our data (Kokka and George, unpublished data) and other reports[113,117] which show that radioimmunoassayable plasma growth hormone in several species is not elevated in response to a hypoglycemia dose of insulin.

Benzodiazepines

The principal compounds of this group that have been studied for their actions on endocrine systems are chlordiazepoxide and diazepam. The following discussion will be in reference only to these two agents.

Pituitary-adrenal Axis

Acute administration of diazepam has been shown to significantly elevate corticosterone levels in rats 1 to 2 hours after administration of a dose between 2.5 to 5.0 mg/kg; lower doses were ineffective.[118] In the rabbit, it has been shown that chlordiazepoxide inhibits stress-induced eosinopenia.[119] In man, chlordiazepoxide (20 mg) accentuates the early evening fall in plasma cortisol levels.[120]

Chronic administration of diazepam, thrice daily for three and eight-day periods, maintains elevated corticosterone levels in rats, indicative of lack of tolerance to this effect of the drug.[118] In another study using rats, Superstein and Sulman[121] injected their animals with diazepam or chlordiazepoxide over 100 days with doses ranging from 5 to 50 mg/kg/day. Both drugs increased 17-ketosteroid excretion and adrenal weights, but did not affect thyroid and gonadal function. At high doses there was a slight increase in prolactin secretion. Both drugs also retarded growth in male rats, but chlordiazepoxide increased the body weight of females.

Pituitary-thyroid Axis

Diazepam has been reported to depress thyroid function as measured by ^{131}I uptake in man.[122] However, this effect has not been confirmed in animals and other human studies. Schindler et al.[123] found that neither diazepam nor chlordiazepoxide altered various parameters of thyroid function in mice. Clark et al.[124,125] failed to note any differences during chlordiazepoxide and diazepam treatment in ^{131}I uptake or thyroid hormone release in their psychiatric patients; it also made no difference whether they were euthyroid or mildly thyrotoxic. In a double-blind placebo controlled study using normal subjects, Mazzaferri and Skillman[126] also failed to find any alterations in thyroid activity following a 12 to 18 weeks' course of diazepam administration.

Growth Hormone

In our laboratory we have found that acute injections of low doses of diazepam (5 to 10 mg/kg) into the rat elevate immunoreactive plasma levels of growth hormone without influencing plasma corticosterone levels. Acute administration of a higher dose of diazepam (20 mg/kg) reverses these effects, i.e., plasma corticosterone levels become elevated, while growth hormone levels are decreased (Kokka and George, unpublished data).

AMPHETAMINES

Although the amphetamines (dextro-, hydroxy-, and methyl-amphetamine) are widely used, it is surprising that their effects on neuroendocrine function have not been investigated very extensively. Thus, very few data on this subject have been reported.

Pituitary-adrenal Axis

Amphetamine and hydroxyamphetamine acutely administered lower the ascorbic acid content of rat adrenals.[127,128] Similarly, acute administration of amphetamine to rats significantly elevates plasma corticosterone levels.[129,130] However, the results of Marks, et al.[84] indicate that amphetamine not only reduces the resting level of plasma corticosterone, but that amphetamine also reduces the rise in corticosterone in response to stress. The studies of Besser and his associates[120,131,132] also have shown that oral administration of *d*-amphetamine (10 mg) or intravenous injection of methylamphetamine (15 mg) causes an increase in plasma cortisol levels both in the morning (9 a.m.) and the evening (6 p.m.) of normal human subjects. Placebo administration was without effect. This effect of methylamphetamine is inhibited by thymoxamine, an α-adrenergic blocker, but is facilitated by propranolol, a β-blocker.

The effect of amphetamines on ACTH secretion in the dog appears to be at variance with the results reported above. Lorenzen and Ganong[133] found that amphetamine (1.5 to 4.0 mg/kg) and methamphetamine (3.0 to 5.0 mg/kg) inhibited the rise in adrenal venous output of 17-hydroxycorticoids in response to surgical stress. However, they noted that this type of inhibition was usually associated with a prolonged pressor response to these drugs. The indoles, α-ethyltryptamine and α-methyltryptamine, also blocked ACTH release in response to surgical stress while they simultaneously elevated the blood pressure.

Pituitary-gonad Axis

The only suggestion that amphetamines may influence pituitary-gonadal activity comes from the report by Stoffer[134] that in five of seven patients abusing large doses of amphetamine, there was an increase in flow and duration of the menses associated with cramps. In a follow-up study Stoffer et al.[135] investigated the effects of chronic administration of *d*-amphetamine (15 mg daily) on the menstrual cycles of six ex-narcotic addicts. Menstrual function was evaluated by means of basal body temperatures, biweekly cervical and lateral vaginal wall smears, and the quantity of menstrual discharge. They found that *d*-amphetamine did not significantly alter menstruation, based upon these parameters.

Growth Hormone

Acute administration of *d*-amphetamine and methylamphetamine to normal human subjects does not alter immunoreactive growth hormone levels.[131] However, pretreatment with adrenergic blockers, thymoxamine and propranolol, and then followed by methylamphetamine (15 mg) produced significant elevations in plasma hormone levels.[132]

The effect of chronic administration of amphetamine on the body weights of rats has been reported to vary with the age of the animals. Administration of amphetamine (5 mg/kg) to young rats for 20 days did not interfere with body weight increase when compared with saline injected controls.[129] Similar results have been noted in our laboratory after 28 days of amphetamine (10 mg/kg) administration (French and George, unpublished data).

Insulin

Recently, McMahon et al.[136] found that administration of amphetamine or methamphetamine to rats and mice produces a marked and rapid rise in immunoassayable plasma insulin. The increase in insulin secretion was not due, secondarily to a rise in plasma glucose. In rats, methamphetamine (30 mg/kg, i.d.) produced a three-to-fourfold increase in insulin levels within 15 minutes. Methamphetamine (7.5 mg/kg, i.v.) injected into mice elevated the plasma level of insulin within 2.5 minutes. Also, in vitro studies with incubated mouse pancreas showed that methamphetamine was capable of stimulating insulin secretion, indicating that the drug exerts a direct effect on the pancreas.

PSYCHOTOMIMETICS

Few studies of the effects of psychotomimetics on endocrine function have been carried out, and it is only in the case of marihuana that attempts have been made to elucidate the mechanisms of action.

Pituitary-adrenal Axis

Measurements of plasma cortisol levels were carried out in the course of experiments in which human volunteers took doses of Δ^9-tetrahydrocannabinol (Δ^9-THC), ranging from 15 to 70 mg, or synhexyl (50 to 200 mg) by mouth.[137,138] The plasma cortisol levels were unchanged after administration of the drugs, except when psychological stress was clinically in evidence. Although psychological stress, with accompanying pituitary-adrenal activation, is to be expected after administration of psychotomimetics, the clinical impression was that the euphoric and sedative effects of the drugs mitigated such psychotomimetic phenomena.[138]

In studies in the rat Δ^9-THC was found to stimulate ACTH secretion, as evidenced by depletion of adrenal ascorbic acid.[139] This effect was enhanced by anesthetic doses of pentobarbital. In this respect Δ^9-THC is different from morphine (see above). No evidence of tolerance was seen in these experiments after five daily injections of Δ^9-THC (5 mg/kg). Assays of plasma corticosterone 45 minutes after injection of Δ^9-THC into rats revealed marked pituitary-adrenal activation which persisted after repeated administrations for 8 days. The maximum elevation of plasma corticosterone levels occurred with doses between 4 and 16 mg/kg. Hypophysectomy, six days before testing, completely abolished the response to Δ^9-THC, indicating that the drug is not acting at the level of the adrenal gland. Premedication of the animals with pentobarbital (50 mg/kg) and morphine (20 mg/kg), which blocks the release of CRF in response to stressful stimuli,[10] prevented the rise in plasma corticosterone induced by Δ^9-THC (8 mg/kg). These last experiments indicate that hypothalamic stimulation is involved in the pituitary-adrenal activation by Δ^9-THC.[140] A hypothalamic locus of action was further supported by the observation that Δ^9-THC doubled the urine output in these rats, suggesting inhibition of release of antidiuretic hormone.[141]

This difference in response between man and the rat could merely reflect the disparity in dosage, rather than a fundamentally different pharmacological action in the two species.

Urinary output of 17-hydroxycorticosteroids, 17-ketogenic steroids, and 17-ketosteroids has been measured in volunteer subjects on consecutive days, before and after oral administration of lysergic acid dethylamide (LSD) (1.5 or 2 μg/kg) or mescaline (5 to 6 mg/kg).[137] These subjects were experienced in the effects of these drugs. The only significant change seen in these studies was an increase in 17-ketogenic steroids following LSD.

In groups of young, male albino mice injection of mescaline (50 or 100 mg/kg s.c. on alternate days for 8 doses) caused significant increases in adrenal weights accompanied by decreases in thymus weights which were dose dependent. These changes were felt to be a reflection of heightened adrenocortical function.[142] These results were similar to those occurring after administration of LSD to male rats.[143]

Pituitary-thyroid Axis

Marihuana has many pharmacological effects that are similar to those of morphine.[144] Included among these is depression of pituitary-thyroid activity. Miras[145] reported that intraperitoneal injection of cannabis resin depresses the uptake of radioactive iodine into the thyroid gland of the rat and a similar inhibition of ^{125}I uptake has been reported after a single dose of Δ^9-THC (10 mg/kg) in this species.[146] Systemic injection of marihuana distillate extract, of which Δ^9-THC was the major single constituent, in a dose equivalent to 2.5 mg/kg Δ^9-THC twice daily, inhibited the release of radioiodine from the thyroid gland of the rat. Thyroid stimulating hormone (TSH) increased the release of radioiodine in rats pretreated with Δ^9-THC, which suggested that reduced TSH secretion is the primary cause of the thyroid inhibition induced by Δ^9-THC. Bilateral electrolytic lesions in the medial mammillary region blocked the inhibitory effect of Δ^9-THC, whereas lesions in the rostral hypothalamus were without effect on this response. These results were interpreted as indicating that Δ^9-THC inhibits pituitary-thyroid function through an action on neurons in the caudal hypothalamus.[147] It is possible that the decreased thyroid activity is due to stimulation of specific inhibitory centers in the hypothalamus, rather than to depression of neurons concerned with tonic release of TSH. This action of marihuana appears to be analogous to that of morphine (see above).

SUMMARY AND CONCLUSIONS

It is apparent from the data described above that many drugs that produce dependence are capable of altering endocrine function. In general, the changes in endocrine activity are due to the actions of these drugs on the central nervous system, with the hypothalamus serving as a nodal point between the midbrain and limbic system. The mechanisms by which these agents can influence the hypothalamic-pituitary system are, probably, through a direct action on the neurosecretory cells, which contain releasing factors, or through an action on the "transmitters" (norepinephrine; dopamine; 5-hydroxytryptamine; and acetylcholine) that are released at nerve terminals and which are in a presynaptic position to the neurosecretory cells. Of these two possible mechanisms, the latter seems to be the more likely one since the "transmitters" are found in the hypothalamus and their turnover rates or concentrations in the brain may be altered by some of the drugs which produce dependence (see Way and Shen[148] and Weinstock[149]). In addition, there is evidence suggesting the existence of a serotonergic[150,151] and a cholinergic link[152,153] for the control of ACTH, a catecholaminergic control system for gonadotropin and prolactin secretion,[154] and for growth hormone secretion.[155] Also, there are striking similarities of some of the drugs in their actions on both endocrine activity and their effects on transmitter release at nerve terminals. For example, acute morphine or chlorpromazine administration increases ACTH, TSH, and prolactin secretion while LH and FSH secretion is inhibited; chronic administration of these two agents suppresses ACTH, TSH, and gonadotropin secretion.

Data have also been described above which lend some support to the view that these drugs exert their actions on endocrine activity through a peripheral mechanism. Evidence has been cited, particularly, for a peripheral action by the barbiturates and phenothiazines.

REFERENCES

1. Green, J. D. and Harris, G. W., The neurovascular link between the neurohypophysis and adenohypophysis, *J. Endocr.*, 5, 136, 1947.

2. Saffran, M. and Schally, A. V., The release of corticotrophin by anterior pituitary tissue *in vitro, Canad. J. Biochem. Physiol.*, 33, 408, 1955.

3. MacLean, P. D., The limbic system with respect to self preservation of species, *J. Nerv. Ment. Dis.*, 127, 1, 1958.

4. MacLean, P. D., The limbic brain in relation to the psychoses, in *Physiological Correlates of Emotion*, Black, P., Ed., Academic Press, New York, 1970, 129.

5. George, R., Hypothalamus: Anterior pituitary gland, in *Narcotic Drugs Biochemical Pharmacology*, Clouet, D. H., Ed., Plenum Press, New York, 1971, 283.

6. Sloan, J. W., Corticosteroid hormones, in *Narcotic Drugs Biochemical Pharmacology*, Clouet, D. H., Ed., Plenum Press, New York, 1971, 262.

7. George, R. and Way, E. L., Studies on the mechanism of pituitary-adrenal activation by morphine, *Brit. J. Pharmacol.*, 10, 260, 1955.

8. Nasmyth, P. A., Factors influencing the effect of morphine sulfate on the ascorbic acid content of rats' adrenal glands, *Brit. J. Pharmacol.*, 9, 95, 1954.

9. Van Peenen, P. F. D. and Way, E. L., Effect of certain central nervous system depressants on pituitary-adrenal activating agents, *J. Pharmacol.*, 120, 261, 1957.

10. Briggs, F. N. and Munson, P. L., Studies on the mechanism of stimulation of ACTH secretion and the aid of morphine as a blocking agent, *Endocrinology*, 57, 205, 1955.

11. Nikodijevic, O. and Maickel, R. P., Some effects of morphine on pituitary-adrenocortical function in the rat, *Biochem. Pharmacol.*, 16, 2137, 1967.

12. Lotti, V. J., Kokka, N., and George, R., Pituitary-adrenal activation following intrahypothalamic microinjection of morphine, *Neuroendocrinology*, 4, 326, 1969.

13. Burdette, B. H., Leeman, S., and Munson, P. L., The reversal by nalorphine of the inhibitory effect of morphine on the secretion of adrenocorticotrophic hormones in stress, *J. Pharmacol.*, 132, 323, 1961.

14. Oliver, J. T. and Troop, R. C., Plasma corticosterone levels in stressed rats following the administration of pentobarbital, morphine and dephenylhydantoin, *Steroids*, 1, 670, 1963.

15. Slusher, M. A. and Browning, B., Morphine inhibition of plasma corticosteroid levels in chronic venous-catheterized rats, *Amer. J. Physiol.*, 200, 1032, 1961.

16. Suzuki, T., Yamashita, K., Zinnouchi, S., and Mitamura, T., Effect of morphine upon the adrenal 17-hydroxycorticosteroid secretion in the dog, *Nature*, 183, 825, 1959.

17. Sobel, H., Schapiro, S., and Marmorston, J., Influence of morphine on urinary corticoid excretion by guinea pigs following exposure to cold and administration of Pitressin, *Amer. J. Physiol.*, 195, 147, 1958.

18. Eisenman, A. J., Fraser, H. F., Sloan, J., and Isbell, H., Urinary 17-ketosteroid excretion during a cycle of addiction to morphine, *J. Pharmacol. Exp. Ther.*, 124, 305, 1958.

19. Munson, P. L. and Briggs, F. N., The mechanism of stimulation of ACTH secretion, *Recent Progr. Hormone Res.*, 11, 83, 1955.

20. McDonald, R. K., Evans, F. T., Weise, V. K., and Patrick, R. W., Effect of morphine and nalorphine on plasma hydrocortisone levels in man, *J. Pharmacol.*, 125, 241, 1959.

21. MacKay, E. M. and MacKay, L. L., Resistance to morphine in experimental uremia, *Proc. Soc. Exp. Biol. Med.*, 24, 129, 1926.

22. George, R. and Way, E. L., The role of the hypothalamus in pituitary-adrenal activation and antidiuresis by morphine, *J. Pharmacol.*, 125, 111, 1959.

23. Tanabe, T. and Cafruny, E. J., Adrenal hypertrophy in rats treated chronically with morphine, *J. Pharmacol.*, 122, 148, 1958.

24. Sloan, J. W., Brooks, J. W., Eisenman, A. J., and Martin, W. R., The effect of addiction to and abstinence from morphine on rat tissue catecholamine and serotonin levels, *Psychopharmacologia*, 4, 261, 1963.

25. Sloan, J. W. and Eisenman, A. J., Long persisting changes in catecholamine metabolism following addiction to and withdrawal from morphine, *Res. Publ. Ass. Ment. Dis.*, 46, 96, 1968.

26. Paroli, E. and Melchiorri, P., Urinary excretion of hydroxysteroids, 17-ketosteroids and aldosterone in rats during a cycle of treatment with morphine, *Biochem. Pharmacol.*, 6, 1, 1961.

27. Eisenman, A. J., Fraser, H. F., and Brooks, J. W., Urinary excretion and plasma levels of 17-hydroxycorticosteroids during a cycle of addiction to morphine, *J. Pharmacol.*, 132, 226, 1961.

28. Cushman, P., Jr., Bordier, B., and Hilton, J. G., Hypothalamic-pituitary adrenal axis in methadone-treated heroin addicts, *J. Clin. Endocr.*, 30, 24, 1970.

29. Redding, T. W., Bowers, C. Y., and Schally, A. V., The effects of morphine and other narcotics on thyroid function in mice, *Acta Endocr.*, 51, 391, 1966.

30. Schreiber, V., Zbuzek, V., and Zbuzková-Kmentová, V., Effect of codeine on thyroid function in the rat, *Physiol. Bohemoslov.*, 17, 253, 1968.

31. Hohlweg, V. W., Knappe, G., and Dörner, G., Tierexperimentelle Untersuchungen über den Einfluss von Morphin auf die gonadotrope und thyreotrope Hypophysenfunktion, *Endokr. Bd.*, 40, 152, 1961.

32. George, R. and Lomax, P., The effects of morphine, chlorpromazine and reserpine on pituitary-thyroid activity in rats, *J. Pharmacol.*, 150, 129, 1965.

33. Sámel, M., Blocking of the thyrotrophic hormone secretion by morphine and chlorpromazine in rats, *Arch. Int. Pharmacodyn.*, 117, 151, 1958.

34. Greer, M. A., The role of the hypothalamus in the control of thyroid function, *J. Clin. Endocr.*, 12, 1259, 1952.

35. Harris, G. W. and Woods, J. W., The effect of electrical stimulation of the hypothalamus or pituitary gland on thyroid activity, *J. Physiol.* (London), 143, 246, 1958.

36. Lomax, P. and George, R., Thyroid activity following administration of morphine in rats with hypothalamic lesions, *Brain Res.*, 2, 361, 1966.

37. Lomax, P., Kokka, N., and George, R., Thyroid activity following intracerebral injection of morphine in the rat, *Neuroendocrinology*, 6, 146, 1970.

38. Vertes, M., Vertes, Z., and Kovacs, S., Effect of hypothalamic stimulation on pituitary-thyroid function, *Acta Physiol. Acad. Sci. Hung.*, 27, 229, 1965.

39. Lotti, V. J., Lomax, P., and George, R., Temperature responses in the rat following intracerebral microinjection of morphine, *J. Pharmacol.*, 150, 135, 1965.

40. Barraclough, C. A. and Sawyer, C. H., Inhibition of the release of pituitary ovulatory hormone in the rat by morphine, *Endocrinology*, 57, 329, 1955.

41. Sawyer, C. H., Neuroendocrine blocking agents: Discussion, in *Advances in Neuroendocrinology*, Nalbandov, A. V., Ed., University of Illinois Press, Urbana, 1963, 444.

42. Menninger-Lerchenthal, E., Schwanguschaft und Geburt morphinistischer Frauen, *Zbl. Gynaek.*, 58, 1044, 1934.

43. Rennels, E. G., Effect of morphine on pituitary cytology and gonadotrophic levels in the rat, *Tex. Rep. Biol. Med.*, 19, 646, 1961.

44. Kokka, N., Garcia, J. F., Morgan, M., and George, R., Immunoassay of plasma growth hormone in cats following fasting and administration of insulin, arginine, 2-deoxyglucose and hypothalamic extract, *Endocrinology*, 88, 359, 1971.

45. Müller, E. E. and Pecile, A., Studies on the neural control of growth hormone secretion, in *Growth Hormone*, Pecile, A. and Müller, A. A., Eds., Excerpta Medical Foundation, Milan, 1968, 253.

46. Meites, J., Control of mammary growth and lactation, in *Neuroendocrinology*, Vol. 1, Martini, L. and Ganong, W. F., Eds., Academic Press, New York, 1966, 669.

47. Gold, E. M. and Ganong, W. F., Effects of drugs on neuroendocrine processes, in *Neuroendocrinology*, Vol. 2, Martini, L. and Ganong, W. F., Eds., Academic Press, New York, 1967, 377.

48. Greer, M. A. and Rockie, C., Inhibition by pentobarbital of ether-induced ACTH secretion in the rat, *Endocrinology*, 83, 1247, 1968.

49. Cohen, A. and Pernot, J-C., Réponse des surrénales feetales du rat à une aggression dans différentes conditions expérimentales; effet du nembutal, *C. R. Soc. Biol.*, 162, 1675, 1968.

50. Pohujani, S. M., Chittal, S. M., Raut, V. S., and Sheth, U. K., Studies in stress induced changes on rat's adrenals. Part 1. Effect of central nervous depressants, *Indian Jour. Med. Res.*, 57, 1081, 1969.

51. Japundžić, M. M. and Kulić-Japundžić, I. P., The stimulation of compensatory adrenal growth in rats by propylthiouracil, *Acta Anat.*, 77, 50, 1970.

52. Conney, A. H., Jacobson, M., Schneidman, K., and Knutzman, R., Introduction of liver microsomal cortisol 6β-hydroxylase by diphenylhydantoin or phenobarbital: An explanation for the increased excretion of 6-hydroxy-cortisol in humans treated with these drugs, *Life Sci.*, 4, 1091, 1965.

53. Marc, V. and Morselli, P. L., Metabolism of exogenous cortisol in the rat in various experimental conditions, *J. Pharm. Pharmacol.*, 21, 864, 1969.

54. Southern, L., Gordon, G. G., Tochimoto, S., Krikun, I., Kreiger, D., Jacobson, M., and Kuntzman, R., Effect of *N*-phenylbarbital (Phetbarbital) on the metabolism of testosterone and cortisol in man, *J. Clin. Endocr.*, 29, 251, 1969.

55. Morselli, P. L., Marc, V., Garratini, S., and Zaccala, M., Metabolism of exogenous cortisol in humans. Influence of phenobarbital treatment on plasma cortisol disappearance rate, *Rev. Europ. Etudes Clin. Biol.*, 15, 195, 1970.

56. Berman, M. L. and Green, O. C., Acute stimulation of cortisol metabolism by pentobarbital in man, *Anesthesiology*, 34, 365, 1971.

57. Kröner, von H., Bojar, H. -E., Hollmann, S., and Staib, W., Wirkung von Barbital auf Enzyminduktionen in der Ratleber, *Z. Klin. Chem.*, 8, 45, 1970.

58. Schwartz, H. L., Kozyreff, V., Surks, M. I., and Oppenheimer, J. H., Increased deiodination of L-thyroxine and L-triiodothyronine by liver microsomes from rats treated with phenobarbital, *Nature* (London), 221, 1262, 1969.

59. Schwartz, H. L., Bernstein, G., and Oppenheimer, J. H., Effect of phenobarbital administration on the subcellular distribution of ^{125}I-thyroxine in rat liver: Importance of microsomal binding, *Endocrinology*, 84, 270, 1969.

60. Oppenheimer, J. H., Shapiro, H. C., Schwartz, H. L., and Surks, M. I., Dissociation between thyroxine metabolism and hormonal action in phenobarbital-treated rats, *Endocrinology*, 88, 115, 1971.

61. Harbison, R. D. and Becker, B. A., Barbiturate mortality in hypothyroid and hyperthyroid rats, *J. Pharm. Sci.*, 58, 183, 1969.

62. Gillespie, F. C., Harland, W. A., and Orr, J. S., A new technique for thyroxine secretion rate demonstrating the effect of phenobarbitone in rats, *J. Physiol.* (London), 211, Suppl. 45P, 1970.

63. Ying, S. -Y. and Meyer, R. K., Effect of coitus on barbiturate-blocked ovulation in immature rats, in *Fertility and Sterility*, 20, 772, 1969.

64. Ying, S. -Y. and Meyer, R. K., Effects of steroids on neuropharmacologic blockade of ovulation in pregnant mare's serum (PMS)-primed immature rats, *Endocrinology*, 84, 1466, 1969.

65. Toyoda, Y. and Chang, M. C., Delayed ovulation and embryonic development in the rat treated with pentobarbital sodium, *Endocrinology*, 84, 1456, 1969.

66. Brown-Grant, K., The effects of progesterone and of pentobarbitone administered at the dioestrous stage on the ovarian cycle of the rat, *J. Endocr.*, 43, 539, 1969.

67. Doane, T. A. and Parlow, A. F., Periovulatory patterns of rat serum follicle stimulating hormone and luteinizing hormone during the normal estrous cycle: Effects of pentobarbital, *Endocrinology*, 88, 653, 1971.

68. Weick, R. F., Smith, E. R., Dominquez, R., Dhariwal, A. P. S., and Davidson, J. M., Mechanism of stimulatory feedback effect of estradiol benzoate on the pituitary, *Endocrinology*, 88, 293, 1971.

69. Wenzel, M. and Stahl, H. -J., Verstärkte-Hydroxylierung von Östrogen beim Menschen nach Arzneimittelgabe Nachweis durch HTO-Analyse des Körperwassers, *Hoppe Seyler Z. Physiol. Chem.*, 351, 761, 1970.

70. Fahim, M. S., Dement, G., Hall, D. G., and Fahim, Z., Induced alterations in the hepatic metabolism of androgens in the rat, *Amer. J. Obstet. Gynec.*, 107, 1085, 1970.

71. Wuttke, W. and Meites, J., Effects of ether and pentobarbital on serum prolactin and LH levels in proestrous rats, *Proc. Soc. Exp. Biol. Med.*, 135, 648, 1970.

72. Wilson, J. T., Identification of sonatotrophin as the hormone in a mixture of somatotrophin, adrenocorticotrophic hormone and prolactin which decreased liver drug metabolism in the rat, *Biochem. Pharmacol.*, 18, 2029, 1969.

73. Wilson, J. T., Alteration of normal development of drug metabolism by injection of growth hormone, *Nature*, 225, 861, 1970.

74. Takahashi, K., Doughaday, W. H., and Kipnis, D. M., Regulation of immunoreactive growth hormone secretion in male rats, *Endocrinology*, 88, 909, 1971.

75. Kokka, N., Garcia, J. F., and George, R., unpublished data.

76. Krusins, F. E., Vartia, K. O., and Forsander, O., Biological action of alcohol. II. Adrenocortical function, *Ann. Med. Exp. Biol. Fenn.* (Helsinki), 36, 424, 1958.

77. Bliss, E. L., Migeon, C. J., Eik-Nes, K., Sandberg, A. A., and Samuels, L. T., The effects of insuiin, histamine, bacterial pyrogen, and the antabuse-alcohol reaction upon the levels of 17-hydroxycorticosteroids in the peripheral blood of man, *Metab. Clin. Exp.*, 3, 493, 1954.

78. Steer, P., Marnell, R., and Werk, E. E., Clinical alcohol hypoglycemia and isolated adrenocorticotrophic hormone deficiency, *Ann. Intern. Med.*, 71, 343, 1969.

79. Bellet, S., Roman, R., Debastro, O., and Herrera, M., Effect of acute ethanol intake on plasma 11 hydroxycorticosteroid levels, *Metabolism*, 19, 664, 1970.

80. Merry, J. and Marks, V., Plasma hydrocortisone response to ethanol in chronic alcoholics, *Lancet*, 1, 921, 1969.

81. Kissin, B., Schenker, V., and Schenker, A. C., Adrenal cortical function and liver disease in alcoholics, *Amer. J. Med. Sci.*, 238, 344, 1959.

82. Kieffer, J. D. and Ketchel, M. M., Blockade of ovulation in the rat by ethanol, *Acta Endocr.*, 65, 117, 1970.

83. De Wied, D., Chlorpromazine and endocrine function, *Pharmacol. Rev.*, 19, 251, 1967.

84. Marks, B. H., Hall, M. M., and Bhattacharya, A. N., Psychopharmacological effects and pituitary-adrenal activity, *Prog. Brain Res.*, 32, 57, 1970.

85. Sasaki, Sh., Studies on the central regulation of the pituitary-adrenocortical system, *Acta Med. Biol.*, 11, 185, 1963.

86. Egdahl, R. H. and Richards, J. B., Effect of chlorpromazine on pituitary ACTH secretion in the dog, *Amer. J. Physiol.*, 185, 235, 1956.

87. Betz, D. and Ganong, W. F., Effect of chlorpromazine on pituitary-adrenal function in the dog, *Acta Endocr.*, 43, 264, 1963.

88. Harwood, C. T. and Mason, J. W., Effects of tranquilizing drugs on the anterior pituitary-ACTH mechanism, *Endocrinology*, 60, 239, 1957.

89. Olling, Ch. C. J. and De Wied, D., Inhibition of the release of corticotrophin from the hypophysis by chlorpromazine, *Acta Endocr.*, 22, 283, 1956.

90. Christy, N. P., Longson, D., Horwitz, W. A., and Knight, M. M., Inhibitory effect of chlorpromazine upon the adrenal cortical response to insulin hypoglycemia in man, *J. Clin. Invest.*, 36, 543, 1957.

91. Fotherby, K., Forrest, A. D., and Laverty, S. G., The effect of chlorpromazine on adrenocortical function, *Acta Endocr.*, 32, 425, 1959.

92. Arvay, A., Lampé, L., Kertész, L., and Medveczky, L., Changes of thyroid function in response to severe nervous stimulation, *Acta Endocr.*, 35, 469, 1960.

93. von Brauchitsch, H., Endokrinologische Aspekte des Wirkungsmechanismus neuroplegischer Medikamente, *Psychopharmacologia*, 2, 1, 1961.

94. Sulman, F. G., The mechanism of the "Push and Pull" principle, *Arch. Int. Pharmacodyn.*, 118, 298, 1959.

95. Aleshin, B. V. and Us, L. A., L'effect de la chlorpromazine sur les fonctions de la structure du lobe antérieur de l'hypophyse dans certaines conditions expérimentales, *Prob. Endokr. Gormonater*, 6, 32, 1960.

96. Meidinger, F., Action comparée sur l'hypophyse d'antihistaminiques, de neuroplégiques et d'anti-inflammatoires, *C. R. Soc. Biol.* (Paris), 148, 1086, 1954.

97. Blumberg, A. G. and Klein, D. F., Chlorpromazine-procyclidine and imipramine-effects on thyroid function in psychiatric patients,*Clin. Pharmacol. Ther.*, 10, 350, 1969.

98. Yamashita, K., Bloom, G., Rainard, B., Zor, U., and Field, J. B., Effects of chlorpromazine, propranolol and phospholipase C on thyrotropin and prostoglandin stimulation of adenyl cyclase-cyclic AMP system in dog thyroid slices, *Metabolism*, 19, 1109, 1970.

99. Wolff, J. and Jones, A. B., Inhibition of hormone-sensitive adenyl cyclase by phenothiazines, *Proc. Nat. Acad. Sci.*, 65, 454, 1970.

100. Onaya, T. and Solomon, D. H., Effects of chlorpromazine and propranolol on in vitro thyroid activation by thyrotropin, long-acting thyroid stimulator and dibutyryl cyclic-AMP, *Endocrinology*, 85, 1010, 1969.

101. Williams, J. A. and Wolff, J., Thyroid secretion in vitro: Multiple actions of agents affecting secretion, *Endocrinology*, 88, 206, 1971.

102. Py, O. and Mathieu, P., Galactorrhée et troubles du cycle menstruel au cours de tractements neuroleptiques, *Presse Méd.*, 68, 765, 1960.

103. Zarrow, M. X. and Brown-Grant, K., Inhibition of ovulation in the gonadotrophin-treated immature rat by chlorpromazine, *J. Endocr.*, 30, 87, 1964.

104. Bourrillon, R., Marcy, R., and Got, R., Die Wirkung des Chlorpromazins auf die Hypophyso-gonaden Achse, *Endokrinologie*, 37, 285, 1959.

105. Whitelaw, M. J., Delay in ovulation and menstruation induced by chlorpromazine, *J. Clin. Endocr.*, 16, 972, 1956.

106. Grönroos, M., Kalliomäki, J. L., Keyriläinen, T. O., and Marianen, P., Effects of reserpine and chlorpromazine on the mammary glands of the rat, *Acta Endocr.*, 31, 154, 1959.

107. Ciro, C., Peripheral nervous system and susceptibility of the tissues for hormoneal action: effect of prolactin and chlorpromazine on the peripheral nerves in the mammary gland of the rat, *Acta Neuroveg.* (Wien), 22, 333, 1961.

108. Barraclough, C. A. and Sawyer, C. H., Induction of pseudopregnancy in the rat by reserpine and chlorpromazine, *Endocrinology*, 65, 563, 1959.

109. Ben-David, M., Danon, A., and Sulman, F. G., Acute changes in blood and pituitary prolactin after a single injection of perphenazine, *Neuroendocrinology*, 6, 336, 1970.

110. Bryant, G. D., Connan, R. M., and Greenwood, F. C., Changes in plasma prolactin induced by acepromazine in sheep, *J. Endocr.*, 41, 613, 1968.

111. Bryant, G. D. and Greenwood, F. C., Plasma prolactin level in the goat: physiological experimental modification, *J. Endocr.*, 40, IV, 1968.

112. Danon, A. and Sulman, F. G., Storage of prolactin-inhibiting factor in the hypothalamus of perphenazine-treated rats, *Neuroendocrinology*, 6, 295, 1970.

113. Glick, S. M., The regulation of growth hormone secretion, in *Frontiers in Neuroendocrinology*, Ganong, W. F. and Martini, L., Eds., Oxford University Press, New York, 1969, 141.

114. Kipnis, D. M., Hertelendy, F., and Machlin, J. L., Studies of growth hormone secretion, *Progress in Endocrinology*, 3rd Int. Cong. Endocrinol., Mexico City, Excerpta Medica Foundation, Amsterdam, 1968, 601.

115. Cranston, E. M. and Segal, M. S., Effect of tranquilizer and other agents on sexual cycle of mice, *Proc. Soc. Exp. Biol. Med.*, 98, 320, 1958.

116. Meyer, V. and Knobil, E., Growth hormone secretion in the unanesthetized Rhesus monkey in response to noxious stimuli, *Endocrinology*, 80, 163, 1967.

117. Schalch, D. S. and Reichlin, S., Stress and growth hormone release, in *Growth Hormone*, Pecile, A. and Müller, E. E., Eds., Excerpta Medica Foundation, Milan, 1968, 211.

118. Marc, V. and Marselli, P. L., Effect of diazepam on plasma corticosterone levels in the rat, *J. Pharm. Pharmacol.*, 21, 784, 1969.

119. Dasgupta, S. R. and Mukherjee, B. P., Effect of chlordiazepoxide on eosinopenia of stress in rabbits, *Nature*, 213, 199, 1967.

120. Butler, P. W. P., Besser, G. M., and Steinberg, H., Changes in plasma cortisol induced by dexamphetamine and chlordiazepoxide given alone and in combination in man, *J. Endocr.*, 40, 391, 1968.

121. Superstein, E. and Sulman, F. G., The mechanism of the push and pull principle VII. Endocrine effects of chlordiazepoxide, diazepam, and guanethidine, *Arch. Int. Pharmacodyn.*, 1, 160, 1966.

122. Harvey, R. F., Drugs and thyroid function tests, *Brit. Med. J.*, 2, 52, 1967.

123. Schindler, W. J., Matthews, M. G., and McHorse, T. S., Influence of centrally acting drugs on pituitary TSH release and thyroid activity in the mouse, *Fed. Proc.*, 25, 380, 1966.

124. Clark, F. and Hall, R., Chlordiazepoxide (Librium®) and tests of thyroid function, *Brit. Med. J.*, 2, 266, 1970.

125. Clark, F., Hall, R., and Ormston, B. J., Diazepam and tests of thyroid function, *Brit. Med. J.*, 1, 585, 1971.

126. Mazzaferri, E. L. and Skillman, T. G., Diazepam (Valium®) and thyroid function: A double-blind placebo controlled study in normal volunteers showing no drug effect, *Amer. J. Med. Sci.*, 257, 388, 1969.

127. Nasmyth, P. A., The effect of some sympathomimetic amines on the ascorbic acid content of rats' adrenal glands, *J. Physiol.* (London), 110, 294, 1950.

128. Ohler, E. A. and Sevy, R. W., Effect of Paredrine and adrenergic blockade on ACTH discharge, *Amer. J. Physiol.*, 171, 753, 1952.

129. Zeim, M., Coper, H., Broermann, I., and Strauss, S., Vergleichende Untersuchungen über einige Wirkungen des Amphetamines bei Ratten verschiedenen Alters, Naunyn-Schmiedebergs, *Arch. Pharmak.*, 267, 208, 1970.

130. Naumenko, E. V., Role of adrenergic and cholinergic structures in the control of the pituitary-adrenal system, *Endocrinology*, 80, 69, 1967.

131. Besser, G. M., Butler, P. W. P., Landou, J., and Rees, L., Influence of amphetamines on plasma corticosteroid and growth hormone levels in man, *Brit. Med. J.*, 4, 528, 1969.

132. Rees, L., Butler, P. W. P., Gosling, C., and Besser, G. M., Adrenergic blockade and the corticosteroid and growth hormone responses to methylamphetamine, *Nature*, 228, 565, 1970.

133. Lorenzen, L. C. and Ganong, W. F., Effect of drugs related to *a*-ethyl-tryptamine on stress-induced ACTH secretion in the dog, *Endocrinology*, 80, 889, 1967.

134. Stoffer, S. S., A gynecologic study of drug addicts, *Amer. J. Obstet. Gynec.*, 101, 779, 1968.

135. Stoffer, S. S., Sapira, J. D., Tweeddale, D. N., and Meketon, B. F., Effect of d-amphetamine on menstruation, *Amer. J. Obstet. Gynec.*, 105, 989, 1969.

136. McMahon, E. M., Andersen, D. K., Feldman, J. M., and Schanberg, S. M., Methamphetamine-induced insulin release, *Science*, 174, 66, 1971.

137. Hollister, L. E., Steroids and moods: Correlations in schizophrenics and subjects treated with lysergic acid diethylamide (LSD), mescaline, tetrahydrocannabinol, and synhexyl, *J. Clin. Pharmacol.*, 9, 24, 1969.

138. Hollister, L. E., Moore, F., Kanter, S., and Noble, E., Δ^1-tetrahydrocannabinol, synhexyl and marijuana extract administered orally in man: Catecholamine excretion, plasma cortisol levels and platelet serotonin content, *Psychopharmacologia*, 17, 354, 1970.

139. Dewey, W. L., Peng, T-C., and Harris, L. S., The effect of 1-trans-Δ^9-tetrahydrocannabinol on the hypothalamo-hypophyseal-adrenal axis of rats, *Europ. J. Pharmacol.*, 12, 382, 1970.

140. Kubena, R. K., Perhach, J. L., and Barry, H., Cortisone elevation mediated centrally by Δ^1-tetrahydrocannabinol in rats, *Europ. J. Pharmacol.*, 14, 89, 1971.

141. Barry, H., Perhach, J. L., and Kubena, R. K., Δ^1-tetrahydrocannabinol activation of pituitary-adrenal function, *Pharmacologist*, 12, 258, 1970.

142. Weltman, A. S., Sackler, A. M., and Schwartz, R., Mescaline hydrochloride effects on the endocrine activity of male albino mice, *Exp. Med. Surg.*, 26, 187, 1968.

143. Weltman, A. S. and Sackler, A. M., Metabolic and endocrine effects of lysergic acid diethylamide (LSD-25) on male rats, *J. Endocr.*, 34, 81, 1966.

144. Lomax, P., Animal pharmacology of marihuana, *Proc. West. Pharmacol. Soc.*, 14, 10, 1971.

145. Miras, C. J., Some aspects of cannabis action, in *Hashish: Its Chemistry and Pharmacology*, Wolstenholme, G. E. W. and Knight, J., Eds., Little, Brown and Co., Boston, 1965.

146. Kaymakcalan, S. and Deneau, G. A., Some pharmacological effects of synthetic Δ^9-tetrahydrocannabinol (THC), *Pharmacologist*, 13, 247, 1971.

147. Lomax, P., The effect of marihuana on pituitary-thyroid activity in the rat, *Agents and Actions*, 1, 252, 1970.

148. Way, E. L. and Shen, F-H., Catecholamines and 5-hydroxytryptamine, in *Narcotic Drugs Biochemical Pharmacology*, Clouet, D., Ed., Plenum Press, New York, 1971, 229.

149. Weinstock, M., Acetylcholine and cholinesterase, in *Narcotic Drugs Biochemical Pharmacology*, Clouet, D., Ed., Plenum Press, New York, 1971, 254.

150. Naumenko, E. V., Hypothalamic chemoreactive structures and the regulation of pituitary-adrenal functions. Effects of local injections of norepinephrine, carbachol and serotonin into the brain of guinea pigs with intact brains and after mesencephalic transection, *Brain Res.*, 11, 1, 1968.

151. Krieger, D. T. and Rizzo, F., Serotonin mediation of circadian periodicity of plasma 17-hydroxycorticosteroids, *Amer. J. Physiol.*, 217, 1703, 1969.

152. Hedge, G. A. and Smelik, P. G., Corticotropin release: Inhibition by intrahypothalamic implantation of atropine, *Science*, 159, 891, 1968.

153. Krieger, D. T., Silverberg, A. I., Rizzo, F., and Krieger, H. P., Abolition of circadian periodicity of plasma 17-OHCS levels in the cat, *Amer. J. Physiol.*, 215, 959, 1968.

154. Donoso, A. O., Bishop, W., Fawcett, C. P., Kruhlich, L., and McCann, S. M., Effects of drugs that modify brain monoamine concentrations on plasma gonadotropin and prolactin levels in the rat, *Endocrinology*, 89, 774, 1971.

155. Blackard, W. G. and Heidingsfelder, S. A., Adrenergic control mechanism for growth hormone secretion, *J. Clin. Invest.*, 47, 1407, 1968.

THEORETICAL BIOCHEMICAL MECHANISMS FOR DRUG DEPENDENCE

D. H. Clouet

TABLE OF CONTENTS

INTRODUCTION

Drugs which produce dependence in man have one characteristic in common: in effective doses, they induce an alteration in behavior.* This characteristic does not define drug dependence, however, since other drugs modify behavior without inducing drug dependence. The responses to drug use in behavioral parameters do designate the central nervous system as the target organ in which the ultimate chemical intervention by the drug

*Since the introductory description of the central nervous system and the exposition of the various theories on the mechanism of drug dependence are based on the studies, research, writings, and speculation of many neurobiologists and pharmacologists, the author wished to acknowledge her debt to these scientists as a group, and reserve documentation for statements describing experimentally-derived evidence. Throughout the chapter, 'drug' is used as an abbreviation for 'drugs which induce dependence'.

occurs. The basic mechanisms of neural function will be described briefly in order to provide the orientation needed in the discussion of the particular biochemical sites of intervention by specific drugs.

The nervous system is a communication machine and deals in information. It gathers information, transforms it, stores it, retrieves the information from the stores, distributes it, and integrates it. The information gathered by the nervous system is produced outside the nervous system in the form of various physical and chemical stimuli which come into contact with receptor areas in the peripheral nervous system such as sound waves, light waves, pressure, temperature, and gustatory and olfactory chemovectors. At the receptor site the stimulus is transformed into nerve impulse, an electrochemical wave which can move from the receptor sensory locus to the appropriate loci in the central nervous system. The transformed information can, at other levels of function in the nervous system, be combined with on-going impulses to increase, decrease, or abolish on-going activity. Information also arises within the central nervous system as on-going spontaneous activity and built-in patterns derived from learning or genetic development interact with environmental events to generate streams of information. The once-transformed information undergoes many further internal transformations at many stages and levels in the central nervous system before output is generated in the form of afferent impulses which activate motor or vegetative function or behavior.

The transmission of the message may be examined experimentally at many levels of integration. *Subcellular* levels are the cytological and biochemical aspects of the generation of the impulse and its transmission. *Cellular* levels are the location of the cell structures where transmission of the message from cell to cell occurs. *Electrochemical* levels include physicochemical aspects of the movement of the electrical impulse through fibers and its dimension. *Specific control systems* include mechanisms and pathways, such as the autonomic nervous system, which function below the level of consciousness in the regulation of respiration, circulation, digestion, body temperature, etc. *Higher levels of integration* are the mechanisms and pathways of conscious behavior such as cognition, problem solving, or the use of language. Some behavioral responses are automatic, either genetically endowed or learned responses. Other behavioral responses are not automatic, but are generated through a complex system of reward, punishment mechanisms, etc.

The nerve impulse can convey specific meanings by anatomical localization since the pathway of the impulse is limited by the interneuronal connections to existing pathways. However, in complex interlocking systems, pathway localization is inadequate and is supplemented by a system of codes. The nerve impulse as an electrochemical wave has certain dimensions such as potential and amplitude, frequency, and sequence. The neural codes rely on properties of impulses such as frequency of firing, increment above background, latency between firings, phase differences in sequence, etc., and can best be examined by computer analysis. In ensemble activity where there is integration at many levels, one can relate topography and phasing to amplitude and potential of the impulse.

On the neuronal level, the propagation of the nerve impulse from the dendritic receptor to the cell body and out through the axon to the nerve ending is well understood chemically in the peripheral nervous system and presumed to be similar in the central nervous system. At the receptor a depolarization is initiated by membrane leakage of potassium ions. The difference in potential across the cell membrane maintains the depolarization wave until it reaches the axonal nerve endings. The transmission of the impulse from cell to cell involves a chemical transmission at the synapse, where the two neurons are in close proximity, involving the group of compounds called neurotransmitters or neurohormones, which are secreted by the transmitting neuron into the synaptic cleft between the neurons where they react with the receptor cell membrane of the receiving neuron. The putative chemical transmitters in the central nervous system include acetylcholine, serotonin, norepinephrine, and dopamine. All of these compounds are synthesized in the nerve ending from precursor molecules through enzymatic activity, are secreted from the nerve ending, or stored in storage vesicles, or destroyed by catabolic enzyme activity. The importance of these reactions is that at each step the normal sequence is open to interference by certain drugs, and that these drugs belong to the categories of drugs which act on brain function, altering mood and behavior and often inducing dependence. The response to the changes in data input is controlled in two temporal modes: *short-time* modes in which shifts in the rate or direction of basic metabolic reactions produce new metabolic equilibrium situations capable of handling the changed input or altering the input itself peripherally, and *long-time* modes in which a major change in the patterns of data input brings into play the superregulatory systems of adaptation. Steroid and peptide hormones as well as the neurotransmitters play a role in adaptation acting both as modifiers in the central nervous system and as messengers of target organs.

The immediate effects of drug administration in an acute dose may be ascribed to alterations in some step in synaptic transmission at some site in the central nervous system, as a primary or secondary response. However, information accrual and storage, learning and memory in some biochemical mode, must be implicated in the development of drug dependence, particularly physical dependence and tolerance. There are a number of hypotheses describing the molecular basis of memory which include the formation of an 'engram' in response to the afferent informational impulse. The engram is defined as the physiochemical change in brain which reflects the long-lasting acquired behavioral change and is variously described as: (1) short-term coding of the afferent impulse by RNA which is translated into protein for long-term storage; (2) an allosteric change in a neuronal membrane component such as a glyco- or lipo-protein which permanently records the information; (3) the elaboration of new interneuronal connections through chronic stimulation; (4) the development of a new code 'word' characterized by a new combination of phasing and amplitude of the nerve impulse; or (5) the elaboration of an immunological protein, an antibody, in response to an antigen formed by drug-protein interaction. Whether the biological correlates so far discovered during the formation of long-term memory are relevant or merely epiphenomena is not clear at the present time. Progress in the definition of neuronal memory (and, perhaps, of immunological memory) will clarify the definition of the effects of dependence-producing drugs by such phenomena. The involvement of an informational storage mechanism of the CNS in the mechanisms of dependence is presumed in most of the hypotheses concerning the molecular basis of dependence.

It follows that when a drug intervenes to disturb the dynamic equilibrium of the nervous system, the expression of normal functioning, i.e., behavior may also be altered. A panoply of neurochemical responses may be produced in sites in the CNS and elsewhere in the body by a single drug, acting either directly or indirectly. For theoretical and therapeutic reasons it is important to distinguish the 'initial biochemical lesion' produced by the drug from consequential secondary responses, although most of the pharmacological responses to drug use are likely to be produced through secondary mechanisms. It is even more important to distinguish between the biochemical mechanisms underlying the initial pharmacological responses to drugs of dependence, and the reactions whereby tolerance and dependence are produced by chronic drug use.

Instead of reviewing systematically the kinds of biological interference produced by each category of dependence-producing drugs, I plan to discuss the types and possible sites of intervention together with the pertinent evidence that a major drug effect is produced through, or accompanied by, an alteration at the metabolic site.

The drugs that produce dependence are classified as *Morphine-type, Barbiturate-alcohol type, Amphetamine-type, Hallucinogen-type, Cocaine-type* and *Cannabis-type.*[1] These drug categories reflect the differences in behavioral changes, and pharmacological responses produced by the drugs, as well as the physicochemical properties of the common structure of the drugs in each category. The pharmacological and chemical characteristics of the classes of drug dependence have already been described in earlier chapters. Some of the basic biochemical mechanisms underlying pharmacological action and dependence production may be common to drugs in all classes. However, it is logical to assume that there are also basic mechanisms unique for each class. Certainly, the biochemical effects of drugs which produce psychic dependence without tolerance or physical dependence would be expected to differ from those produced by the opiates.

Although the central nervous system is the primary site of drug intervention by mind-altering drugs, the action of a drug is limited by its level in the CNS. Therefore, factors affecting brain levels of drugs such as the absorption, distribution, transport, plasma binding, metabolism, and excretion of the drugs must be considered as additional possible sites of alteration during chronic drug use.

MECHANISMS IN TISSUES OTHER THAN THE CENTRAL NERVOUS SYSTEM

Liver

The importance of the conversion of active drugs to less active catabolites through the metabolism of drugs in the liver lies in the ability of such reactions to alter the effective drug levels in plasma and in tissue. There are many instances in the recent literature of an altered metabolism of a dependence-producing drug by the prior administration of the same drug or of another drug. For most classes of drugs which induce dependence, alteration in the rate of drug metabolism in the liver may be considered of minimal importance in mechanisms for the development of dependence and tolerance.

Barbiturates

The role played in the development of tolerance to barbiturates by an increased rate of drug metabolism has been examined in experimental animals by Remmer.[2] The catabolism of hexobarbital was measured by following the decline in blood levels of the drug for a period of 4 hours after each administration of the drug to dogs. Daily treatment with hexobarbital resulted in a faster disappearance of hexobarbital from the blood. Pretreatment with phenobarbital or tolbutamide also resulted in a faster decline of blood levels of hexobarbital. A corresponding decrease in a pharmacological response (ataxia) indicated that this response was related to the levels of the drug in circulating blood.

Similar results were obtained in other species such as rats, rabbits and mice,[3] and man.[4] Earlier studies from several laboratories related the pharmacological responses after hexobarbital administration to the activity of the catabolic drug-metabolizing enzymes in the liver, showing that the drug-induced increase in drug-metabolizing enzyme activity was correlated to the decrease in sleeping-time after hexobarbital.[5] Thus, in experimental situations, the phenomena of tolerance to the chronic use of short-acting barbiturates can be ascribed entirely to an increased catabolism of the drugs by induced liver enzymes.

The mechanisms of the induction of microsomal drug-metabolizing enzymes (DMEs) in liver are not clearly understood. A proliferation of the liver endoplasmic reticulum is accompanied by an increase in protein synthesis[6] and an increase in RNA synthesis,[7] and by a decrease in RNA breakdown due to the progressive inhibition of RNAase activity during induction.[8,9] The specificity in induction of the synthesis of the protein enzyme involved in the microsomal respiratory system is quite distinct from the general increase in protein synthesis induced by hepatectomy or by anabolic steriod hormones such as nortestosterone.[10] In addition to the effect of the induction of the DMEs by inducer drugs, there is a direct competition between drugs for the DMEs in liver. In in vitro systems, many drugs can be shown to be competitive inhibitors for other drugs.[11] In the intact animal, however, there are requirements of similarity of Km and Vmax values before one drug can have an important effect on the metabolism of another drug.[12] Thus, ethylmorphine and codeine which have similar kinetic properties to hexobarbital inhibit hexobarbital metabolism in vivo while morphine and norcodeine do not.[13]

Ethanol

Ethanol is metabolized in the soluble cytoplasm of the liver cell by alcohol dehydrogenase coupled with an NADH or NADPH oxidase. In in vitro systems catalase and a peroxide-generating system can replace the dehydrogenase-oxidase system in the conversion of ethanol to acetaldehyde. However, this reaction does not seem to be important in vivo, since an examination of the relative ratios of reduced to oxidized forms of NAD and NADP in liver after ethanol administration indicated that the soluble NADH oxidase functioned as the usual cofactor for alcohol dehydrogenase.[14] However, during chronic alcohol administration, NADPH oxidase is induced at the same time as cytochrome P450 and NADPH cytochrome c reductase.[15] Thus, it is possible that the liver microsomal DMEs assume importance during chronic alcohol use. If this is so, the cross tolerance between alcohol and barbiturates may be related to the mutual induction of the activity of liver DMEs by each drug.

Opiates

As is true for other classes of drugs, the effective levels of opiates in plasma and tissue are related to the rate of drug catabolism. Inducers such as phenobarbital can increase the conversion of opiates to dealkylated or hydroxylated metabolites.[16] This effect, however, plays a minimal effect in the development of tolerance to opiates in experimental animals.[17]

In male rats, the chronic administration of opiates decreases the level of liver DMEs.[18] The pharmacological responses to opiates decrease simultaneously with the liver DME activity.[19] However, this phenomenon is peculiar to the liver of male rats, since the morphine-induced decrease in DME activity is not found in other species.[20] In rats there is a sex difference in the liver DME activity which is responsive to sex hormones.[21] Specifically, the magnitude of the spectral change due to ethyl-morphine binding is greater in the male rat liver indicating higher binding to oxidized cytochrome P450.[22] The involvement of the adrenal steroid hormones in this sex difference in rats is indicated by the greater decrease in DME activity after adrenalectomy in the male, reversible by cortisone administration.[23] This suggests that the effect of opiates on DME activity in male rat liver may be effected through adrenal mechanisms.[24]

Amphetamines

The metabolism of amphetamine is altered by induction of the liver DME.[25] An inducer drug such as imipramine competes with amphetamine as a substrate for oxidized P450, slowing the catabolism of amphetamine, and thus potentiating the pharmacological response.[26] Such effects, however, are related more to the toxic effects of the drug than to its ability to induce psychic dependence.

Other Tissues

There are many physiological reactions occurring outside the CNS which alter the effective levels of drug in blood (such as plasma protein binding and changes in blood flow and excretory rates) for which there is no evidence of involvement in dependence. These reactions will not be discussed here. Other types of reactions such as the immune response or the formation of transfer factors, which have been suggested as possible mechanisms for the development of tolerance, will be considered briefly.

Immune Response

The possibility that some form of antigen-antibody reaction can be induced by drug administration leading to the production of circulating antibodies to the drug was suggested many years ago by Gioffredi as an explanation of opiate tolerance.[27] Evidence in favor of an immunological response comes from experiments in which serum from morphine-tolerant animals was shown to attenuate the pharmacological response to the drug in naïve animals.[28] However, potentiation rather than attenuation of the morphine effect resulted from the injection of serum from morphine-tolerant animals to naïve recipients in other experiments.[29] Such results are not mutually exclusive because the temporal dimensions of an immune response would be directly related to the duration of effective tissue levels of the drug and thus the dose schedule during chronic drug treatment. Other unknown factors in the demonstration of antibodies to drugs can be related to the site of antibody formation, the nature of the stimulus which releases the antibodies into blood, and the stability of the antibodies in blood. The effect of cyclophoramide, an immunosuppressive drug, in inhibiting the development of tolerance to morphine has reinforced the impression that an immune response may be involved.[30]

Recently, Spector and his colleagues have been successful in preparing antibodies to opiates, barbiturates, and tetrahydrocannabinols by injecting suitable conjugates of the drug and protein into rabbits and isolating antibodies to the drugs.[31] Such antibodies have proved useful as tools in the microdetection of drugs in biological specimens.[32] It should be possible with modern immunochemical techniques to establish whether or not antibodies are formed during chronic treatment with dependence-producing drugs. The development of tolerance to drug use could be directly related to such antibodies. Drug dependence, however, would be involved only if the immune response occurs in the CNS.

MECHANISMS IN THE CENTRAL NERVOUS SYSTEM

Psychic dependence and at least some of the symptoms of physical dependence are centrally mediated phenomena with underlying biochemical mechanisms. In some types of dependence, especially opiate-induced, it is possible that these mechanisms are not directly related to the drug action at the receptor sites which is responsible for invoking pharmacological responses. If there are, indeed, separate biochemical mechanisms leading to the expression of pharmacological responses, or to dependence, it is also possible that in simpler types of dependence such as cocaine-induced, an adaptation at the receptor site is all that is necessary to produce the symptoms of psychic dependence.

In the preceding sections, we have discussed some factors which can alter blood levels of drugs, and thereby also alter the drug levels in the central nervous system. The extracerebral changes in the levels of drugs entering the CNS seem to be important only in the development of tolerance to short-acting barbiturates, and possibly alcohol. There is no evidence that dependence on drugs is related to the changes in brain levels of the drugs during chronic treatment. There is also no evidence that an altered transport of drugs into brain is involved in either tolerance or dependence. The disposition of drugs in brain regions during chronic drug treatment has been compared with that in untreated animals in numerous studies, particularly with opiate treatment. A general conclusion derived from these studies is that there is no significant change in drug levels in nervous tissue, and no change in the rate of uptake or disappearance of drugs from brain during chronic treatment.[33] However, any changes in the amount of drug at the cellular level, or alterations in the drug:receptor ratio would not be detected in measurements of drug concentrations in gross tissue areas, or even in subcellular fractions from regions of the brain.

Although no changes in the catabolism of drugs in brain during chronic drug treatment have been shown, the possibility of such change cannot be eliminated from consideration because an altered catabolism of that amount of drug which is acting pharmacologically may be undetected in the presence of much larger amounts of non-metabolized, inactive drug. Thus, alterations *at the tissue level* in drug disposition in the CNS can be dismissed as a mechanism for the development of tolerance and dependence, and changes *at the neuronal or subcellular level* retained as an option. There has been some speculation concerning the need for the conversion of opiates, tetrahydrocannabinol, dimethyltryptamine, and barbiturates to 'active' metabolites before interaction with CNS receptors.[34-36] There is a fine line of distinction between drug metabolism to an 'active' form and structural changes in the drug molecule during receptor binding. There is no evidence to date of the need for conversion to an 'active' metabolite for the simple prototype drugs which produce dependence.

In this section, we shall first consider sites in the process of neurotransmission where drugs act, or are suspected of acting, and then consider the kinds of macromolecular biosynthesis which would be necessary to support the metabolic adaptation to chronic drug stimulation.

Neurotransmission

Competitive Inhibition

There is little evidence that drugs which induce dependence compete as a general phenomenon with naturally-occurring precursors and intermediates as substrates for the enzymes that catalyze the sequential steps in the biosynthetic pathways of the neurotransmitters in the CNS. One drug which does serve as a competitive substrate is *d*-amphetamine, a substrate for dopamine β-hydroxylase. In vivo *d*-amphetamine is *p*-hydroxylated, presumably through the liver microsomal cytochrome system, and β-hydroxylated to *p*-hydroxynorephedrine.[37] This metabolite is responsible for some of the cardiovascular effects of amphetamine,[38] but does not play an important role in CNS effects. Evidence for this last statement comes from experiments in which *l*-amphetamine, which is not a substrate for dopamine β-hydroxylase, is shown to cause a release of brain catecholamines similar to that evoked by the *d*-isomer;[39] and from experiments in which the conversion of *d*-amphetamine to *p*-hydroxynorephedrine was blocked by desmethylimipramine with an enhancement of its CNS effects.[40] However, some of the persistent effects of amphetamine on the levels of brain catecholamines are attributed to the presence of *p*-hydroxynorephedrine in the CNS, since this metabolite persists in brain for six or seven days after a single injection of amphetamine.[41]

Another drug metabolite, acetaldehyde, formed by the oxidation of ethanol, serves as a competitive substrate for aldehyde oxidase, leading to a decreased production of oxidized catabolites of catecholamines in subjects consuming large amounts of alcohol.[42] This competitive inhibition of catecholamine metabolism may also occur in the CNS since aldehyde reductase isolated from bovine brain is inhibited by a number of barbiturates,[43] although $C^{14}O_2$ is not evolved when C^{14}-ethanol is incubated with brain tissue.[44]

Synaptic Phenomena

The important role played by neuroamines and their rates of biosynthesis, release, re-uptake and degradation in affecting the action of CNS-active drugs is emphasized by the results of the many studies which demonstrate an interference by drugs at some step in neurotransmission at the synaptic level.

The uptake of biogenic amines from the synaptic cleft into the nerve ending, or into synaptic vesicles, is inhibited by many classes of drugs which induce dependence. Both isomers of amphetamine are active in blocking the uptake of catecholamines in brain regions.[45] The *d*-form is a more potent inhibitor of the uptake of both norepinephrine and dopamine by norepinephrinergic neurons, but the two isomers are equally active in inhibiting the uptake into the dopaminergic neurons of the striatum.[46] These differences in the activity of the isomers are reflections of the differences in pharmacological responses to the administration of each isomer.[47] Many of the neurochemical effects attributed to a direct action of amphetamine are actually responses to a decrease in *intra*synaptic catecholamines and an increase in *extra*synaptic amines. Thus, the increase in extrasynaptosomal norepinephrine after amphetamine administration can be interpreted as an increase in amine release rather than as an inhibition of re-uptake; and the catabolism of norepinephrine by extrasynaptic catechol-O-methyltransferase instead of intrasynaptic monoamine oxidase can be interpreted as an inhibition of monoamine oxidase rather than a decreased availability of norepinephrine to monoamine oxidase.[48] Similarly, an amphetamine-induced increase in norepinephrine turnover can be attributed to a stimulatory effect on tyrosine hydroxylase rather than a release of feedback inhibition of the enzyme by norepinephrine.[49] Amphetamine also enhances the release of serotonin.[50] Some substituted amphetamines such as bis(3,4-dichlorophenylethyl)amine are more active as catecholamine and serotonin depleters than amphetamine, and some, such as the *p*-chloro derivatives, act specifically on serotonin depletion.[51] *P*-chloroamphetamine is a competitive inhibitor of tryptophan hydroxylase with effects similar to *p*-chlorophenylalanine.[52]

Cocaine interferes with neurotransmission at the same site as amphetamine, inhibiting the re-uptake of norepinephrine into the nerve ending. After cocaine administration there is a shift to the extrasynaptic catabolism of norepinephrine to normetanephrine rather than to intracellular oxidation by monoamine oxidase, for the same reason that amphetamine administration shifts norepinephrine metabolism to nonoxidized catabolites.[53]

Reserpine interferes with catecholamine re-uptake into the nerve ending, but at the synaptic vesicular membrane rather than at the nerve ending membrane as cocaine and amphetamines do.[54] The storage of neuroamines inside the nerve ending is inhibited by reserpine administration because the amines are transported through the cell membrane but not enclosed in vesicles, and thus are available for monoamine oxidase action in the cytoplasm within the nerve ending.[55] In the adrenal gland, the uptake of amine into the medullary granules in the presence of ATP and Mg is inhibited by reserpine,[56] and in the CNS, a similar inhibition in the process whereby biogenic amines are stored in vesicles is postulated.[57] The storage of other putative neurotransmitters such as histamine, aminobutyric acid, and acetylcholine is also altered by resperine treatment.[58]

The most consistent biochemical effect of LSD and similar drugs is a decrease of turnover rate of serotonin in the brain.[59] However, since catecholamine levels in the CNS are also depressed, the specificity of the response and the mechanism at the synaptic level are still largely unexplored.[59]

The opiates can effect changes in neurotransmitter levels in the CNS. An acute dose of morphine produces a transient decrease in brain dopamine and norepinephrine, an effect to which tolerance develops.[60] The turnover of dopamine in rat brain is increased shortly after the administration of morphine,[61,62] presumably to replenish the dopamine pool. Although this effect can be produced after each daily injection of morphine in the rat, tolerance develops in this biochemical parameter if there is a more constant supply of drug by multiple daily injections or by morphine pellet implantation.[62,63]

The complexity of the interrelationships among the neurotransmitters makes it difficult to ascribe a temporal primacy of drug reaction to adrenergic, serotonergic, or cholinergic systems. Cholinergic pathways control some of the locomotor activity, autonomic activity, and adrenal medullary responses which are among the pharmacological symptoms of drug administration.[64] In addition, a number of behavioral responses such as the altering effect and the enhancement of learning are controlled through cholinergic pathways in the hippocampus,[64] and other behavioral effects such as conditioned learning are attributed to extra-hippocampal muscarinic pathways, since they are inhibited by atropine.[65] A number of drugs that induce dependence alter the level of acetylcholine in the brain. After the administration of barbiturates or reserpine, the levels of acetylcholine rise.[66,67] Morphine and other narcotic drugs also produce an increase in acetycholine levels.[68] The release of acetylcholine from the cortical surface of the living cat is decreased by morphine, meperidine, pentazocine, and many other agonists, as well as by partial antagonists:agonists such as levallorphan and nalorphine.[69] It is possible that there is an inhibition of acetylcholine release from the neuron, since narcotic drugs and acetylcholine have been shown to compete for membrane transport.[70] This surplus of acetylcholine may account for the decrease in choline acetyltransferase activity seen in the caudate nucleus of morphine-treated rats.[71]

Ionic Membrane Phenomena

The transmission of the nerve impulse is accompanied by a depolarization of the neuronal membrane, reversing the polarity from its resting negative potential difference. An essential requirement for the generation of the action potential is a concentration gradient of ions between the inner and outer sides of the membrane. The gradient of Na^{++} between the inner and outer surfaces of the membrane is maintained by the operation of a K^+,Na^+ exchange pump which actively extrudes Na^+ from the cell. The membrane components responsible for the ion transport include Na^+, K^+, Mg^{++}-activated ATPase, and binding and transport macromolecules, some possibly enzymes. Many anionic components are able to bind the monovalent cations; among these membrane components are lipids, proteins, peptides, and glyco- and lipo- proteins.

At the synaptic junction Ca^{++} ions are prerequisite for the transmission of the nerve impulse. Recent evidence suggests that the release of Ca^{++} at the synapse is similar to the release of Ca^{++} from the adrenal medullary granules by emiocytosis upon stimulation.[72] By analogy, the entire contents of the synaptic vesicle including neurotransmitters and Ca^{++} would be extruded after a fusion of the vesicular and neuronal membranes.

It is to be expected that changes in the excitatory state in the central nervous system during drug administration would be accompanied by changes in the location or amount of these ions in brain, and some such changes have been described.

Phenothiazines have an effect on the structural integrity of the cell, since high doses cause cell lysis.[73] In lower doses the drugs produce a decrease in membrane permeability.[74] This effect is possibly an indirect one, since the phenothiazines uncouple oxidative phosphorylation in the mitochondria, thereby altering ATP availability and membrane ATPase activity.[75] Ethanol, too, has an effect on active ion transport. Brain ATPase activity is inhibited by ethanol. Since this inhibition is limited to K^+-stimulated ATPase activity, the net accumulation of K^+ by cortex slices is inhibited by ethanol.[76] An antagonism between Ca^{++} and ethanol at the surface has been observed in peripheral nerve.[77]

The effect of local anesthetics on ion permeability has been extensively studied.[78] The primary action of this class of drugs is limited to the membrane of the nerve fiber, probably with an interaction of the drugs with anionic charged sites in the membranes. A functional alteration of the membrane results in a decreased movement of K^+, Na^+, and Ca^{++} across the membrane.[79]

Cocaine alters the influx of Na^+ and the efflux of K^+ through the cerebral cortex cell membrane.[80] The transport of Ca^{++} in either direction is also inhibited by cocaine.[80] Morphine also inhibits the influx of Ca^{++} into the nerve cell, but only in a low Ca^{++} medium.[81] The activity of morphine seems to be related to depolarization, in contrast to cocaine which seems to inhibit active transport.[82] The administration of morphine produces a decrease in total brain Ca^{++} in mice, a biochemical effect to which tolerance develops.[83]

The involvement of prostaglandins and cyclic AMP in the interaction of hormones with cellular membranes suggests that these "second messengers" may be mediators or substrates in the interaction of drugs and plasma membranes. There is little evidence to support this hypothesis at the moment. In the isolated guinea pig ileum preparation, morphine in very low doses inhibits the effect of prostaglandin PGE_1 in eliciting a contraction. Nalorphine and etoniazine have similar effects in antagonizing this prostaglandin action.[84] This antagonism is incomplete and probably results from an inhibition by morphine of a neural component of the prostaglandin-induced stimulation.[85] In brain, the rate of biosynthesis of c-AMP is increased after acute morphine administration, and the effect to which tolerance develops during chronic morphine treatment.[86] Second messenger mediation suggests that there is primary action preceding its effects such as a release of neurotransmitters in synaptic transmission.

This discussion would not be complete without briefly mentioning the effect of narcotic analgesics on membrane integrity in single cell systems. The incubation of bacterial cells, or mammalian cells in tissue culture, in the presence of narcotics results in an inhibition of many metabolic pathways.[87,88] The primary effect of the drugs seems to be on the cell membranes with a change in membrane permeability as an early consequence, leading to a loss of many small molecular weight molecules including ATP.[89]

Macromolecular Synthesis

The various theories concerning the mechanisms for the development of tolerance and dependence have been discussed in greater detail elsewhere. In many of the hypotheses, there is a requirement for the biosynthesis of macromolecules, either an increase in the levels of substances already present, or the synthesis of new molecules such as an 'induction' of the enzymes involved in neurotransmitter biosynthesis,[90,91] or a 'memory' molecule,[92] or the synthesis of new receptors,[93] an increased protein synthesis following derepression of DNA by the opiate,[94] or a 'hypertrophy' of redundant pathways.[95] Experimental evidence supporting such macromolecular biosynthesis is both scanty and usually indicative of an indirect effect.

Single Proteins

The induction of an enzyme (or enzymes) involved in neurotransmitter synthesis by a derepression of the nucleic acid template has been suggested as the mode of biochemical adaptation to chronic stimulation by continuing drug administration. Induction, the synthesis of new protein, is sometimes difficult to differentiate from enzyme activation, since both processes are characterized by an increased enzyme activity in tissue. When the observed increase in enzyme activity is prevented by the administration of an inhibitor of protein or RNA synthesis, the increased enzyme activity can be ascribed to induction.

Tyrosine hydroxylase, as the rate-limiting enzyme in the biosynthesis of catecholamines, has seemed a suitable enzyme candidate for induction by drugs. The repeated stimulation of the superior cervical ganglion produces an induction of this enzyme in the ganglion,[96] and electroconvulsive shock to the whole animal has induced an increase in tyrosine hydroxylase in the rat brain stem and cortex.[97] Similar neurally-mediated increases in tyrosine hydroxylase have been induced by reserpine in sympathetic ganglia and in brain stem.[98] These latter responses have been shown to be true enzyme induction since they are inhibited by the administration of cycloheximide or actinomycin D.[99] In the adrenal gland, not only reserpine but also amphetamine, methadrine, and 6-hydroxydopamine induced tyrosine hydroxylase activity.[100] These responses are probably inductions since similar responses seen in the adrenal medulla were prevented by the administration of inhibitors of protein synthesis.[101]

The biochemical adaptation in tolerant animals to the effect of acute morphine treatment in eliciting an increased turnover of brain dopamine suggested that tyrosine hydroxylase induction in the neuron might be the mechanism of the adaptation. In our laboratory, we have examined the levels of tyrosine hydroxylase in six areas of rat brain by both in vivo and in vitro techniques after treatment with various regimens of morphine dosage. We found that the actual rate of catecholamine biosynthesis in the brain regions varied widely during drug administration, but that the tyrosine hydroxylase activity in the isolated tissue preparations from the same regions did not vary significantly between responsive and tolerant animals.[102] However, we did find an absolute increase in the enzyme level in the striatum of rats injected for more than ten days with morphine.[103] These temporal parameters of enzyme induction are consistent with the estimated half-life of brain proteins.

Another rate-limiting enzyme in the biosynthesis of a neurotransmitter, tryptophan hydroxylase, has also been suggested as a possible candidate for enzyme induction in the CNS during chronic morphine treatment.[104] This enzyme is induced in developing rat brain, but has not been examined in drug-treated animals.[105]

The biosynthesis of antibodies to administered conjugated opiates, marihuana, and barbiturates is surely an example of new protein synthesis. These antibodies have been produced recently in rabbits by the administration of protein-drug conjugates to the animals.[31,32] As yet, the presence of circulating antibodies or of CNS-antibodies in animals treated with unconjugated drugs has not been reported. The earlier reports of 'transfer' factors extractable from blood or brain of morphine-tolerant animals which transfer tolerance when given to naive animals[28,29] may be related to antibody development.

Membranes

The biosynthesis of receptor molecules in the neuronal or plasma membranes is suggested in several hypotheses of the mechanism by which dependence is induced. In animals, there has been no direct evidence of an increased synthesis of membranal components after chronic drug treatment, although in bacterial systems, an increased synthesis of cardiolipin is found in cells grown in the presence of levorphanol.[106] It is possible that the changes in the relative rates of biosynthesis of the various classes of brain phospholipids seen in guinea pig brain after morphine treatment may be an indication that membranal phospholipid synthesis is being induced by the drug.[107]

Protein and Nucleic Acid Synthesis

The effect of the administration of inhibitors of protein or nucleic acid synthesis in inhibiting the development of tolerance to chronic morphine treatment has been taken as an indication that protein synthesis is required in order for tolerance to develop. This conclusion is not necessarily true since a general inhibition of macromolecular synthesis in an animal can be expected to cause many important deficiencies in metabolism and function which may disrupt the development of tolerance. An inhibition of overall protein synthesis has been seen in the brains of rats treated acutely with morphine.[108] This is a transient effect which is followed by a recovery to above control levels. In other studies in which the turnover of various fractions of brain proteins isolated from mice treated either acutely or chronically with morphine was compared with those from control animals, no difference in turnover was found for the water-soluble proteins.[109] In bacterial systems and in mammalian cells grown in tissue culture, the addition of an opiate to the medium has a pronounced inhibitory effect of protein synthesis.[110,111] As in the intact animal, the inhibition of protein synthesis may be a reflection of a prior inhibition of RNA synthesis. In single cell systems, an inhibition of RNA synthesis precedes, and is larger than, the inhibition of protein synthesis.[110] In rat brain, there is a transient decrease in the rate of overall RNA synthesis after acute morphine treatment, perhaps due to an observed decrease in brain polyribosomal stability.[112] The involvement of RNA synthesis in the development of tolerance to opiates in animals is supported experimentally by the abolition or delay in tolerance development which is seen in animals also treated with actinomycin D, azoguanine, or other inhibitors[113-115] of RNA synthesis.

The need for macromolecular synthesis in the development of psychic dependence to morphine, or in the development of dependence to non-opiates has been largely unexplored. Overall protein synthesis in mouse brain is decreased 1 to 3 hours after an injection of ethanol, and increased after 7 or 14 days of ethanol administration.[116] This increase in the capacity for brain protein synthesis was related to higher plasma corticosterone levels, and ascribed to a nonspecific stress effect. The control of protein synthesis by steroid hormones is dependent on a selective association of the steroid hormone and cellular RNA.[117] Many alkaloids related structurally to phenanthrene-steroids bind to nucleic acids in a specific way and inhibit protein synthesis.[118] An interaction has been seen between morphine and other opiates and DNA and RNA.[119] The primary effect may be a drug interference with protein:RNA binding rather than a direct drug:RNA interaction, since various neuropharmacological agents inhibit the interaction of nucleic acids with histones or other basic proteins; among the drugs are opiates, tranquilizers, and anticholinergic agents.[120] It has been suggested that the proper functioning of repression or expression of the translation or transcription process is interrupted by the presence of psychotropic drugs in the CNS.

CONCLUSIONS

The correlations of manifest behavior with molecular interactions at specific sites in the nervous system are obscured by the exquisite intricacies of the brain. The relations between a neurochemical reaction and its behavioral consequences have many dimensions: among them, time, magnitude and phasing, location (both of the neurochemical event and the means of expressing the behavior), and another parameter which might be termed circuitry potential (the existence of a connection in the neural organization between the two events). Multidisciplinary explorations of behavior have resulted in a fairly accurate notion of its physiological basis, but little detailed information upon the chain of events linking the entrance of information into the CNS to its translation into behavior. Studies of the behavioral effects of drugs have been particularly useful in identifying relationships between molecular reactions in the CNS and behavior, and, conversely, behavioral phenomena have been useful in classifying the psychoactive drugs. It has become obvious that there are common biochemical mechanisms in the nervous system through which many different behavioral alterations are effected, and that various drug-induced behavioral responses are effected through these common mechanisms. For example, although stereotyped behavior is ordinarily induced by amphetamine in the rat, it can also be induced by LSD, morphine, methyltryptamine, cocaine, and apomorphine.[121] The stereotyped behavior induced by these various drugs is correlated with an accumulation of O-methylated derivatives of dopamine in brain.[121] A dopaminergic meditation at specific neuronal sites will be the common mechanism for drug-induced stereotyped behavior, if the biochemical effects at specific dopamine synapses continue to be quantitatively related to the degree of alteration in this behavior.

Drug-seeking behavior, or psychic dependence, is presumably also mediated through central neurohormonal mechanisms. The psychophysiological responses to the initial exposure to an effective level of drug are the reinforcers for the resulting drug-seeking behavior, modified by the functional status of the system upon which the drug-induced responses are imposed. An open question is whether prior alterations of the neuronal milieu provide a more or less amenable substrate for effective reinforcement of drug-seeking behavior. A relative unimportance of environmental and genetic factors in the evocation of this behavior is suggested by the ease of establishing drug-seeking by self-administration techniques in experimental animals, although it can be argued that the relatively few strains and species of animals involved in these studies may happen to be both genetically suitable and environmentally deprived. In any case, the basic biochemical mechanisms underlying psychic dependence on drugs are related to the central mediation and regulation of behavior through the synaptic events described earlier in the chapter.

Physical dependence and tolerance are more tangible aspects of drug dependence because these phenomena can be evoked and quantitated in experimental animals by chronic drug administration. The basic riddles of dependence are (1) the identity, or lack of it, between the molecular sites and pathways which mediate acute responses to drugs and those underlying the biochemical adaptations in CNS tolerance to drugs and (2) are psychic and physical dependence expressions of the same neurochemical alterations in different modalities. A tentative yes to the question of identity of pathways for acute and chronic effects is supported by the evidence of biochemical adaptation in the pituitary-adrenal responses and in the release of neurotransmitters in the CNS, although a fine distinction may be made on the identity of normal and adapted membranes, of induced and uninduced enzymes, or of normal and 'expanded' receptors. The separation of dependence-producing drugs into two categories: (1) those which induce physical dependence and tolerance as well as psychic dependence and (2) those which induce only psychic dependence, argues for a no to question two. One alternative suggestion is that the basic mechanisms underlying the psychic dependence produced by cocaine are different from those underlying the psychic dependence produced by opiates: the latter then could be another manifestation of the central alterations which produce physical dependence to these drugs. The fact that the dose of drug and the time between doses controls the rate of tolerance development adds another possible solution to the riddle: all drugs which induce psychic dependence also are capable of inducing physical dependence and tolerance if suitable dose:schedules are employed. Choosing among these alternative solutions to the riddle of drug dependence would be a foolhardy undertaking particularly since some of the questions asked are amenable to experimental solutions.

REFERENCES

1. Eddy, N. B., Halbach, H., Isbell, H. and Seevers, M. H., Drug dependence: its significance and characteristics, *Bull. W.H.O.*, 37, 1, 1965.

2. Remmer, H., Gewöhnung on Hexobarbital durch beschleunigten Abbau, *Arch. Int. Pharmacodyn.*, 152, 346, 1964.

3. Remmer, H., Tolerance to barbiturates by increased breakdown, in *Scientific Basis of Drug Dependence,* Steinberg, H., Ed., J. & A. Churchill, London, 1965.

4. Morselli, P. L., Rizzo, M., and Garattini, S., Interaction between phenobarbital and diphenylhydantoin in animals and man, *Ann. N.Y. Acad. Sci.*, 179, 88, 1971.

5. Conney, A. H. and Burns, J. J., Factors influencing drug metabolism, *Advances Pharmacol.*, 1, 31, 1962.

6. Nebert, D. W. and Gelboin, H. V., Cellular responses during enzyme induction, *J. Biol. Chem.*, 243, 6250, 1968.

7. Nebert, D. W. and Gelboin, H. V., The role of RNA and protein synthesis in microsomal aryl hydroxylase in mammalian cell culture, *J. Biol. Chem.*, 245, 160, 1970.

8. Mycek, M. J., Microsomal nucleic acid breakdown in livers of phenobarbital treated rats, *Biochem. Pharmacol.*, 20, 325, 1971.

9. Louis-Ferdinand, R. T. and Fuller, G. C., Suppression of hepatic ribonuclease during phenobarbital stimulation of drug metabolism, *Biochem. Biophys. Res. Commun.*, 38, 811, 1970.

10. Booth, J. and Gillette, J. R., The effect of anabolic steroids on drug metabolism by liver microsomal enzymes in rat liver, *J. Pharmacol. Exp. Ther.*, 137, 374, 1962.

11. Dayton, P. G. and Perel, J. M., Physiological and physicochemical bases of drug interactions in man, *Ann. N. Y. Acad. Sci.*, 179, 67, 1971

12. McMahon, R. E., The competitive inhibition of the *N*-demethylation of butynamine by 2,4-dichloro-6-phenylphenoxyethylamine (DPEA), *J. Pharmacol. Exp. Ther.*, 138, 382, 1962.

13. Rubin, A., Tephley, T. R., and Mannering, G. J., Inhibition of hexobarbital metabolism by ethylmorphine and codeine in the intact rat, *Biochem. Pharmacol.*, 13, 1053, 1964.

14. Slater, T. F., Sawyer, B. C., and Strauli, U. D., Changes in liver nucleotide concentrations in experimental liver injury, *Biochem. J.*, 93, 267, 1964.

15. Carter, E. A. and Isselbacher, K. J., The role of microsomes in the hepatic metabolism of ethanol, *Ann. N. Y. Acad. Sci.*, 179, 282, 1971.

16. Mannering, G. J. and Takemori, A. E., Effect of repeated doses of levorphan, dextrorphan and morphine on the capacity of rat liver preparations to demethylate, *J. Pharmacol. Exp. Ther.*, 127, 187, 1959.

17. Clouet, D. H. and Ratner, M., The effect of altering liver microsomal *N*-demethylase activity on the development of tolerance to morphine in rats, *J. Pharmacol. Exp. Ther.*, 144, 362, 1964.

18. Axelrod, J., Possible mechanisms of tolerance to narcotic drugs, *Science*, 124, 263, 1956.

19. Cochin, J. and Axelrod, J., Biochemical and pharmacological changes in rat following chronic administration of morphine, nalorphine and normorphine, *J. Pharmacol. Exp. Ther.*, 125, 105, 1959.

20. Kato, R. and Onodo, R., Effect of morphine administration on the activities of microsomal drug metabolizing enzymes in liver of different species, *Jap. J. Pharmacol.*, 16, 217, 1966.

21. Quinn, G. P., Axelrod, J., and Brodie, B. B., Species, Strain and sex differences in metabolism of hexobarbitone, amidopyrine and aniline, *Biochem. Pharmacol.*, 1, 152, 1958.

22. Gillette, J. R., Factors affecting drug metabolism, *Ann. N.Y. Acad. Sci.*, 179, 43, 1971.

23. Kato, R. and Gillette, J. R., Sex differences in the effects of abnormal physiological states on the metabolism of drugs by rat liver microsomes, *J. Pharmacol. Exp. Ther.*, 150, 285, 1965.

24. Bousquet, W. F., Rupe, B. D., and Miya, T. S., Morphine inhibition of drug metabolism in the rat, *Biochem. Pharmacol.*, 13, 123, 1964.

25. Benakis, A. and Thomasset, M., Metabolism of amphetamines and their interaction with barbiturates and SKF-525A, in *Amphetamines and Related Compounds*, Costa, E. and Garattini, S., Eds., Raven Press, New York, 1970.

26. Sulser, F., Owens, M. L., and Dingell, J. V., On the mechanism of amphetamine potentiation by desipramine, *Psychopharmacologia*, 5, 198, 1966.

27. Gioffredi, C., L'immunizzazione per gli alcaloidi vegetali tentativi di sieroterapia negli avvelenamenti richerche sperimentali, *Gior. Internaz. Sci. Med.*, 19, 829, 1897.

28. Cochin, J., Role of possible immune mechanisms in the development of tolerance, in *Narcotic Drugs: Biochemical Pharmacology*, Clouet, D. H., Ed., Plenum Press, New York, 1971.

29. Kornetsky, C. and Kiplinger, G. F., Potentiation of an effect of morphine in the rat by sera from morphine-tolerant and abstinent dogs and monkeys, *Psychopharmacologia*, 4, 66, 1963.

30. Feinberg, M. and Cochin, J., Effect of cyclophosphamide on tolerance to morphine, *Pharmacologist*, 10, 188, 1968.

31. Spector, S. and Parker, C. W., Morphine: radioimmunoassay, *Science*, 168, 1347, 1970.

32. Spector, S. and Vesell, E. S., Disposition of morphine in man, *Science*, 174, 421, 1971.

33. Mulé, S. J., Redman, C. M., and Flesher, J. W., Intracellular distribution of H^3-morphine in the brain and liver of tolerant and non-tolerant guinea-pigs, *J. Pharmacol. Exp. Ther.*, 157, 459, 1967.

34. Mechoulam, R., Marihuana chemistry, *Science*, 168, 1159, 1970.

35. Szara, S., Discussion of the fate and metabolism of some hallucinogenic indolealkylamines, *Advances Pharmacol.*, 6, 230, 1968.

36. Beckett, A. H., Analgesics and their antagonists: some steric and chemical considerations, *J. Pharm. Pharmacol.*, 8, 848, 1956.

37. Goldstein, M. and Anagnoste, B., The conversion *in vivo* of *d*-amphetamine to *p*-hydroxynorephedrine, *Biochim. Biophys. Acta*, 107, 166, 1965.

38. Schmitt, H. and Schmitt, H., Interactions between reserpine and amphetamine on blood pressure, in *Amphetamines and Related Compounds*, Costa, E. and Garattini, S., Eds., Raven Press, New York, 1970.

39. Sulser, F. and Sanders-Bush, E., Effect of drugs on amines in the CNS, *Ann. Rev. Pharmacol.*, 11, 209, 1971.

40. Groppetti, A. and Costa, E., Tissue concentrations of *p*-hydroxynorephedrine in rats injected with *d*-amphetamine, *Life Sci.*, 8, 653, 1969.

41. Lewander, T., Urinary excretion and tissue levels of catecholamines during chronic amphetamine intoxication, *Psychopharmacologia,* 13, 394, 1968.

42. Davis, V. E., Brown, H., Huff, J. A., and Cashaw, J. L., Ethanol induced alterations in norepinephrine metabolism in man, *J. Lab. Clin. Med.,* 69, 787, 1967.

43. Erwin, B. G., Tabakoff, B., and Bronaugh, R. L., Inhibition of a reduced nicotinamide adenine dinucleotide phosphate-linked aldehyde reductase from bovine brain by barbiturates, *Molec. Pharmacol.,* 7, 169, 1971.

44. Wallgren, H., Effects of alcohol on biochemical processes in the central nervous system, *Psychosomat. Med.,* 28, 431, 1966.

45. Coyle, J. T. and Snyder, S. H., Catecholamine uptake by synaptosomes in homogenates of rat brain: stereospecificity in different areas, *J. Pharmacol. Exp. Ther.,* 170, 221, 1969.

46. Taylor, K. T. and Snyder, S. H., Amphetamines: differentiation by *d* and *l* isomers of behavior involving brain norepinephrine or dopamine, *Science,* 168, 1487, 1970.

47. Strada, S. J., Sanders-Bush, E., and Sulser, F., *p*-Chloroamphetamine-temporal relationship between psycho motor stimulation and metabolism of brain norepinephrine, *Biochem. Pharmacol.,* 19, 2621, 1970.

48. Glowinski, J., Axelrod, J., and Iversen, L., Regional studies of catecholamines in the rat brain, I., *J. Pharmacol. Exp. Ther.,* 153, 30, 1966.

49. Glowinski, J., Effects of amphetamine on various aspects of catecholamine metabolism in the central nervous system of the rat, in *Amphetamines and Related Compounds,* Costa, E. and Garattini, S., Ed., Raven Press, New York, 1970.

50. Fuxe, K., Hökfelt, T., and Ungerstedt, U., Localization of indolealkylamines in CNS, *Advances Pharmacol.,* 6, 235, 1968.

51. Pletscher, A., DaPrada, M., and Burkard, W. P., The effect of substituted phenylethylamines on the metabolism of biogenic amines, in *Amphetamines and Related Compounds,* Costa, E. and Garattini, S., Eds., Plenum Press, New York, 1970.

52. Fuller, R. W., Serotonin oxidation by rat brain monoamine oxidase. Inhibition by 4-chloroamphetamine, *Life Sci.,* 5, 2247, 1966.

53. Schildkraut, J. J., Schanberg, S. M., Breese, G. R., and Kopin, I. J., Norepinephrine metabolism and drugs used in the affective disorders: a possible mechanism of action, *Amer. J. Psychiat.,* 124, 600, 1967.

54. Glowinski, J., Iversen, L., and Axelrod, J., Storage and synthesis of norepinephrine in the reserpine-treated rat brain, *J. Pharmacol. Exp. Ther.,* 151, 385, 1966.

55. Kopin, I. J. and Gordon, E. K., Metabolism of administered and drug-released norepinephrine-H^3 in the rat, *J. Pharmacol. Exp. Ther.,* 140, 207, 1963.

56. Carlsson, A., Hillorp, N. A., and Waldeck, B., A Mg^{++}-ATP-dependent storage mechanism in the amine granules of the adrenal medulla, *Med. Exp.,* 6, 47, 1962.

57. Hamberger, B., Reserpine-resistant uptake of catecholamines in isolated tissue of the rat, *Acta Physiol. Scand.,* Suppl. 295, 1967.

58. Crossland, J., Psychotropic drug and neurohumoral substances in the central nervous system, *Progr. Med. Chem.,* 5, 251, 1967.

59. Szara, S. I., Hallucinogens, in *Handbook of Neurochemistry,* Vol. 6, Lajtha, A., Ed., Plenum Press, New York, 1971. 441.

60. Maynert, E. W., Catecholamine metabolism in the brain and adrenal medulla during addiction to morphine and in the early abstinence period, in *The Addictive States,* Wikler, A., Ed., Williams & Wilkins, Baltimore, 1968.

61. Clouet, D. H. and Ratner, M., Catecholamine biosynthesis in brains of rats treated with morphine, *Science,* 168, 854, 1970.

62. Smith, C. B., Villarreal, J. E., Bednarczyk, J. H., and Sheldon, M. I., Tolerance to morphine-induced increases in C^{14}-catecholamine synthesis in mouse brain, *Science,* 170, 1106, 1970.

63. Clouet, D. H. and Ratner, M., The biosynthesis of catecholamines in the brains of morphine-treated rats, reported to the Committee on Problems of Drug Dependence, NRC-NAS Meeting, 1970.

64. Izquierdo, I. and Izquierdo, J. A., Effects of drugs on deep brain centers, *Ann. Rev. Pharmacol.,* 11, 189, 1971.

65. White, R. P., Nash, C. B., Westubeke, E. J., and Possanza, G. J., Phylogenetic comparison of central actions produced by different doses of atropine and hyoscine, *Arch. Int. Pharmacodyn.,* 132, 349, 1961.

66. Mazel, P. and Bush, M., Brain barbital levels and anethesia as influenced by physostigmine and epinephrine, *Biochem. Pharmacol.,* 18, 579, 1969.

67. Giarman, N. J. and Pepeu, G., Drug-induced changes in brain acetylcholine, *Brit. J. Pharmacol.,* 19, 226, 1962.

68. Jhamandas, K., Phillis, J. W., and Pinsky, C., Effects of narcotic analgesics and antagonists on the *in vivo* release of acetylcholine from the central cortex of the cat, *Brit. J. Pharmacol.,* 43, 53, 1971.

69. Weinstock, M., The effect of narcotic analgesic drugs on acetylcholine and cholinesterase, in *Narcotic Drugs: Biochemical Pharmacology,* Clouet, D. H., Ed., Plenum Press, New York, 1971.

70. Schuberth, J. and Sundwall, A., Effects of some drugs on the uptake of acetylcholine in cortex slices of mouse brain, *J. Neurochem.,* 14, 807, 1967.

71. Datta, K., Thal, L., and Wajda, I. J., Effects of morphine on choline acetyltransferase levels in the caudate nucleus of the rat, *Brit. J. Pharmacol.,* 41, 84, 1971.

72. Diamond, I. and Goldberg, A. L., Uptake and release of ^{45}Ca by brain microsomes, synaptosomes and synaptic vesicles, *J. Neurochem.,* 18, 1419, 1971.

73. Agrawal, R. P. and Guha, A., Lytic action of chlorpromazine HC1 on *E. coli* G cells, *Brit. J. Pharmacol.,* 24, 466, 1965.

74. Freeman, A. R. and Spirtes, M. A., Effects of chlorpromazine on biological membranes. II. Chlorpromazine induced changes in human erythrocytes, *Biochem. Pharmacol.,* 12, 47, 1963.

75. Kaul, C. L., Lewis, J. J., and Livingston, S. D., Influence of chlorpromazine on the levels of adenine nucleotides in the rat brain and hypothalamus *in vivo, Biochem. Pharmacol.,* 14, 165, 1965.

76. Israel-Jacard, Y. and Kalant, H., Effect of ethanol on electrolyte transport and electrogenesis in animal tissues, *J. Cell. Comp. Physiol.,* 65, 127, 1965.

77. Rosenberg, P. and Bartels, E., Drug effects on the spontaneous electrical activity of the squid giant axon, *J. Pharmacol. Exp. Ther.,* 155, 532, 1967.

78. Mullins, L. J., Anesthetics, in *Handbook of Neurochemistry,* Vol. 6, Lajtha, A., Ed., Plenum Press, New York, 1971, 395.

79. Dettbarn, W.-D., Local Anesthetics, in *Handbook of Neurochemistry,* Vol. 6, Lajtha, A., Ed., Plenum Press, New York, 1971, 423.

80. Kakunaga, T., The effect of morphine and other drugs on the efflux of calcium ions from rat brain cortex slices, *Folia Pharmacol. Jap.,* 62, 40, 1966.

81. Fairhurst, A. S., Macri, J., and Herliky, N., Methadone inhibition of calcium uptake by muscle and brain fractions, *Life Sci.,* 10, 1133, 1971.

82. Kaneto, H., The role of calcium in the mechanism of action of opiates, in *Narcotic Drugs: Biochemical Pharmacology,* Clouet, D. H., Ed., Plenum Press, New York, 1971.

83. Shikimi, T., Kaneto, H., and Hano, K., Changes in brain Ca^{++} Content in normal and morphinized mice after administration of morphine, *Jap. J. Pharmacol.,* 17, 135, 1967.

84. Jaques, R., Morphine as an inhibitor of prostaglandin in isolated guinea pig intestine, *Experientia,* 25, 1059, 1969.

85. Sanner, J., Prostaglandin inhibition with a dibenzoxazepine hydrazide derivative and morphine, *Ann. N.Y. Acad. Sci.,* 180, 396, 1971.

86. Chou, W. S., Ho, A. K. S., and Loh, H. H., Effect of acute and chronic morphine and norepinephrine on brain adenyl cyclase activity, *Proc. West. Pharmacol. Soc.,* 14, 42, 1971.

87. Simon, E. J. and VanPraag, D., Inhibition of RNA synthesis in *E. coli* by levorphanol, *Proc. Nat. Acad. Sci.,* 51, 877, 1964.

88. Noteboom, W. D. and Mueller, G. C., Inhibition of cell growth and the synthesis of RNA and protein in hela cells by morphinans and related compounds, *Molec. Pharmacol.,* 5, 38, 1969.

89. Green, R. and Magasanik, B., The mode of action of levallorphan as an inhibitor cell growth, *Molec. Pharmacol.,* 3, 453, 1967.

90. Shuster, L., Repression and de-repression of enzyme synthesis as a possible explanation of some aspects of drug action, *Nature,* 189, 314, 1961.

91. Goldstein, D. B. and Goldstein, A., Possible role of enzyme inhibition and repression in drug tolerance and addiction, *Biochem. Pharmacol.,* 8, 48, 1961.

92. Ungar, G. and Galvan, L., Conditions of transfer of morphine tolerance by brain extracts, *Proc. Soc. Exp. Biol. Med.,* 130, 287, 1969.

93. Collier, H. O. J., Supersensitivity and dependence, *Nature,* 220, 228, 1968.

94. Cox, B. M. and Osman, O. H., The role of protein synthesis inhibition in the prevention of morphine tolerance, *Brit. J. Pharmacol.,* 35, 373, 1969.

95. Martin, W. R., A homeostatic and redundancy theory of tolerance to and dependence on narcotic analgesics, in *The Addictive States,* Wikler, A., Ed., Williams and Wilkins, Baltimore, Maryland, 1968.

96. Thierry, A. M., Javoy, F., Glowinski, J., and Kety, S. E., Effects of stress on the metabolism of norepinephrine, dopamine and serotonin in the central nervous system of the rat, *J. Pharmacol. Exp. Ther.,* 163, 163, 1968.

97. Musacchio, J. M., Julou, L., Kety, S. S., and Glowinski, J., Increase in rat brain tyrosine hydroxylase activity produced by electroconvulsive shock, *Proc. Nat. Acad. Sci.,* 63, 1117, 1969.

98. Thoenen, H., Mueller, R. A., and Axelrod, J., Increased tyrosine hydroxylase activity after drug-induced alteration of sympathetic transmission, *Nature,* 221, 1264, 1969.

99. Mueller, R. A., Thoenen, H. and Axelrod, J., Inhibition of trans-synaptically increased tyrosine hydroxylase activity by cycloheximide and actinomycin D, *Molec. Pharmacol.,* 5, 463, 1969.

100. Mandell, A. J. and Morgan, M., Amphetamine-induced increase in tyrosine hydroxylase activity, *Nature,* 227, 75, 1970.

101. Weiner, N., Regulation of norepinephrine biosynthesis, *Ann. Rev. Pharmacol.,* 10, 273, 1970.

102. Clouet, D. H. and Ratner, M., Effect of morphine on brain tyrosine hydroxylase activity, *Fed. Proc.,* 30, 501, 1971.

103. Clouet, D. H. and Ratner, M., Tyrosine hydroxylase activity in areas of the brains of morphine-treated rats, reported to the *Committee on Problems of Drug Dependence* (Feb. 17, 1971), 728, 1971.

104. Way, E. L., Loh, H. H., and Shen, F.-H., Morphine tolerance, physical dependence and the synthesis of brain serotonin, *Science*, 162, 1290, 1968.

105. Schmidt, M. J. and Sanders-Bush, E., Tryptophan hydroxylase in developing rat brain, *J. Neurochem.*, 18, 2549, 1971.

106. Wurster, N., Elsbach, P., Rand, J., and Simon, E. J., Effects of levorphanol on phospholipid metabolism and composition in *E. coli*, *Biochim. Biophys. Acta*, 248, 282, 1971.

107. Mulé, S. J., Morphine and the incorporation of P^{32} into brain phospholipids of non-tolerant, tolerant and abstinent guinea-pigs, *J. Pharmacol. Exp. Ther.*, 154, 370, 1966.

108. Clouet, D. H. and Ratner, M., The effect of the administration of morphine on the incorporation of C^{14}-leucine into the proteins of rat brain *in vivo*, *Brain Res.*, 4, 43, 1967.

109. Hahn, D. L. and Goldstein, A., Amounts and turnover rates of brain proteins in morphine-tolerant mice, *J. Neurochem.*, 18, 1887, 1971.

110. Simon, E. J., Inhibition of synthesis of RNA in *E. coli* by the narcotic drug, levorphanol, *Nature*, 198, 794, 1963.

111. Noteboom, W. D. and Mueller, G. C., Inhibition of protein and RNA synthesis in *Hela* cells by levallorphan and levorphanol, *Molec. Pharmacol.*, 2, 534, 1966.

112. Cohen, M., Keats, A. S., Krivoy, W., and Ungar, G., Effect of actinomycin-D on morphine tolerance, *Proc. Soc. Exp. Biol. Med.*, 119, 381, 1965.

113. Spoerlein, M. T. and Scrafani, J., Effects of time and 8-azaguanire on the development of morphine tolerance, *Life Sci.*, 6, 1549, 1967.

114. Yamamoto, S., Inoki, R., Tamari, Y., and Iwatsubo, K., Inhibitory effect of 8-azaguanire on the development of tolerance in the analgesic action of morphine, *Jap. J. Pharmacol.*, 17, 140, 1967.

115. Smith, A. A., Karmin, M., and Gavitt, J., Blocking effect of puromycin, ethanol and chloroform on the development of tolerance to an opiate, *Biochem. Pharmacol.*, 15, 1877, 1966.

116. Kuriyama, K., Sze, P. Y., and Rauscher, G. E., Effects of acute and chronic ethanol administration ribosomal protein synthesis in mouse brain and liver, *Life Sci.*, 10, 181, 1971.

117. Chin, R. C. and Kidson, C., Selective association of hormonal steroids with amino acyl transfer RNAs and control of protein synthesis, *Proc. Nat. Acad. Sci.*, 68, 2448, 1971.

118. Grollman, A. P., Structural basis for inhibition of protein synthesis by emetine and cycloheximide based on an analogy between ipecac alkaloids and glutarimide antibiotics, *Proc. Nat. Acad. Sci.*, 56, 1867, 1966.

119. Clouet, D. H., The effect of morphine on protein and ribonucleic acid metabolism in brain, in *Drug Abuse: Social and Psychopharmacological Aspects*, Cole, J. O. and Wittenborn, J. R., Eds., Charles C Thomas, Springfield, Ill., 1969.

120. Kubinski, H. and Kornguth, S., The effects of various neuropharmacological agents on the interactions of RNA with proteins, reported to Second National Meeting, Amer. Soc. Neurochem., March, 1971. (Bis. Conference Report # 11).

121. Randrup, A. and Munkvad, I., Biochemical, anatomical and psychological investigations of stereotyped behavior induced by amphetamines, in *Amphetamines and Related Compounds*, Costa, E. and Garattini, S., Eds., Raven Press, New York, 1970.

CRC PRESS Publications in Toxicology and Related Subjects

"INSTRUMENTAL AND RADIOCHEMICAL ACTIVATION ANALYSIS"

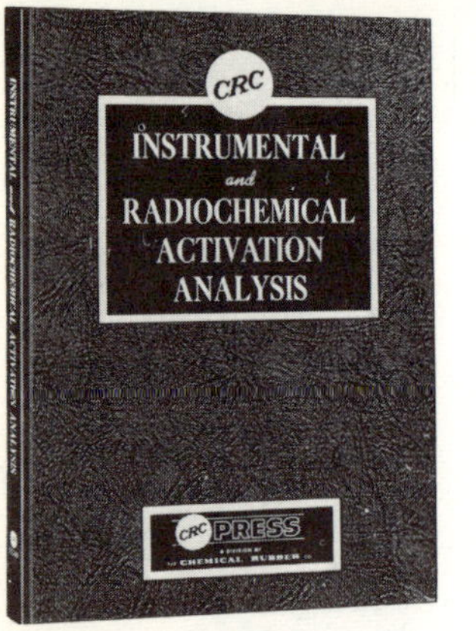

Authors: F. ADAMS, J.P. OP DE BEECK, P. VAN DEN WINKEL, R. GIJBELS, D. DE SOETE and J. HOSTE. All at the University, Department of Chemistry, Ghent, Belgium. Approx. 150 pages, 7½ x 10½. Hard cover. Well documented with 566 references.

The development and diversification of activation analysis has been quite spectacular in recent years, so that it could be expected that a critical review will be welcomed even by scientists with a broad experience in this field. However a choice had to be made among the numerous subjects to keep the monograph within reasonable limits.

It seemed obvious that instrumental methods had to be treated, as the use of semi-conductor detectors and associated equipment caused a real revolution in non-destructive activation analysis. The high resolution of these detectors simultaneously created a need for computer handling of the data, so that this topic can in fact not be separated from the previous one.

Although germanium-lithium detectors and computer treatment of the data now allow purely instrument techniques, it is obvious that not all the problems can be solved in this way. Chemical separations are not likely to disappear, but are to be adapted to the new instrumentation and also, of course, to the specific analytical problem. Automation of chemical separations is also a field developing rapidly for routine analysis of large series.

Activation analysis with other means as nuclear reactors are also of increasing interest. Among these, the so called neutron generator is perhaps the most important one for the time being. High intensities of 14 MeV neutrons now allow trace determinations of many elements, whereas "sealed tubes" provide impressively long and constant outputs. Precise analyses are also possible here, as sources of errors are better understood, due to flux gradients and neutron removal in the sample to mention only these.

MAIN CONTENT HEADINGS

I. Instrumental Neutron Activation Analyses. II. Computer Applications. III. Radiochemical Separations. IV. Activation Analysis with Neutron Generators. V. Photon and Charged Particle Activation Analysis. Addendum I: Recent Advances in Instrumental Neutron Activation Analysis. Addendum II: Computer Applications. References. Errata.

CAT. NO. 109 (Add 50¢ Outside U.S.A.—U.S. Currency Only) **Each $14.00**

"ACTIVATION ANALYSIS"

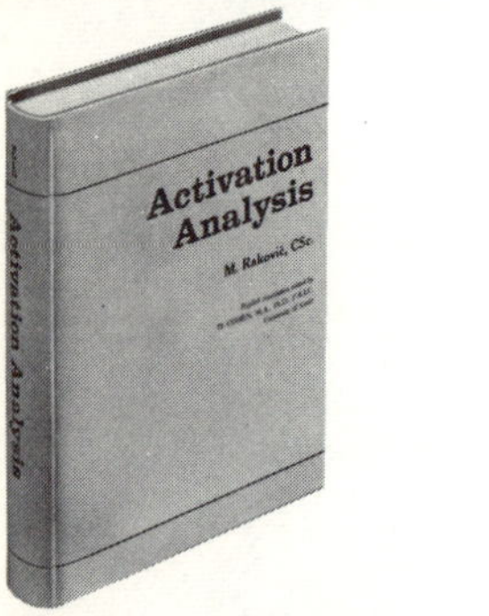

By M. RAKOVIC, D.Sc., Czechoslovakia
Translation edited by D. COHEN, Ph.D., University of Keele, England
326 pp., 5½ x 8½, 1970

Activation analysis has become one of the most important methods of elemental analysis. Its extreme sensitivity makes it indispensable in areas ranging from chemistry and biology, to forensic science and archeology. As a result of the extremely rapid development of knowledge in this field, only a few monographs are now available; this book is intended to help fill the void.

CONTENTS

PART I, GENERAL PRINCIPLES AND PHYSICAL PROCESSES: Neutron Activation Analysis, Activation Analysis by Charged Particles and Gamma Rays. PART II, ANALYTICAL PROCEDURES: Metals and Alloys, Non-Metallic Elements, Inorganic Compounds, Organic Materials, Reactor Materials, Meteorites, Minerals, Rocks, Sediments, Water, Human and Animal Tissues, Plant Material, Foods, Forensic Use, Archeological Use. PART III, TABLES FOR THE PRACTICAL APPLICATION OF ACTIVATION ANALYSIS.

CAT. NO. 892 (Add 50¢ Outside U.S.A. — U. S. Currency Only) **Each $32.90**

"PRACTICAL TOXICOLOGY OF PLASTICS"

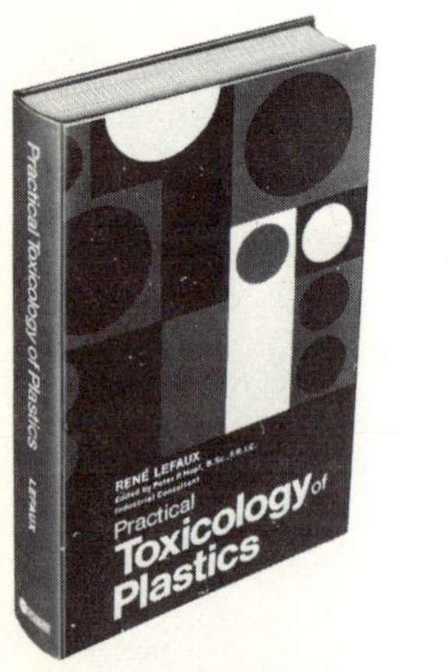

PROBLEMS ENCOUNTERED IN MANUFACTURE, FABRICATION AND USE

By Rene Lefaux, France, translation edited by Peter P. Hoff, Industrial Consultant. 584 pp., 6¼ x 10, 1968.

This book distinguishes between the knowledge that has to be available to the manufacturer of resins and additives, to the fabricator, and to the user. It should be an invaluable manual to all responsible people engaged in the plastics and allied industries, including those engaged on the commercial and administrative sides.

CONTENTS: Introduction. Formation of the Macromolecule. Cohesive Forces—Structure. Properties of Macromolecular Compounds. Principal Organic High Polymers: Plastics, Elastomers, Textiles. Toxicology of the Macromolecule: Oral Intake, Implants, Intravenous Route, Cutaneous Action. **INDUSTRIAL HYGIENE:** Principles of Manufacture of Plastics, Elastomers, and Synthetic Textiles. Industrial Toxicology of Monomers, Solvents, Plasticizers, Phosphoric Esters, Phthalic Esters, Other Plasticizers, Catalysts. Occupational Dermatoses: General Characteristics, Irritants and Sensitizers, Dermatitis in Plastic, Elastomer, and Textile Manufacturing. Dermatitis Through Use of the Finished Product: Plastics and Varnishes. Elastomers. Textiles. Health and Safety: Large Industrial Concerns, Conversion Workshops, Protection of the Worker. Inflammability and Combustibility of Plastics. Appendix I: Toxic Gases and Vapors. Appendix II: Toxic Dusts, Smokes, and Fogs. **MEDICAL AND SURGICAL APPLICATIONS:** Medical and Surgical Plastics: Reaction of Tissues to Various Plastics. Carcinogenic Properties of Plastics. Medical and Surgical Applications: Synthetic Ligatures. Sounds, Drains, and Catheters. Surgical Prostheses. Transfusion and Perfusion Equipment. Macromolecular Compounds Suitable for Injection into the Human Body. **FOOD TOXICOLOGY:** Monomers. Plasticizers. Phosphoric Esters. Phthalic Esters. Adipic, Sebacic, and Azelaic Esters. Stearic, Oleic, and Ricinoleic Esters. Citric Esters. Chlorinated Organic Derivatives. Glycols and Their Compounds. Esters of Glycerine. Sulfamide Derivatives. Plastic Polymers. Stabilizers. Antioxidents. Surface-Active Compounds. Lubricants. Vulcanization Accelerators. Polycondensation Catalysts. Plastics in the Food Industry: Physical and Chemical Compatibility of Plastics with Food Products. Extraction and Liquid Foodstuffs. Regulating the Use of Plastics.

CAT. NO. 857 (Add 50¢ Outside U.S.A.—U.S. Currency Only) **Each $38.00**

"CHEMICAL SYNONYMS AND TRADE NAMES"

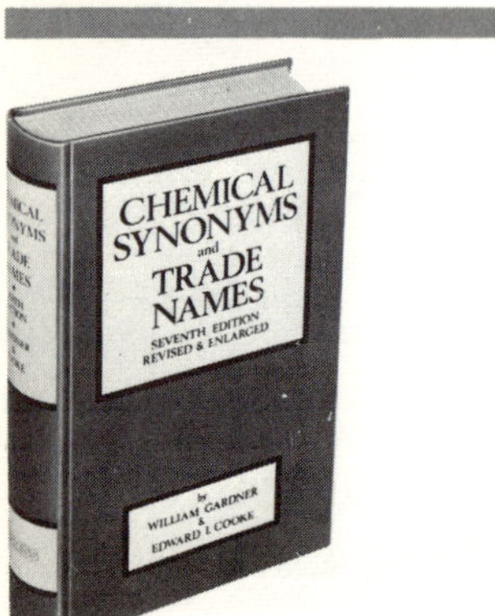

A DICTIONARY AND COMMERCIAL HANDBOOK • 4600 NEW ENTRIES

Edited by EDWARD I. COOKE, M.A., B.Sc., Associate of the Royal Institute of Chemistry. Based on work originally compiled by the late William Gardner. Approx. 650 pp., 9½ x 6, 1971.

This volume provides approximately 30,000 definitions and cross references on minerals, dyestuffs, explosives, pigments, drugs, alloys, commercial chemicals, plastics, pharmaceuticals, and other materials in common use. Continuing a practice begun in the 6th edition, all new entries known to the Editor to be proprietary trade names have been distinguished by a reference number appearing in brackets after the definition itself. Such numbers refer to a list of manufacturers appearing at the back of the book and are used to identify those claiming proprietary rights to the name in question. Special care has been devoted to bringing as nearly possible up to date the list of trade names and synonyms used in the pharmaceutical industry.

Listings are alphabetical by their generic names or proprietary trade names and followed by applicable information such as synonyms, chemical formulation, description and application.

CAT. NO. 916 (Add 50c Outside U.S.A.—U.S. Currency Only) **Each $38.50**

CRC PRESS A Division of THE CHEMICAL RUBBER CO., 18901 Cranwood Parkway • Cleveland, Ohio 44128